Cartilage Injury in the Athlete

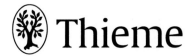

Cartilage Injury in the Athlete

Raffy Mirzayan, M.D.
Co-Director of Sports Medicine
Director of Cartilage Regeneration and Repair
Kaiser Permanente
Baldwin Park, California

Clinical Associate Professor
Department of Orthopaedic Surgery
Keck School of Medicine
University of Southern California
Los Angeles, California

Thieme
New York • Stuttgart

Thieme Medical Publishers, Inc.
333 Seventh Ave.
New York, NY 10001

Consulting Editor: Esther Gumpert
Associate Editor: Owen Zurhellen
Vice-President, Production and Electronic Publishing: Anne T. Vinnicombe
Production Editor: Becky Dille
Sales Director: Ross Lumpkin
Chief Financial Officer: Peter van Woerden
President: Brian D. Scanlan
Compositor: Thomson Digital Services
Printer: Maple-Vail Book Manufacturing Group

Library of Congress Cataloging-in-Publication Data

Cartilage injury in the athlete / [edited by] Raffy Mirzayan.
    p. ; cm.
   Includes bibliographical references and index.
   ISBN 1-58890-305-2 (alk. paper) – ISBN 3-13-140321-7 (alk. paper)
   1. Sports injuries. 2. Cartilage–Wounds and injuries.   I. Mirzayan,
Raffy.
   [DNLM: 1. Athletic Injuries. 2. Cartilage–injuries.   WE 300
C32715 2006]
RD97.C368 2006
617.1'027–dc22
                              2005031421

Important note: Medical knowledge is ever-changing. As new research and clinical experience broaden our knowledge, changes in treatment and drug therapy may be required. The authors and editors of the material herein have consulted sources believed to be reliable in their efforts to provide information that is complete and in accord with the standards accepted at the time of publication. However, in the view of the possibility of human error by the authors, editors, or publisher of the work herein or changes in medical knowledge, neither the authors, editors, or publisher, nor any other party who has been involved in the preparation of this work, warrants that the information contained herein is in every respect accurate or complete, and they are not responsible for any errors or omissions or for the results obtained from use of such information. Readers are encouraged to confirm the information contained herein with other sources. For example, readers are advised to check the product information sheet included in the package of each drug they plan to administer to be certain that the information contained in this publication is accurate and that changes have not been made in the recommended dose or in the contraindications for administration. This recommendation is of particular importance in connection with new or infrequently used drugs.

Some of the product names, patents, and registered designs referred to in this book are in fact registered trademarks or proprietary names even though specific reference to this fact is not always made in the text. Therefore, the appearance of a name without designation as proprietary is not to be construed as a representation by the publisher that it is in the public domain.

Printed in the United States of America

5 4 3 2 1

TMP ISBN 1-58890-305-2

GTV ISBN 3 13 140321 7

Dedication

I dedicate this book to my wife, Armena, whom I have known and loved since junior high school. Since the first day I met her, she has known of my desire to become a physician. She has stood beside me and supported me with unwavering devotion. More importantly, she has given me three wonderful boys, Zareh, Andre, and Raymond, who make all the hard work worthwhile and rewarding.

Contents

Dedication v

Foreword ix

Preface xi

Acknowledgments xiii

Section I   **Basic Science** 1

Chapter 1   Structure and Function of Cartilage Biology 3
               Michael A. Schwartz and Michael G. Ciccotti

Chapter 2   Biomechanics of Synovial Joints 10
               Thay Q. Lee, Stefan Fornalski, Tomoyuki Sasaki, and Savio L.-Y. Woo

Chapter 3   Response of Articular Cartilage to Injury 24
               Vahé R. Panossian

Chapter 4   Effects of Electrothermal Energy on Cartilage 31
               Yan Lu, Ryland B. Edwards, and Mark D. Markel

Section II   **Assessment** 45

Chapter 5   Clinical Evaluation of the Patient with a Chondral Injury 47
               Raffy Mirzayan

Chapter 6   Imaging Techniques of Cartilage Injury 50
               Christine B. Chung, Aurea Mohana-Borges, and Donald L. Resnick

Chapter 7   Classification of Articular Cartilage Injury and Repair 60
               Bert R. Mandelbaum, Ralph A. Gambardella, and Jason M. Scopp

Section III   **Nonoperative Treatment** 71

Chapter 8   Analgesics and Antiinflammatory Medications 73
               Orrin M. Troum

Chapter 9   Glucosamine and Chondroitin Sulfate 86
               Ronald A. Navarro

Chapter 10   Hyaluronic Acid Injections: Viscosupplementation 92
               Ronald A. Navarro and Julian Paul Ballesteros

Section IV   **Operative Treatment** 97

Chapter 11   Arthroscopic Management of the Early Arthritic Joint 99
               Steven S. Goldberg, Raffy Mirzayan, and C. Thomas Vangsness, Jr.

Chapter 12   Electrothermal Chondroplasty 109
            Amir M. Khan and Gary S. Fanton

Chapter 13   Microfracture Technique 116
            Paul Sethi, Raffy Mirzayan, and F. Daniel Kharrazi

Chapter 14   Osteochondral Autograft Transplantation (OATS/Mosaicplasty) 124
            Jason L. Koh, László Hangody, and Gabor Kristof Ráthonyi

Chapter 15   Autologous Chondrocyte Implantation 141
            Jeffrey W. Wiley, Tim Bryant, and Tom Minas

Chapter 16   Osteochondral Allograft Transplantation 158
            William D. Bugbee and Michael J. Ostempowski

Section V   **Joint-Specific Treatment** **169**

Chapter 17   Osteochondral Lesions of the Talus 171
            Mark E. Easley, Steven D. Sides, and Alison P. Toth

Chapter 18   Acute Osteochondral Defects in the Knee 187
            John G. Costouros, Marc R. Safran, and Gregory B. Maletis

Chapter 19   Osteochondral Defects in the Elbow 202
            Russell S. Petrie and James P. Bradley

Chapter 20   Cartilage Injuries in the Shoulder 217
            Jeff A. Fox, Brian J. Cole, Tamara K. Pylawka, and Anthony A. Romeo

Chapter 21   Cartilage Injury in the Skeletally Immature 232
            Christopher Iobst and Mininder S. Kocher

Section VI   **Adjunctive Treatments with Cartilage Restoration** **247**

Chapter 22   Corrective Osteotomies Around the Knee 249
            Gregory J. Adamson, Jennifer R. Miller, and Pierre Durand Jr.

Chapter 23   Meniscal Transplantation 263
            Wayne K. Gersoff

Chapter 24   Surgical Management of Patellofemoral Disease 273
            Tom Minas

Section VII   **Future Directions** **287**

Chapter 25   Future Directions in the Treatment of Cartilage Injury in the Athlete 289
            Constance R. Chu, Volker Musahl, and Freddie H. Fu

Chapter 26   Gene Therapy in the Treatment of Cartilage Injury 297
            Andre F. Steinert, Glyn D. Palmer, Steven C. Ghivizzani, and Christopher H. Evans

Chapter 27   Hyaluronian-Based Autologous Chondrocyte Implantation 309
            *Stefano Zaffagnini, Elizaveta Kon, Leonardo Marchesini, Maria Pia Neri, Francesco Iacono,
            and Maurilio Marcacci*

Index 317

Foreword

From an almost nihilistic view on the possibility of treatment of articular cartilage injuries established over the past two thousand years, three important manuscripts published in the mid-1990's have raised some hope and optimism. These include works on the microfracture technique whereby bone marrow stem cells are mobilized to the repair area, the osteochondral autograft transfer technique whereby osteochondral autologous cylinders are transferred into the repair area, and autologous chondrocyte implantation, which attempts to create hyaline cartilage by the use of isolated, cultured autologous chondrocytes implanted into a cartilage defect.

The medium- to long-term results of these treatment techniques are promising and include the possibility of returning to the pre-injury level for top athletes and to sports for middle-aged recreational athletes. This is a significant step forward compared to previous treatments. There is, however, still no gold standard for the treatment of cartilage injuries, although the ongoing basic research and clinical developments are very encouraging for the future. As the new techniques offer acceptable treatment results, the interest and need for further education and information on cartilage repair is increasing on the research and orthopaedic communities. Today most international meetings, symposia, and instructional courses include an update on progress in basic research and clinical treatment techniques in articular cartilage repair.

This new book edited by Raffy Mirzayan is a great contribution to physicians, educating them in the present status of research and clinical development. It includes 27 chapters divided into seven appropriate sections: Basic Science, Assessment, Nonoperative Treatment, Operative Treatment, Joint-Specific Treatment, Adjunctive Treatments with Cartilage Restoration, and Future Directions. The comprehensive chapters cover the whole field of cartilage repair and regeneration at the present and are a valuable contribution to the education of treating physicians.

Lars Peterson, M.D., Ph.D.
Gothenburg, Sweden

Preface

The poor inherent ability of cartilage injuries to heal was recognized as early as 1743 by Hunter[1]. He noted that ulcerations of articular cartilage do not have the capacity to repair themselves. Injury to articular cartilage can lead to acute and chronic symptoms, which can lead to functional limitations in daily and sporting activities. If left untreated, the lesions can lead to degenerative arthrosis of the joint. In older patients, joint arthroplasty can reliably eliminate the pain. Since arthroplasty is not a viable option in younger and more athletic populations, numerous regenerative, reparative, and restorative procedures have been described over the last two centuries to treat articular cartilage injuries. These include lavage, debridement, drilling, microfracture, periosteum transplantation, allografts, autograft transfer, and autologous chondrocyte implantation. Earlier procedures yielded mostly regenerated fibrocartilage tissue with low durability. Newer techniques have been able to regenerate hyaline-like tissue. To date, normal hyaline cartilage has not been reliably reproduced with any technique. The reproduction of articular hyaline cartilage still remains the "Holy Grail" of orthopaedic surgery.

This book describes the normal anatomy and function of hyaline cartilage and its response to injury. The diagnosis, classification, imaging, nonoperative and operative management, including surgical techniques for various reparative and restorative procedures, in young, athletic patients with cartilage injury is covered in detail. Joint specific treatments for the shoulder, elbow, knee, and ankle as well as future directions in the treatment of cartilage injury including gene therapy are also discussed.

REFERENCE

1. Hunter W. On the structure and diseases of articulating cartilages. Philos Trans Roy Soc. 42B:514-521, 1743.

Acknowledgments

I would like to thank many people who were instrumental in the completion of this book. Esther Gumpert, Senior Editor at Thieme Medical Publishers, who believed in this project and supported me in editing this book. Thanks for the opportunity to work with you again. J. Owen Zurhellen, Associate Editor at Thieme Medical Publishers, who was extremely helpful in the day-to-day operations of completing this book. Judith Tomat, Editorial Assistant at Thieme Medical Publishers, who made sure that all the "i's" were dotted and the "t's" were crossed before submitting the manuscript for production. Rebecca Dille, Senior Production Editor, was instrumental in getting our work to the point where it could reach the market.

I would like to thank one of my patients, KP, who was a young dancer and presented with an acute cartilage injury and gave me the idea for this book. I would like to thank all the contributors and co-contributors who have worked hard and diligently in submitting high-quality chapters. They did it for the love of the topic and to help improve our patients' quality of life. Without their hard work, this book would not have come to fruition.

Lastly, but definitely not least, I would like to thank my family who sacrificed so much to allow me to pursue my dreams, who understood what it took to reach my goals, and who supported me along the way. I especially wish to thank my parents, Janet and Dr. Leon Mirzayan, who made sacrifices their whole lives in order for me to succeed; my brother Dr. Armen Mirzayan, his wife Jeannie and daughter Mia; my sister Adrineh; my in-laws, Alex and Lilly Andranian, who have been like parents to me; my brother-in-law Armond, his wife, Annie, and boys, Alec and Arsen; lastly, my grandmother, Armenouhi (Armik mom), who dedicated her life to raise six children by herself, helped to raise me, and instilled in me the value of hard work, without which I would not have been able to persevere my medical training.

Contributors

Gregory J. Adamson, M.D.
Clinical Professor
Department of Orthopaedic Surgery
University of Southern California
Keck School of Medicine
Los Angeles, California

Congress Medical Associates
Pasadena, California

Julian Paul Ballesteros, M.D.
Chief Resident
Department of Orthopaedic Surgery
Harbor–University of California at
Los Angeles Medical Center
Torrance, California

James P. Bradley, M.D.
Associate Clinical Professor
Department of Orthopaedic Surgery
University of Pittsburgh Medical Center
Pittsburgh, Pennsylvania

Tim Bryant, B.S.N., R.N.
Cartilage Repair Center at Brigham and
Women's Hospital
Harvard Medical School
Chestnut Hill, Massachusetts

William D. Bugbee, M.D.
Associate Professor
Department of Orthopaedic Surgery
University of California–San Diego
La Jolla, California

Constance R. Chu, M.D.
Assistant Professor of Orthopaedic Surgery
Division of Joint Replacement
University of Pittsburgh Medical Center
Head, Cartilage Injury and Repair Division
Ferguson Laboratory
University of Pittsburgh
Pittsburgh, Pennsylvania

Christine B. Chung, M.D.
Assistant Professor
Department of Radiology
University of California–San Diego
Veterans Administration Healthcare System
La Jolla, California

Michael G. Ciccotti, M.D.
Chief, Division of Sports Medicine
Director, Orthopaedic Sports Medicine Fellowship
Associate Professor of Orthopaedic Surgery
Department of Orthopaedics
Rothman Institute
Thomas Jefferson University
Philadelphia, Pennsylvania

Brian J. Cole, M.D., M.B.A.
Associate Professor
Department of Orthopaedics and Anatomy
and Cell Biology
Director
The Rush Cartilage Restoration Center
Rush University Medical Center
Chicago, Illinois

John G. Costouros, M.D.
Clinical Instructor
Department of Orthopaedic Surgery
Harvard Medical School
Harvard Shoulder Service
Boston, Massachusetts

Pierre Durand Jr., M.D.
Private Practice
Thousand Oaks, California

Mark E. Easley, M.D.
Assistant Professor
Department of Orthopaedic Surgery
Duke University Medical Center
Durham, North Carolina

Ryland B. Edwards, D.V.M., M.S., Ph.D.
Clinical Assistant Professor
Department of Surgical Sciences
University of Wisconsin–Madison
School of Veterinary Medicine
Madison, Wisconsin

Christopher H. Evans, Ph.D., D. Sc.
Robert Lovett Professor of Orthopaedic Surgery
Harvard Medical School
Boston, Massachusetts

Gary S. Fanton, M.D.
Chief
Division of Sports Medicine
Department of Orthopaedics
Stanford University
Palo Alto, California

Stefan Fornalski, M.D.
Orthopaedic Biomechanics Laboratory
Long Branch Veterans Administration Hospital
University of California, Irvine, Medical Center
Orange, California

Jeff A. Fox, M.D.
Central States Orthopaedic Specialists
Tulsa, Oklahoma

Freddie H. Fu, M.D.
David Silver Professor and Chairman
Department of Orthopaedic Surgery
University of Pittsburgh Medical Center
Pittsburgh, Pennsylvania

Ralph A. Gambardella, M.D.
Clinical Associate Professor
University of Southern California School of Medicine
Kerlan-Jobe Orthopaedic Clinic
Los Angeles, California

Wayne K. Gersoff, M.D.
Chairman
Department of Orthopaedic Surgery
Skyride Medical Center
Highlands Ranch, Colorado

Steven C. Ghivizzani, Ph.D.
Associate Professor of Orthopaedic Surgery
Department of Orthopaedics and Rehabilitation
University of Florida College of Medicine
Gainesville, Florida

Steven S. Goldberg, M.D.
Associate Staff Physician
Department of Orthopaedic Surgery
Cleveland Clinic Florida
Naples, Florida

László Hangody, M.D., Ph.D., D.S.C.
Professor
Department of Orthopaedics
Uzsoki Hospital
Budapest, Hungary

Francesco Iacono, M.D.
Assistant Professor
Department of Orthopaedic and Sports Traumatology
Rizzoli Orthopaedic Institute
Bologna, Italy

Christopher Iobst, M.D.
Department of Orthopaedic Surgery
Miami Children's Hospital
University of Miami School of Medicine
Miami, Florida

Amir M. Khan, M.D.
Texas Institute of Orthopaedic Surgery and Sports
    Medicine
Coppell, Texas

F. Daniel Kharrazi, M.D.
Orthopaedic Surgeon
Kerlan-Jobe Orthopaedic Clinic
Los Angeles, California

Mininder S. Kocher, M.D., M.P.H.
Assistant Professor of Orthopaedic Surgery
Department of Orthopaedic Surgery–Children's
    Hospital
Harvard Medical School
Boston, Massachusetts

Jason L. Koh, M.D.
Assistant Professor
Department of Orthopaedic Surgery
Northwestern University
Feinberg School of Medicine
Chicago, Illinois

Elizaveta Kon, M.D.
Assistant Professor
Department of Orthopaedic and Sports Traumatology
Rizzoli Orthopaedic Institute
Bologna, Italy

Thay Q. Lee, Ph.D.
Research Career Scientist
Orthopaedic Biomechanics Laboratory
Veterans Administration Long Beach
Healthcare System
Professor and Vice Chairman for Research
Department of Orthopaedic Surgery
Professor
Department of Biomedical Engineering
University of California Irvine
Long Beach, California

Yan Lu, D.V.M., Ph.D.
Scientist
Department of Medical Sciences
University of Wisconsin–Madison
School of Veterinary Medicine
Madison, Wisconsin

Gregory B. Maletis, M.D.
Assistant Chief
Department of Orthopaedic Surgery
Director of Sports Medicine
Kaiser Permanente
Baldwin Park, California

Bert R. Mandelbaum, M.D.
Director, Fellowship Program
President, Research and Education Foundation
Santa Monica Orthopaedic and Sports
Medicine Group
Santa Monica, California

Maurilio Marcacci, M.D.
Professor of Medicine
Department of Orthopaedic and Sports Traumatology
Rizzoli Orthopaedic Institute
Bologna, Italy

Leonardo Marchesini, M.D.
Assistant Professor
Department of Orthopaedic and Sports Traumatology
Rizzoli Orthopaedic Institute
Bologna, Italy

Mark D. Markel, D.V.M., Ph.D.
Professor and Chair
Department of Medical Sciences
University of Wisconsin–Madison
School of Veterinary Medicine
Madison, Wisconsin

Jennifer R. Miller, M.D.
Idaho Sports Medicine Institute
Boise, Idaho

Tom Minas, M.D.
Director
Cartilage Repair Center
Brigham and Women's Hospital

Associate Professor
Harvard Medical School
Chestnut Hill, Massachusetts

Raffy Mirzayan, M.D.
Co-Director of Sports Medicine
Director of Cartilage Regeneration and Repair
Kaiser Permanente
Baldwin Park, California

Clinical Associate Professor
Department of Orthopaedic Surgery
Keck School of Medicine
University of Southern California
Los Angeles, California

Aurea Mohana-Borges, M.D.
Department of Radiology
University of California–San Diego
Veterans Administration Healthcare System
La Jolla, California

Volker Musahl, M.D.
Department of Orthopaedic Surgery
University of Pittsburgh Medical Center
Pittsburgh, Pennsylvania

Ronald A. Navarro, M.D.
Chief of Orthopaedic Surgery
Southern California Permanente Medical Group

Regional Lead, Cartilage Studies
Department of Orthopaedics
South Bay Medical Center
Kaiser Permanente
Harbor City, California

Maria Pia Neri, M.D.
Assistant Professor
Department of Orthopaedic and Sports Traumatology
Rizzoli Orthopaedic Institute
Bologna, Italy

Michael J. Ostempowski, M.D.
Orthopaedic Surgeon–Private Practice
Amherst Orthopaedics
Depew, New York

Glyn D. Palmer, Ph.D.
Instructor
Department of Orthopaedic Surgery
Harvard Medical School
Boston, Massachusetts

Vahé R. Panossian, M.D.
Attending Physician
Department of Orthopaedic Surgery
Huntington Memorial Hospital
Pasadena, California

Russell S. Petrie, M.D.
Department of Orthopaedic Surgery
Hoag Memorial Hospital
Newport Beach, California

Tamara K. Pylawka, B.S., M.S.
Rush University Medical Center
Chicago, Illinois

Gabor Kristof Ráthonyi, M.D.
Department of Orthopaedics and Traumatology
Uzsoki Hospital
Budapest, Hungary

Donald L. Resnick, M.D.
Professor
Department of Radiology
University of California–San Diego
Veterans Administration Healthcare System
La Jolla, California

Anthony A. Romeo, M.D.
Associate Professor
Department of Orthopaedics
Rush Medical College
Rush–Presbyterian–St. Luke's Medical Center
Chicago, Illinois

Marc R. Safran, M.D.
Associate Professor
Chief, Sports Medicine Service
Department of Orthopaedic Surgery
University of California, San Francisco
San Francisco, California

Tomoyuki Sasaki, M.D.
Assistant Professor
Department of Orthopaedic Surgery
Hirosaki University School of Medicine
Hirosaki, Aomori, Japan

Michael A. Schwartz, M.D.
Clinical Instructor, Orthopaedic Surgery
Division of Sports Medicine
Department of Orthopaedics
Rothman Institute
Thomas Jefferson University
Philadelphia, Pennsylvania

Jason M. Scopp, M.D.
Orthopaedic Surgeon
Sports Medicine and Cartilage Restoration
Peninsula Orthopaedic Associates
Salisbury, Maryland

Paul Sethi, M.D.
Orthopaedic Surgeon
Orthopaedic and Neurosurgery Specialists
Greenwich, Connecticut

Steven D. Sides, M.D.
Chief
Department of Orthopaedic Foot and
    Ankle Surgery
Orthopaedic Surgeon Service
Madigan Army Medical Center
Fort Lewis, Washington

Andre F. Steinert, M.D.
Department of Orthopaedic Surgery
Julius Maximilians University Würzburg
Würzburg, Germany

Alison P. Toth, M.D.
Director
Duke Women's Sports Medicine Program
Assistant Professor
Department of Orthopaedic Surgery
Duke University Medical Center
Durham, North Carolina

Orrin Troum, M.D.
Keck School of Medicine
University of Southern California
Los Angeles, California

C. Thomas Vangsness, Jr., M.D.
Professor
Department of Orthopaedic Surgery
Keck School of Medicine
University of Southern California
Los Angeles, California

Jeffrey W. Wiley, M.D.
Concord Orthopaedics, P.A.
Concord, New Hampshire

Savio L.-Y. Woo, Ph.D., D.Sc.
W. K. Whiteford Professor and Director
Musculoskeletal Research Center
Department of Bioengineering
University of Pittsburgh
Pittsburgh, Pennsylvania

Stefano Zaffagnini, M.D.
Associate Professor
Biomechanics Laboratory
Department of Orthopaedic and Sports Traumatology
Rizzoli Orthopaedic Institute
Bologna, Italy

Basic Science

1

Structure and Function
of Cartilage Biology

MICHAEL A. SCHWARTZ AND MICHAEL G. CICCOTTI

Articular cartilage is a highly specialized tissue, exhibiting unique biomechanical properties. It is specifically organized to allow for the complex movements performed by synovial joints. With its specialized structure, articular cartilage has the benefit of excellent load-bearing characteristics, as well as friction, lubrication, and wear characteristics. This design enables articular cartilage to withstand many cycles of stress, a resiliency that is unique to the tissue.

■ Composition

The makeup of articular cartilage is ~95% extracellular and 5% cellular, exclusively chondrocytes.[1] The vast extracellular space is ~75% water, 20% collagen, 5% proteoglycans, and less than 1% other proteins, such as various growth factors, adhesive proteins, enzymes, and lipids.

Extracellular

Interstitial fluid is distributed more densely at the surface of articular cartilage, with a superficial concentration of 85%, and a its deep concentration of 65%.[2] This high surface water concentration allows for deformation in response to external stress, by shifting of the fluid in and out of cartilage. In addition, water plays a pivotal role in joint nutrition and lubrication.

The collagen of articular cartilage is primarily type II (90–95%), with small contributions from types IX and XI.[3–5] Under electron microscopy, collagen is noted to have a cross-banded fibrillar structure. Three α chains intertwine into a triple helix, forming a procollagen molecule. After the N- and C- terminal ends are cleaved off, the collagen fibrils are fashioned in a quarter-stagger overlapping configuration, producing the cross-banded appearance.[6–13] Covalent interfibrillar cross-links form, connecting the collagen molecules. This collagen imparts to the cartilage its mechanical properties of tensile stiffness, strength, and mechanical stability. The individual fiber diameter and orientation, the density of collagen fibers, and the amount of collagen interfibrillar cross-links all contribute to these unique characteristics.[4,11–17] In addition, collagen type XI functions as an adhesive that holds the collagen latticework together.[18–20]

Proteoglycans are glycosaminoglycan aggregates that are produced by the chondrocytes and secreted into the matrix. They are primarily responsible for the compressive strength of cartilage, by regulating the matrix hydration via trapping and holding water. The structure of the proteoglycan aggrecan molecule resembles a test-tube brush with keratin and chondroitin sulfate (glycosaminoglycan) side chains bound to a protein core. Multiple proteoglycan aggrecans are attached to a hyaluronic acid (HA) backbone via a link protein, forming a proteoglycan aggregate (**Fig. 1–1**). The concentrations of proteoglycans are highest in the articular cartilage middle zones and lowest in the more superficial zone.

Cartilage synthesis is regulated by various protein growth factors. Of these, transforming growth factor-β

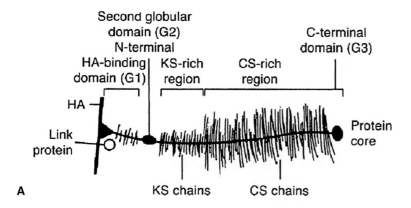

A

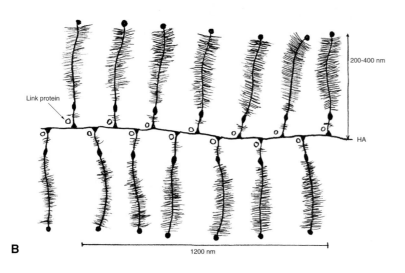

B

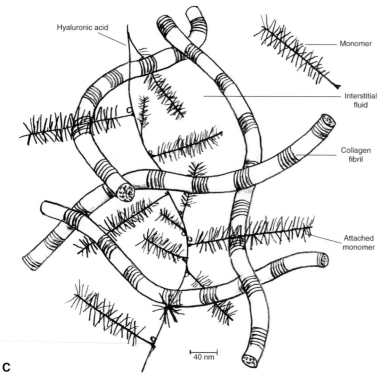

C

FIGURE 1–1 The structure of aggregating proteoglycans and their association with the collagen matrix. **(A)** The glycosaminoglycans keratin sulfate (KS) and chondroitin sulfate (CS) attach to aggrecan, which in turn binds to hyaluronic acid (HA) via its N-terminal globular domain through interaction facilitated by link protein. **(B)** HA is a large polysaccharide composed of repeats of a disaccharide of N-acetylglucosamine and glucuronic acid. **(C)** The negative charge associated with the proteoglycans trapped in a collagen matrix attracts cations and water into the matrix. (A and B by permission from Mankin HJ, Mow VC, Buckwalter JA, Iannotti JP, Ratcliffe A. Articular cartilage structure, composition, and function. In: Buckwalter JS, Einhorn TA, Simon SR, eds. Orthopaedic Basic Science: Biology and Biomechanics of the Musculoskeletal System, 2nd ed. Rosemont, IL: American Academy of Orthopaedic Surgeons, 2000:449–450. C by permission from Mow VC, Proctor CS, Kelly MA: Biomechanics of articular cartilage. In: Nordin M, Frankel VH, eds. Basic Biomechanics of the Musculoskeletal System, 2nd ed. Philadelphia: Lea and Febiger, 1989:31–57.)

(TGF-β), fibroblast growth factor (FGF), insulin-like growth factor-I (IGF-I), and platelet-derived growth factor (PDGF) are best understood. It is believed that TGF-β can stimulate proteoglycan synthesis and inhibit type II collagen synthesis. FGF stimulates DNA synthesis in adult articular chondrocytes. IGF-I stimulates DNA and matrix synthesis in both adult articular cartilage and immature growth plate cartilage. PDGF functions to promote proliferative responses on many mesenchymal cell types, including various connective tissues.

Minimal information is available on the various adhesives and other proteins in articular cartilage. The best understood is link protein, which helps stabilize the proteoglycan aggregates.[21,22] Anchorin and chondronectin are examples of other adhesive molecules that are known to exist in articular cartilage. There are also several major and minor cartilage matrix proteins that function to transduce signals from the extracellular environment to the cells via integrins and other similar cell-surface receptors.

Cellular

In mature articular cartilage, chondrocytes occupy only ~5% of the total volume. As a result of this comparatively low cell volume, chondrocytes are considered to be very metabolically active cells (**Fig. 1–2**).[1] They function to regulate the synthesis, maintenance, and turnover of the extracellular matrix proteins.

■ Structure

Articular cartilage is arranged in a highly stratified fashion, with four distinct but adjoining layers. Within each layer, there is a specific cellular organization and morphology, as well as varied degrees of tensile strength and stiffness. This ultrastructure is designed to enable each individual layer to fulfill its mechanical role. The four zones are (1) the tangential (superficial) zone, (2) the transitional (intermediate) zone, (3) the radial (deep) zone, and (4) the zone of calcified cartilage (**Fig. 1–3**).

Tangential (Superficial) Zone

The tangential zone forms the surface of the articular cartilage. It consists mainly of densely packed collagen fibrils, which are secreted by elongated chondrocytes and oriented parallel to the surface. Its high collagen-to-proteoglycan ratio correlates with its particularly high tensile strength and its lack of swelling properties seen in other zones. This imparts to this zone the ability to function against shear.

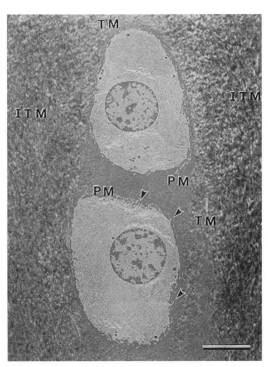

FIGURE 1–2 Electron micrograph of a pair of radial zone chondrocytes embedded in extracellular matrix. The chondrocytes show organelles necessary for matrix synthesis, including endoplasmic reticulum and Golgi's membranes. The extracellular matrix is compartmentalized into the pericellular matrix (PM), the territorial matrix (TM), and the interterritorial matrix (ITM). Arrowheads: fine cellular processes. Original magnification ×3500; bar = 5 μm. (By permission from Hunziker E, Michel M, Studer D. Ultrastructure of adult human articular cartilage matrix after cryotechnical processing. Microsc Res Tech 1997;37:271.)

Transitional (Intermediate) Zone

The transitional zone has structural and biomechanical properties between those of the superficial and underlying deep zones. The chondrocytes are smaller and more spherical, and the fibrils are organized obliquely. When seen under electron microscopy, these fibrils appear to bend over and form arcades (**Fig. 1–4**).[23] In addition, there is a relatively higher proteoglycan and lower collagen content when compared with the superficial zone. Its function transitions between resisting both shearing and compressive forces.

Radial (Deep) Zone

The chondrocytes are the largest and most synthetically active in this zone. Also, the proteoglycan content is highest in the upper radial zone, giving compressive properties to the articular cartilage. In addition, the collagen fibers are oriented perpendicular to the subchondral bone plate, providing the attachment to

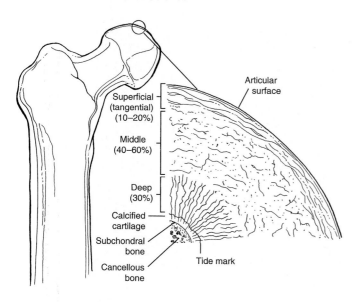

FIGURE 1–3 Articular cartilage layers. (By permission from Brinker MR, Miller MD. Fundamentals of Orthopaedics. Philadelphia: WB Saunders, 1999:9.)

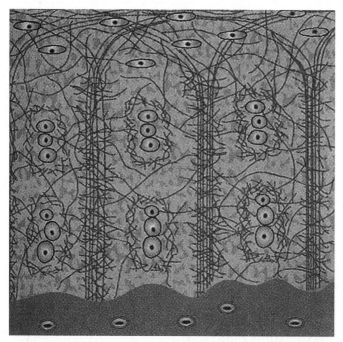

FIGURE 1–4 Adult articular cartilage. The collagen fibrils (black lines) give articular cartilage its overall structure. In the radial zone, the collagen fibrils are predominantly oriented perpendicular to the bone plate and provide anchorage to the subchondral bone. In the transitional zone, the fibrils bend over to form arcades. In the superficial zone, the fibrils run parallel to the surface. (By permission from Hunziker E, Michel M, Studer D. Ultrastructure of adult human articular cartilage matrix after cryotechnical processing. Microsc Res Tech 1997;37:271.)

the underlying calcified cartilage and subchondral bone.[24] The function of this zone is primarily to resist compression.

Calcified Cartilage Zone

This layer helps anchor the cartilage into the underlying bone. Specifically, it attaches the articular cartilage to the subchondral bone via interdigitated contours and type X collagen. Within the calcified cartilage zone is the tidemark layer, which bridges the border between the calcified and overlying uncalcified cartilage.

Matrix Compartmentalization

In addition to the four distinct zones, the extracellular matrix is also compartmentalized into three separate divisions, known as the pericellular, the territorial, and the interterritorial matrices (**Fig. 1–2**). The pericellular matrix surrounds the chondrocytes and is in close contact with their cell membranes.[5,25–28] It contains mainly proteoglycans, as well as glycoproteins and other noncollagenous proteins. The territorial matrix abuts the pericellular matrix and contains primarily collagen, forming a basket-like meshwork around the cells. It is thicker than the pericellular matrix and possibly functions to protect the cells during loading. The largest of the three matrix compartments is the interterritorial matrix, which also has the largest collagen fibrils. It is the orientation of these collagen fibers that accounts for the differences seen in the four distinct cartilage layers, that is, parallel in the superficial zone and perpendicular in the deep zone.[25-29] Hence, the interterritorial matrix is most likely predominantly responsible for the mechanical properties of the tissue.

■ Function of Normal Articular Cartilage

Human articular cartilage is required to withstand loads greater than five times body weight during walking and jogging. While sustaining such high loads, articular cartilage minimizes the stresses and strains on the matrix. More specifically, as a load is imparted to a joint, an elaborate distribution of tensile, shear, and compressive stresses are produced within the articular cartilage.[30-33] In response to such a load, articular cartilage behaves biphasically: (1) the solid matrix deforms, resulting in amplified contact areas and reduced contact stresses, and (2) fluid film lubrication is enhanced at the articular surface, by fluid exudation and redistribution.[30-32,34,35] This lubrication permits the relative movement of opposing joint surfaces, while limiting friction and wear. After the load has been removed, the tissue is allowed to recover by resorption of the fluid that had been extruded.

The intimate relationship between the collagen matrix and the proteoglycans is essential to the function of articular cartilage. Each aggrecan molecule has a large negative charge from the sulfate groups derived from the two types of glycosaminoglycan chains, chondroitin sulfate and keratin sulfate. The entrapment of these large, negatively charged aggregating proteoglycans within the collagen matrix attracts cations, which in turn generate an increase in the osmolality of the tissue. This attracts water, which then decreases the osmolality and causes a high tissue pressure. There is no associated swelling, as the highly interconnected type II collagen maintains the integrity of the tissue.[36]

Compression

When cartilage is subject to a constant compression force, fluid is extravasated from the solid matrix and redistributed until an equilibrium state, where no more fluid flow occurs, is reached. Such behavior is known as compressive creep. As a result, this process is dependent on both the permeability of the tissue and its compressive stiffness in the equilibrium state, where the deformed solid matrix supports the entire load. The egress of water from the cartilage during compression delivers a thin film of liquid that minimizes friction and smooths the gliding of opposing articular surfaces.[36]

When a compressive force is suddenly applied and then held constant, articular cartilage behaves according to a stress-relaxation model. In this paradigm, the stress initially peaks and then declines, until an equilibrium is attained.

Shear

Articular cartilage responds to shearing stresses mainly by stretching of the collagen and proteoglycan molecules. Because no interstitial fluid flow occurs in the pure shear state, the inherent viscoelastic properties of cartilage are utilized. This is a consequence of motions of both the proteoglycan and collagen molecules, and not from the frictional dissipation of fluid flow, as in compression. A proteoglycancollagen structure is more elastic in shear than a pure proteoglycan solution alone and more viscoelastic and more dissipative than a homogeneous collagen matrix alone.

Tension

The tension stress-strain curve of articular cartilage is similar to that of other soft tissues. It shows an initial curved "toe region," during which the collagen network is straightened, followed by a straight region, in which the collagen network is stretched, and then a failure point (**Fig. 1-5**). Young's modulus, the proportionality constant

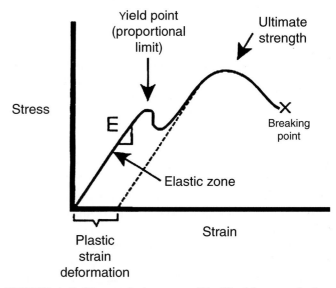

FIGURE 1-5 Stress-strain curve. (Modified by permission from Miller MD. Review of Orthopaedics, 3rd ed. Philadelphia: WB Saunders, 2000:121.)

in the linear stress-strain portion, is illustrative of the stiffness of the proteoglycan-collagen matrix in tension. As the tensile properties of articular cartilage correlate well with both the collagen content and the collagen/proteoglycan ratio, the different zones of articular cartilage have variable degrees of stiffness.[11-15] Specifically, the surface layer is stiffer than the deep layer, because of its high collagen/proteoglycan ratio, the highly oriented arrangement of the collagen fibrils, and, possibly, a high cross-linking density in this zone.[5,37-39] From various studies,[40-42] it has been learned that proteoglycans alone likely have little intrinsic tensile stiffness but do interact with collagen to resist the initial straightening when the tissue is pulled in tension. The collagen network alone, however, does resist the tensile load at equilibrium, providing cartilage with tensile strength and stiffness. The coupling of proteoglycans with collagen to produce a proteoglycan-collagen meshwork regulates the time-dependent behavior of articular cartilage in tension.[43]

■ Structure-Function Relationships of Articular Cartilage

Chondrocyte nutrition relies on periodic mechanical force, as the fluid flow under compression provides cell and tissue metabolites from the matrix. Variable loads promote matrix synthesis, which is influenced by the frequency and amplitude of the load.[44] Specifically, cyclic hydrostatic pressure triggers proteoglycan synthesis, whereas static compression results in an inhibition of metabolic activity.[45-48] Studies correlating mechanical and biochemical properties have enhanced our knowledge of the inherent structure-function relationships exhibited by articular cartilage. In vivo, areas of high weight-bearing and physical activity contained increased proteoglycan content. In contrast, decreased proteoglycan content was noted in response to reduced loading. Furthermore, it is now understood that static compression of articular cartilage results in a heterogeneous strain pattern, that is, considerably higher strains are found in the superficial layer relative to the deeper layers.[45]

■ Conclusion

Articular cartilage contains a highly organized architecture that is composed of a specific distribution of extracellular matrix components, mainly collagen, proteoglycans, and other proteins, which, in turn, are maintained by the highly specialized chondrocytes. It is this organization that enables articular cartilage to perform its function of facilitating the synovial joints' ability to carry out intricate movements by way of its excellent load-bearing, friction, lubrication, and wear characteristics.

REFERENCES

1. Hunziker EB. Articular cartilage structure in humans and experimental animals. In: Kuettner KE, Schleyerbach R, Peyron JG, Hascall VC, eds. Articular Cartilage and Osteoarthritis. New York: Raven Press, 1992:183
2. Lipshitz H, Etheredge R III, Glimcher MJ. Changes in the hexosamine content and swelling ratio of articular cartilage as functions of depth from the surface. J Bone Joint Surg Am 1976;58A:1149–1153
3. Nimni ME. Collagen: structure, function, and metabolism in normal and fibrotic tissues. Semin Arthritis Rheum 1983;13:1–86
4. Nimni ME, Harkness RD. Molecular structure and functions of collagen. In: Nimni ME, ed. Collagen. Boca Raton, FL: CRC Press, 1988:1–78
5. Buckwalter J, Hunzicker E, Rosenberg L, et al. Articular cartilage: composition and structure. In: Woo SL-Y, Buckwalter JA, eds. Injury and Repair of the Musculoskeletal Soft Tissues. Park Ridge, IL: American Academy of Orthopaedic Surgeons, 1988:405–425
6. Mow VC, Zhu W, Ratcliffe A. Structure and function of articular cartilage and meniscus. In: Mow VC, Hayes WC, eds. Basic Orthopaedic Biomechanics. New York: Raven Press, 1991:143–198
7. Muir IHM. The chemistry of the ground substance of joint cartilage. In: Sokoloff L, ed. The Joints and Synovial Fluid, vol 2. New York: Academic Press, 1980:27–94
8. Eyre DR, Grynpas MD, Shapiro FD, et al. Mature crosslink formation and molecular packing in articular cartilage collagen. Semin Arthritis Rheum 1981;11:46–47
9. Eyre DR, Apon S, Wu JJ, et al. Collagen type IX: evidence for covalent linkages to type II collagen in cartilage. FEBS Lett 1987;220:337–341
10. Eyre DR, Dickson IR, Van Ness K. Collagen cross-linking in human bone and articular cartilage: age-related changes in the content of mature hydroxypyridinium residues. Biochem J 1988;252:495–500
11. Kempson GE, Muir H, Pollard C, et al. The tensile properties of the cartilage of human femoral condyles related to the content of collagen and glycosaminoglycans. Biochim Biophys Acta 1973;297:456–472
12. Kempson GE. Mechanical properties of articular cartilage. In: Freeman MAR, ed. Adult Articular Cartilage, 2nd ed. Tunbridge Wells, England: Pitman Medical, 1979:333–414
13. Woo SL, Akeson WH, Jemmott GF. Measurements of nonhomogeneous, directional mechanical properties of articular cartilage in tension. J Biomech 1976;9:785–791
14. Roth V, Mow VC. The intrinsic tensile behavior of the matrix of bovine articular cartilage and its variation with age. J Bone Joint Surg. 1980;62A:1102–1117
15. Akizuki S, Mow VC, Müller F, et al. Tensile properties of human knee joint cartilage: I. Influence of ionic conditions, weight bearing, and fibrillation of the tensile modulus. J Orthop Res 1986;4:379–392
16. Schmidt MD, Schoonbeck JM, Mow VC, et al. Effects of enzymatic extraction of proteoglycans on the tensile properties of articular cartilage. Trans Orthop Res Soc 1986;11:450
17. Schmidt MD, Schoonbeck JM, Mow VC, et al. The relationship between collagen crosslinking and the tensile properties of articular cartilage. Trans Orthop Res Soc 1987;12:134
18. Eyre D, We JJ. Type IX of 123 collagen. In: Mayne R, Burgeson RE, eds. Structure and Function of Collagen Types. Orlando, FL: Academic Press, 1987
19. van der Rest M, Mayne R. Type IX collagen proteoglycan from cartilage is covalently cross-linked to type ii collagen. J Biol Chem 1988;263:1615–1618
20. Mayne R, Irwin MH. Collagen types in cartilage. In: Kuettner KE, Schleyerback R, Hascall VC, eds. Articular Cartilage Biochemistry. New York: Raven Press, 1986:23–38

21. Hardingham TE. The role of link-protein in the structure of cartilage proteoglycan aggregates. Biochem J 1979;177:237–247

22. Mow VC, Zhu WB, Lai TE, et al. The influence of link protein stabilization on the viscometric properties of proteoglycan aggregate solutions. Biochim Biophys Acta 1989;992:201–208

23. Hunziker E, Michel M, Studer D. Ultrastructure of adult human articular cartilage matrix after cryotechnical processing. Microsc Res Tech 1997;37:271–284

24. Redler I, Mow VC, Zimny M, et al. The ultrastructure and biomechanical significance of the tidemark of articular cartilage. Clin Orthop 1975;112:357–362

25. Clarke IC. Articular cartilage: a review and scanning electron microscope study. 1. The interterritorial fibrillar architecture. J Bone Joint Surg 1971;53B:732–750

26. Lane JM, Weiss C. Review of articular cartilage collagen research. Arthritis Rheum 1975;18:553–562

27. Poole CA, Flint MH, Beaumont BW. Morphologic and functional interrelationships of articular cartilage matrices. J Anat 1984;138: 113–138

28. Clarke JM. The organization of collagen in cryofractured rabbit articular cartilage: a scanning electron microscopic study. J Orthop Res 1985;3:17–29

29. Redler I, Zimny ML. Scanning electron microscopy of normal and abnormal articular cartilage and synovium. J Bone Joint Surg 1970;52A:1395–1404

30. Mow VC, Lai WM. Recent developments in synovial joint biomechanics. SIAM Rev 1980;22:275–317

31. Hou JS, Lai Wm, Holmes MH, et al. Boundary conditions and fluid flow through cartilage under squeeze film action. ASME Adv Bioeng 1988;14:181–182

32. Hou JS, Holmes MH, Lai WM, et al. Effects of changing cartilage stiffness, Poisson's ratio and permeability on squeeze film lubrication. ASME Adv Bioeng 1989;15:103–104

33. Askew MJ, Mow VC. The biomechanical function of the collagen fibril ultrastructure of articular cartilage. J Biomech Eng 1978; 100:105–115

34. Dowson D, Unsworth A, Cooke AF, et al. Lubrication of joints. In: Dowson D, Wright V, eds. An Introduction to the Biomechanics of Joints and Joint Replacement. London: Mechanical Engineering Publications, 1981:120–145

35. Mow VC, Mak AF. Lubrication of diarthrodial joints. In: Skalak R, Chien S, eds. Handbook of Bioengineering. New York: McGraw-Hill, 1987:5.1–5.34

36. Ulrich-Vinther M, Maloney MD, Schwarz EM, et al. Articular cartilage biology. J Am Acad Orthop Surg 2003;11(6): 421–430

37. Kempson G. Mechanical properties of articular cartilage and their relationship to matrix degradation and age. Ann Rheum Dis 1975;34 suppl. 2:111–113

38. Roth V, Mow V. The intrinsic tensile behavior of the matrix of bovine articular cartilage and its variation with age. J Bone Joint Surg 1980;62A:1102–1117

39. Schmidt M, Schoonbeck J, Mow V. The relationship between collagen crosslinking and the tensile properties of articular cartilage. Trans Orthop Res Soc 1987;12:134

40. Schmidt MB, Schoonbeck JM, Mow VC, et al. Effects of enzymatic extraction of proteoglycans on the tensile properties of articular cartilage. Trans Orthop Res Soc 1986;11:450

41. Schmidt MB, Mow VC, Chun LE, et al. Effects of proteoglycan extraction on the tensile behavior of articular cartilage. J Orthop Res 1989;7:771–782

42. Schmidt MB, Schoonbeck JM, Mow VC, et al. The relationship between collagen crosslinking and the tensile properties of articular cartilage. Trans Orthop Res Soc 1987;12:134

43. Ratcliffe A, Mow VC. The structure, function, and biologic repair of articular cartilage. In: Friedlaender GE, Goldberg VM, eds. Bone and Cartilage Allografts: Biology and Clinical Applications. Park Ridge, IL: American Academy of Orthopaedic Surgeons, 1991:123–154

44. Kim YJ, Sah RLY, Gordzinsky AJ, et al. Mechanical regulation of cartilage biosynthetic behavior: physical stimuli. Arch Biochem Biophys 1994;311:1–12

45. Wong M, Wuethrich P, Buschmann M, et al. Chondrocyte biosynthesis correlates with local tissue strain in statistically compressed adult articular cartilage. J Orthop Res 1997;15: 189–196

46. Hall A, Urban J, Gehl K. The effects of hydrostatic pressure on matrix synthesis in articular cartilage. J Orthop Res 1991;9: 1–10

47. Gray ML, Pizzanelli AM, Grodzinsky AJ, et al. Mechanical and physicochemical determinants of the chondrocyte biosynthetic response. J Orthop Res 1988;6:777–792

48. Schneiderman R, Keret D, Maroudas A. Effects of mechanical and osmotic pressure on the rate of glycosaminoglycan synthesis in the human adult femoral head cartilage: an in vitro study. J Orthop Res 1986;4:393–408

2

Biomechanics of Synovial Joints

THAY Q. LEE, STEFAN FORNALSKI, TOMOYUKI SASAKI,
AND SAVIO L.-Y. WOO

Human movement is possible due to the unique design and function of the synovial joint. Whether it is activities of daily living such as walking or high-performance activity in a sporting event, the synovial joint depends on complex interactions that occur between connective tissue structures. These structures include ligaments, tendons, menisci, subchondral bone, fibrous capsule, synovium, and hyaline articular cartilage. Articular cartilage is an integral component in this nearly frictionless system.

Articular cartilage functions under high loads with good tissue integrity into the seventh or eighth decade of life. This is due to the unique structural and biomechanical properties of articular cartilage. The intricate biomechanical behavior of articular cartilage is the result of its multiphasic material property, consisting of both a liquid and solid phase, unique viscoelastic properties, and swelling properties.[1] Articular cartilage and synovial joint lubrication allows a large range of joint loading conditions throughout life with minimal cartilage wear. Cartilage injury may occur over time as seen in chronic degenerative osteoarthritis or from acute athletic injuries. Athletic cartilage injuries may occur from acute direct trauma with excessive joint loading or from chronic altered joint biomechanics as observed in the sequelae of anterior cruciate ligament injuries.[2] In the elderly, failed nonsurgical management of osteoarthritis is addressed with joint replacement such as total hip or total knee arthroplasty. In the younger, active, athletic patient, joint arthroplasty is not the first line of surgical management. Some of the surgical treatments for the younger athletic patient include arthroscopic joint debridement, abrasion arthroplasty, subchondral drilling, osteochondral allografts, autologous chondrocyte implantation, and autologous osteochondral transplantation.[3]

This chapter discusses basic biomechanics, the composition and biomechanics of synovial joints with a focus on articular cartilage and joint lubrication, the effects of joint loading and altered biomechanics on articular cartilage, and the biomechanics of current cartilage repair including the surgical procedures of autologous chondrocyte implantation and autologous osteochondral transplantation.

■ Biomechanics

Newton's Laws

Newton's first law states that if a zero net external force is applied to a body, that body will remain in constant motion or at rest (sum of external forces applied to body equals zero). Newton's second law states that the acceleration of an object with a mass is directly proportional to the force applied to the object. Newton's third law states that for every action there is an equal and opposite reaction.[4] Biomechanics applies Newton's laws of motion to biologic systems to describe the function as well as the mechanical and structural integrity of the system.

Forces, including joint reaction force, are important parameters in understanding joint stability and function. Forces are vector quantities, which have both direction and magnitude. The length of the vector equals magnitude, the tail of the vector is the point of force application, the head of the vector is the direction, and the orientation of the vector is the line of action. Force, velocity, acceleration, and moment are also vector quantities. When a person is standing, a force exists between the foot and floor according to Newtons's third law (action with opposite reaction).[5] The joint forces usually considered are *compression* and *tension* in a perpendicular orientation to the articular surface and *shear force* in a parallel orientation to the articular surface. The principle of the "parallelogram of forces" allows vectors to be added, producing a resultant vector. By the same principle, vectors can also be broken down into component forces such as compression and shear force, which exist in different planes.

Moment is the rotational effect of a force on a body about an axis. A force acting at a distance from an axis produces a *moment* or *torque* about the point. For example, the biceps muscle acts at a defined perpendicular distance from the center of elbow rotation. Moment equals the force multiplied by the perpendicular distance to a specified axis of rotation (moment arm). An important concept for understanding muscle forces around joints is the force couple. A couple is a moment created by equal, parallel, but opposite directed forces. The force created by the couple is zero at equilibrium.[1,5]

Statics

Statics is the study of the action of forces on a joint or body at rest or in equilibrium. Although most biologic systems are normally not in complete equilibrium, the concept of static equilibrium is helpful in determining unknown forces or moments about synovial joints. Assumptions made with this model are that the bodies are completely rigid and that the sum of all forces and moments equal zero.[1,5,6] Free body diagrams use the concept of equilibrium and the known forces and moments to solve for unknown forces and moments.

Dynamics

Dynamics is the study of nonequilibrium conditions. An unopposed force acting on a body changes the velocity of the object. This may mean a change in direction or acceleration or deceleration. Acceleration produced by a linear force is termed linear acceleration and that about an axis of rotation with torque is termed angular acceleration. An example of linear deceleration is a basketball player landing from a jump. The downward velocity is being acted upon by the upward ground reaction force. This linear deceleration is proportional to the ground reaction force. By decreasing the deceleration by bending the knees and wearing shock-absorbing tennis shoes, the person can decrease the impact or ground reaction force.[1,5] An example of angular acceleration is a baseball pitcher throwing from the late cocking phase to the release phase of throwing.

Kinematics

Kinematics is the study of joint or body motion in terms of displacement, acceleration, and velocity without consideration of forces or moments on the moving body. Range of motion in a joint is constrained by the shape of the articulation (e.g., ball-and-socket or hinge joint), overall osseous architecture, active muscle forces, and by passive soft tissue constraints. To describe joint motion, a reference frame must be assumed. In a three-dimensional coordinate system of x, y, and z axes, the joint motion of translation and rotation occurs in six degrees of freedom. In a two-dimensional reference frame, only two coordinates (i.e., x and y) are required to define the position vector. In three dimensions a total of three coordinates (i.e., x, y, and z) and three orientation angles relative to the reference frame are required to define the position vector.[1,5,6]

Velocity vectors are defined as the change in displacement with respect to time. Synovial joint motion consists of both translational (sliding) and rolling motion. The amount of translation and rolling motion varies from joint to joint. If two points on a rigid body are moving in the same direction, pure translation is occurring. If two points are moving in different directions, both translation and rotation are occurring.[1,5]

The instant center of rotation is the point at which the joint rotates. In the knee, the instant center of rotation changes due to the added translation of the joint. The instant center of rotation normally lies on a line perpendicular to the tangent of the joint surface at all contact points. Pure translation has no angular changes and as such no instant center of rotation.[1,5,6]

■ Structural Properties

When an object is subjected to an external load, it will give a deformation response that is dependent on the magnitude and direction of the applied load, the materials that make up the object, and the shape and size of the object. The load-deformation curve is similar to the stress-strain curve and is derived by plotting the force applied by the deformation produced. The load-deformation curve relates to the structural properties of materials, that is, it is being affected by the size, shape, and intrinsic material properties. The slope in the linear elastic region of the load-deformation curve is referred to as the stiffness of the structure (**Fig. 2–1**).

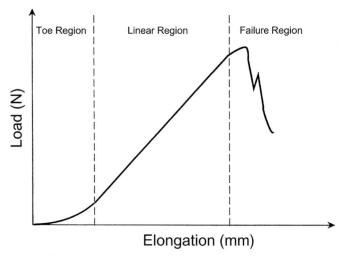

FIGURE 2–1 Load-elongation curve for tendon showing distinct response regions.[1]

Material Properties

Stress-strain curves relate to material properties. Stress is a physical quantity defined as force per unit area. This concept can be applied to an elderly patient with osteoarthritis. In degenerative joint disease, joint surface congruity is decreased, producing decreased contact area, increased stress on articular cartilage, and in turn the predisposition for degenerative changes. Compressive and tensile stresses refer to the stresses that are perpendicular to the surface, whereas shear stress refers to the stresses that are parallel to the surface. Strain is a relative measure of deformation. It is equal to the change in length of an object divided by the original length of the object. A stress-strain curve is simply the relationship of stress versus strain. In the elastic region of the curve (linear portion) the stress and strain are directly proportional and the elastic deformation is fully recoverable (strain is completely recovered on stress removal). This linear region, calculated as a slope, is known as Young's modulus of elasticity and represents the ability of a material to resist deformation.[1,5] The proportional limit (P) refers to a point at the end of the elastic range where stress-strain is no longer proportional. Past this point a small amount of plastic deformation occurs, and when the force is released a small permanent deformation exists (all of strain is not recovered) due to damage of the internal structure of the tissue. The yield strength (Y) is the point at which a nonrecoverable strain starts to occur, typically 0.2% strain past the proportional limit. Ultimate tensile strength (U) is the point of specimen failure. Stress at failure is usually thought of as the strength of the material. The area beneath the stress-strain curve is the intrinsic material toughness. The

stress-strain curves can typically be used to characterize the intrinsic material properties.

Linear elasticity has three important fundamental principles: (1) stress and strain are directly proportional, (2) strain produced is reversible once stress is removed, (3) the material response is insensitive to the rate of loading.[1,5,6] In living connective tissue, linear elasticity does not represent a true model, and the property of viscoelasticity must be recognized.

Viscoelasticity

In musculoskeletal tissue, linear elastic behavior is not frequently observed. Muscles, tendons, ligaments, cartilage, and bone exhibit the property of *viscoelasticity*.[1,5–7] Viscoelastic behavior is time dependent and is the manifestation of the internal friction within a biologic material. The stress-strain relationship is dependent on the strain rate, where the force response increases with the increasing rate of deformation.

Viscoelastic materials exhibit the unique behavior of *creep* and *stress relaxation*.[7,8] Creep is seen when a constant force is applied to a material causing increasing deformation until an equilibrium state is reached. *Stress-relaxation* is seen with a constantly held deformation, where force decreases over time until some equilibrium is reached.[1,5–8] Synovial joints display the viscoelastic properties of creep and stress relaxation.

Isotropy/Anisotropy

Biologic materials also have directional properties termed isotropy and anisotropy. Isotropic materials have intrinsic material properties independent of the direction of loading. Such materials include cancellous bone, plastic, and metals. Isotropic materials have a random internal structure. In contrast, anisotropic materials have intrinsic material properties that are dependent on the result of the direction of loading. An example of this is the trabecular pattern seen in the proximal femur. Anisotropic materials include bone, meniscus, ligaments, tendon, and articular cartilage. Anisotropic materials usually have an organized internal structure.[1,5]

■ Synovial Joints

Joint Composition

The proper function of a synovial joint, such as the knee, requires intricate function and coordination of multiple connective tissues. Synovial joint connective tissue structures include ligaments, tendons, meniscus, subchondral bone, the fibrous capsule, synovium, and articular cartilage. Both intraarticular and extraarticular ligaments are important for providing physical restraints, for both joint stability and limiting joint range of motion. Tendons provide a mechanism for transfer of muscle forces to bony insertions and across synovial joints to produce movement. The meniscus functions in force dispersion and in creating an improved functional congruity within a joint. The fibrous capsule and synovial lining constitute the boundaries of the synovial joint and are bathed in synovial fluid. Hyaline articular cartilage lines the subchondral bone of synovial joints, and functions to provide a lubricated and nearly frictionless weight-bearing surface, to protect subchondral bone, and to more evenly distribute forces to subchondral bone.[9] Articular cartilage functions under high loads with good tissue integrity into the seventh and eighth decade of life. The following sections discuss the unique composition of articular cartilage, the biomechanics of articular cartilage, and synovium/lubrication theories.

Articular Cartilage Composition

Articular cartilage lines the load-bearing surfaces in synovial joints. Through its unique biomechanical and structural properties, it functions to minimize friction between articulating surfaces, to absorb mechanical loads, and to spread joint loads over larger surface areas and to subchondral bone. Articular cartilage is avascular, aneural, and alymphatic, and it receives nutrients through diffusion in synovial fluid. In turn, cartilage shows poor healing capacity. Both the unique structural and biomechanical properties of articular cartilage allow synovial joints to function in a variety of loading conditions throughout life.[1]

Structurally cartilage is composed of a large extracellular matrix (ECM) interspersed with specialized cartilage cells called the chondrocytes. The components of the ECM primarily include water (60–80%), collagen type II (10–20%), proteoglycans (4–7%), and other proteins and glycoproteins (<5%). Collagen and proteoglycans are the two major structural macromolecules in the articular cartilage ECM.[1,5,10,11]

Water

Water makes up about 60 to 80% of the wet weight of articular cartilage. This includes intracellular (chondrocytes) water, although the majority of water in articular cartilage is in the molecular pores of the ECM. Dissolved in water are sodium, calcium, potassium, and chloride. The relative water concentration decreases from the superficial to deeper zones in articular cartilage.[10,11] Water moves through the ECM by mechanical compression of the ECM and also due to a pressure

gradient. The permeability of articular cartilage is low. As water moves through the molecular pores in the ECM, high frictional resistance is encountered. Pressurization within the ECM, with mechanical loading and frictional resistance of water movement, are critical to articular cartilage biomechanics and its load-bearing capacity. Water flow is also important for nutrient flow within the tissue. In addition, as described in the lubrication section, water is important in the weeping effect of lubrication.[12-14] An important quality of articular cartilage is its hydrophilic nature. This is mostly due to the proteoglycans. The interaction among water, proteoglycans, and collagen is critical in forming a solid resilient cartilage matrix.[11,15]

Chondrocytes

Chondrocytes are specialized cartilage cells derived from mesenchymal cells. They occupy less than 10% of the cartilage volume. Chondrocytes maintain the ECM and produce collagen, proteoglycans, and glycoproteins. These cells respond to growth factors, interleukins, medications, and physical stimulation such as mechanical and hydrostatic pressure changes.[5,16,17]

Collagens

The major structural component of the ECM is the collagen macromolecule. There are numerous types of collagen in bone, tendon, skin, blood vessels, ligaments, and cartilage. Characteristically collagen consists of a triple-helical structure composed of three polypeptide chains (α chains) (**Fig. 2–2**).[1,16] In articular cartilage, over

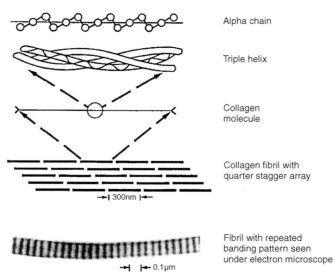

Alpha chain

Triple helix

Collagen molecule

Collagen fibril with quarter stagger array

├─┤ 300nm ├─┤

Fibril with repeated banding pattern seen under electron microscope

├─┤ ├─ 0.1μm

FIGURE 2–2 Illustration showing hierarchical organization and photomicrograph of collagen fibril.[1]

50% of the dry weight is collagen. Type II collagen is the predominant (95%) collagen in articular cartilage. Other types in articular cartilage include types V, VI, IX, X, and XI.[1,10,15,16] Collagen provides the shear and tensile properties of articular cartilage and also anchors proteoglycans within the ECM. Other collagen functions include type VI in anchoring chondrocytes in the matrix, type X in mineralization in the deeper cartilage layers, and types IX and XI may function to form cross-links between type II collagen fibers.[5] Collagen cross-linking increases the insolubility of collagen in the ECM and likely is involved with the tensile properties of articular cartilage.[1,6,17]

Proteoglycans

Proteoglycans are large ECM molecules composed of a protein core and covalently bound glycosaminoglycan (GAG) chains. Proteoglycans are hydrophilic, producing the water affinity of articular cartilage.[1,14,15] GAGs are long unbranched disaccharide units. The three types most often found in articular cartilage are keratan sulfate, dermatan sulfate, and chondroitin 4- and 6-sulfate. The chondroitin sulfates are the most prevalent and account for over 50% of the GAG.[5] GAG chains have repeating sulfate (SO_4) and/or carboxyl (COOH) groups that become ionized in solution and in the physiologic environment. These negative charges require positive counter-ions such as calcium and sodium ions (positive ions in solution). These free ions give rise to an osmotic pressure also known as the Donnan effect. In addition, the negative GAG charges result in charge-to-charge repulsive forces. As will be described in later sections both the osmotic pressure and charged repulsive forces are important for maintaining the structural integrity of articular cartilage.[5,10,11,14,15]

The majority of proteoglycans in articular cartilage are of the aggrecan type. These are composed of a long protein core molecule with up to 100 GAGs covalently bound to the protein core **(Fig. 2–3).**[1,5] Hyaluronate is an unusual GAG that is very large in size, not bound to a protein core, and without sulfate groups. Hyaluronate and numerous aggrecan molecules binding to hyaluronate form large macromolecular complexes similar in structure to that of a bottle brush **(Fig. 2–4).**[1] This large macromolecular size likely aids in stabilizing the aggrecan molecules in the ECM.[1,10,11,16] Smaller proteoglycan molecules in articular cartilage include decorin, biglycan, and fibromodulin. The role of these smaller molecules is not as well understood as that of the aggrecan type.[1]

Structural Matrix

The macromolecular organization of the proteoglycan-collagen and the proteoglycan-proteoglycan interaction

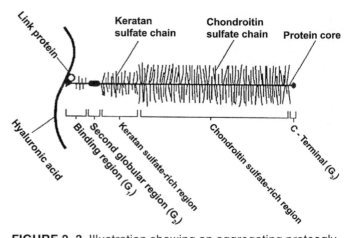

FIGURE 2–3 Illustration showing an aggregating proteoglycan monomer, the protein core with branches of glycosaminoglycan chains (keratan and chondroitin sulfate), link protein, and hyaluronic acid.[34]

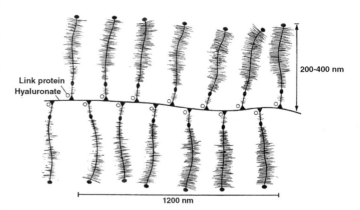

FIGURE 2–4 Depiction of many proteoglycan monomers attached to a chain of hyaluronate via link protein.[6]

and water content within the ECM combine to produce a solid and rigid matrix.[1,10] The large proteoglycans trapped within the ECM attract water, creating a swelling pressure. This swelling pressure expands and is countered in force by the cross-linked collagen network **(Fig. 2–5).** To simplify the discussion, collagen and proteoglycan interact to form a porous resilient matrix and trap water molecules to give cartilage its unique swelling properties. This unique structural organization creates the dynamic biomechanical properties seen in articular cartilage.[1,10,11,15]

Zones of Articular Cartilage

Articular cartilage varies by depth and can be divided into four main layers or zones **(Fig. 2–6).** These zones, from superficial (articular surface) to deep (subchondral bone), are the superficial zone, the middle (transitional) zone, the deep zone, and the zone of

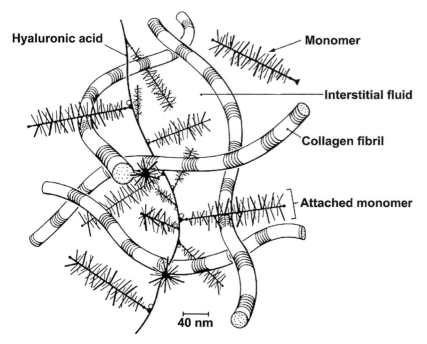

Hyaluronic acid

Monomer

Interstitial fluid

Collagen fibril

Attached monomer

40 nm

FIGURE 2–5 Depiction of articular cartilage matrix, collagen, and proteoglycan interact to form a porous resilient matrix and trap water molecules to give cartilage its unique swelling properties.[6]

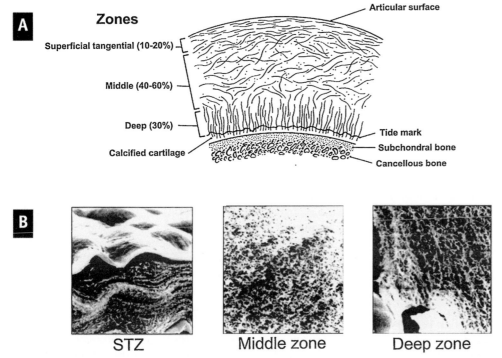

A

Zones

Superficial tangential (10-20%)

Middle (40-60%)

Deep (30%)

Calcified cartilage

Articular surface

Tide mark
Subchondral bone
Cancellous bone

B

STZ   Middle zone   Deep zone

FIGURE 2–6 Illustration and electromicrograph (×3000) showing zones of articular cartilage (see text for explanation).[35]

calcification.[1] The amount and orientation of collagen, proteoglycans, water, and cells varies according to the level or zone **(Fig. 2–6).** In the *superficial zone* (upper 10–20%) collagen is oriented parallel to the surface, and chondrocytes are elongated and parallel to collagen. This collagen orientation likely functions during shear stress to the articular surface.[1] Collagen and water content is highest, and proteoglycan content is lowest compared with other layers. In the *middle (transitional) zone* (40–60%) collagen fibers are thicker and more randomly oriented and chondrocytes have a more rounded shape. This layer likely functions in compression.[1,5] The *deep zone* (30%) has the lowest water content, the highest proteoglycan content, and spherical-shaped chondrocytes arranged with collagen in columnar arrays perpendicular to joint surface. This

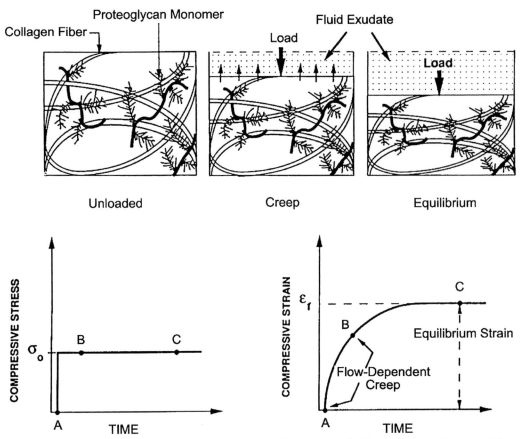

FIGURE 2–7 Nonlinear strain-dependent permeability property of articular cartilage serves to prevent excessive and rapid fluid exudation from articular cartilage. Regulation of fluid exudation is important for support in compression loads and also in energy dissipation.[1]

vertical collagen orientation likely functions in compression.[1,5] The *tide mark* is the border between the *deep zone* and the *zone of calcification*. It represents the uppermost border of mineralization. The *zone of calcification* consists of a calcified ECM and is the border between cartilage and subchondral bone.[1,5,6,10]

Auricular Cartilage Biomechanics

Biphasic Nature of Articular Cartilage

Articular cartilage is a viscoelastic tissue that is exposed to a spectrum of loading conditions in everyday life and in competitive athletics. It consists of a hydrated proteoglycan-collagen matrix functioning as a low-friction, shock-absorbing system. The matrix structure in articular cartilage includes proteoglycans, collagen, and water that are all organized into a resilient, tough tissue that is able to sustain tremendous stress and strain during joint loading.[1,5,10] The biomechanics of articular cartilage can be understood by viewing articular cartilage as a biphasic material consisting of both a solid and liquid phase.[18,19] The solid phase is the proteoglycan-collagen matrix. The liquid phase is the water and associated dissolved ions.[1,18,19]

Articular cartilage biomechanical properties are due to the swelling pressure and resistance to water flow through the matrix. As previously described, water makes up 60 to 80% of articular cartilage and flows through the matrix by mechanical compression or pressure gradient.[1,10,11] High pressures are required to move water through cartilage. With articular cartilage compression, volume is decreased and tissue pressure is increased. Water flow through the low permeable matrix causes high frictional forces, creating high hydrodynamic forces.[1,10–14] In normal short-duration cartilage compressive loading, fluid pressure provides the support, and the solid (collagen-proteoglycan) phase is protected in a type of stress shielding.[5] Articular cartilage permeability is nonlinear, decreasing with increasing compression **(Fig. 2–7)**.[1,20] With compression, this property allows the prevention of rapid water exit from articular cartilage. In turn, increased hydrodynamic forces are created for load bearing. This nonlinear effect occurs with cartilage compression, because porosity is reduced and the density of the negative charge contribution is increased due to increased concentration of proteoglycans. Both the decreased porosity and increased negative charge density will make it harder for water to exit the articular cartilage matrix, in turn increasing the hydrodynamic forces and load-bearing capacity.[1,10,20]

Swelling of Articular Cartilage

Articular cartilage swelling is due to the biphasic nature of articular cartilage.[1,7,18] The unique mechanical properties of articular cartilage arise from the swelling pressure created by the interaction of proteoglycans, water, and ions.[10,11] The large proteoglycans are trapped in the collagen matrix, attracting and trapping water. This in turn causes swelling and a swelling pressure. This swelling pressure is due to the negative charge of the proteoglycan molecules and counterbalancing by positive ions (sodium and calcium).[1,10,11] This overall increase in tissue/matrix ion concentration and larger relative ion concentration, as compared with that outside of the tissue, drives water into the matrix and creates the *Donnan osmotic pressure*.[1] In addition, the closely spaced negative charges cause charge repulsion and matrix expansion in what is termed *chemical expansion stress*.[5] The total swelling pressure in articular cartilage is the sum of the Donnan osmotic pressure and the chemical expansion stress.[5] This overall swelling pressure is resisted by the tensile properties of the collagenous matrix and exists in constant physiologic equilibrium. The matrix can be thought of as being "inflated" by the swelling pressures and limited by the collagenous reinforced matrix.[1,6,10]

Flow Dependent and Independent Viscoelastic Properties of Auricular Cartilage

Articular cartilage is a viscoelastic material with time-dependent behavior.[1,7,18] Viscoelasticity and concepts of creep and stress relaxation were previously reviewed. Creep occurs with a constant compressive stress causing tissue deformation until an equilibrium is reached.[1,8] Stress-relaxation occurs with a constant tissue deformation, causing stress to rise to a maximum and then decrease over time until some equilibrium is reached.[1,8] Articular cartilage compression, shear, and tensile forces can be described by two mechanisms: *flow-dependent viscoelasticity* and *flow-independent viscoelasticity*.[1,5,18,19]

Flow-dependent viscoelasticity describes articular cartilage under compressive forces. With a constant compressive force applied to articular cartilage, creep is observed, and with a constant tissue deformation, stress decreases over time. These properties are based on hydrostatic pressure and fluid flow within the tissue.[1,5,6,8] With constant compression the load is initially supported by the hydrostatic pressure within the articular cartilage matrix. Creep occurs over time as the fluid exits the tissue, decreasing the hydrostatic pressure.[1,12–14,18] Fluid flow out of tissue and permeability is nonlinear as previously reviewed (**Fig. 2–7**).[20] Over time, the load applied is transferred from the fluid phase (hydrostatic pressure) to the solid phase (proteoglycan-collagen matrix). For normal articular cartilage, this equilibration takes from 2.5 to 6 hours. At equilibrium the hydrostatic fluid pressure is gone and the load is completely supported by the collagen-proteoglycan matrix.[1,5,7,10,12,19] In normal dynamic joint loading this equilibrium is never reached and hydrostatic fluid pressure is the dominant load support system in synovial joints.[1,5]

Flow-independent viscoelasticity describes articular cartilage under a *pure shear force*.[1,5,6] Under this condition, no fluid flow or tissue volume change occurs. The main contributor of articular cartilage properties under pure shear conditions is the collagen organization in the middle zone. Under shear forces the collagen fibers are stressed and provide the tissue resistance.[1,6,16,17] With a nearly frictionless synovial joint it would seem that shear forces do not effect articular cartilage. This is not true, due to the concept of Poisson's ratio effect. Poisson's ratio is a measure of how much a material will expand in the plane perpendicular to the applied compressive force, and any material with a ratio other than zero will expand in this plane.[1,6] Articular cartilage is attached to subchondral bone. With compressive loading the articular cartilage cannot expand at this attachment point (subchondral bone–cartilage interface), and in turn a shear force is experienced by the cartilage tissue. With excessive compressive loading, as in trauma or high impact, the shear forces can overcome the cartilage–bone interface and detach cartilage from the bone.[1,5,10]

The *tensile properties* of articular cartilage are the result of both flow-dependent and flow-independent viscoelastic mechanisms.[1,5,17] With articular cartilage placed under tension at equilibrium conditions (i.e., creep and stress-strain equilibrium) or at extremely slow stretching conditions, the collagen matrix response to tensile force can be tested independent of viscoelasticity. The intrinsic tensile properties of the collagen matrix, under the above-described equilibrium conditions, can be shown with a stress-strain curve (**Fig. 2–8**).[1] This is a similar curve obtained with tendons and ligaments. A curved toe region is seen where collagen fibers are aligning themselves under a tensile force (**Fig. 2–8**). The linear region represents the tensile modulus for articular cartilage. This reflects the stiffness of the articular cartilage in tension. This varies depending on the zone of articular cartilage sampled, with the superficial zone having the highest stiffness.[1]

■ Synovium and Lubrication Theories

Synovium

Synovial joints are exposed to a variety of loading conditions during activities of daily living and athletic activities. Human hip and knee joints often are exposed to

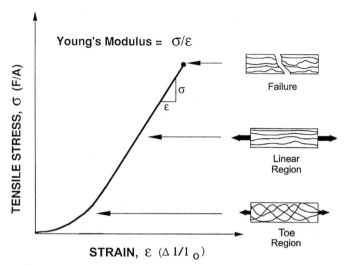

Young's Modulus = σ/ε

FIGURE 2–8 Stress-strain curve for articular cartilage. The toe region shows an increasing slope until parallel collagen fiber orientation is reached. Linear portion of curve has a slope equal to the Young's modulus.[6]

forces of 5 to 10 times body weight.[9] Throughout a person's life there is generally little wear in synovial joints. This minimal wear is made possible by the interaction of synovial fluid and articular cartilage in synovial joints. The articular lined bone ends are enclosed by the tough fibrous joint capsule and inner synovial lining.[21] The synovium mediates the exchange of nutrients between blood and the joint and also secretes synovial fluid into the joint.[1,9] This fluid is highly viscous and exhibits non-Newtonian flow characteristics.[22] The viscosity coefficient is not constant and synovial fluid viscosity is nonlinear. Viscosity increases as shear rate decreases or vice versa.[1,9,22] Synovial fluid is an ultrafiltrate or dialysate of blood plasma containing no clotting factors, erythrocytes, or hemoglobin. Synovial fluid does contain hyaluronic acid (glycosaminoglycan), proteinases, collagenases, and glycoprotein (lubricin). Hyaluronic acid is a glycosaminoglycan molecule that forms an elastic network of macromolecules that can be deformed by energy and act as an elastic solid at higher forces.[5] Degradation of hyaluronic acid, as in rheumatoid arthritis, results in synovial fluid losing its non-Newtonian properties and in turn losing its biomechanical protective properties. Lubricin is a glycoprotein that functions as a key component in lubrication. Normally, the amount of synovial fluid within synovial joints is minimal; there is about 1 to 5 mL of synovial fluid in the human knee joint.[5,9]

Several lubrication theories have been developed to explain the almost frictionless and minimal wear characteristics produced by the interaction of synovial fluid and articular cartilage. These theories can be divided into two categories: fluid-film lubrication and boundary lubrication theories.[1]

Cartilage Lubrication Theories

Fluid-film lubrication models include hydrodynamic, elastohydrodynamic, squeeze-film, weeping, and boosted. Synovial fluid is the lubricant in fluid-film lubrication. Fluid-film lubrication functions mostly under short loading durations and submaximal joint loading conditions. Under severe, prolonged synovial joint loading conditions, the fluid film is depleted and boundary lubrication becomes the primary mode of lubrication.[1,16]

Hydrodynamic lubrication occurs with a thin film of fluid on the bearing surfaces that is able to withstand an applied load. In this condition the bearing surfaces do not come into contact. The hydrodynamic theory is not an accurate model for synovial joints; rather, it is for example, for ball bearings. This model is accurate for low loads and with high speeds between bearing surfaces. Assumptions made with this model include the following: the lubricant displays Newtonian (constant) properties, bearing surfaces are rigid, loads are low and the relative speed of two bearing surfaces is high, and the fluid forms a wedge-shaped gap.[5] With excessive joint reaction force, the fluid film is overcome and boundary lubrication occurs. This model may be analogous to a rapid swing phase at the knee joint with no joint loading.[1,5,6]

Elastohydrodynamic lubrication considers the unique biomechanical properties and elastic deformation of articular cartilage. A thin fluid film along with cartilage deformation creates a low friction system that is the dominant mechanism for lubrication in synovial joints. Articular cartilage deformation spreads the joint load over a larger surface area. Synovial fluid displays non-Newtonian properties including its shear rate dependent viscosity and elastic energy spring secondary to the internal macromolecular network (hyaluronic acid).[1,5,6,22]

Weeping lubrication occurs during dynamic synovial joint loading. Fluid shifts out of cartilage and into areas of loading. This "weeping" effect is created during articular cartilage compression and serves to form the fluid film between the two joint surfaces.[1,5,6,16]

In squeeze-film lubrication the two bearing surfaces approach each other with no sliding motion. The resistance of the lubricant between the two surfaces causes increased pressure and fluid film that can withstand large loads for short periods (a few seconds). Synovial joint lubrication during human gait may be a combination of elastohydrodynamic lubrication during the unloaded/fast swing phase and squeeze-film lubrication during the foot strike phase of gait.[1,5,16]

Boosted lubrication involves fluid entrapment and increasing the concentration of hyaluronic acid at the articulating surfaces. The two weight-bearing surfaces approach each other in a squeeze-film manner. Water passes into articular cartilage through small pores, leaving behind a large concentration of protein hyaluronic acid molecules. Articular cartilage pores are normally smaller than hyaluronic acid molecules. The increased hyaluronic acid concentration at the articulation increases the viscosity of the synovial fluid, in turn "boosting" the load-carrying capacity of the synovial fluid.[5]

With prolonged and maximal joint loading, fluid-film lubrication is not maintained and boundary lubrication becomes the primary mode of lubrication. In boundary lubrication the fluid film has been depleted and a thin layer of a glycoprotein, known as lubricin, is on the articular surfaces. This minimizes friction and abrasion. During synovial joint loading, likely a combination of both fluid-film and boundary lubrication act to minimize friction and wear at the articular surface.[1,5]

Effects of Joint Loading and Altered Biomechanics on Articular Cartilage

Synovial joint motion and articular cartilage loading occurs on a daily basis. Running and walking may load articular cartilage with 2 to 4 times the body weight and with excessive loading may be up to 8 to 10 times the body weight.[5,9] Regular daily joint loading is required to maintain normal healthy articular cartilage. Articular cartilage is aneural, alymphatic, and avascular.[5] Normal joint loading circulates synovial fluid, produces the weeping effect at the articular cartilage surface, provides dynamic compression of and flow through the cartilage matrix, and provides movement of nutrients to articular cartilage via synovial fluid.[1,5,9,13]

Increased joint loading can be due to increased magnitude or high-frequency use. This can be in the form of a single traumatic injury or chronic use. With loss of soft tissue restraints (e.g., knee cruciate ligaments and meniscus) within synovial joints the stress distribution and motion within the joint are altered. In experimental animal models, transection of the anterior cruciate ligament and meniscectomy produce articular cartilage degenerative changes including fibrillation, a change in proteoglycan amount, and increased hydration.[5]

Immobilization of a joint leads to articular cartilage atrophy and degenerative changes. In models using rigid fixation, immobilization can be divided into noncontact and contact conditions relative to joint articular surface.[5] Rigid fixation and static constant pressure between two articular surfaces produces chondrocyte death and severe degenerative changes at areas of contact. Rigid immobilization with noncontact of articular surfaces results in decreased proteoglycan content and tissue fibrillation. Inhibiting both the function of normal joint motion and the delivery of nutrients to articular cartilage via synovial fluid is likely an important factor in the observed articular cartilage changes. Biomechanical changes, likely secondary to alteration in proteogycan, include increased fluid efflux and increased tissue deformation with a compressive force.[5] Tensile properties are dependent on collagen, and in turn are mostly unchanged.[5,17] The biochemical and biomechanical changes seen are reversible with remobilization. A recent animal study found that after 11 weeks of immobilization knee articular cartilage thickness decreased by 9% and deformation rate increased up to 42%.[23] Recovery of cartilage properties is inversely related to time and amount of immobilization.

In animal models, normal running exercise may increase stiffness and proteoglycan content, decrease water efflux, and increase cartilage thickness.[5] With articular cartilage injury, continuous passive motion (CPM) is believed to aid in cartilage repair.[24] It is believed that joint loading and motion affect chondrocyte function by electrical, mechanical, and physiochemical signals.[16,17] Changing matrix ion concentration may function in electrical signal transduction. Hydrostatic pressure within the matrix may mechanically deform chondrocyte cellular membranes and produce intracellular signaling, in turn causing production or degradation of products. Fluid movement through tissue matrix may be a transport mechanism for growth factors and other cell mediators.[16,17] Further research is required to determine the effects of these signals on chondrocytes.

■ Biomechanics of Current Articular Cartilage Repair Techniques

Treatment of isolated traumatic knee articular cartilage injury remains a difficult challenge. These can be debilitating lesions, especially in the younger athlete. In addition, these lesions are also considered a risk factor for more extensive joint injury including osteoarthritis.[3] Articular cartilage is a unique tissue that is avascular, aneural, and alymphatic, with slow chondrocyte turnover.[5] This gives articular cartilage poor healing and repair capacities. Articular cartilage has a unique architecture with an elaborate interaction among chondrocytes, water, proteoglycans, and collagen.[1,5,6,10] This elaborate interaction gives articular cartilage its unique biomechanical properties, which are difficult to reproduce in damaged cartilage. For isolated articular cartilage injuries, several surgical treatments exist including arthroscopic joint debridement, abrasion arthroplasty, subchondral drilling, microfracture technique, osteochondral allografts, autologous chondrocyte implantation, and autologous osteochondral transfer.[3,9]

With acute traumatic articular cartilage injury, the goal must be to repair the lesion with hyaline-like material and attempt to reproduce the biomechanical properties of hyaline articular cartilage. Subchondral drilling and microfracture involve bone marrow cell stimulation and fibrin clot formation in the articular cartilage lesion.[3,9] These procedures utilize the available cartilage precursors in bone marrow. Unfortunately, with these procedures a fibrous cartilage usually fills the lesion and lacks the unique biomechanical and biochemical characteristics of hyaline articular cartilage.[3,9]

One of the great challenges is to repair the articular cartilage defect with hyaline-type cartilage that has the biomechanical properties of normal articular cartilage. Two techniques focused on this effort are autologous chondrocyte implantation and autologous osteochondral transplantation.[9] There have been several recent studies involving the biomechanics of the surgical treatments of autologous chondrocyte implantation and autologous osteochondral transplantation. They are reviewed in the following section.

Autologous Chondrocyte Implantation

Autologous chondrocyte implantation (ACI) can be used with larger cartilage lesions of 2.5 cm or larger. ACI is a two-stage surgical procedure. Step 1 involves arthroscopically harvesting the patient's own articular cartilage cells and expanding them in in vivo cell culture for 2 to 3 weeks. Step 2 involves taking the cultured chondrocyte cells and implanting them under an autologous periosteal tissue flap at the articular cartilage defect.[3,9]

Autologous chondrocyte implantation was studied in animal models in the 1980s. Implantation of harvested cultured chondrocytes into articular cartilage lesions produced hyaline-like cartilage by histology.[25] Much of the early clinical work with ACI was done in Sweden. Over the past 5 to 7 years, ACI has been widely used throughout the United States and Europe. Although studies have shown histologically a hyaline-like cartilage following ACI, there is sparse information regarding the biomechanics of this graft tissue. Peterson et al[26] evaluated the clinical, histologic, and biomechanical characteristics of the grafted tissue following ACI. ACI was conducted in 61 human subjects for isolated cartilage defects on the femoral condyle or patella. Mean follow-up of the patients was 7.4 years (range 5–11 years). For clinical evaluation patients were followed up at two different time intervals: at 2 years and between 5 and 11 years. At 2 years 50 of 61 patients had good to excellent clinical results. At the later stage of 5- to 11-year follow-up, 51 of 61 patients had good to excellent results. From these 61 patients, 11 patients were taken back for a second-look arthroscopy, during which the biomechanical properties of the grafted areas were evaluated with an electromechanical probe (average follow-up 54.3 months). Indentation measurements with the electromechanical probe were done in the center of the grafted site and also at the surrounding normal hyaline articular cartilage of the same femoral condyle (control value). In addition, biopsy samples from these 11 patients were taken as 2-mm biopsies from the center of the graft site. Eight out of 12 biopsy specimens were of hyaline-like tissue, and the other 4 were fibrous-type cartilage. Overall, stiffness in grafted areas was 2.4 ± 0.3 N (mean ± SD) compared with 3.2 ± 0.3 N for control cartilage. The mean measured stiffness in the grafted area with hyaline cartilage-type tissue was twice that of the grafted site with fibrous tissue, 3.0 ± 1.1 N stiffness compared with 1.5 ± 0.35 N, respectively. In the eight out of 12 specimens with graft-site hyaline cartilage-type tissue, the measured stiffness was 90% or more compared with the normal adjacent control hyaline articular cartilage.[26]

Autologous Osteochondral Transfer

Autologous osteochondral transfer involves transplanting an osteochondral tissue plug, consisting of intact hyaline articular cartilage attached to underlying subchondral bone, into an articular cartilage defect. The harvest graft or osteochondral plug is taken from a minimal weight-bearing area of the femoral condyle such as the intercondylar notch or superolateral femoral condyle ridge above the sulcus terminalis. This is a one-stage surgical procedure, and is usually used for cartilage lesions of less than 2 cm². The procedure is done either arthroscopically or open. The grafts are immediately transferred to the lesion site, and an attempt is made to restore the articular surface geometry at the lesion site.[3,9]

Lane et al[27] conducted an animal study to determine the morphologic, biochemical, and biomechanical effects of autologous osteochondral transfer in goats. This study evaluated the short-term effects over a 12-week period. Six goats were used in the study. Two 4.5-mm osteochondral plugs were harvested from the superolateral femoral trochlea and transferred to a central weight-bearing portion of the medial femoral condyle. Postoperative survival time for the animals was 12 weeks. Postmortem studies were done on both the experimental and contralateral knees. Results showed no gross morphologic changes in the operative/experimental knee. The tibial plateau and patella showed no increased degenerative changes postsurgery. Synovial DNA was analyzed, showing no increased inflammatory response. Histologic evaluation at the transferred graft site showed increased glycosaminoglycan upregulation, probably due to a repair response. Biomechanical properties of the osteochondral regions of the transferred/repaired sites from postmortem tissue were compared against corresponding contralateral femoral condyle areas (control). Again a special indentation device was used to determine a calculated stiffness. Stiffness of the experimental tissue was six to seven times stiffer than the contralateral control tissue. Stiffness in experimental and control specimens were 5.29 ± 1.04 N/mm and 0.79 ± 0.15 N/mm, respectively. Lee et al[28] found the harvested cartilage to have up to three times the stiffness in a canine knee model. Questions regarding the reason for increased stiffness and long-term outcome of these transferred autologous osteochondral grafts remain unanswered.[27]

Other recent biomechanical studies addressing the donor site/recipient sites, the stability of implanted osteochondral grafts, and the importance of orientation of the transferred osteochondral graft have been published over the past 2 years. Ahmad et al[29] conducted a biomechanical study with five cadaver knees to determine quantitative biomechanical and topographic aspects of donor and recipient sites to optimize the transfer of autologous osteochondral plugs. Kinematic data was obtained from cadaver specimens at different knee flexion angles. Surface curvature, cartilage thickness, and contact pressures were determined using a stereophotogrammetry method. The lateral trochlea, medial trochlea, and intercondylar notch were shown to have non-load-bearing areas. However, the lateral trochlea, intercondylar notch, and proximal medial trochlea non-load-bearing areas were small and close to load-bearing areas. Donor sites at the distal medial trochlea were completely non-load-bearing and larger in size than other donor sites. Cartilage thickness at different donor sites was determined. Donor sites had similar cartilage thickness of a 2.1-mm average compared with recipient sites of average 2.5 mm. Topography showed the curvature of the lateral and medial trochlea donor sites to best match the curvature of recipient sites on the femoral condyle. The donor site of intercondylar notch better matched the shape of the recipient sites of the central trochlea.[29] These data may assist surgeons in reconstructing the most optimal femoral articular surface.

Duchow et al[30] biomechanically evaluated the primary strength of press fit implanted osteochondral grafts with respect to graft size, harvesting conditions of graft, and repeated insertion after pullout. Porcine femurs and the Osteochondral Autograft Transfer System (OATS) (Arthrex, Naples, FL) were used in the study. Pullout forces were determined under multiple conditions. Results showed failure loads to be significantly lower with 10-mm-long grafts (mean 47 N) as compared with 15-mm- (mean 93 N) or 20-mm- (mean 110 N) long grafts. Pullout and reinsertion of a 15-mm graft resulted in a load to failure from 93 N to 44 N. Failure load of 8-mm diameter (15-mm length) graft compared with

11-mm diameter (15-mm length) was significantly lower at 41 N and 92 N, respectively. The incorrect technique of levering the chisel during harvest (mean 32 N) significantly lowered the pullout strength compared with when the correct technique of simple chisel turning was done (mean 52 N).[30] These findings show that graft size is an important consideration in maximizing the stability of the graft. Planning the graft placement, so that pullout and reinsertion are avoided, and proper technique are also important factors for successful autologous osteochondral transfer.

Proper alignment and placement of autologous osteochondral plugs are important for optimal results. Below et al[31] conducted a study determining the surface collagen orientation of the distal femur and created a cartilage split line map of the distal femur. The study used eight cadaveric knee joints to show a consistent collagen orientation of the load-bearing regions of the distal femoral articular cartilage (**Fig. 2–9**). The orientation of these split lines is likely the direction in which the articular cartilage experiences shear stress. It is hypothesized that placement and orientation of autologous grafts with

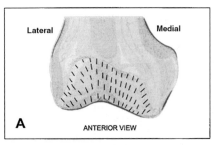

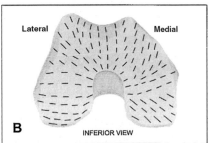

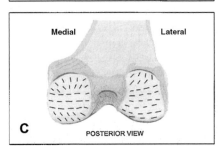

FIGURE 2–9 Illustration showing the **(A)** anterior, **(B)** inferior, and **(C)** posterior split-line patterns of distal femur articular cartilage.[31]

respect to the split line direction may minimize wear forces and maximize durability of the transferred graft.[31]

The most current study to date by Horas et al[32] involves a prospective trial comparing the clinical and histologic outcomes of ACI and autologous osteochondral transfer. This prospective clinical trial involved 40 patients and investigated 2-year outcomes. The 40 patients were randomly assigned to either the ACI group or the autologous osteochondral transfer group. There were 20 patients in each group. All patients had a femoral articular cartilage lesion. Patients were clinically evaluated with a standard scoring system at 6, 12, and 24 months. All patients had improvement, but ACI patients had significantly ($p < .05$) slower recovery compared with autologous osteochondral transfer at 6, 12, and 24 months. At 24 months arthroscopy and biopsy were done on six of the ACI patients and five of the autologous osteochondral transfer patients. Histologic and electron microscopy evaluation were done. The ACI biopsy results consisted mostly of fibrocartilage, whereas the osteochondral transfer biopsies revealed no difference compared with the surrounding original articular cartilage. In the osteochondral transfer group, a gap was consistently seen between the transfer site and the original surrounding cartilage.[32]

■ Conclusion

This chapter has reviewed basic biomechanics of synovial joints, synovial joint lubrication, the biomechanical and structural properties of articular cartilage, and the biomechanics of cartilage repair techniques. A properly functioning synovial joint is an elegant, nearly frictionless system. The tissues compromising the synovial joint are closely linked in form and function. One example is hyaline articular cartilage. The unique structural and biomechanical properties of hyaline articular cartilage allow for complex human movement throughout life with minimal joint wear under normal circumstances. With acute traumatic impaction of joint surfaces, isolated cartilage lesions can occur. These can be debilitating and may lead to osteoarthritis. Articular cartilage histology, biology, and biochemistry, biomechanics, and the treatment of articular cartilage lesions has gained much interest over the past decade. Currently the ability to re-create hyaline articular cartilage with exact preinjury biomechanical properties is lacking. There are several surgical options to address these lesions that utilize stimulation of chondrocyte progenitor cells, osteochondral transfer, and implantation of autologous harvested cultured chondrocytes. Questions remain about which is the better technique and how we might re-create the unique biomechanical properties of hyaline cartilage. It must be remembered that biomechanics exists and affects systems on all levels, ultimately down to the molecular level. Joint loading may increase the hydrostatic pressure within the articular cartilage matrix, providing supported load bearing, and may at the same time deform chondrocyte cellular membranes setting off intracellular signaling cascades to the nucleus that may alter the production of molecules.[28,33] The idea of biomechanics affecting and altering cellular nuclear function is an intriguing concept. With the added realm of genetic engineering, articular cartilage science and repair should prove to be a very interesting subject over the next decade. Understanding the biomechanical properties of articular cartilage and articular cartilage repair are critical for the scientist and treating surgeon. This will allow scientists to do further research and the surgeon to choose the appropriate surgical procedure and techniques for cartilage repair.

REFERENCES

1. Mow VC, Hayes WC. Basic Orthopaedic Biomechanics. New York: Raven Press, 1991
2. Buckwalter JA. Articular cartilage injuries. Clin Orthop 2002;402: 21–37
3. Sgaglione NA, Miniaci A, Gillogly SD, Carter TR. Update on advanced surgical techniques in the treatment of traumatic focal articular cartilage lesions in the knee. Arthroscopy 2002;18:9–32
4. Newton SI. The Principia: Mathematical Principles of Natural Philosophy. Los Angeles: University of California Press, 1999
5. Buckwalter JA, Einhorn TA, Simon SR. Orthopaedic Basic Science: Biology and Biomechanics of the Musculoskeletal System. Orlando, FL: American Academy of Orthopaedic Surgeons, 2000
6. Mow VC, Ratcliffe A, Woo SL. Biomechanics of Diarthrodial Joints. New York: Springer-Verlag, 1990
7. Woo SL, Simon BR, Kuei SC, Akeson WH. Quasi-linear viscoelastic properties of normal articular cartilage. J Biomech Eng 1980;102:85–90
8. Mow VC, Kuei SC, Lai WM, Armstrong CG. Biphasic creep and stress relaxation of articular cartilage in compression? Theory and experiments. J Biomech Eng 1980;102:73–84
9. Insall JN, Scott WN. Surgery of the Knee. New York: Churchill Livingstone, 2001
10. Buckwalter JA, Mankin HJ. Articular cartilage I: tissue design and chondrocyte-matrix interactions. Instr Course Lect 1998;47: 477–486
11. Roughley PJ, Lee ER. Cartilage proteoglycans: structure and potential functions. Microsc Res Tech 1994;28:385–397
12. Mansour JM, Mow VC. The permeability of articular cartilage under compressive strain and at high pressures. J Bone Joint Surg Am 1976;58:509–516
13. Mow VC, Holmes MH, Lai WM. Fluid transport and mechanical properties of articular cartilage: a review. J Biomech 1984;17: 377–394
14. Torzilli PA. Influence of cartilage conformation on its equilibrium water partition. J Orthop Res 1985;3:473–483
15. Zhu W, Iatridis JC, Hlibczuk V, Ratcliffe A, Mow VC. Determination of collagen-proteoglycan interactions in vitro. J Biomech 1996;29:773–783
16. Mow VC, Ratcliffe A, Poole AR. Cartilage and diarthrodial joints as paradigms for hierarchical materials and structures. Biomaterials 1992;13:67–97

17. Roth V, Mow VC. The intrinsic tensile behavior of the matrix of bovine articular cartilage and its variation with age. J Bone Joint Surg Am 1980;62:1102–1117

18. DiSilvestro MR, Zhu Q, Wong M, Jurvelin JS, Suh JK. Biphasic poroviscoelastic simulation of the unconfined compression of articular cartilage: I. Simultaneous prediction of reaction force and lateral displacement. J Biomech Eng 2001;123:191–197

19. Mak AF, Lai WM, Mow VC. Biphasic indentation of articular cartilage–I. Theoretical analysis. J Biomech 1987;20:703–714

20. Lai WM, Mow VC, Roth V. Effects of nonlinear strain-dependent permeability and rate of compression on the stress behavior of articular cartilage. J Biomech Eng 1981;103:61–66

21. Mow VC. Lubrication of diarthrodial joints. In: Skalak R, ed. Handbook of Bioengineering. New York: McGraw-Hill, 1987

22. Schurz J, Ribitsch V. Rheology of synovial fluid. Biorheology 1987;24:385–399

23. Vanwanseele B, Lucchinetti E, Stussi E. The effects of immobilization on the characteristics of articular cartilage: current concepts and future directions. Osteoarthritis Cartilage 2002;10:408–419

24. Salter RB, Simmonds DF, Malcolm BW, Rumble EJ, MacMichael D, Clements ND. The biological effect of continuous passive motion on the healing of full-thickness defects in articular cartilage. An experimental investigation in the rabbit. J Bone Joint Surg Am 1980;62:1232–1251

25. Grande DA, Pitman MI, Peterson L, Menche D, Klein M. The repair of experimentally produced defects in rabbit articular cartilage by autologous chondrocyte transplantation. J Orthop Res 1989;7:208–218

26. Peterson L, Brittberg M, Kiviranta I, Akerlund EL, Lindahl A. Autologous chondrocyte transplantation. Biomechanics and long-term durability. Am J Sports Med 2002;30:2–12

27. Lane JG, Tontz WL Jr, Ball ST, et al. A morphologic, biochemical, and biomechanical assessment of short-term effects of osteochondral autograft plug transfer in an animal model. Arthroscopy 2001;17:856–863

28. Lee CR, Grodzinsky AJ, Hsu HP, Martin SD, Spector M. Effects of harvest and selected cartilage repair procedures on the physical and biochemical properties of articular cartilage in the canine knee. J Orthop Res 2000;18:790–799

29. Ahmad CS, Cohen ZA, Levine WN, Ateshian GA, Mow VC. Biomechanical and topographic considerations for autologous osteochondral grafting in the knee. Am J Sports Med 2001;29:201–206

30. Duchow J, Hess T, Kohn D. Primary stability of press-fit-implanted osteochondral grafts. Influence of graft size, repeated insertion, and harvesting technique. Am J Sports Med 2000;28:24–27

31. Below S, Arnoczky SP, Dodds J, Kooima C, Walter N. The split-line pattern of the distal femur: a consideration in the orientation of autologous cartilage grafts. Arthroscopy 2002;18:613–617

32. Horas U, Pelinkovic D, Herr G, Aigner T, Schnettler R. Autologous chondrocyte implantation and osteochondral cylinder transplantation in cartilage repair of the knee joint: a prospective, comparative trial. J Bone Joint Surg Am 2003;85-A:185–192

33. Lee DA, Bader DL. Compressive strains at physiological frequencies influence the metabolism of chondrocytes seeded in agarose. J Orthop Res 1997;15:181–188

34. Heinegard D, Paulsson M, Inerot S, Carlstrom C. A novel low-molecular weight chondroitin sulphate proteoglycan isolated from cartilage. Biochem J 1981;197(2):355–366

35. Mow VC, Kelly M. Biomechanics of articular cartilage. In: Nordin M, ed. Basic Biomechanics of the Locomotor System. Philadelphia: Lea and Febiger, 1989

3

Response of Articular Cartilage to Injury

VAHÉ R. PANOSSIAN

Articular cartilage is a homogeneous connective tissue that caps the articulating ends of synovial joints. Composed of primarily type II collagen, it is avascular and without innervation. It consists of a relatively small number of cells (chondrocytes) embedded in an abundance of extracellular matrix, composed of collagen, protein polysaccharides (proteoglycans), and water[1,2] **(Fig. 3–1).** The physical properties of articular cartilage are determined by the chemical nature and arrangements of these constituents.[3,4]

Chondrocytes are responsible for the synthesis of the extracellular matrix. In the skeletally immature individual, chondrocytes control the growth and remodeling of the articular cartilage. In the adult, however, chondrocytes are oriented into four transitional zones, which include the tangential zone, transitional zone, radial zone, and the calcified zone **(Fig. 3–2).** The cells within these zones differ in spatial orientation, morphology, and force transduction.[5–7]

Since the beginnings of early orthopaedics, the perplexing nature of articular cartilage defects have been well recognized as difficult to treat.[8–10] In 1743, Hunter[11] stated that "from Hippocrates down to the present age, we shall find that ulcerated cartilage is universally allowed to be a very troublesome disease, that it admits of a cure with more difficulty than a carious bone, and that when destroyed, it is never recovered." Later in 1853, Paget[12] noted, "There are, I believe, no instances in which a lost portion of cartilage has been restored, or a wounded portion repaired, with new and well-formed permanent cartilage in the human subject." Today, traumatic injuries of articular cartilage are becoming more frequent in comparably younger age groups, largely due to the increasing involvement in sports. The secondary posttraumatic changes of cartilage and bone seen in young, healthy athletes are becoming more frequent than the primary arthritic injuries seen with degeneration.

Clinical experience has demonstrated that when left untreated, these lesions usually fail to heal, and defects that involve a significant portion of the articular surface may progress to symptomatic joint degeneration. Therefore, treatment of selected isolated chondral and osteochondral defects may delay or even prevent the development of osteoarthritis.

A few studies have shown that under certain conditions articular cartilage is able to initiate a reparative process in the adult. Unfortunately, its common response is to form a repair tissue that lacks the composition, mechanical properties, structural organization, and durability that is unique to articular cartilage and vital for its normal function.[8,13] Despite our knowledge, amassed over the past several hundred years, of the limited healing capacity of chondral lesions, the fundamental understanding required for the reliable treatment of articular cartilage defects has advanced little.

■ Replication Process

The ability of the chondrocyte to replicate is an important consideration when evaluating the potential of cartilage to proliferate or repair itself. It has been shown that in the immature individual, cell replication occurs

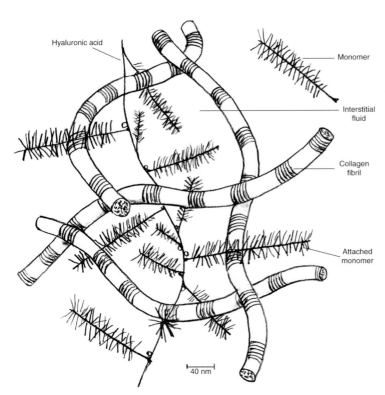

Hyaluronic acid

Monomer

Interstitial fluid

Collagen fibril

Attached monomer

40 nm

FIGURE 3–1 Collagen matrix composition consisting of collagen fibrils, hyaluronic acid, and water.

in the superficial zone beneath the tangential layer and a deeper zone adjacent to the calcified layer. However, at the time of epiphyseal closure, the chondrocyte becomes quiescent and the mitotic index decreases. At maturity, with the development of the tidemark, all evidence of mitotic activity ceases. This finding suggests that there is no compensatory mechanism to replace the cells lost to normal cell death and attrition. As such, one would expect a decrease in the number of chondrocytes with age. In reality, however, there is little or no decrease in cell count with advancing age.[6] This apparent paradox has been explained by the intrinsic response and the ability of the mature chondrocyte to be able to revert to a more primitive chondroblastic state and begin the replication of its own DNA to form new cells.[13]

In experimental animal models, it has been shown that following superficial lacerative articular injuries, the chondrocytes adjacent to the wound margins die or undergo apoptosis. D'Lima et al[14] have shown that 34% of chondrocytes undergo apoptosis, as opposed to a baseline rate of 1%. Twenty-four hours thereafter, the adjacent cells demonstrate an increase in mitotic activity. This proliferation is associated with increased rates of synthesis of matrix components and various enzymes. Although such parameters of synthetic and degradative activity increase over the first few days following injury, they subsequently return to their preinjury levels in 1 to 2 weeks.[13] As such, it appears that healing process is short-lived and does not continue to progress with time.

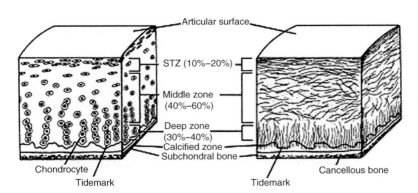

Articular surface

STZ (10%–20%)

Middle zone (40%–60%)

Deep zone (30%–40%)

Calcified zone
Subchondral bone

Chondrocyte

Tidemark

Tidemark

Cancellous bone

FIGURE 3–2 Chondrocyte orientation into four transitional zones, which include the tangential zone, transitional zone, radial zone, and the calcified zone. (From Buckwalter JA, Mow VC, Ratcliffe A. Restoration of injured or degenerated articular cartilage J Am Acad Orthop Surg 1994;2: 192–201, with permission of the American Academy of Orthopaedic Surgeons.)

■ Response to Injury

An intrinsic response has been observed in the cells of adult articular cartilage following lacerative injury and continuous mild compression. This "intrinsic" response refers to the limited ability of mature chondrocytes to revert to their primitive chondroblastic state and replicate DNA to form new cells. Experimental studies have also shown that chondrocytes of immature and mature articular cartilage demonstrate increased rates of proteoglycan synthesis in response to a wide variety of stimuli.[13] Despite numerous studies aimed at stimulating DNA synthesis in an effort to induce chondrocyte replication and increase matrix synthesis, this intrinsic reparative response is deemed clinically inadequate. Therefore, current studies have now been directed to the "extrinsic" factors, which may enhance the reparative process.

A normal response of vascularized tissues to injury is dependent on its supplying vascular network, which in turn provides the initial stages of the inflammatory response to ultimately establish a fibrin clot.[9] Although cartilage is avascular, its subchondral bone has an excellent blood supply. As a result, the response of articular cartilage to a defect largely depends on the nature of the injury, that is, whether the subchondral bone has been disrupted to access the medullary vascular supply.

Superficial Articular Lesions

By lacking access to the nutrients of the subchondral bone, it follows that articular lesions which are confined within cartilage matrix fail to heal spontaneously.[15-18] In contrast, articular lesions that penetrate the underlying layer of subchondral bone demonstrate a limited reparative process. In addition to accessing a plentiful vascular supply, this phenomenon has also been attributed to primitive mesenchymal cells accessing the lesion from the bone marrow and vascular networks.[17,19,20] This reparative response is highly variable with respect to the quantity and quality of the tissue formed.

The repair of superficial cartilage defects depends on the response of chondrocytes at the site of injury. Numerous animal studies have demonstrated that the local response to lacerated cartilage lesions may involve some initial stages of necrosis and loss of proteoglycans[18,21] that are subsequently followed by a short-lived increase in the synthesis of matrix components.[18,22] In an experimental model, D'Lima et al[14] have shown that the use of caspase inhibitors, which inhibit the enzymes that cause apoptosis, reduced cell death and the loss of glycosaminoglycans. This holds promise for the future, in that inhibition of apoptosis may play a role in reducing cartilage tissue damage after a traumatic injury. However, at present, there is little evidence to suggest that these lesions progress to degenerative processes within articulating joints.

Articular Lesions of Subchondral Bone

A different response is seen when the articular defect penetrates the subchondral bone. Originally, the penetration of subchondral bone was the first method used to stimulate the formation of new articular cartilage.[23,24] In areas with full-thickness loss or advanced degeneration of articular cartilage, penetration of the subchondral bone (via microfracture technique, abrasion arthroplasty, or drilling) was shown to disrupt subchondral blood vessels and lead to the formation of a fibrin clot over the bony surface, which later formalizes itself into fibrocartilage **(Fig. 3–3)**. With the surface protected from excessive loading, this fibrin clot is invaded by undifferentiated mesenchymal fibroblast-like cells.[25] The subsequent release of growth factors and other proteins that influence multiple cell functions, including migration, proliferation, differentiation, and matrix synthesis, simultaneously occurs. As a result, a fibroblastic repair tissue forms that can rapidly fill the defect with cartilaginous tissue types.

Within as little as 2 weeks, primitive mesenchymal cells have assumed the rounded form of chondrocytes and have begun to produce reparative tissues consisting of chondrocyte-like cells and a large extracellular matrix of glycosaminoglycans. As determined through immunohistochemical protocols, the tissue appears to contain a significant proportion of type I and type II collagens. At 6 to 8 weeks after injury, the tissue within the chondral portion of the defects contains a relatively high

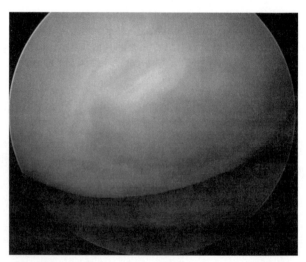

FIGURE 3–3 Fibrocartilage filling a defect after microfracture procedure.

proportion of the chondrocyte-like cells and a matrix composed of type I and II collagen and proteoglycans. Concurrently, cells within the bony segment of the defect form immature bone, fibrous tissue, and cartilage with a hyaline matrix. The bone formation restores the original level of subchondral bone. It rarely progresses into the chondral portion of the defect. At 6 months after injury, the subchondral bone defect has been repaired with a tissue that consists primarily of bone, but also contains some regions of fibrous tissue and hyaline cartilage.[10] In contrast, however, the chondral defect is rarely completely healed.

With time, the proteoglycan content is lost from this tissue, allowing fibrillation to occur and giving the tissue a fibrocartilaginous appearance.[8,22,26] The remaining cells usually have the appearance of fibroblasts, and the surrounding matrix consists of densely packed collagen fibrils. Most studies have shown the formation of fibrocartilage with little evidence of the formation of hyaline cartilage. Ultimately, the repair tissue that fills the defect can be of a variable, sometimes mixed, histologic pattern that fails to restore an articular surface.[27] Occasionally, the repair tissue persists, remodels, and functions satisfactorily as an articular surface for a prolonged period of time.

The ability to heal full-thickness chondral defects may also be related to the size of the defect.[9] It has been shown that small defects produce repair tissue that is superior to that from the reparative process observed in larger defects.[4] Other factors to be considered include age[28] and the location of the site of injury[29,30] on the articulating surface. At present, there are no known studies that have consistently demonstrated the restoration of native articular cartilage following injury.

Articular Cartilage Response to Impact

Several studies have described the differences in articular cartilage after either a single excessive high-impact load or multiple moderate impact loads. It has become apparent that either type of loading process can injure cartilage. Chondrocyte death, matrix damage, surface fissuring, bony injury, and thickening of the tidemark have all been described.[10] At a certain threshold level, the cartilage may become sheared off of the subchondral bone. This observation has been widely regarded as the cause of basal layer degeneration of articular cartilage, which in turn, leads to remodeling of the deep zones of cartilage.

Histologically, repetitive multiple injuries lead to thickening of the calcified zone and advancement of the tidemark at the expense of articular cartilage thickness. Thus, by stiffening of the cartilage–bone junction, changes in these morphologic parameters lead to

alterations in the stresses and strains acting within cartilage during normal function,[10] and with time, arthritic changes follow.

■ Durability of Repair Cartilage

Effective repair requires the maintenance of optimal functional characteristics over time. The difference in material properties between repair cartilage and native cartilage may help explain the frequent deterioration of repair cartilage over time. In normal cartilage, the collagen lattice gives the tissue its form and tensile strength as it resists swelling and compression. Repair cartilage lacks organization of the collagen network, often having a random orientation relative to the articular surface. Furthermore, the repair tissue fails to establish the normal relationships between proteoglycans and the native collagen network due to formation of different types of collagen, lack of organization, insufficient concentration of adhesive molecules, or the dysfunctional assembly of the cartilage matrix.

On the macroscopic level, these biochemical differences result in cleft formation and fibrillation (**Fig. 3–4**). The cleft between the repair and adjacent native cartilage adversely influences the long-term quality of the repair. The persisting cleft acts as a theoretic stress riser, thereby initiating a degenerative process in both the repair tissue and the adjacent native cartilage. Even in areas without cleft formation, the border between the repair cartilage and the native cartilage is usually obvious as a result of the inferior morphologic quality and insufficient production of proteoglycans. Thus, the marked difference in stiffness and deformation between the repair tissue and native cartilage increases the force

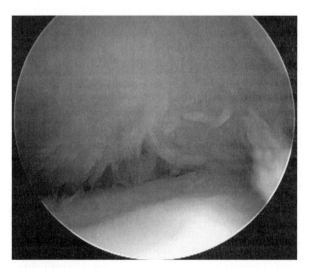

FIGURE 3–4 Fibrillation of cartilage with a "crabmeat" appearance.

gradients across the interface and subsequently induces shear stresses, causing the propagation of clefts into large splits.[10] To date, this phenomenon has not been adequately addressed as it continues to compromise the reparative process.

■ Effect of Motion on Cartilage Repair

The role of motion in the formation and development of cartilage in embryos was clearly demonstrated in 1966.[31] Later, the clinical role for motion in cartilage repair was described by DePalma and associates,[19] who suggested that weight bearing and motion could improve the healing of cartilage defects. Subsequently, Salter and associates[32] studied the influence of continuous passive motion on cartilage healing. In numerous studies of the formation of new cartilage in rabbit knees from periosteal grafts, continuous passive motion was found to enhance repair activity more than immobilization[33,34] or normal cage activity.[35] It is believed that these changes, in part, are due to differences in nutritive transport to cartilage from the synovial fluid by means of diffusion and convection. Therefore, as expected, these biochemical changes are partly reversible on remobilization of the joint.

The mechanical environment of a joint is known to influence the phenotypic expression and activity of chondrocytes within the matrix. Although the mechanism of signal transduction to the nucleus of a chondrocyte is unknown, it is thought that integrins are involved in the signaling pathway, as they connect the intracellular cytoplasm to the matrix. As a result, a given chondrocyte may detect hydrostatic pressure, shear, compression, and tension. Bassett et al[36] have demonstrated that compression and low oxygen tension caused primitive pleuripotential mesenchymal cells to produce cartilage. Furthermore, rates of deformation and interstitial fluid flow, along with streaming electrical potentials, have also demonstrated promising results. Numerous reports suggest that articular cartilage remodels quickly following alteration of mechanical stimuli to the tissue in vivo while changing its metabolic activities in vitro. Hence, changes in loading, unloading, or movement of the joint appear to stimulate different biochemical pathways in the cartilage and, ultimately, affect its biomechanical properties.

Before the development of artificial joints, surgeons found that resection of degenerated joint surfaces followed by decreased loading and joint motion resulted in the formation of fibrocartilaginous tissue over raw bony ends.[8,37] Specifically, it was noted that the surface between the bony surfaces filled with a fibrin clot and then granulation tissue. While allowing for joint motion,

Aldegheri et al[38] studied the effects of joint distraction to treat 80 patients with a variety of hip disorders. Twenty-four patients who either had inflammatory joint disease or were older than 45 years old had poor results, leaving only four patients older than 45 years old who had good results with joint distraction. However, 42 patients (72%) younger than 45 years old with osteoarthritis, hip dysplasia, avascular necrosis, or chondrolysis had good outcomes. These results suggested, that in patients younger than 45 years, decreased contact pressures and continued motion of the damaged hip joint can improve painful symptoms. Van Valburg et al[39] detailed a similar finding in patients having undergone joint distraction for ankle arthritis. Cumulatively, these studies suggest that both age and a decrease in joint reactive forces play vital functions in symptomatic improvement and, ultimately, the healing process. To date, however, the major factors that influence the development of new articular cartilage remain to be determined.

■ Potential Practical Remedies

Currently, there exists no pharmacologic therapy that initiates and promotes the healing of partial- or full-thickness articular cartilage lesions. As a result, surgical intervention is the only known practical remedy. Several surgical paradigms have been developed in an effort to induce functionally competent and enduring repair tissue to form within articular cartilage lesions. These efforts have included the introduction of cells with chondrogenic potential,[40] the introduction of genetically manipulated chondrocytes,[41] the deposition of osteochondral tissues,[30,42–46] and the local administration of signaling substrates.[47]

Such interventions may prove beneficial for patients with focal or localized lesions of the articular cartilage due to trauma or early osteoarthritis. However, they are not recommended in patients who have complementing lesions on articulating surfaces. They are also not recommended in patients having large areas of the joint surface involvement as seen in the advanced stages of osteoarthritis. Such patients will unequivocally benefit from arthroplasty.

Autologous Chondrocyte Implantation

Autologous chondrocyte implantation (ACI) was initiated in the early 1980s. Animal studies demonstrated the production of hyaline-like repair tissue when cultured chondrocytes were implanted beneath a periosteal patch.[44,48] Pioneered in Sweden, the clinical use of ACI was demonstrated in 1987 and is now commercially available (Genzyme Corporation, Cambridge, MA). A hyaline cartilage biopsy sample from the patient's trochlear notch is harvested, and a primitive pluripotential cell population is expanded through cell culture technology. The new expanded population is subsequently reimplanted into the defect and covered with a periosteal flap.

Clinical reports in 1994 demonstrated that 14 of 16 patients with injuries to the femoral condyles had good or excellent results and that 11 of 15 biopsy samples from the patients demonstrated hyaline-like cartilage.[49] However, only 2 of 7 patients with patellar injuries had good function after treatment, and only 1 of 7 had cartilage with a hyaline-like appearance.[49] Since then, numerous investigators demonstrated similar encouraging early clinical results.[50-52] Together, these studies have demonstrated improvement in 85% of femoral lesions with short to medium-length follow-up.

Recently, Peterson et al[53] characterized the histologic, biomechanical, functional, and long-term outcomes of 61 consecutive patients who underwent ACI. They demonstrated that the grafted area contained hyaline cartilage that was indistinguishable from surrounding cartilage and that the grafted area was well anchored to the subchondral bone. However, it was noted that most biopsy specimens had a superficial fibrous surface resulting from the incorporation of the periosteal remnant. The authors stated that the remnant had no effect on either the immediate clinical effectiveness of the ACI or its long-term durability. Their results further suggested that a reliable indicator of future outcome was related to the patient's status at 2 years following transplantation. Patients who returned to the normal activities of daily living and sports by 2 years after transplantation are able to continue these activities through the long term, whereas patients with graft failure demonstrated poor outcome within the first 2 years after implantation. Moreover, they noted that graft survival was close to 100% in patients who were functional at 3 to 8 years following implantation.

Although it may be based on sound scientific theory, ACI is still in its infancy. The functional and morphologic results are mixed. On return arthroscopy, a hypertrophic fibrocartilaginous-type tissue often overlays the defect. Although it may provide for coverage of the articular defect, this reparative tissue grossly lacks the structural integrity, matrix composition, and the biomechanical properties of hyaline cartilage.

■ Conclusion

The effective treatment of articular cartilage lesions continues to challenge modern orthopaedics. Cur-

rently, there exists no satisfactory solution to this long-standing perplexing problem. Despite much thought and research, our understanding of the reparative process within articular lesions remains insufficient, leaving the orthopaedic community without the necessary scientific foundation to build and develop effective regimens for the treatment of articular cartilage lesions.

REFERENCES

1. Arnoczky SP, Torzilli PA. The biology of cartilage. In: Hunter LY, Funk FJ, eds. Rehabilitation of the Injured Knee. St. Louis: CV Mosby, 1984:148–209
2. Barnett CH, Davies DV, MacConaill MA. Synovial Joints: Their Structure and Mechanics. Springfield, IL: Charles C Thomas, 1982
3. Bullough PG. Cartilage. In: Owen R, Goodfellow J, Bullough PG, eds. Scientific Foundations of Orthopaedics and Traumatology. Philadelphia: WB Saunders, 1980:11–17
4. Convery FR, Akeson WH, Keown GH. The repair of large osteochondral defects: an experimental study in horses. Clin Orthop 1972;82:253–262
5. Cheung HS, Lynch KL, Johnson RP, Brewer BJ. In vitro synthesis of tissue specific type II collagen by healing cartilage. Short term repair of cartilage by mature rabbits. Arthritis Rheum 1980;23:211–219
6. Stockwell RA. Cell density of human articular cartilage and costal cartilage. J Anat 1967;101:753–763
7. Weiss C, Rosenberg L, Helfet AJ. An ultrastructural study of normal young adult human articular cartilage. J Bone Joint Surg 1968;50A:663–674
8. Buckwalter JA, Mow VC, Hunzinker EB. Cartilage repair in osteoarthritis. In: Moskowitz RW, Howell DS, Goldberg VM, Mankin HJ, eds. Osteoarthritis: Diagnosis and Medical/Surgical Management, 3rd ed. Philadelphia: WB Saunders, 2001:101–111
9. Buckwalter J, Roseberg L, Couts R, et al. Articular cartilage: injury and repair. In: Woo SL-Y, Buckwalter JA, eds. Injury and Repair of the Musculoskeletal Soft Tissues. Park Ridge. IL: American Academy of Orthopaedic Surgeons, 1988:465–482
10. Mankin HJ, Mow VC, Buckwalter JA, Iannotti JP, Racliffe A. Form and function of articular cartilage. In: Simon SR, ed. Orthopedic Basic Science. Rosemont, IL: American Academy Orthopaedic Surgeons, 1994:3–45
11. Hunter W. On the structure and diseases of articulating cartilage. Philos Trans R Soc Lond B Biol Sci 1743;9:267
12. Paget J. Healing of injuries in various tissues. Lect Surg Pathol T 1853:262
13. Mankin HJ. 2: The response of articular cartilage to mechanical injury. J Bone Joint Surg 1982;64A:460–466
14. D'Lima DD, Hashimoto S, Chen PC, Colwell CW Jr, Lotz MK. Impact of mechanical trauma on matrix and cells. Clin Orthop 2001;391(suppl):S90–S99
15. Hunziker EB, Rosenberg LC. Repair of partial thickness articular cartilage defects. Cell recruitment from the synovium. J Bone Joint Surg 1996;78A:721–733
16. Kim HKW, Moran ME, Salter RB. The potential for regeneration of articular cartilage in defects created by chondral shaving and subchondral abrasion—an experimental investigation in rabbits. J Bone Joint Surg 1994;73A:1301–1315
17. Mankin HJ. 1: The reaction of articular cartilage to injury and osteoarthritis (first of two parts). N Engl J Med 1974;291:1285–1292

18. Meachim G. The effect of scarification on articular cartilage in the rabbit. J Bone Joint Surg 1963;45B:150–161

19. DePalma AF, McKeever CD, Subin DK. Process of repair of articular cartilage demonstrated by histology and autoradiography with tritiated thymidine. Clin Orthop 1966;48:229–242

20. Harada K, Oida S, Sasaki S. Chondrogenesis and osteogenesis of bone marrow-derived cells by bone inductive factor. Bone 1988;9: 177–183

21. Mankin HJ. Localization of tritiated thymidine in articular cartilage of rabbits: II. Repair in immature cartilage. J Bone Joint Surg 1962;44A:688–698

22. Mitchell N, Shepard N. The resurfacing of adult rabbit articular cartilage by multiple perforations through subchondral bone. J Bone Joint Surg 1976;58A:230–233

23. Buckwalter JA, Lohmander S. Operative treatment of osteoarthrosis: current practice and future development. J Bone Joint Surg 1994;76A:1405–1418

24. Johnson LL. 1. Arthroscopic abrasion arthroplasty. In: McGinty JB, ed. Operative Arthroscopy. Philadelphia: Lippincott-Raven, 1996:427–446

25. Shapiro F, Koide S, Glimcher MJ. Cell origination and differentiation in the repair of full-thickness defects of articular cartilage. J Bone Joint Surg 1993;75:532–553

26. Furukawa T, Eyre DR, Koide S, et al. Biochemical studies on repair cartilage resurfacing in healing and normal rabbit articular cartilage. J Bone Joint Surg 1980;62A:79–89

27. Johnson LL. 2. The sclerotic lesion: pathology and the clinical response to arthroscopic abrasion arthroplasty. In: Ewing JW, ed. Articular Cartilage and Knee Joint Function. Basic Science and Arthroscopy. New York: Raven Press, 1990:319–333

28. Huibregtse BA, Johnstone B, Caplan AI, Goldberg VM. Natural repair of full-thickness osteochondral defects in growing and mature rabbits. Trans Orthop Res Soc 1998;23:796

29. O'Driscoll SW, Delaney JP, Salter RB. Experimental patellar resurfacing using periosteal autografts: reasons for failure. Trans Orthop Res Soc 1989;14:145

30. Wakitani S, Goto T, Pineda SJ, et al. Mesenchymal cell-based repair of large, full-thickness defects of articular cartilage. J Bone Joint Surg 1994;76A:579–592

31. Drachman DB, Sokoloff L. The role of movement in embryonic joint development. Dev Biol 1966;14:401–420

32. Salter RB, Simmonds DF, Malcolm BW, et al. The biological effect of continuous passive motion on the healing of full-thickness defects in articular cartilage: an experimental investigation in the rabbit. J Bone Joint Surg 1980;62A:1232–1251

33. O'Driscoll SW, Salter RB. The induction of neochondrogenesis in free intra-articular periosteal autografts under the influence of continuous passive motion: an experimental investigation in the rabbit. J Bone Joint Surg 1984;66A:1248–1257

34. O'Driscoll SW, Salter RB. The repair of major osteochondral defects in joint surfaces by neochondrogenesis with autogenous osteoperiosteal grafts stimulated by continuous passive motion: an experimental investigation in the rabbit. Clin Orthop 1988;208:131–140

35. O'Driscoll SW, Keeley FW, Salter RB. The chondrogenic potential of free autogenous periosteal grafts for biological resurfacing of major full-thickness defects in joint surfaces under the influence of continuous passive motion: an experimental investigation in the rabbit. J Bone Joint Surg 1986;68A:1017–1035

36. Bassett CA. Current concepts of bone formation. J Bone Joint Surg 1962;44A:1217

37. Hass J. Functional arthroplasty. J Bone Joint Surg 1944;26:297–307

38. Aldegheri R, Trivella G, Saleh M. Articulated distraction of the hip. Clin Orthop 1994;301:94–101

39. van Valburg AA, van Roermund PM, Lammens J, et al. Can Ilizarov joint distraction delay the need for an arthrodesis of the ankle? A preliminary report. J Bone Joint Surg 1995;77A:720–725

40. Baragi VM, Renkiewics RR, Qui LP, et al. Transplantation of adenovirally transduces allogeneic chondrocytes into articular cartilage defects in vivo. Osteoarthritis Cartilage 1997;5:275–282

41. Kang R, Marui T, Ghivizzani SC, et al. Ex vivo gene transfer to chondrocytes in full-thickness articular cartilage defects: a feasibility study. Osteoarthritis Cartilage 1997;5:139–143

42. Bobic V. Arthroscopic osteochondral autograft transplantation in anterior cruciate ligament reconstruction: a preliminary clinical study. Knee Surg Sports Traumatol Arthrosc 1996;3:262–264

43. Girdler NM. Repair of articular defects with autologous mandibular condylar cartilage. J Bone Joint Surg 1993;75B:710–714

44. Grande DA, Pitman MI, Peterson L, Menche D, Klein M. The repair of experimentally produced defects in rabbit articular cartilage by autologous chondrocyte transplantation. J Orthop Res 1989;7:208–218

45. Itay S, Abramovici A, Nevo Z. Use of cultured embryonal chick epiphyseal chondrocytes as grafts for defects in chick articular cartilage. Clin Orthop 1987;220:284–303

46. Yamashita F, Sakakida K, Suzu F, Takai S. The transplantation of autogeneic osteochondral fragment for osteochondritis dessicans of the knee. Clin Orthop 1985;201:43–50

47. Hunzinker EB, Rosenberg LC. Biologic basis for repair of superficial articular cartilage lesions. In: Friedlander GE, Jared KJ, eds. Transaction of 38th Annual Meeting. Washington, DC: Orthopaedic Research Society, 1992;231:1

48. Brittberg M, Nilsson A, Lindahl A, et al. Rabbit articular cartilage defects treated with autologous cultured chondrocytes. Clin Orthop 1996;326:270–283

49. Brittberg M1, Lindahl A, Nilsson A, et al. Treatment of deep cartilage defects in the knee with autologous chondrocyte transplantation. N Engl J Med 1994;331:889–895

50. Bahuaud J, Maitrot R, Bouvet R, et al. Implantation of autologous chondrocytes for cartilaginous lesions in young patients. A study of 24 cases. Chirurgie 1998;123:568–571

51. Gillogly SD, Voight M, Blackburn T. Treatment of articular cartilage defects of the knee with autologous chondrocyte implantation. J Orthop Sports Phys Ther 1998;28:241–251

52. Minas T. The role of cartilage repair techniques, including chondrocyte transplantation, in focal chondral knee damage. Inst Course Lect 1999;48:629–643

53. Peterson L, Brittberg M, Kivianta I, Akerlund E, Lindahl A. Autologous chondrocyte transplantation: biomechanics and long-term durability. Am J Sports Med 2002;30:2–12

4

Effects of Electrothermal Energy on Cartilage

YAN LU, RYLAND B. EDWARDS, AND MARK D. MARKEL

Articular cartilage lesions, including softening, delamination, and fibrillation, are common findings during arthroscopic evaluation of joints. The management of these disease conditions remains controversial. Some lesions are silent and neither progress nor produce symptoms. Others may produce significant discomfort and progress to severe osteoarthritis and dysfunction. Multiple methods of treatment, including mechanical debridement, microfracture, osteochondral autografts and allografts, chondral autografts, and chondrocyte cell cultures, attempt to provide a more stable and smooth articular surface. Each of these modalities has its drawbacks. Electrothermal energy for chondroplasty is a relatively new treatment option that aims to contour and seal the articular cartilage surface with minimal local damage to chondrocytes and cartilage matrix.

The first time heat (thermal energy) was used in the medical field was by Papyrus in ~3000 BC. In 1514, Giovanni da Vigo stated, "Wounds that are not curable by iron are curable by fire." In 1540, Johannes Wechtlin began to use a cauterizing "probe" for treatment of patients' wounds. With the passage of time and technique advancement, electrocautery, laser, and radiofrequency energy (RFE) devices designed for musculoskeletal applications have been increasingly used for the treatment of cartilage lesions.

In 1985, Rand and Gaffey evaluated the effects of electrocautery on fresh human cartilage. Results of this study demonstrated that electrocautery at the lowest setting (27 W) did not cause excessive damage to cartilage. Recently, Stein et al[2] determined the clinical effect of electrocautery for arthroscopic chondroplasty of chondromalacic cartilage. This study demonstrated that electrocautery did not produce a significant benefit compared with mechanical chondroplasty alone for the treatment of chondromalacic lesions. Electrocautery appeared to have a deleterious effect on chondromalacic lesions of grade III and higher.

In 1989, Miller et al[3] compared the effects of the neodymium:yttrium-aluminum-garnet (Nd:YAG) laser with electrocautery and mechanical debridement on articular cartilage lesions and concluded that lasers had biologic advantages over mechanical resurfacing and electrocautery in arthroscopic procedures. In 1990, Raunest and Lohnert[4] reported on the use of the excimer laser for chondromalacic cartilage of Outerbridge grade II and III. The results of this study demonstrated significant pain relief and reduction of reactive synovitis in treated patients. In 1994, Grifka et al[5] also reported that the use of excimer laser on chondromalacic cartilage of Outerbridge grade II produced a smooth cartilaginous surface via scanning electron microscopy. Despite these encouraging results, the laser has fallen out of favor in arthroscopic surgery because of high cost, inconvenience, and most importantly, safety concerns about the modality, resulting in osteonecrosis, cartilage loss, and avascular necrosis after laser chondroplasty.[6–11] Recently, Lane et al[12] and Mainil-Varlet et al[13] demonstrated that chondroplasty with laser energy caused significant proteoglycan loss and chondrocyte death.

Before RFE was used for thermal chondroplasty, it was used to correct cardiac electrical conduction pathway abnormalities, to ablate local tumors and cancers, to combat chronic sleep disorders, and to shrink joint capsular tissue and ligaments. It began to be investigated and used for thermal chondroplasty in 1996 to 1997.[14] Currently, there are two basic RFE systems available for clinical application: monopolar RFE (mRFE) and bipolar RFE (bRFE). In addition, temperature-controlled RFE probes/generators are available for clinical application with both mRFE and bRFE systems. RFE has the potential advantages of being safe, relatively inexpensive, and simple to use via arthroscopy. It can rapidly contour and smooth fibrillated regions associated with chondromalacic cartilage compared with conventional mechanical debridement, but there are limited in vivo reports regarding its effects on articular cartilage, and the peer-reviewed literature currently provides conflicting results with regard to its safety and efficacy.[15,16]

■ Articular Cartilage

Articular cartilage in diarthrodial joints has two primary functions: (1) to distribute joint loads over a wide area, thus decreasing the stresses sustained by the contacting joint surfaces, and (2) to allow relative movement of the opposing joint surfaces with minimal friction and wear. There are three types of cartilage in the human body: hyaline cartilage, fibrocartilage, and elastic cartilage. Healthy or normal hyaline cartilage appears glassy, smooth, and glistening and covers long bones and growth plates; fibrocartilage consists of dense tissue and is located in intervertebral disks and menisci; elastic cartilage is yellowish or opaque and is located in the epiglottis and the eustachian tube.

Cartilage is composed of chondrocytes and matrix. Chondrocytes are sparsely distributed cells in articular cartilage and account for less than 10% of the cartilage's volume. Chondrocytes also manufacture, secrete, and maintain the organic components of cartilage matrix. The cartilage matrix is composed of a dense network of fine collagen (type II) enmeshed in a concentrated solution of proteoglycans. Collagen and proteoglycans account for 10 to 40% of the matrix, with the remaining 60 to 90% being water, inorganic salts, and small amounts of other matrix proteins, glycoproteins, and lipids. Articular cartilage is unique in that it is devoid of lymphatic, neural, and vascular components. The avascular nature of articular cartilage establishes an environment of low oxygen concentration where chondrocytes rely on anaerobic metabolism.

Chondrocytes are divided into three zones (superficial tangential, middle, and deep) from the cartilage surface to the tidemark (the demarcation between the calcified and noncalcified cartilage). In the superficial tangential zone, chondrocytes are oblong with their long axes aligned parallel to the articular surface. In the middle zone, the chondrocytes are round and randomly distributed. In the deep zone, chondrocytes are arranged in columnar fashion oriented perpendicular to the tidemark. Chondrocytes are the sole cell type in articular cartilage and receive nutrition from synovial fluid flow into the matrix through compression and relaxation during normal joint motion. An important feature of chondrocytes is that they lack direct cell-to-cell contact, and therefore communication between cells must occur via the extracellular matrix. If chondrocytes are injured or damaged, they have very little ability to regenerate.

Collagen in articular cartilage has a high level of structural organization that provides the fibrous ultrastructure to cartilage. Type II collagen is the principal molecular component in cartilage, but collagens III, VI, IX, X, XI, XII, and XIV all contribute to the mature matrix. In developing cartilage, the core fibrillar network is a cross-linked copolymer of collagens II, IX, and XI. The function of collagen IX and XI in this heteropolymer are not yet fully defined, but evidently they are critically important because mutations in collagen IX and XI genes result in chondrodysplasia phenotypes that feature precocious osteoarthritis. Collagens XII and XIV are thought also to be bound to fibril surfaces but not covalently attached. Collagen VI polymerizes into its own type of filamentous network that has multiple adhesion domains for cells and other matrix components. Collagen X is normally restricted to the thin layer of calcified cartilage that interfaces articular cartilage with bone. The collagen in articular cartilage is inhomogeneously distributed, giving the tissue a layered character. Collagens are also divided into three zones (superficial tangential, middle, and deep) within the full thickness of cartilage. In the superficial tangential zone, which represents 10 to 20% of the total thickness, there are sheets of fine, densely packed fibers randomly woven in planes parallel to the articular surface. In the middle zone (40 to 60% of the total thickness), the randomly oriented and homogeneously dispersed fibers are less densely packed to accommodate the high concentration of proteoglycans and water. In the deep zone (~30% of the total thickness), the fibers come together, forming larger, radially oriented fiber bundles; these bundles then cross the tidemark to enter the calcified cartilage, forming an interlocking "root" system that anchors the cartilage to the subchondral bone. This layering inhomogeneity appears to serve an important biomechanical function by distributing the stress more uniformly across the loaded regions of the joint. The most important mechanical properties of collagen fibers are their tensile stiffness and strength.

Cartilage proteoglycans are large protein-polysaccharide molecules that exist as either monomers or aggregates. Proteoglycan monomers consist of an

~200-nm-long protein core to which ~150 glyco-saminoglycan chains and both O-linked and N-linked oligosaccharides are covalently attached. In native cartilage, most proteoglycan monomers associate with hyaluronate to form proteoglycan aggregates. Proteoglycan aggregation promotes immobilization of the proteoglycans within the collagen meshwork, adding the structural rigidity to the extracellular matrix. The function of proteoglycans is to resist compression. The proteoglycan and collagen also interact with each other. A small portion of the proteoglycans has been shown to be closely associated with collagen and may serve as a bonding agent between collagen fibrils.

■ Chondromalacic Cartilage

Chondromalacia is a softening or wearing away and cracking of the articular cartilage. Chondromalacia describes the changes that occur in cartilage covering the ends of bones as it breaks down and degenerates. This condition is not the same as osteoarthritis, and one does not necessarily lead to the other. Osteoarthritis results from long-term wear that causes the lining of the joints to become rough and painful. Chondromalacia results from an injury to otherwise healthy cartilage or as a response to abnormal pressure on the cartilage. An accepted grading scale of chondromalacia by Outerbridge is as follows: grade I, cartilage is softening and swelling; grade II, fibrillation or superficial fissures of cartilage; the fissures in the cartilage are no greater than 1.3 cm^2 in area and the fissures do not extend into subchondral bone at this stage; grade III, deep fissuring of the cartilage without exposed subchondral bone; the cartilage has a "crab-meat-like" appearance; and grade IV, erosion changes that extend into subchondral bone and involve more than half of the patellar surface.[17] Histologically, chondromalacic cartilage has a fibrillated surface with reduced proteoglycan and collagen staining (Fig. 4–1A). Additionally, chondrocyte clones are found in the middle and deep zones and at the junction of normal and chondromalacic cartilage (Fig. 4–1B).

Because chondromalacia causes discomfort and restricts movement, it usually requires medical evaluation to determine its cause and corresponding treatment. The treatment includes conservative and surgical approaches. Recently, a highly controversial study published by Moseley et al[18] demonstrated that conventional treatment for osteoarthritis and chondromalacia using mechanical debridement did not yield a better outcome compared with a placebo procedure.

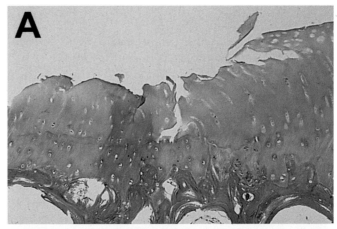

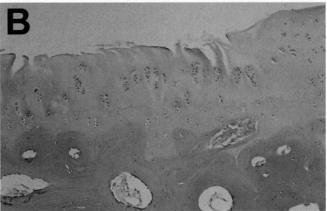

FIGURE 4–1 (A) Safranin O–stained chondromalacic articular cartilage of grade II or III with surface irregularities, fissures, and reduced proteoglycan concentration (×100). **(B)** Hematoxylin and eosin (H&E) stained chondromalacic articular cartilage of grade II with surface irregularities, fibrillation, and chondrocyte cloning (×100) (See Color Plate 4–1).

■ Principles and Techniques of Electrothermal Treatment of Cartilage

The devices used for medical application of thermal energy mainly refer to electrocautery, laser, and radiofrequency modalities. The use of thermal cautery to stop bleeding is an ancient practice. As early as 3000 B.C., tools heated in a fire were used to reduce hemorrhage in accidental injuries. The first units to utilize electrical energy for the heating of cautery instruments date back to the early 1900s. The thermal cautery unit (also called electrocautery) is now a well-established surgical instrument. Electrocautery is a device in which an electric current is used to heat a treatment instrument or probe. When the cautery tip is applied to tissue for coagulation, several changes occur: cells vaporize, removing water from the tissue, causing the tissue to shrink and the blood vessels to contract, or causing the protein from the blood cells and the tissue to form a coagulum. This device does not transfer electric current to the patient. The heat source is the probe tip.

Laser energy is similar in principle to an electrocautery device, but employs laser energy to cut, vaporize, and simultaneously coagulate a targeted area without disrupting adjacent tissue. "Laser" is an acronym for light amplification by stimulated emission of radiation. When applied to any tissue, light energy can be reflected, transmitted, scattered, or absorbed. In principle, the greater the absorption of light by the target tissue, the more precise and efficient the intended effect. The evolution of laser technology has been based on developing lasers with wavelengths that are optimally absorbed by the musculoskeletal tissue, including the carbon dioxide (CO_2), the neodymium, and the holmium lasers. To be clinically useful in sports medicine, lasers must be delivered by reliable fiberoptic technology in an arthroscopic environment. The first clinical studies of laser-assisted arthroscopic surgery were performed with CO_2 lasers in the 1970s.[19] The main disadvantage of CO_2 lasers was that they could not be transmitted through flexible optical fibers. Later, the neodymium:yttrium-aluminum-garnet (Nd:YAG) laser was used in combination with intraarticularly administered fluid for chondroplasty. The wavelength (1.06 µm) of the Nd:YAG lasers allows both the use of quartz fibers and laser treatment under water. Due to the Nd:YAG's absorption spectrum, significant collateral thermal damage of the tissue can occur during clinical application of the device, diminishing its usefulness.

Arthroscopic laser systems must cut tissue deeply enough and quickly. The cut edges must be exact, not ragged. Thermal damage and other side effects must be kept to a minimum. There should be no carbonization. The system must be easy to use with a simple laser beam guidance system. These requirements should be met for laser treatment of all tissues, not only for joint cartilage, but also for meniscus, tendons, and even bony tissues. The Nd:YAG laser, therefore, did not fulfill many of these requirements.

Named for the rare element holmium, into which crystals of yttrium, argon, and garnet have been incorporated, the Ho:YAG laser generates a wavelength of 2.1 µm, and fulfills all of the above mentioned requirements, and also has sufficient ablation capabilities to be useful for orthopaedic procedures. Lasers are small in comparison to mechanical instruments and can be used not only in arthroscopic procedures but also for endoscopic procedures. Since the late 1980s, the Ho: YAG laser has been the definitive laser tool used in arthroscopic surgery. Currently, the erbium:YAG (Er:YAG) laser emitting at 2.94 µm appears to have superior effect attributes compared with the Ho:YAG laser for chondroplasty. The Er:YAG laser is known for very shallow optical penetration, in the range of a few micrometers,

and for precise ablation with minimal thermal damage to the surrounding tissue.[19]

The use of RFE for the treatment of fibrillated cartilage has increased tremendously over the past 8 years. The safety and efficacy of this technique is dependent on an understanding of the physics behind RFE. First, RFE is not electrocautery. During RFE application, a high-frequency alternating current flows from the uninsulated probe tip into the tissue. Ionic agitation is produced in the tissue or the irrigation solution about the probe tip as the ions attempt to follow the changes in direction of the alternating current. This agitation results in frictional heating so that the tissue or the irrigation solution about the probe tip, rather than the probe tip itself, is the primary source of heat. The heat produced during RFE application is the difference between the heat generated by RFE current flow through the tissue surrounding the probe tip and the heat lost from this region. The heat generated in the tissue about the probe tip is governed by three factors: (1) distance from the tip; (2) RFE current intensity; and (3) duration of application of the RFE current.

The heat generated in the tissue varies as $1/r^4$ (where r is the distance between the tissue surface and the probe tip). This implies that tissue-heating changes rapidly with the distance from the probe tip. Physically, a RFE lesion is a prolate spheroid aligned along the electrode tip.

For RFE current intensity, the lesion size generated varies as the intensity is squared. Current intensity, if it is too high and applied too rapidly, will have one of two effects. First, heating of the tissue around the probe tip may be so intense that solidification and char formation will quickly limit further current flow and heating. The lesion size, therefore, will be much smaller than expected. Second, too rapid spread of heat produces scattered areas of explosive water vaporization, resulting in an irregularly shaped lesion larger than the desired size.

Lesion size also depends on the RFE treatment time. For current intensity I, and treatment time T, the RFE heat varies as I^2T. Therefore increasing current intensity has a much greater effect on lesion size than increasing treatment time. However, a minimum time is required before a treatment effect will be reached.

Heat loss is a very important factor during RFE application. RFE heat is lost by conduction and by convection via the circulation. At equilibrium, heat generated by the RFE equals heat loss, and lesion temperature remains constant during the remainder of lesion creation. Lesions different in size and shape from those expected result from heat loss by convection in relatively vascularized areas. An indirect form of heat loss can be caused by impaired heat generation through the shunting away of RFE current from a lesion site by the presence of low resistance electrical paths such as cerebrospinal fluid. In this case, the anticipated level of RFE current will be inadequate because of loss of the heating effect caused by the shunted current.

The size of the RFE probe tip affects lesion size in the expected manner, larger tips producing larger lesions. The effect of increasing the length of the uninsulated tip is a direct result of the $1/r^4$ attenuation of the heat effect.

Currently, there are three major RFE device systems available for clinical arthroscopic application in thermal chondroplasty. These include the Vulcan EAS™ coupled with a TAC-C probe (Smith & Nephew Endoscopy, Menlo Park, CA), Mitek VAPR™ System coupled with a Flexible Side Effect Electrode (Mitek Surgical Products, Inc., Westwood, MA), and ArthroCare 2000 System™ coupled with CoVac probe (ArthroCare Corp., Sunnyvale, CA) **(Fig. 4–2).** The Smith & Nephew device is mRFE, whereas the latter two are bRFE devices.

Electrosurgical RFE devices usually use frequencies between 300 kHz and 13 MHz. RFE oscillates the electrolytes in the intracellular and extracellular solutions, producing molecular friction. RFE devices are selected to act at greater than 300 kHz to avoid muscle fasciculation and nerve stimulation observed at lower frequencies.[20] During mRFE heating, the alternating electric current passes from the RFE generator through the connecting cable, through the probe (positive electrode), through the patient's body to the negative electrode (grounding plate).

The mRFE system currently used in clinical application (Vulcan EAS™ RFE generator) is a temperature-controlled device. The mRFE system uses delivered power to control the tissue temperature reflected by a thermocouple within the mRFE probe tip. At the beginning of treatment, the RFE generator delivers full preset power to cause tissue heating. The thermocouple within the mRFE probe tip is subsequently heated, reaching the preset temperature relatively quickly. After reaching

the preset temperature, the mRFE algorithm reduces the power to prevent tissue/probe-tip temperature from continuing to increase and then uses bursts of power output to maintain the tissue temperature near the preset temperature. This may result in the mRFE generator delivering mean powers that are significantly less than preset powers to maintain the preset temperatures. The current mRFE (Smith & Nephew, Endoscopy, Menlo Park, CA) setting for chondroplasty is 70°C/15 W. The mRFE chondroplasty should be applied in light contact using a paintbrush pattern.

In the bRFE heating, the alternating electric current passes from the RFE generator through the connecting cable, through the probe, through the positive electrode to the negative electrode, where both positive and negative electrodes are in the probe tip. The conduction pass of the bRFE is within the irrigation fluid, resulting in vaporization of the physiologic saline in the joint. Therefore, the tissue effects with bRFE are secondary to thermal and ionic modification of the tissue.

Most bRFE systems such as Mitek VAPR™ System (Mitek Surgical Products, Inc.) and ArthroCare 2000 System™ (ArthroCare Corp.) are power-controlled devices. These devices produce uniform and direct power output or a variable amplitude sinusoidal waveform while the bRFE probes are activated. No thermocouples are embedded in the probe tips to monitor and adjust the temperature at the interface between the probe tip and treated tissue. Recently, the manufacturer of Mitek introduced a new bRFE (VAPR II Electrosurgical System and VAPR TC Electrode) with temperature-controlled mode for thermal chondroplasty. Shellock[21] reported that this new bRFE maintained the temperature at the RFE electrode–tissue interface relatively close to the RFE preset temperature and may be useful for thermal-assisted chondroplasty. The manufacturer of the ArthroCare RFE device also claims an added benefit for thermal chondroplasty using a process they call coblation (cooler,

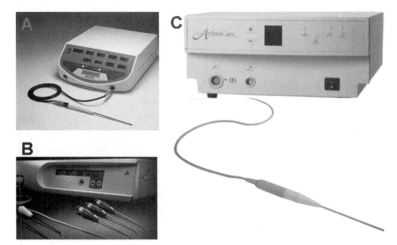

FIGURE 4–2 (A) Smith & Nephew, Endoscopy, Vulcan EAS™ monopolar radiofrequency energy (mRFE) system. **(B)** Mitek VAPR™ bipolar RFE (bRFE) system. **(C)** ArthroCare 2000™ bRFE system.

controlled ablation), which the company claims is a non-heat-driven process. Instead, bRFE is applied to a conductive medium (usually saline), causing a highly focused plasma field to form around the electrodes. The plasma field is composed of highly ionized particles. These ionized particles have sufficient energy to break organic molecular bonds within the tissue. Currently, the setting for Mitek bRFE system is V40 and the setting for ArthroCare is setting 2. The bRFE devices should be applied in noncontact using a paintbrush pattern.

Electrothermal Effects on Articular Cartilage

Electrothermal energy devices such as electrocautery, lasers, and RFE have been used to ablate and contour roughened or irregular cartilaginous surface since the 1980s. The results of both experimental and clinical studies have been variable and contradictory.[14-16,22,23] Articular cartilage has a poor and limited capability of regeneration after it is injured. In 1743, Hunter[24] stated, "From Hippocrates to the present age, it is universally allowed that ulcerated cartilage is a troublesome thing and that, once destroyed, it is not repaired."[24] When using electrothermal energy to treat articular cartilage, it is important to understand the temperature threshold that causes chondrocyte death. When chondrocytes located within the cartilage matrix reach the temperature threshold, the cells may undergo necrosis. If located along the margin of this threshold zone, they may be stimulated to undergo apoptosis, and may affect adjacent chondrocytes through extracellular signaling pathway. In a study performed by Li et al,[25] the investigators demonstrated that temperatures between 48° and 52°C were critical for causing irreversible cellular necrosis and apoptosis of osteoblasts. Züger et al[26] demonstrated that the temperature threshold for chondrocyte death was 54°C after osteochondral sections were heated for 5 minutes in phosphate buffer solution (PBS).

By thermally sealing and contouring fibrillated or degenerated articular cartilage, it has been hypothesized that electrothermal devices may be able to retard the degenerative process of cartilage delamination and fretting. This is not a reparative or stimulatory effect but rather focuses on sealing and smoothing the surface of the lesion. The purpose of this treatment is to retard the continued breakdown of cartilage and thereby minimize the chemical by-products and enzymes that are closely associated with synovitis, effusion, and pain.[27]

The effect of electrocautery on articular cartilage has been assessed since the 1980s. Initially, electrocautery devices were used for lateral retinacular release as well as meniscal surgery. Miller et al[28] evaluated 51 patients who had arthroscopic partial meniscectomies with electrocautery between 1982 and 1985. They reported that the average depth of damage was 0.29 mm as determined by histologic analysis, and newly developed electrocautery devices did not appear to decrease the depth of damage. Stein et al[2] evaluated the effectiveness of electrocautery for treating chondromalacic lesions. The study demonstrated that electrocautery used for chondroplasty did not produce a significant benefit and appeared to have a detrimental effect on chondromalacic lesions of grade III or higher. The possible reason for this negative result may be due to high temperatures in excess of 400°C reached during electrocautery application. This high temperature may cause not only chondrocyte death but also matrix loss.

The ability to excise abnormal articular cartilage with precision made the laser a potentially valuable tool in orthopaedic surgery. However, avascular necrosis and osteonecrosis that were presumed to be due to the pulsing effect of laser energy have been reported.[6,7,8,10] Several investigators have reported that the Ho:YAG laser resulted in significant chondrocyte death and the injury of subchondral bone while smoothing the cartilaginous surface.[7,12] Compared with Ho:YAG laser, the Er:YAG laser demonstrated superior ablation effectiveness while causing less acute collateral tissue damage.[13] The long-term outcomes of Er:YAG laser chondroplasty need to be investigated.

During thermal chondroplasty, it has been reported that laser energy not only reshapes articular cartilage but also may possibly stimulate chondrocyte metabolism. Several researchers have conducted these studies on arthritis models, but the results have been contradictory. Pullin et al[29] reported chondrocyte cloning close to a location treated by the Ho:YAG laser in articular cartilage in vivo in the horse, but regeneration of cartilage was not reported. Lane et al[12] demonstrated substantial reduction of proteoglycans compared with control, with cell viability greatly reduced in the treated area when an articular lesion was treated with the Ho:YAG laser. Ebert et al[30] performed a study to determine whether irradiation with a low-intensity diode laser, which produces radiation at a wavelength of 810 nm, would induce nonthermal enhancement of chondrocyte metabolism. This study demonstrated that minimal thermal increases in cartilage explants with use of a low-intensity diode laser resulted in no change in proteoglycan metabolism of chondrocytes. Torricelli et al[31] studied the effect of a new gallium-aluminum-arsenic diode laser on chondrocyte cultures derived from rabbit and human cartilage and reported a positive biostimulatory effect on cell proliferation as compared with the control group. Currently, the mechanism of laser irradiation's effect on chondrocytes is not yet fully understood. It has been postulated that laser irradiation may influence the pore structure, water permeability of extracellular matrix, and the rate and efficacy of chondrocyte nutrition.

Radiofrequency energy has the ability to smooth and contour the surface of articular cartilage, ablate cartilage delaminating flaps, trim and stabilize the loose edges of chondromalacic cartilage, and stop bleeding from subchondral bone after debridement, but surgeons must be aware that RFE uses heat to accomplish these effects, and overtreatment or inappropriate treatment will result in thermal injury.[22] During RFE chondroplasty, because the settings recommended by manufacturers for both mRFE and bRFE produce higher treatment temperatures than the threshold temperature for chondrocyte death, RFE will result in chondrocyte death and collagen denaturation. The extent of thermal injury caused by RFE depends on the treatment speed, the power output, or temperature settings selected, the probe design used, the treatment duration and location, the temperature of the lavage solution used, the RFE probe tip pressure, and the treatment modes or patterns applied.[32] There is a direct relationship between treatment power output and depth of thermal effect; the higher the treatment power output, the deeper the thermal effect.[32]

Different tissues have different electrical impedances. The impedance of articular cartilage is 400 to 500 ohms and the subchondral bone is 900 to 1000 ohms. This high impedance discourages the conduction of RFE (especially for mRFE) into cartilage. During treatment, mRFE energy will flow away from the cartilage to the surrounding low-impedance saline, creating a relatively superficial thermal effect.[33]

Chondrocytes are highly sensitive to temperature, and chondrocyte viability after RFE treatment is of great concern. Conventional analysis of cell viability depends on histologic staining such as hematoxylin and eosin (H&E) or safranin O. Several researchers have demonstrated that standard histology using these stains underestimate chondrocyte death compared with vital staining using confocal laser microscopy (CLM).[13,23,26]

Confocal laser microscopy has been used to determine chondrocyte viability following electrothermal treatment since 1996.[15] CLM uses a laser source to stimulate the fluorescent-labeled sample and projects the resulting image on a monitor through computer-controlled software. CLM with double cell staining is recognized as an accurate and sensitive method of determining cell viability. This technique uses Calcein-AM to label live cells and ethidium homodimer-1 (EthD-1) for dead cells. Calcein-AM is an uncharged, nonfluorescent substrate that freely diffuses into live cells and is enzymatically converted to the intensely fluorescent calcein by an esterase. The polyanionic calcein is charged and only retained in live cells, producing green fluorescence on excitation (excitation/emission $\approx$495 nm/ $\approx$515 nm). EthD-1 has low cell membrane permeability and is excluded by the intact membrane of live cells. The molecular size of EthD-1 is ~100 times the size of molecules that normally move by osmosis through cell membranes (such as sodium or potassium). Cell membranes that allow EthD-1 to enter are significantly damaged. Once passing through damaged membranes, EthD-1 undergoes a 40-fold enhancement of fluorescence upon binding nucleic acids, producing a strong red fluorescence in nonviable cells.[23]

Electrothermal Energy Application in Cartilage

Both experimental and clinical studies regarding electrocautery and laser energy for chondroplasty have indicated that they have more detrimental than beneficial effects.[2,12] RFE has the potential advantage of being safe, relatively inexpensive, and easy to use via arthroscopy. In addition, numerous RFE manufacturers now provide an array of probes designed for multiple arthroscopic applications. Over the past 8 years, RFE has gained widespread use in the field of sports medicine and orthopaedics. Both mRFE and bRFE have become frequently used arthroscopic techniques for thermal chondroplasty. It has been hypothesized that the smoothing and contouring of the cartilage surface using RFE may also reduce the release of collagen and proteoglycan epitopes into the synovial fluid and reduce the cycle of cartilage degradation, synovial inflammation, and further articular degeneration. However, ex vivo and in vivo studies regarding RFE for chondroplasty provide conflicting results.[14–16,21,22]

Turner et al[16] did one of the first studies describing the in vivo effects of a bRFE ablative device on ovine articular cartilage (Bipolar Arthroscopic Probe, Electroscope, Inc., Bolder, CO). The investigators proposed that this bRFE device would allow surface contouring without damaging adjacent normal articular cartilage and would not produce the surface irregularities previously reported with the use of mechanical shavers during chondroplasty.[5] In this study, sheep were sacrificed at four time points: immediately after surgery, and 6, 12, and 24 weeks after surgery. Routine histologic methods (H&E and safranin-O staining) were used to analyze osteochondral samples. The authors concluded that the bRFE device destroyed fewer chondrocytes and produced a better histologic appearance of the cartilage than traditional mechanical debridement. This study stimulated the orthopedic community to pursue the use of RFE for chondroplasty. The main shortcoming of this study was that the investigators did not evaluate chondrocyte viability after RFE treatment.

In 2000, Lu et el[15] reported the effect of mRFE (ElectroThermal System ORA-50™, Oratec Interventions Inc., Mountain View, CA) on partial-thickness defects of articular cartilage. At that time, no studies had evaluated the effect of mRFE on articular cartilage and the investigators hypothesized that mRFE would smooth and stabilize the articular surface in a partial-thickness cartilaginous defect, thereby interrupting the cascade that leads to osteoarthritis and joint dysfunction. In this in vivo ovine model, the investigators evaluated the effects of mRFE on partial-thickness defects of articular cartilage and also the outcome of partial-thickness defects treated with mRFE to treatment by conversion of partial-thickness defects to full-thickness defects by curettage and microfracture. The settings for the mRFE generator were 55°C/15 W. The sheep were euthanized immediately after surgery (time 0), and at 2, 12, or 24 weeks. The treated regions were evaluated with routine histologic analysis (H&E and safranin-O staining) for general morphology and proteoglycan concentration, scanning electron microscopy (SEM) for cartilage surface analysis, and CLM for cell viability. This was the first study to use CLM to determine chondrocyte viability after mRFE chondroplasty.

Confocal laser microscopy and vital cell staining (calcein-AM and EthD-1) demonstrated that mRFE caused immediate chondrocyte death with a clear dead zone present in the treated site at time 0. This zone of chondrocyte death progressed to full-thickness death at 2 weeks after surgery **(Fig. 4–3).** At 12 and 24 weeks, all chondrocytes were dead in the mRFE-treated sites. Histologic analysis demonstrated that mRFE treatment caused detrimental effects to proteoglycan concentrations that progressed over time. SEM showed that the mRFE-treated defect surface appeared to be contoured and sealed at time 0, and remained smooth for up to 24 weeks after surgery. This study was the first to report negative effects of RFE for chondroplasty. The authors concluded that mRFE for chondroplasty caused immediate chondrocyte death and thus influenced proteoglycan concentration. On the contrary, mechanical debridement and microfracture produced better histologic healing than mRFE chondroplasty. The results of this study did not demonstrate the beneficial effect of mRFE reported in Turner et al's[16] study. This study cautioned surgeons against using RFE for chondroplasty.

Kaplan et al[14] examined the acute effects of bRFE (ArthroCare 2000™ System coupled with the right-angle ArthroWand™ 3.0 mm, 90 degrees, ArthroCare Corp., Sunnyvale, CA) on human osteochondral explants with naturally occurring chondromalacia. The proposed goal of this ex vivo study was to determine chondrocyte viability adjacent to treated areas, and the depths of penetration and ablation at three different power settings (S2, S4, and S6). The treatment pattern was applied in light contact, and the treatment time for each sample was 3 seconds. After bRFE treatment, the samples were processed for evaluation using histology via light microscopy (LM). The authors reported that the bRFE probe ablated and smoothed the fibrillated cartilage surface. The ablative depths are 120 ± 20 µm for setting 2, 230 ± 50 µm for setting 4, and 370 ±

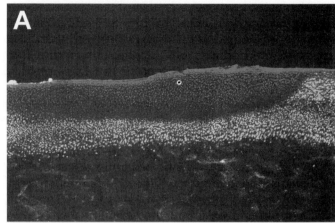

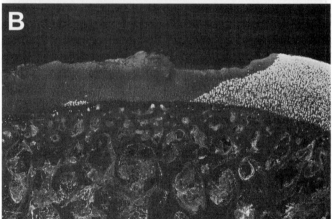

FIGURE 4–3 Confocal microscopic image demonstrating RFE-treated cartilage surface (top of each image) and subchondral bone (bottom of each image) following a paintbrush pattern application (×20). The green dots indicate viable chondrocytes, and the red dots indicate dead chondrocytes. **(A)** 0 time, RFE treatment caused immediate chondrocyte death and a clear "dead zone" appeared. Cartilaginous surface was contoured. **(B)** Two-week group. By 2 weeks after RFE treatment, all chondrocytes were dead and the cartilaginous surface appeared relatively smooth (See Color Plate 4–3).

170 µm for setting 6. The chondrocytes adjacent to the treated areas did not show evidence of nuclear, cytoplasmic, or perilucunar alterations in structure and appeared to be viable at all bRFE settings. The authors concluded that bRFE was safe for chondroplasty, even at the highest power settings. This study supported the findings of the study performed by Turner et al.[16] The limitation of this study was that cell viability was analyzed by an insensitive method, that is, LM with H&E. The viability of cells using histology via LM is inferred from the appearance of the cell cytoplasm, organelles, and the nucleus. Fixation, dehydration, embedding, and staining techniques each affect the cellular appearance within the tissue. Under certain conditions, especially for acute injury, cell membranes may be damaged or broken while maintaining the nucleus and general cell morphology intact. For this acute injury, it is relatively

difficult for routine histologic analysis via LM to differentiate whether cells are alive or dead.

To verify the findings of Kaplan et al's[14] study, Lu et al[23] repeated the study using CLM combined with cell vital staining (in addition to LM) to determine chondrocyte viability after bRFE acute ablation. The authors hypothesized that CLM would show significant chondrocyte death that was not apparent using standard LM techniques. Twelve fresh osteochondral sections from 12 patients undergoing total or partial knee arthroplasty were used in this study. Under arthroscopic visualization, bRFE (ArthroCare 2000™ System, Arthro-Care Corp., Sunnyvale, CA) coupled with the right-angle ArthroWand™ 3.0 mm, 90 degrees, or CoVac™ 50-degree probe (currently used for clinical patients; ArthroCare, Corp., Sunnyvale, CA) was used to treat cartilage samples in noncontact at one of three settings: S2 (133–147 kHz), S4 (160–179 kHz), or S6 (190–210 kHz). The bRFE treatment time for each single probe pass was 3 seconds. Each treated area was processed for analysis by LM, using H&E and safranin O, and by CLM using vital cell staining after treatment. Histologic analysis via LM demonstrated normal morphology of chondrocytes in the bRFE-treated regions compared with the control at all treatment settings and for both probes tested. The depth and width of chondrocyte death increased along with the higher settings used for both probes **(Fig. 4–4);** however, the increase in chondrocyte death with increased settings was significant only for the ArthroWand probe ($p < .05$). There was a trend for the CoVac 50-degree probe to kill more chondrocytes to a greater depth than the ArthroWand ($p = .08$). In some instances, thermal injury extended to the level of subchondral bone for both probes. The results of this work contradicted Kaplan et al's[14] study performed in a similar fashion. The authors concluded that (1) bRFE delivered through the probes investigated created significant chondrocyte death in chondromalacic human articular cartilage in vitro, posing a great danger for creating full-thickness chondrocyte death and subchondral bone necrosis clinically, and

(2) CLM is a sensitive technique for demonstrating this finding whereas LM is not.

Concerns raised by some researchers regarding the Lu et al study,[15,23,34] were that some chondrocytes may not actually have been killed after RFE treatment, but had been temporarily impaired or in "heat shock" following bRFE thermal chondroplasty. There are many bodies of work that support the validity of CLM and the fact that thermal treatment results in irreversible chondrocyte death.[13,26] In Lu et al's previous sheep study with partial-thickness cartilage defects, chondrocyte death was identifiable at time 0 and persisted until the termination of the project 6 months after surgery.[15] In no case, did the investigators observe return of cell viability in areas where previous cell death had been demonstrated. In addition, treatment temperatures for both mRFE and bRFE for chondroplasty are always above 65°C.[34]

To evaluate RFE effects on articular cartilage, Lu et al[34] compared three commonly used RFE devices in the field of sports medicine using bovine articular cartilage. Two bRFE devices and a mRFE device were compared in this ex vivo study. The purpose of this study was to assess the effects of mRFE and bRFE on articular cartilage at the manufacturers' recommended settings for thermal chondroplasty. The authors hypothesized that thermal smoothing of the articular cartilage could be achieved with these devices, but that unacceptable thermal injury to the chondrocytes would occur with these devices. Three different treatment patterns were used in this study to compare the acute effects of these RFE devices on articular cartilage. In the first pattern, the RFE probe was applied to the surface with a motorized jig that applied 50 g of weight through the probe tip at a velocity of 1 mm/sec to simulate a single, controlled pass across the cartilage with contact (single pass contact mode). The second treatment was performed with a motorized jig that maintained the probe tip 1 mm/sec from the cartilage surface at a velocity of 1 mm/sec (single pass noncontact mode). The third treatment was designed to mimic the clinical application of RFE for thermal chondroplasty of abraded articular cartilage (paintbrush

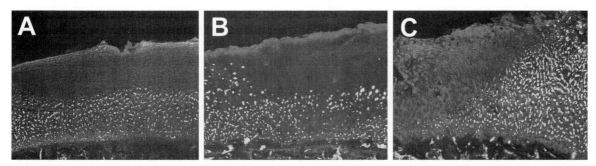

FIGURE 4–4 Confocal images indicated thermal damage with clear demarcation in ArthroCare bRFE treatment group. **(A)** Setting 2. **(B)** Setting 4. **(C)** Setting 6 (×20). Thermal penetration increased with higher bRFE settings (See Color Plate 4–4).

clinical pattern). The osteochondral sections were treated using the manufacturers' recommended settings: ElectroThermal System ORA-50 coupled with TAC-C probe at 55°C/25 W (Oratec Interventions Inc., Menlo Park, CA); Mitek VAPR™ System coupled with Flexible Side Effect Electrode at V2: 40 W (Mitek Products, Inc., Westwood, MA); and Arthroscopic Electrosurgery System™ coupled with 3.0 mm × 90 degree ArthroWand at controller setting of 2 (ArthroCare Corp., Sunnyvale, CA). The results of this study demonstrated that bRFE contoured the articular surface significantly faster than mRFE. The paintbrush clinical pattern resulted in penetration to the level of subchondral bone in all sections treated with bRFE and none of the sections treated with mRFE. The depth of chondrocyte death was greater for the bRFE systems than mRFE in all tested treatment modes. bRFE devices produced both visual and SEM-demonstrated smoothing of the articular cartilage surface compared with the control in contact and noncontact modes, whereas the mRFE smoothed the surface only in contact mode. Limitations of this study included the following: (1) the three RFE devices' settings were not equal to each other based on different RFE generators' designs and algorithms; therefore, direct comparison among the three systems cannot be made regarding power settings; (2) the probe diameters of each system were not uniform, and therefore may contribute to variation in the chondrocyte death produced; and (3) the osteochondral sections used were normal bovine cartilage samples that were abraded to simulate human chondromalacia, resulting in prolonged treatment times because of the large fissures or flaps created and the cartilage being firmer than naturally diseased cartilage. The authors concluded that both bRFE and mRFE, at the manufacturers' recommended settings, produced immediate chondrocyte death, especially bRFE systems that created chondrocyte death extending to the subchondral bone in many instances. The authors further concluded that RFE should not be used for thermal chondroplasty until further work established consistent methods for limiting chondrocyte death while still achieving a smooth articular surface.

To verify the RFE devices' effects on chondromalacic human cartilage, Edwards et al[22] compared the three most commonly utilized RFE devices (two bRFE and one mRFE) for thermal chondroplasty using human naturally occurring chondromalacic cartilage. In this ex vivo study, the authors hypothesized that CLM combined with vital cell staining would demonstrate significant chondrocyte death after RFE chondroplasty as reported in the previous bovine study by Lu et al.[34] Chondromalacic cartilage samples (grade II and III) harvested from 22 patients undergoing knee arthroplasty were used in this study. A circular area of 1.5 cm in diameter was marked on the cartilage surface and treated with one of three RFE devices: ArthroCare 2000™ with CoVac™ 50 probe, setting of 2 (ArthroCare Corp., Sunnyvale, CA); Mitek VAPR™ version 2.1 with 3.5-mm side effect probe, setting of V2–40 (Mitek Corp., Anondale, MA); and Vulcan EAS™ version 3.12, with a TAC-C probe, temperature control setting at 70°C/30 W (Oratec Interventions Inc., Menlo Park, CA). All samples were treated using a custom-designed jig to simulate arthroscopic surgery with an irrigation flow rate of 120 mL/min of saline at 22°C. The results of this study demonstrated that all three RFE devices successfully smoothed the chondromalacic cartilaginous surface at the following mean treatment times: 24 seconds for Arthrocare, 23 seconds for Mitek, and 39 seconds for Oratec. The bRFE devices resulted in significantly greater chondrocyte death than mRFE, and the chondrocyte death extended to the level of subchondral bone in over 50% of the tested samples with both bRFE devices, whereas none extended to the subchondral bone with the mRFE device. This study confirmed the findings of the previous bovine study and emphasized that both bRFE and mRFE were unsafe for human clinical thermal chondroplasty. One of the limitations for this study was that RFE treatments were performed in an ex vivo environment and may not reflect actual effects of RFE in in vivo conditions. Further research in this field should be focused on limiting chondrocyte death to a level consistently less than 250 to 300 μm, the depth of chondrocyte death that usually occurs following mechanical debridement.

Chondrocytes are known to be thermal sensitive, and excessive temperatures may cause chondrocyte death and promote the degeneration of articular cartilage. Therefore, it is imperative to determine the lowest possible RFE settings that will produce the desired thermal effect. Shellock and Shields[35] determined the temperature changes associated with the use of bRFE at different settings to bovine articular cartilage. The bRFE device used in this investigation was the VAPR System coupled with a Side Effect Thermal Electrode (Mitek Products, Westwood, MA). The bRFE device was set at both ablative and desiccation modes (V2–20, 40, 60, and 120). To accurately measure the RFE tip temperature, a fluoroptic thermometry system (Model 3100, Luxtron, Santa Clara, CA) was used in this study. Fresh bovine cartilage samples were placed in a temperature-controlled bath at 37°C. The bRFE probe was positioned so that the centermost portion of the active probe was directly over the fluoroptic thermometry probe. In this way, the temperature of the electrode-tissue interface was recorded. Temperatures were recorded at 1-second intervals for a baseline period of 5 seconds, during the delivery of bRFE for 2 seconds, and for a period of 3 seconds after RFE delivery. The findings of this study indicated that three of the four settings used (V2–40,

60, and 120) produced observable changes in the appearance of the articular cartilage, corresponding to temperatures ranging between 58° and 80°C in both ablative and desiccation modes. The authors recommended that V2–40 should be used initially, increasing to higher settings only if necessary to achieve the desired changes, and that bRFE was safe to use for chondroplasty as Kaplan et al[14] and Turner et al[16] reported previously.

To evaluate the temperatures reached in the cartilage matrix caused by both bRFE and mRFE during thermal chondroplasty, Edwards et al[36] compared matrix temperatures at three depths below the articular surface and also determined the effect of irrigation flow during RFE chondroplasty. The authors hypothesized that cartilage matrix temperatures would be significantly higher to greater depths for bRFE application than mRFE application, and that irrigation fluid flow would reduce thermal penetration. Sixty fresh bovine osteochondral sections were used in this study. The sections were placed in a device that guided fluoroptic thermocouples (SFF-2, Luxtron Corp., Santa Clara, CA) tangentially and parallel to the cartilage surface at one of the following depths for each application: 200, 500, and 2000 μm below the articular surface. The cartilage surface was treated with one of two devices: bRFE (ArthroCare 2000™, CoVac 50 probe, setting of 2, ArthroCare Corp., Sunnyvale, CA) or mRFE (Vulcan EAS™, TAC-C probe, 70°C/30 W, Oratec Interventions Inc., Menlo Park, CA) with flow or no flow of 22°C lavage solution. Temperatures were recorded for 5 seconds of baseline, for 20 seconds of probe activation, and then for a 15-second period after RFE activation. A circular area (10-mm diameter) of each section was treated by bRFE in noncontact or mRFE in light contact using a paintbrush pattern. The temperatures recorded by fluoroptic thermometry demonstrated that cartilage temperatures were significantly higher in the bRFE group than the mRFE group at all depths. For the bRFE device, the temperatures recorded exceeded 75°C at all three measured depths. For the mRFE device, the temperatures exceeded 50°C only at 200 μm and 500 μm. Lavage solution flow did not have significant effects on cartilage matrix temperatures during bRFE application, whereas it resulted in higher temperatures in the cartilage matrix during mRFE application. The investigators concluded that bRFE caused significantly greater and deeper temperature rises within the cartilage matrix than mRFE during thermal chondroplasty. Even at 2000 μm below the cartilage surface, the measured temperature caused by bRFE exceeded 75°C, higher than the temperature threshold that results in chondrocyte death. This study further demonstrated that bRFE posed great danger for creating full-thickness chondrocyte death and subchondral bone necrosis and that bRFE devices were not safe for thermal chondroplasty.

To investigate the effects of RFE treatment time on articular cartilage for clinicians who use RFE to treat chondromalacic cartilage, Lu et al[37] investigated the effects of RFE treatment time on chondrocyte viability and surface contouring. The purpose of this study was to evaluate both chondrocyte viability and cartilaginous surface contouring using CLM and SEM, respectively, during different treatment time intervals with mRFE and bRFE at the manufacturers' recommended settings. Forty-two fresh osteochondral sections from 17 patients undergoing total or partial knee arthroplasty were used for this study. Each of 36 sections was divided into two distinct 1-cm² regions, which were treated with either bRFE or mRFE. Only chondromalacic cartilage of grade II was selected for use in this study. Each specimen was placed on a custom designed jig maintaining a lavage fluid temperature of 22°C. No fluid flow was used during mRFE treatment based on information from a previous study that determined the effect of irrigation fluid flow on cartilage matrix temperatures reached during chondroplasty.[36] This study demonstrated that with flow, mRFE delivered more output power (more heat than during no flow conditions) to maintain the probe tip temperature close to the preset temperature because the probe tip was cooled by the lavage flow. A flow rate of 120 mL/min was used when applying the bipolar RFE device, approximating the irrigation flow rate used clinically. This flow rate prevents air bubble accumulation within the treatment field and has no positive or negative effect on cartilage matrix temperature as previously reported.[36] The ArthroCare 2000™ bRFE System coupled with a CoVac™ 50° angle probe (ArthroCare Corp., Sunnyvale, CA) was used to deliver bRFE in noncontact (1 mm above cartilage surface) over a 1.0-cm² area in the treatment pattern at a generator setting of 2 (133–147 kHz). The Vulcan EAS™ coupled with a TAC-C probe (Smith & Nephew, Endoscopy, Menlo Park, CA) was used to deliver mRFE in light contact over a 1.0-cm² area in a treatment pattern identical to the bipolar device at a generator setting of 70°C and 15 W. Six RF treatment time intervals were evaluated: 5, 10, 15, 20, 30, and 40 seconds. For each RFE generator/treatment time combination, six independent samples were used (total, 36 treatments/RFE generator). Another sham-operated group of six specimens served as control. In addition, margins of each treated section served as its own control. Following RFE treatment, each treated area was processed for analysis by CLM and SEM. Arthroscopic examination showed that mRFE melted the fine fronds but could not do so for the contour-thickened fissures and clefts in the 5- and 10-second treatment time groups, while 15-second treatment produced a smooth and light gray cartilaginous surface. Continued treatment times up to 40 seconds resulted in discoloration of the treated area to light yellow. bRFE treatment for 5 and 10 seconds melted the fine fronds, and macroscopic smoothing was achieved at 15 seconds. Continued treatment from 20 to 40 seconds produced a smooth cartilaginous surface that changed from yellow to brown in color. CLM demonstrated that mRFE caused significantly less depth of chondrocyte death than bRFE at each treatment time interval. In the mRFE group, there were no significant differences in the depth of chondrocyte death among the 10-, 15-, and 20-second treatment time groups. Thirty- and 40-second treatment time groups caused significantly more depth of chondrocyte death than the 10-, 15-, and 20-second groups. After bipolar RFE treatment, the 15-, 20-, and 30-second groups caused significantly more depth of chondrocyte death than the 5- and 10-second groups. The 40-second group caused significantly more depth of chondrocyte death than the 15-second groups. SEM demonstrated that both mRFE and bRFE contoured rough chondromalacic surfaces dependent on the treatment time. Analysis of SEM images revealed that both mRFE and bRFE required a minimum of 15 seconds to smooth the cartilage surface sufficiently to reach the SEM score of 2 (relatively smooth with melted fronds) **(Fig. 4–5)**. mRFE created a smoother surface than bRFE at the 5-second treatment time. There were no significant differences in surface smoothing between bRFE and mRFE at the remaining treatment time intervals. This study demonstrated that bRFE caused significantly greater chondrocyte death than mRFE at identical treatment time intervals, confirming the findings of previous studies.[22,34,36] This study also demonstrated that it took 15 seconds for both bRFE and mRFE to contour a

1-cm^2 chondromalacic cartilaginous surface to a relatively smooth surface as demonstrated by SEM. When applying thermal chondroplasty clinically, a broad treatment time range may result in variable degrees of cartilage smoothness and potentially, significant chondrocyte death.

Lu et al[32] performed the first study to determine a method to limit chondrocyte death for temperature controlled mRFE. The purpose of this study was to evaluate the thermal penetration and surface smoothing of chondromalacic articular cartilage after mRFE treatment at one of two lavage temperatures: 22°C and 37°C. Based on the mRFE device's temperature-controlled design, it was hypothesized that thermal chondroplasty with mRFE in 37°C lavage solution would reduce chondrocyte death compared with 22°C lavage solution and result in greater smoothing of the articular cartilage surface. Sixteen fresh osteochondral sections from 16 patients undergoing total or partial knee arthroplasty were used to complete this study. To avoid experimental bias, only chondromalacic cartilage of grade II was selected for use in this study and each graded osteochondral section was cut into two sections. One section was treated with mRFE in physiologic saline at 22°C (room temperature), whereas the other section was treated at 37°C. An area 2 cm distant from the RFE treated area on each specimen served as control. The Vulcan EAS™ coupled with a TAC-C II probe (Smith & Nephew, Endoscopy, Menlo Park, CA) was used to deliver mRFE in a light contact fashion over a 1.0-cm^2 area on each section in a paintbrush treatment pattern at a generator

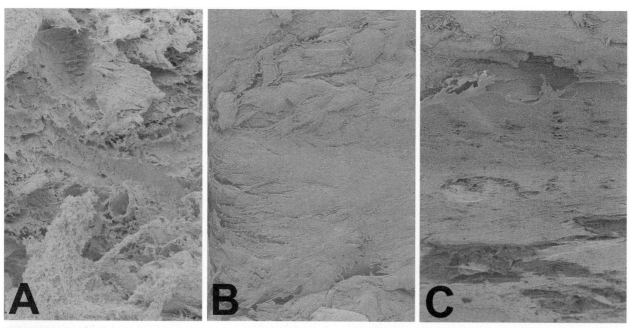

FIGURE 4–5 **(A)** Scanning electron microscopy (SEM) image demonstrating sham-operated control cartilage with fibrillated and rough surface. **(B)** Fifteen-second mRFE treatment produced relatively smooth cartilaginous surface with melted fronds. **(C)** Fifteen-second bRFE treatment produced relatively smoothed cartilaginous surface with melted fronds (×1000).

setting of 70°C and 15 W. RFE treatment times of 10 seconds and 15 seconds were evaluated in this study. For each treatment time/lavage temperature combination, eight sections were tested (total, 32 treatments, four groups, $n = 8$). Ten- and 15-second treatment times were selected based on the results of a previous study.[37] After RFE treatment, each treated area was processed for analysis by vital cell staining/CLM and SEM. CLM demonstrated that the depth of chondrocyte death in 37°C lavage solution was significantly less than that in 22°C solution at both 10- and 15-second treatment times. SEM demonstrated that cartilage surfaces were smoothed in both 37°C and 22°C lavage solutions treated for both the 10-second and 15-second treatment times compared with the control specimens. The mean mRFE treatment temperatures in 37°C lavage solution was higher than in 22°C lavage solution for both the 10-second and 15-second treatment times ($p < .05$), whereas RFE delivery power in 37°C was lower than 22°C lavage solution for both treatment times ($p < .05$). The authors concluded that thermal chondroplasty performed with mRFE in 37°C lavage solution caused significantly less chondrocyte death than in 22°C lavage solution. Increasing the lavage solution temperature allowed the probe tip to reach preset temperature more rapidly and resulted in less total power (energy) delivery while still effectively smoothing the cartilaginous surface. Based on the results of this study, when thermal chondroplasty with mRFE is performed, lavage solution temperature may have a significant influence on chondrocyte viability.

■ Conclusion

Thermal chondroplasty with electrothermal energy is still a controversial and contradictory topic for both experimental and clinical investigators. Theoretically, benefits of electrothermal chondroplasty include the ability to stabilize the articular surface through a melting process that reduces the cyclic inflammation caused by release of collagen and proteoglycan epitopes, to quickly and accurately smooth the cartilaginous surface compared with mechanical debridement, and to deliver RFE via an arthroscopic approach.

Recently, RFE has increasingly played a major role in thermal chondroplasty because of its advantages over electrocautery and laser, such as its simple and easy use, temperature-controlled RFE delivery, inexpensive cost, and accurate ablation of diseased cartilage without damaging surrounding healthy cartilage. However, two clinical studies have reported contradictory outcomes regarding bRFE on chondromalacic cartilage.[38,39] In 2001, Hogan and Diduch[38] reported on an individual patient who developed progressive cartilage loss following bRFE treatment at 1 year after surgery. Owens et al[39] compared mechanical shaving and bRFE for the management of chondromalacia (grade II or III) in 39 patients. The authors concluded that bRFE provided clear evidence of superior clinical outcome following debridement of chondromalacic patellar grade II or III chondral lesions compared with a mechanical shaver. Currently, there is no clinical study regarding mRFE chondroplasty reported in peer-reviewed journals.

Based on the previous experimental studies, the thermal penetration for the mRFE devices currently used clinically range from 400 to 800 μm, whereas the thermal penetration for bRFE devices currently used clinically range from 1500 to 2500 μm.[22,23,34,37] The depths of thermal penetration caused by both mRFE and bRFE are still greater than that caused by mechanical debridement (i.e., 250–300 μm), although both types of RFE can create a smoother cartilaginous surface than mechanical debridement.

Radiofrequency energy should be used for chondroplasty cautiously if at all, especially bRFE. When surgeons plan thermal chondroplasty with RFE, determining and understanding the cartilage thickness of the treated area will help to prevent full-thickness chondrocyte death or subchondral bone necrosis.

Electrothermal chondroplasty is not a mature and completely safe technique for clinical application at this time. Long-term clinical follow-up studies regarding both mRFE and bRFE applications should continue. Future research should focus on how to improve RFE devices and enhance their safety parameters, for instance, minimizing the depth of chondrocyte death to consistently less than 250 μm while smoothing irregular and rough cartilaginous surfaces.

Acknowledgments   The authors would like to acknowledge John Bogdanske, Vicki Kalscheur, Susan Linden, Rajesh K. Uthamanthil, M.V.Sc., Shane Nho, John Heiner, M.D., and Brian J. Cole, M.D., Ph. D., for assistance with the research studies described; and Smith & Nephew, Endoscopy, the NFL Medical Charities, and the National Institutes of Health for research support.

REFERENCES

1. Rand JA, Gaffey TA. Effect of electrocautery on fresh human articular cartilage. Arthroscopy 1985;1:242–246
2. Stein DT, Ricciardi CA, Viehe T. The effectiveness of the use of electrocautery with chondroplasty in treating chondromalacic lesions: a randomized prospective study. Arthroscopy 2002;18:190–193
3. Miller DV, O'Brien SJ, Arnoczky SS, Kelly A, Fealy SV, Warren RF. The use of the contact Nd:YAG laser in arthroscopic surgery: effects on articular cartilage and meniscal tissue. Arthroscopy 1989;5:245–253
4. Raunest J, Lohnert J. Arthroscopic cartilage debridement by excimer laser in chondromalacia of the knee joint. A prospective

randomized clinical study. Arch Orthop Trauma Surg 1990;109: 155–159

5. Grifka J, Boenke S, Schreiner C, Lohnert J. Significance of laser treatment in arthroscopic therapy of degenerative gonarthritis. A prospective, randomised clinical study and experimental research. Knee Surg Sports Traumatol Arthrosc 1994;2:88–93

6. Fink B, Schneider T, Braunstein S, Schmielau G, Ruther W. Holmium:YAG laser-induced aseptic bone necroses of the femoral condyle. Arthroscopy 1996;12:217–223

7. Fischer R, Krebs R, Scharf HP. Cell vitality in cartilage tissue culture following excimer laser radiation: an in vitro examination. Lasers Surg Med 1993;13:629–637

8. Moller KO, Lind BM, Karcher K, Hohlbach G. [Holmium laser versus mechanical cartilage resection. Comparative studies in the rabbit arthrosis model.] Langenbecks Arch Chir 1994;379:84–94

9. Rozbruch SR, Wickiewicz TL, DiCarlo EF, Potter HG. Osteonecrosis of the knee following arthroscopic laser meniscectomy. Arthroscopy 1996;12:245–250

10. Thal R, Danziger MB, Kelly A. Delayed articular cartilage slough: two cases resulting from holmium:YAG laser damage to normal articular cartilage and a review of the literature. Arthroscopy 1996;12:92–94

11. Trauner KB, Nishioka NS, Flotte T, Patel D. Acute and chronic response of articular cartilage to holmium:YAG laser irradiation. Clin Orthop 1995;310:52–57

12. Lane JG, Amiel MD, Monosov AZ, Amiel D. Matrix assessment of the articular cartilage surface after chondroplasty with the Holmium: YAG laser. Am J Sports Med 1997;25:560–569

13. Mainil-Varlet P, Monin D, Weiler C, et al. Quantification of laser-induced cartilage injury by confocal microscopy in an ex vivo model. J Bone Joint Surg Am 2001;83A:566–571

14. Kaplan L, Uribe JW, Sasken H, Markarian G. The acute effects of radiofrequency energy in articular cartilage: an in vitro study. Arthroscopy 2000;16:2–5

15. Lu Y, Hayashi K, Hecht P, et al. The effect of monopolar radiofrequency energy on partial-thickness defects of articular cartilage. Arthroscopy 2000;16:527–536

16. Turner AS, Tippett JW, Powers BE, Dewell RD, Hallinckrodt CH. Radiofrequency (electrosurgical) ablation of articular cartilage. A study in sheep. Arthroscopy 1998;14:585–591

17. Outerbridge RE. The etiology of chondromalacia patella. J Bone Joint Surg Br 1961;43-B:752–757

18. Moseley JB, O'Malley K, Petersen NJ, et al. A controlled trial of arthroscopic surgery for osteoarthritis of the knee. N Engl J Med 2002;347:81–88

19. Abelow SP. Use of lasers in orthopedic surgery: current concepts. Orthopedics 1993;16:551–556

20. Fanton GS. Arthroscopic electrothermal surgery of the shoulder. Oper Tech Sports Med 1998;6:139–146

21. Shellock FG. Radiofrequency energy-induced heating of bovine articular cartilage: evaluation of a new temperature-controlled, bipolar radiofrequency system used at different settings. J Knee Surg 2002;15:90–96

22. Edwards RB, Lu Y, Kalscheur VL, Nho S, Cole BJ, Markel MD. Thermal chondroplasty of chondromalacic human cartilage: an ex vivo comparison of bipolar and monopolar radiofrequency devices. Am J Sports Med 2001;30:90–97

23. Lu Y, Edwards RB, Kalscheur VL, Nho S, Cole BJ, Markel MD. Effect of bipolar radiofrequency energy on human articular cartilage: comparison of confocal laser microscopy and light microscopy. Arthroscopy 2001;17:117–123

24. Hunter W. Of the structure and diseases of articulating cartilage. Philos Trans 1743;42:514–521

25. Li S, Chien S, Branemark P. Heat shock-induced necrosis and apoptosis in osteoblasts. J Orthop Res 1999;17:891–899

26. Zuger BJ, Ott B, Mainil-Varlet P, et al. Laser solder welding of articular cartilage: tensile strength and chondrocyte viability. Lasers Surg Med 2001;28:427–434

27. Federico DJ, Reider B. Results of isolated patellar debridement for patellofemoral pain in patients with normal patellar alignment. Am J Sports Med 1997;25:663–669

28. Miller GK, Drennan DB, Maylahn DJ. The effect of technique on histology of arthroscopic partial meniscectomy with electrosurgery. Arthroscopy 1987;3:36–44

29. Pullin JG, Collier MA, Das P, et al. Effects of holmium: YAG laser energy on cartilage metabolism, healing, and biochemical properties of lesional and perilesional tissue in a weight-bearing model. Arthroscopy 1996;12:15–25

30. Ebert DW, Bertone AL, Roberts C. Effect of irradiation with a low-intensity diode laser on the metabolism of equine articular cartilage in vitro. Am J Vet Res 1998;59:1613–1618

31. Torricelli P, Giavaresi G, Fini M, et al. Laser biostimulation of cartilage: in vitro evaluation. Biomed Pharmacother 2001;55: 117–120

32. Lu Y, Edwards RB, Nho S, Cole BJ, Markel MD. Lavage solution temperature influences depth of chondrocyte death and surface contouring during thermal chondroplasty with temperature controlled monopolar radiofrequency energy. Am J Sports Med 2002;30:667–673

33. Organ LW. Electrophysiologic principles of radiofrequency lesion making. Appl Neurophysiol 1976;39:69–76

34. Lu Y, Edwards RB, Cole BJ, Markel MD. Thermal chondroplasty with radiofrequency energy: an in vitro comparison of bipolar and monopolar radiofrequency devices. Am J Sports Med 2001;29:42–49

35. Shellock FG, Shields CL. Radiofrequency energy-induced heating of bovine articular cartilage using a bipolar radiofrequency electrode. Am J Sports Med 2000;28:720–724

36. Edwards RB, Lu Y, Rodriguez E, Markel MD. Thermometric determination of cartilage matrix temperatures during thermal chondroplasty: comparison of bipolar and monopolar radiofrequency devices. Arthroscopy 2002;18:339–346

37. Lu Y, Edwards RB III, Nho S, Heiner JP, Cole BJ, Markel MD. Thermal chondroplasty with bipolar and monopolar radiofrequency energy: effect of treatment time on chondrocyte death and surface contouring. Arthroscopy 2002;18:779–788

38. Hogan CJ, Diduch DR. Progressive articular cartilage loss following radiofrequency treatment of a partial-thickness lesion. Arthroscopy 2001;17:E24

39. Owens BD, Stickles BJ, Balikian P, Busconi BD. Prospective analysis of radiofrequency versus mechanical debridement of isolated patellar chondral lesions. Arthroscopy 2002;18:151–155

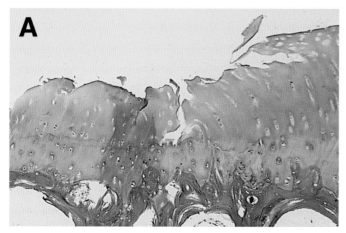

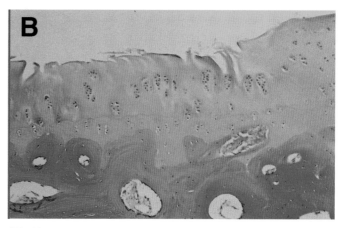

Color Plate 4–1 (A) Safranin O–stained chondromalacic articular cartilage of grade II or III with surface irregularities, fissures, and reduced proteoglycan concentration (×100)

(B) Hematoxylin and eosin (H&E) stained chondromalacic articular cartilage of grade II with surface irregularities, fibrillation, and chondrocyte cloning (×100). See Figure 4–1, page 33.

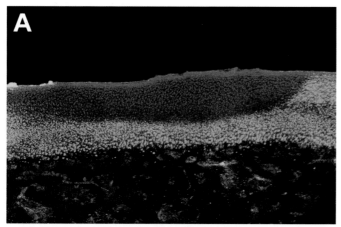

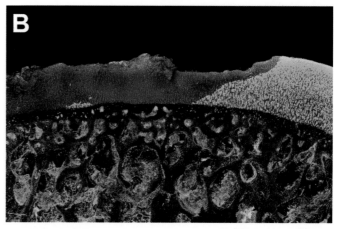

Color Plate 4–3 Confocal microscopic image demonstrating RFE-treated cartilage surface (top of each image) and subchondral bone (bottom of each image) following a paintbrush pattern application (×20). The green dots indicate viable chondrocytes, and the red dots indicate dead chondrocytes.

(A) 0 time, RFE treatment caused immediate chondrocyte death and a clear "dead zone" appeared. Cartilaginous surface was contoured. **(B)** Two-week group. By 2 weeks after RFE treatment, all chondrocytes were dead and the cartilaginous surface appeared relatively smooth. See Figure 4–3, page 38.

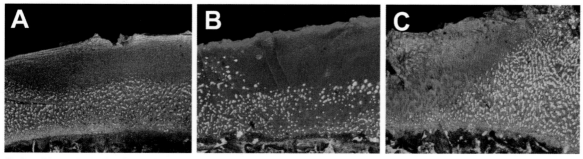

Color Plate 4–4 Confocal images indicated thermal damage with clear demarcation in ArthroCare bRFE treatment group. **(A)** Setting 2. **(B)** Setting 4. **(C)** Setting 6 (×20). Thermal penetration increased with higher bRFE settings. See Figure 4–4, page 39.

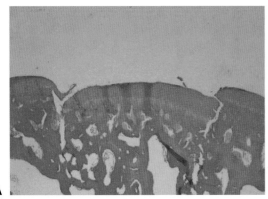 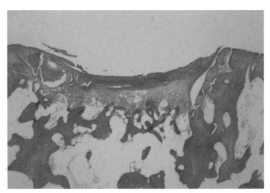

A
B

Color Plate 14–10 (A) Histology of articular cartilage defect treated with OAT at 6 weeks. Note excellent bone–bone healing and maintenance of hyaline cartilage.

(B) Control untreated articular cartilage defect at 6 weeks. Fibrocartilage partially fills the defect, and there is adjacent articular cartilage damage. See Figure 14–10, page 136.

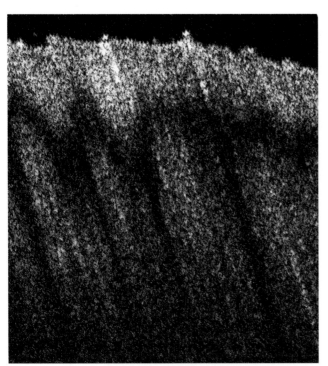

Color Plate 25–1B Cross-sectional OCT image of healthy appearing articular cartilage. See Figure 25–1B, page 290.

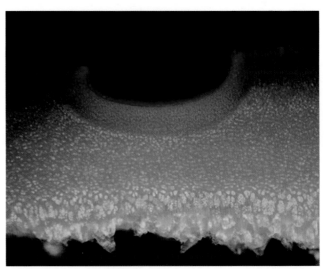

Color Plate 25–2B Computer-controlled treatment stage. See Figure 25–2B, page 292.

Assessment

5

Clinical Evaluation of the Patient with a Chondral Injury

RAFFY MIRZAYAN

Chondral injuries are becoming more frequently recognized. They have an incidence of between 5% and 10% in patients who have experienced acute sporting injuries and present with an acute hemarthrosis.[1] In addition, 20% of anterior cruciate ligament (ACL)-injured knees chronically develop cartilage loss.[2] The diagnosis of a chondral injury is hard to make and is often delayed. It is usually a diagnosis of exclusion and is often made only arthroscopically. Current magnetic resonance imaging (MRI) techniques are not sophisticated enough to appreciate the chondral injuries. However, newer techniques are emerging and will aid in earlier diagnosis. The most important aspect in making an accurate and timely diagnosis is to have a high degree of suspicion.

■ History

Patients with osteochondral injury may present with a variety of symptoms. A detailed history from the patient usually reveals a single traumatic antecedent event associated with the onset of symptoms, which include pain, effusion, locking, and catching. If an acute injury has occurred, ligamentous or meniscal injury should also be suspected. Prior traumatic injuries are common, and a history of the number of traumatic events should be documented. Chondral wear injuries can occur over time due to malalignment of a joint or maltracking of the patella. In these cases, patients may not have a history of an acute injury. If the patient has had a previous surgery of the affected joint, it is crucial to gain as much information from that procedure as possible. It is

extremely helpful to not only have the operative report, but to also obtain video or photographs from the surgery to evaluate the size and location of a cartilage lesion, as well as to assess the cruciate ligaments and menisci. If a partial meniscectomy was performed, the photographs will help to determine how much was removed and if a meniscal transplant may be necessary. If the lesion is an osteochondral defect, the photographs can aid in determining the amount of bony defect.

■ Physical Examination

Physical examination should be performed in a systematic manner, with careful observation of gross morphology, the presence of an effusion and surgical incisions, palpation, range of motion assessment, stability testing, alignment, and use of specialized provocative tests. Tenderness at the joint line may be associated with lesions of the femoral condyles or in the context of underlying meniscal pathology, while focal femoral condylar tenderness or a palpable defect more often indicate the presence of an osteochondral defect. The patient will limit weight bearing. Osteochondral lesions secondary to patellar dislocation can result following avulsion of the medial patellofemoral ligament or due to shear and impaction forces with reduction. This subset of patients will display focal tenderness at the medial epicondyle, along the medial retinaculum, under the medial patellar facet, and at the lateral femoral condyle. Following lateral patellar dislocation, up to 50% of patients show evidence of osteochondral lesions of the lateral femoral condyle, medial patellar facet, or both.[3] Concomitant ligamentous laxity may be present, and ligamentous integrity should be assessed. Despite a thorough history and physical examination, the diagnosis of chondral injury is made by advanced imaging studies and arthroscopic evaluation.

Recurrent effusions may also be associated with chondral injuries. This is particularly true in the case of patellofemoral lesions. Anterior knee pain when ascending and especially descending stairs, as well as anterior knee pain with prolonged sitting ("theater sign"), are indicative of patellofemoral chondral wear. Prior patellar dislocations or patellar maltracking may result in chondral injuries. The Q-angle, hypermobility of the patella, and pain with a patellar grind test should be evaluated.

Radiographic Evaluation

Plain radiographs can be helpful in the diagnosis of osteochondral lesions. However, they may not always reveal the underlying fragment, especially if it is purely a chondral injury devoid of underlying bone. A standard series including weight-bearing anteroposterior (AP), 45-degree posteroanterior (PA) (Rosenberg view[4]), lateral, and Merchant views should be obtained. Additional oblique views may be obtained later if there is suspicion [[Q2: Q2]] on the initial series. These views enable the clinician to assess the presence or absence of fractures as well as joint space congruity and narrowing, malalignment, and the presence of osteochondritis dissecans. However, the amount of bone in an osteochondral injury is often small and not detected through the use of routine plain radiographs.

Full-length (54 inch) standing views that include the center of the femoral head, knee, and talus are obtained to assess the anatomic and mechanical axes of the lower extremity. If a cartilage procedure is to be performed, this will also be a useful preoperative tool for any realignment procedure.

Improvements in MRI techniques continue to expand the ability to detect articular cartilage pathology and osteochondral injury. Proton-density imaging of thin (3- to 4-mm) sections, T1-weighted fat-suppressed three-dimensional (3D) gradient echo, and T2-weighted fast spin-echo sequences optimize resolution of the articular cartilage and underlying subchondral bone.[5] The osteochondral fracture may parallel the joint surface or it may present as a periarticular osseous fracture that extends and crosses perpendicular to the articular cartilage. High signal intensity is frequently identified underlying the fracture segment in acute injuries, while intermediate signal intensity in cartilage or fibrous tissue is more characteristic of chronic lesions. Absence of hyperintensity of the fragment in the junctional zone is associated with fracture stability. High-signal-intensity fluid surrounding the fragment indicates instability and loosening. MRI is also especially useful in detecting osteochondral loose bodies and chondral fragments.

Fat-suppressed, 3D, T1-weighted gradient echo images cause the articular cartilage to appear bright compared with the surrounding joint fluid and subchondral bone and bone marrow.[6] This produces a very accurate representation of the cartilage–fluid and cartilage–bone interfaces[7] and is therefore a very good method for determining articular cartilage defects. However, this technique does not adequately assess the menisci or ligaments.[6] Fast spin-echo techniques allow evaluation of the menisci and ligaments, minimize metallic artifact, offer improved image contrast between cartilage and fluid, and assesses the subchondral bone.[6] The images are prone to blurring and partial volume averaging inaccuracies.[6] Magnetic resonance arthrography (MRA) is performed with intraarticular injection of contrast. It has been shown to be an excellent method for articular cartilage evaluation.[8]

Magnetic resonance imaging continues to be a highly effective diagnostic tool for the assessment of ligamentous and meniscal pathology as its role in the diagnosis of osteochondral injury continues to evolve.

Computed tomography (CT) can be a useful adjunct to other imaging methods previously described, especially in defining the degree of bony involvement. CT is able to demonstrate excellent definition of bony fragments and detailed delineation of size, location, and degree of displacement of the fragment. CT, however, is less sensitive than MRI in defining subtle subchondral microfractures and is limited in the assessment of articular cartilage integrity. CT is also helpful in diagnosing trochlear dysplasia.

Diagnostic arthroscopy continues to be the gold standard in the assessment, evaluation, and characterization of osteochondral lesions. However, accurate assessment of size may be difficult arthroscopically.

■ Conclusion

Until advances in MRI are readily available to assist in the diagnosis of chondral injuries, a high degree of clinical suspicion is the most important diagnostic tool. Arthroscopy is still the best way to diagnose, classify, and treat chondral injuries.

REFERENCES

1. Noyes FR, Bassett RW, Noyes FR, et al. Arthroscopy in acute traumatic hemarthrosis of the knee: incidence of anterior cruciate tears and other injuries. J Bone Joint Surg Am 1980;62A:687–695
2. Minas T, Nehrer S. Current concepts in the treatment of articular cartilage defects. Orthopaedics 1997;20:525–538

3. Boden BP, Pearsall AW, Garrett WE Jr, Feagin JA Jr. Patellofemoral instability: evaluation and management. J Am Acad Orthop Surg 1997;5:47–57

4. Rosenberg T, Paulos L, Parker R, et al. The forty-five degree posterior-anterior flexion weight bearing radiograph of the knee. J Bone Joint Surg Am 1988;70A:1479–1483

5. Stoller DW. Magnetic Resonance Imaging in Orthopaedics and Sports Medicine, 2nd ed. Philadelphia: Lippincott-Raven, 1997:419

6. Winalski C, Minas T. Evaluation of chondral injuries by magnetic resonance imaging: repair assessments. Op Tech Sports Med 2000;8:108–119

7. Recht MP, Kramer J, Marcelis S, et al. Abnormalities of articular cartilage in the knee: analysis of available MR techniques. Radiology 1993;187:473–478

8. Vahlensieck M, Peterfy CG, Wischer T, et al. Indirect MR arthrography: optimization and clinical applications. Radiology 1996; 200:249–254

6

Imaging Techniques of Cartilage Injury

CHRISTINE B. CHUNG, AUREA MOHANA-BORGES, AND DONALD L. RESNICK

By the year 2020, arthritis will have the largest increase in number of new patients of any disease in the United States, making the symptomatic degeneration of articular cartilage among the most prevalent chronic conditions encountered. Not only is it a significant cause of morbidity in affected patients, it is second only to heart disease in causing work disability. The direct traditional medical costs and indirect economic and wage loss from arthritis in the United States has reached in excess of $65 billion annually.[1]

Although arthroscopy has been the gold standard for diagnosing and monitoring cartilage damage and repair, this is less than optimal, for several reasons: It is both invasive and expensive. Moreover, this method relies largely on visual inspection of the articular surface to indicate the need for further evaluation by physically probing the cartilage surface to find abnormalities in texture or hidden defects within the midsubstance of the tissue.

Though several imaging methods exist for cartilage evaluation, magnetic resonance imaging (MRI) has emerged as the imaging method of choice due to its excellent soft tissue contrast and multiplanar imaging capabilities. MRI has proven both sensitive and specific in the diagnosis of high-grade cartilage lesions (those involving partial- or full-thickness lesions). The limitations of MRI lie in the detection of early degenerative change in the cartilage that heralds the presence of structural alteration at the macromolecular level. It is detection of abnormality at this level that will ultimately further the understanding of the etiology and progression of cartilage lesions, and begin an era of prevention of osteoarthritis, rather than palliation.

This chapter focuses on existing, widely available MRI techniques, as well as advances in the MRI evaluation of articular cartilage.

■ Magnetic Resonance Imaging of Articular Cartilage

The general goal of imaging is the accurate depiction of the structure and composition of a tissue to evaluate its integrity. The imaging of articular cartilage proves particularly challenging in this respect due to its zonal changes in structure and biochemical composition over the distance of a few millimeters.

It is for these reasons that the normal MRI appearance of articular cartilage remains a controversial and debated issue, particularly with respect to its structure. It is generally accepted that high-resolution MRI of articular cartilage demonstrates a multilaminar appearance. The departure from and subsequent details of this finding become more complex in almost every aspect. There is much variability in both the number of laminar layers that have been reported to occur in articular cartilage and the signal characteristics of those layers. Moreover, the exact designation of what the layer represents is also debated. Although some studies advocate the hypothesis that the layers reflect the zonal anatomy of this tissue, others emphasize the contribution of truncation artifact in producing this multilaminar appearance.[2–5] In either case, the disruption of the multilaminar pattern suggests an irregularity in the structure of the tissue.

The composition of articular cartilage, chondrocytes within an extracellular matrix composed primarily of water, collagen, and proteoglycans, is perhaps less controversial. Although the exact ratio of each of the above demonstrates zonal variability, the overall composition explains the general signal characteristics that will be discussed with the individual imaging sequences.

■ Current Clinical Magnetic Resonance Imaging Applications

T1-Weighted Spin-Echo Images

One common way to evaluate tissue with MRI is by its intrinsic relaxation times, T1 and T2, which are a reflection of the local tissue properties. T1-weighted spin-echo sequences were initially advocated due to their excellent anatomic detail and high contrast between cartilage and subchondral bone.[6] This is an imaging sequence in which the range of contrast is bordered by bright or high signal intensity seen in fatty tissues such as bone marrow, and by dark or low signal intensity seen in osseous cortex. The signal intensity characteristics of articular cartilage are isointense to muscle or intermediate as compared with the internal standards of fat and cortex. Normal cartilage on this imaging sequence demonstrates homogeneous signal intensity with no multilaminar appearance. Though focal defects are identified by intrasubstance signal hypointensity, the suboptimal contrast between joint fluid (also isointense to muscle) and articular cartilage makes identification of surface irregularity and focal defects difficult.

T2-Weighted Spin-Echo Images

In the T2-weighted image, the borders of the range of contrast include fluid-like signal intensity that appears very bright (high in signal intensity) whereas osseous cortex appears dark (low in signal intensity). Both muscle and fat are intermediate in signal. T2-weighted images capitalize on the arthrogram-like effect produced by the high signal intensity of joint fluid, which accentuates any surface irregularity or focal defect in the articular cartilage.[7–9] As with T1-weighted images, the cartilage demonstrates homogeneous signal intensity in its normal state. Signal alterations generally consist of globular regions of increased signal intensity **(Fig. 6–1)**. The disadvantages of T2-weighted images

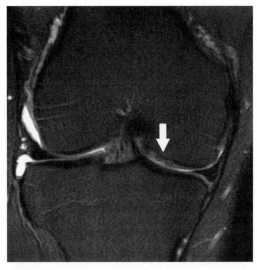

FIGURE 6–1 Coronal T2-weighted [repetition time (TR) 2367, echo time (TE) 90] fat-suppressed fast spin-echo image through the knee demonstrates an area of contour irregularity (arrow) of the lateral aspect of the medial femoral condyle. In addition, there is heterogeneous signal intensity in the cartilage in this region.

include decreased spatial resolution as compared with T1-weighted images, a lack of contrast between cartilage and subchondral cortical bone, and insensitivity to the intrinsically short T2 relaxation time of the zones of cartilage. In addition, T2-weighted sequences are particularly susceptible to an artifact that produces increased signal in highly ordered structures. This artifact is referred to as the magic angle effect and is maximal when the structure imaged is oriented at 55 degrees to the main magnetic field.[5]

Fat Suppression and Fast Spin-Echo Sequences

The application of two techniques in image acquisition for evaluation of articular cartilage has proven quite important in optimizing its evaluation. The first is the utilization of fast spin-echo imaging techniques. These techniques allow improved efficiency in image acquisition with an increase in the signal-to-noise ratio (hence increased spatial resolution) and a decrease in imaging time, which can result in a decrease in motion artifact. Fast spin-echo sequences also introduce the magnetization transfer effect, which results in improved contrast between articular cartilage and adjacent tissues, as well as between normal and abnormal cartilage. With this in mind, it is logical that chondral defects are detected primarily as focal regions of signal abnormality.[10–12]

The second adaptation that has proven quite useful in cartilage evaluation is the addition of fat suppression to T1-weighted images. By suppressing fat, the gray scale of T1-weighted images is reset to include a much narrower range of values, allowing more contrast across the image, hence better delineation between cartilage and synovial fluid. In addition, fat suppression also eliminates chemical-shift artifacts that can distort the cartilage–bone interface.[13,14]

T1-Weighted Fat Suppressed Three-Dimensional Spoiled Gradient Echo Sequences

The augmentation of T1 contrast by fat suppression can be combined with high spatial resolution and a greater signal-to-noise ratio by using a three-dimensional gradient-echo (3D spoiled GRE) technique. This technique allows the acquisition of thin section images with high contrast between bright cartilage and surrounding tissues, which can be reformatted into multiple planes. The cartilage has relatively high signal intensity due to the T1-weighting **(Fig. 6–2)**. The intrinsic signal intensity in the cartilage is homogeneous, with the exception of a midline low signal intensity pseudolamina, believed to be produced by truncation artifact, not the zonal anatomy of cartilage demonstrated on higher resolution

images. This artifact occurs at the junction of two abrupt interfaces such as cartilage and bone, and is the result of undersampling of high spatial resolutions. Chondral defects are detected primarily as regions of altered morphology rather than as areas of signal abnormality. This is currently the most sensitive clinical application for cartilage evaluation readily identifying higher grade lesions.[15,16]

Postarthrography Imaging

Postarthrography imaging capitalizes on the idea that fluid in an articulation can fill cartilage fissures and tears. In this instance, a high image contrast-to-noise ratio between joint fluid and other tissue can be very useful for diagnoses of cartilage damage or injuries. This high image contrast-to-noise has been achieved by both magnetic resonance (MR) arthrography, and more recently computed tomographic (CT) arthrography.

In the case of MR arthrography, a solution of a gadolinium-based contrast agent diluted to a 1 mmol/L concentration with normal saline is placed in the articulation under fluoroscopic guidance. MRI is subsequently performed using T1-weighted fat-suppressed sequences. This distention of the articulation with contrast allows optimal visualization of the articular surface contour **(Fig. 6–3)**. Despite the increase in the dynamic range of

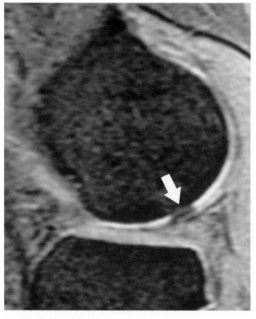
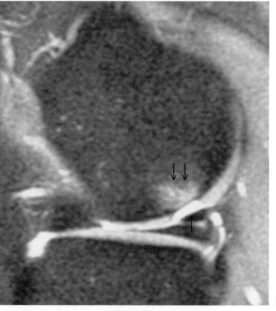

A   **B**

FIGURE 6–2 (A) Sagittal three-dimensional spoiled gradient recalled image (TR 60, TE 5, flip angle 50 degrees, slice thickness 1.5 mm) through the lateral femoral condyle demonstrates a focal full thickness (arrow) chondral defect. **(B)** Corresponding sagittal proton density weighted (TR 4000, TE 15, slice thickness 4 mm) fat-suppressed fast spin-echo image through the lateral femoral condyle also shows the full-thickness (single arrow) chondral defect. The edema (double arrow) in the subchondral bone is more prominent on this image.

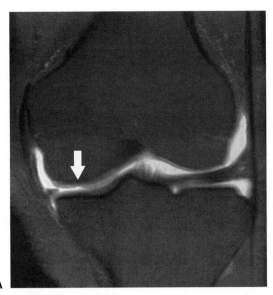

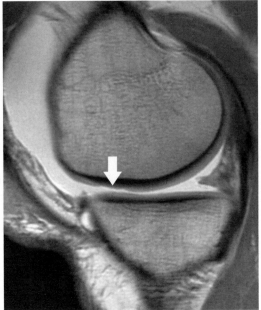

FIGURE 6–3 (A) Coronal T1-weighted (TR 616, TE 16) fat-suppressed fast spin-echo MR arthrogram image of the knee demonstrates a partial-thickness cartilage defect (arrow) in the weight-bearing surface of the medial femoral condyle. **(B)** Corresponding proton density weighted (TR 2900, TE 30) fast spin-echo MR arthrogram image shows the partial-thickness lesion.

contrast in the articular cartilage offered by fat suppression, the T1-weighted image does not allow detection of internal signal changes within the cartilage.[17]

More recently the technique of CT arthrography, using dual-detector spiral scanners, has been introduced for the evaluation of surface cartilage lesions. Similar to MR arthrography, a contrast solution is placed into the articulation. With CT arthrography, the contrast solution is iodine based. A recent study has reported accurate assessment of a surface cartilage lesion **(Fig. 6–4).** Moreover, no statistically significant difference between spiral CT arthrography and MRI in sensitivity and specificity for surface lesions was demonstrated.[18]

The intrinsic benefit of CT with respect to MRI is the superior resolution afforded by CT, as well as its availability for patients who cannot undergo MRI studies because of claustrophobia, a pacemaker, etc. The disadvantage for CT is the relative poor soft tissue contrast as

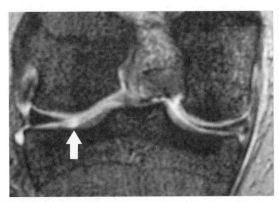

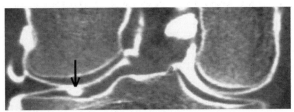

FIGURE 6–4 (A) Coronal three-dimensional spoiled gradient recalled image (TR 600, TE 24, flip angle 30 degrees, slice thickness 3.0 mm) through the knee demonstrates a region of focal high signal intensity (arrow) in the lateral tibial plateau. (Courtesy of Bruno C. Vande Berg, Hopital St. Luc, Brussels, Belgium.) **(B)** Corresponding helical dual detector computed tomographic (CT) arthrogram image better characterizes the focal cartilage lesion (arrow) that involves greater than 50% of the overall cartilage thickness. (Courtesy of Bruno C. Vande Berg, Hopital St. Luc, Brussels, Belgium.)

compared with MRI that precludes evaluation of intrinsic cartilage lesions. The obvious disadvantage of both CT and MR arthrography is the invasive nature of the studies.

Quantitative Imaging Volume Measurement

Several studies have reported the use of 3D reconstruction as a means of articular cartilage quantification and have determined that cartilage volumes can be determined with high accuracy with MRI in large articulations. This process is limited by the fact that global cartilage volume is measured rather than the cartilage defect in isolation. Cartilage thickness maps can combat these difficulties, but are difficult to obtain due to the small thickness of articular cartilage and the unavoidable misregistration. Despite this, measurements of cartilage thickness, topographic maps, and volume analysis can be performed but require more facile and reproducible technique before becoming widely clinically applicable.[19,20]

Parameter Mapping

The mapping of physiologic parameters with MRI has emerged as a promising means for the quantitative assessment of cartilage structure and function in both the normal and pathologic states. The T1 and T2 relaxation times are quantified on a pixel basis, assigned a value, and, if desired, a color to provide a visual assessment of the region of interest. This means of analysis provides an objective way to evaluate changes in signal intensity, and is more practical for evaluation of focal cartilage defects than volumetric analysis. This imaging technique requires high-resolution imaging capabilities in the form of a high field strength magnet or local gradient coils, and does require significant imaging time and postprocess imaging at present.[21]

■ Novel Magnetic Resonance Imaging Applications

Magnetization Transfer Imaging

This method of imaging is based on the concept that a tissue and its components are exposed to the imposed magnetic field. The effect of the imposed field is modified by the interaction and proximity of the separate components, which comprise a local macromolecular environment. Cartilage is particularly suited to evaluation by magnetization transfer as it has a high concentration of macromolecular components to create the desired effect. In other words, the effect of the mag-

netic field on a single component of cartilage in isolation would be different from that of the effect of imaging the tissue as a whole. Cartilage, due to its highly organized nature and macromolecular constituents, demonstrates the effects of magnetization transfer. This appears to be primarily due to the interaction of two components: the collagen matrix and bulk water. Because the intrinsic contrast produced by this effect depends on the exchange between interacting components, any disruption in the ordered structure theoretically would involve a change in that contrast. Generally, when collagen content is diminished, as in cartilage degradation, a decrease in magnetization transfer would occur, resulting in an increase in signal intensity. In its current form, magnetization transfer results in only a moderate contrast-to-noise ratio and its effects in abnormal cartilage are not known. Its sensitivity to the macromolecular environment may prove useful for identifying and monitoring early changes in cartilage.[11,22]

Short Echo-Time–Projection-Reconstruction Imaging

The intrinsic T2 of cartilage shows a zonal variation and increases from the deep to superficial regions. In addition, cartilage demonstrates very short T2 relaxation times likely due to its highly organized structure. These T2 values are on the order of a magnitude less than those normally used in clinical imaging. Projection reconstruction uses an ultrashort echo time to obtain MR signal from those structures with short T2, such as the deep layer of articular cartilage. Cadaveric studies found this imaging sequence superior to magnetization transfer and fat-suppressed 3D spoiled gradient MRI in detection of cartilage lesions. Initial work showed normal cartilage to have high signal intensity and cartilage lesions to be low in signal intensity. Not only was cartilage lesion detection (signal abnormalities) superior with projection reconstruction, but also the determination of cartilage thickness was more precise. Due to its experimental nature at this time, the sequence is not widely available and has not been tested in a clinical population. Because experimental sequences are designed to optimize all imaging parameters, image acquisition is quite long.[23]

Projection-Reconstruction Spectroscopic Imaging

The application of projection reconstruction has been extended to include spectroscopy. Acquisition of a full spectral data set with this technique allows display of images at any spectral frequency. Lipid and water frequency images are acquired as part of the same data set requiring no additional imaging time for the added information. Spectroscopic information is available for each voxel, and in normal cartilage shows variation in line width, which corresponds to the length of the intrinsic T2 value. This may have important implications regarding early detection of subtle abnormalities in the composition of cartilage as well as distinguishing different types of cartilage. It would allow initial detection of an area of potential cartilage abnormality by qualitative means, signal change visualized on images. Subsequently, the area in question could be interrogated by quantitative means, and that area can be compared with an internal control (an area of normal cartilage in the articular surface). The spectral pattern identified on follow-up images theoretically could be identified as to its type (hyaline versus fibrocartilage). This technique requires rather extensive postimaging processing. A limited number of slices can be acquired, restricting application to a specific region of interest.[24]

Driven Equilibrium Fourier Transfer Imaging

The driven equilibrium Fourier transfer (DEFT) sequence produces image contrast that is a function of proton density, intrinsic T1 and T2, as well as echo time and repetition time. Its contrast is well suited to articular cartilage. Synovial fluid is high in signal intensity, and articular cartilage is intermediate in signal intensity. Bone is dark and fat is suppressed, resulting in excellent contrast for cartilage from surrounding tissues. DEFT generates contrast between cartilage and joint fluid by enhancing the signal from joint fluid, rather than by suppressing the cartilage. While maintaining contrast, this sequence succeeds in maintaining a high signal-to-noise ratio as well, and allows visualization of structural elements of cartilage. It does so by requiring the echo time to be as short as possible, rather than using additional echoes to reduce scan time. The benefit of DEFT is that is provides high contrast without loss of cartilage signal. Three-dimensional imaging capabilities have been developed for this sequence and produce scan times that are acceptable for clinical applications.[25]

Diffusion-Weighted Imaging

The basis of diffusion-weighted imaging in cartilage depends on the premise that cartilage is an avascular structure and that transport of small molecular nutrients and waste products occurs primarily by diffusion. This process is presumed to be altered in the early stages of degradation, where overall morphology is grossly intact, but changes in concentration of proteoglycans, water, and organization of collagen may have commenced. Preliminary work has shown that diffu-

sion coefficient maps of water strongly reflect the spatial heterogeneity of cartilage. Moreover, extensive studies of diffusion in cartilage under a variety of circumstances with several small solutes, as well as water, have helped to establish the effect of the macromolecular environment on diffusion. MRI obtained with diffusion-weighted imaging allows the local measurement of diffusion coefficients as well as reveals spatial distribution of diffusion differences. Increases in the available gradient strength on clinical systems will be required to fully evaluate the clinical utility of this imaging sequence.[26]

Contrast-Enhanced Imaging

Gadolinium-enhanced imaging has the potential to monitor glycosaminoglycan content within cartilage, which may have implications for the progression of disease in injured cartilage. The role of glycosaminoglycans in cartilage appears to be primarily that of mechanical support. This component of cartilage appears to be lost early in the course of cartilage degeneration offering a sort of biomarker for early detection.

The theory of gadolinium-enhanced MRI is based on the fact that glycosaminoglycans contribute a strong negative charge to the cartilage matrix. When they are lost due to injury or degeneration, their negative charge is also lost. Consequently, when a negatively charged contrast agent such as gadolinium–diethylenetriamine pentaacetic acid $(Gd-DTPA)^{2-}$ is administered intravenously, it will distribute into the degraded cartilage, no longer repelled by the negative charge of the glycosaminoglycans. The effect of the Gd-DTPA could be assessed visually and quantitatively. This MRI technique could provide assessment of both the morphologic and biochemical status of cartilage. Though it has been used in volunteers, the logistics of this technique have yet to be perfected, and several questions remain as to the optimal imaging protocol.[27]

Sodium Magnetic Resonance Imaging

Another imaging technique has shown promise with respect to evaluation of the biochemical status of cartilage, that of sodium MRI. Similar to the use of ionic gadolinium compounds, this technique allows assessment of the proteoglycan content of cartilage, and has been shown to be both sensitive and specific in detecting small changes. Also based on the charge-related loss paralleling proteoglycan depletion, sodium imaging would depict these regions. Unfortunately, this technique requires the use of sophisticated MRI equipment and long imaging times. In addition, it has a very low inherent signal-to-noise ratio, making it of questionable clinical value in its current form.[28]

High-Resolution Magnetic Resonance Imaging:High Field Strength and Local Gradient Coils

Magnetic resonance imaging has shown great potential in the assessment of articular cartilage because it is possible to obtain relatively high contrast between cartilage and surrounding structures. However, clinical utility is often limited by resolution and the signal-to-noise ratio; the spatial distribution of cartilage structures is small relative to standard imaging resolution, and intrasubstance variations are too small to resolve or are obscured by partial volume effects.

High field systems provide a higher intrinsic signal-to-noise ratio, which is critical when imaging at high resolution. In addition, resolution can be greatly improved with the use of local gradient coils that allow much stronger gradient fields. Moreover, local gradient coils can produce gradients that turn on faster than standard systems, facilitating short echo time techniques like projection reconstruction. Used in concert, high field systems with local gradients will play an increasingly important role in the high-resolution MRI of cartilage.

Magnetic field strength of up to 3 tesla (T) is increasingly being used in the clinical setting, bringing the world of high-resolution imaging close at hand. These high-resolution images are capable of visualizing the fibrous structure of the extracellular matrix and have important implications for early identification of structural alteration. As noted previously, the increased field strength could also prove extremely useful when coupled with certain novel imaging sequences.[29]

Magnetic Resonance Microscopy

To date, MR microscopy has primarily involved the use of very high field strength magnets (7.1 T) equipped with spectrometers and microimaging units for experimental in vitro and ex vivo specimen evaluation. Images are acquired with a pixel resolution on the order of 39 to 78 μm. This imaging tool has been used in conjunction with enzymatic degradation of specimens to determine the role of enzyme exposure to cartilage breakdown. In addition, exciting work has been done with respect to tissue-specific contrast agents that indicate the presence of enzyme-induced damage to cartilage.[30]

An adaptation of this technique has been developed for 1.5-T magnets that utilize an MR microscope with an independent console system (MRMICS). The system results in images with pixel resolution of 100 to 200 μm.[31]

Although these techniques are not practical or necessary for clinical applications at present, they serve to emphasize important concepts with respect to solving the mystery of cartilage degeneration and its role in the development of osteoarthritis. Accurate evaluation of the cartilage surface, its thickness, and its internal structure is of paramount importance in the diagnosis of articular pathology as well as in the assessment of its progression. The utilization of high-resolution imaging in conjunction with tissue-specific contrast agents may provide a functional assessment and a noninvasive means of obtaining information that reflects the histologic composition of cartilage.

Magnetic Resonance Imaging of Postsurgical Cartilage Repair

The imaging of articular cartilage after surgical treatment is increasing in importance as several palliative surgical therapies are now encountered for chondral repair. There are a variety of different surgical cartilage repair techniques, but to date, no randomized studies comparing them have been performed. Two of the more common repair procedures include osteochondral autograft transplantation and autologous chondrocyte implantation.

Osteochondral Autograft Transplantation

Osteochondral autograft transplantation involves the harvesting of osteochondral plugs from a relatively non-weight-bearing portion of the articulation, often the region of the intercondylar notch or the superior edge of lateral or medial femoral condyles. The plugs are then transplanted into the chondral defect while attempting to maintain congruent transition points in the cartilage surface and the subchondral bone. The goals of the procedure are to replace the defect with normal cartilage, to approximate the interface of the graft with the native bone to preserve joint mechanics, and to have incorporation of the graft to the underlying bone **(Fig. 6–5)**.

Magnetic resonance imaging can assess the graft–native bone interface for evidence of loosening, which includes migration or displacement of the graft, as well as fluid surrounding the graft on T2-weighted images **(Fig. 6–6)**. Congruity of the articular surface between the graft and native bone can be measured and designated as either protuberant or depressed. Signal characteristics of the graft cartilage can be assessed for signs of degeneration. Similarly, signal characteristics of the osseous portion of the graft can be readily assessed. Much variability is noted in its signal intensity in the postoperative period. Generally, at 5 months posttransplantation, fatty marrow signal intensity is present to a variable degree within the central portion of the graft, and by 12 months the entire graft should demonstrate fatty marrow. The presence of contrast enhancement can indicate an intact vascular supply to the graft, although

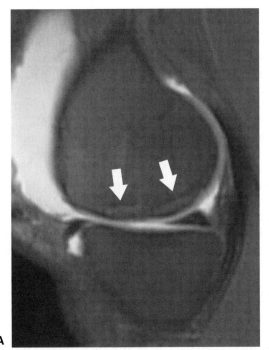
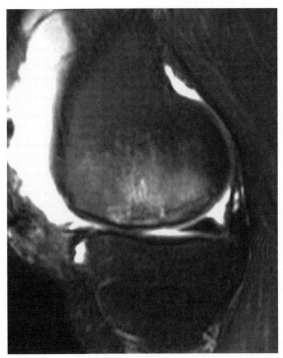

A

B

FIGURE 6–5 (A) Sagittal T1-weighted fat-suppressed (TR 600, TE 15) fast spin-echo MR arthrogram image through the knee in a patient 6 months status post-osteochondral autograft transplantation. Two bone plugs have been placed on the weight-bearing surface of the medial femoral condyle (arrows). The arthrogram image shows a smooth interface between the graft and native bone. **(B)** Corresponding sagittal T2-weighted fat-suppressed (TR 2900, TE 65) fast spin-echo MR arthrogram image demonstrates edema in both the graft and native bone. No areas of abnormal linear high signal or cysts are noted at the graft–native bone interface to suggest graft failure.

enhancement may not occur in the grafts for up to 4 weeks postsurgery. In studies to date, routine clinical MRI protocols have been used for postoperative evaluation that were composed of T2-weighted fat-suppressed fast spin-echo and T1-weighted spin-echo sequences in various imaging planes.[32]

Autologous Chondrocyte Implantation

Autologous chondrocyte implantation is a two-stage surgical procedure that is described in detail in Chapter 15. The first stage includes a diagnostic arthroscopic assessment of the joint, with harvest of cartilage for cell culture. The second stage involves the implantation of cultured chondrocytes. MRI of autologous chondrocyte grafts has proven particularly useful for evaluating the signal of the repair tissue, the degree of defect fill, the integration of the repair cartilage to the subchondral plate, as well as the status of the subchondral bone plate and bone marrow. The imaging protocol utilized incorporates primarily proton density and intermediate-weighted fast spin-echo sequences. Gradient echo sequences were found to introduce excessive susceptibility artifact on the surface of the graft, interfering with graft evaluation. The utilization of arthrographic techniques has also been discussed, particularly for the differentiation between heterogeneous signal intensity within the graft repair cartilage and delamination (separation of the graft from the underlying bone).

The signal intensity of the graft repair tissue can be variable and heterogeneous. Linear fluid-like signal within the graft or at its junction with subchondral bone usually indicates a tear of the periosteal cover or poor integration of the graft. The morphology of the repair tissue should mimic that of the native articular cartilage in its thickness and contour. The margins of the graft should be continuous with the adjacent native cartilage. The subchondral bone plate beneath the graft may appear smooth or slightly irregular. Edema-like signal within the bone marrow subjacent to the graft site is expected in the early postoperative period. However, in mature grafts, the marrow signal abnormalities should be minimal.[33]

Complications encountered in this repair technique have included delamination of the repair tissue. This is most commonly encountered in the early postoperative period (less than 6 months). This can occur in a marginal fashion, with involvement of the junction of graft

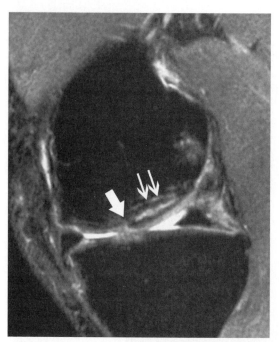

FIGURE 6–6 Sagittal T2-weighted fat-suppressed (TR 3266, TE 45) fast spin-echo image through the knee demonstrates linear high signal intensity (double arrow) between the graft and the native bone. In addition, there appears to be a small focal area of high signal intensity at the interface of the anterior aspect of the graft and the native bone (single arrow). These findings are consistent with graft failure.

and native cartilage, appearing as a fissure. Partial delamination involves separation of a portion of the graft. Complete delamination involves separation of the entire graft from the defect site.

Underfilling of the graft can be visualized at arthroscopy as well as MRI. It is for this reason that the degree of cartilage fill on MRI should be expressed with respect to linear depth and percent of volume of the defect.

Hypertrophy of the periosteal cover can occur in up to 20 to 25% of autologous chondrocyte graft patients. It is commonly encountered between the 3rd and 7th postoperative months. The clinical presentation is that of catching.

■ Conclusion

Both the prevalence of cartilage disease and osteoarthritis and the emergence of several surgical methods of chondral repair emphasize the importance of having a means to detect and follow the progression of cartilage pathology. MRI is currently the most widely accepted noninvasive imaging method for the evaluation of articular cartilage. Current clinical sequences are limited in

their ability to reliably detect early structural abnormalities, but do provide a means to evaluate more than just the articular surface.

As demonstrated in this chapter, the advances in sequence development, coupled with local gradient coils and high field strength imaging, have offered promising results in both the understanding of normal cartilage structure as well as lesion detection. With the perfection of high-resolution imaging and tissue-specific contrast agents, the understanding of the structural failure involved with the development of cartilage lesions and osteoarthritis may become increasingly clear. In addition, the application of these techniques to the analysis of the postsurgical chondral repair may offer some insight into the structural changes surrounding graft behavior.

The ultimate goal in the understanding of cartilage structure, lesion detection, and progression is to enter the realm of prevention, leaving behind that of palliation.

REFERENCES

1. Jackson DW, Simon TM, Aberman HM. Symptomatic articular cartilage degeneration. Clin Orthop 2001;391S:S14–S25
2. Goodwin DW, Zhu H, Dunn JF. In vitro MR imaging of hyaline cartilage: correlation with scanning electron microscopy. AJR Am J Roentgenol 2000;174:405–409
3. Xia Y. Relaxation anisotropy in cartilage by NMR microscopy (muMRI) at 14-microm resolution. Magn Reson Med 1998;39:941–949
4. Frank LR, Brossmann J, Buxton RB, Resnick D. MR imaging truncation artifacts can create a false laminar appearance in cartilage. AJR Am J Roentgenol 1997;168:547–554
5. Erickson SJ, Prost RW, Timins ME. The "magic angle" effect: background physics and clinical relevance [editorial]. Radiology 1993;188:23–25
6. Hayes CW, Sawyer RW, Conway WF. Patellar cartilage lesions: in vitro detection and staging with MR imaging and pathologic correlation. Radiology 1990;176:479–483
7. Hayes CW, Conway WF. Evaluation of articular cartilage: radiographic and cross-sectional imaging techniques. Radiographics 1992;12:409–428
8. McCauley TR, Kier R, Lynch KJ, Jokl P. Chondromalacia patellae: diagnosis with MR imaging [see comments] AJR Am J Roentgenol 1992;158:101–105
9. Spritzer CE, Vogler JB, Martinez S, et al. MR imaging of the knee: preliminary results with a 3DFT GRASS pulse sequence. AJR Am J Roentgenol 1988;150:597–603
10. Rose PM, Demlow TA, Szumowski J, Quinn SF. Chondromalacia patellae: fat-suppressed MR imaging. Radiology 1994;193:437–440
11. Yao L, Gentili A, Thomas A. Incidental magnetization transfer contrast in fast spin-echo imaging of cartilage. J Magn Reson Imaging 1996;6:180–184
12. Broderick LS, Turner DA, Renfrew DL, Schnitzer TJ, Huff JP, Harris C. Severity of articular cartilage abnormality in patients with osteoarthritis: evaluation with fast spin-echo MR vs arthroscopy. AJR Am J Roentgenol 1994;162:99–103
13. Disler DG, McCauley TR, Wirth CR, Fuchs MD. Detection of knee hyaline cartilage defects using fat-suppressed three-dimensional spoiled gradient-echo MR imaging: comparison with standard MR imaging and correlation with arthroscopy. AJR Am J Roentgenol 1995;165:377–382

14. Disler DG, McCauley TR, Kelman CG, et al. Fat-suppressed three-dimensional spoiled gradient-echo MR imaging of hyaline cartilage defects in the knee: comparison with standard MR imaging and arthroscopy [see comments] AJR Am J Roentgenol 1996;167:127–132

15. Recht MP, Piraino DW, Paletta GA, Schils JP, Belhobek GH. Accuracy of fat-suppressed three-dimensional spoiled gradient-echo FLASH MR imaging in the detection of patellofemoral articular cartilage abnormalities. Radiology 1996;198:209–212

16. Disler DG, Peters TL, Muscoreil SJ, et al. Fat-suppressed spoiled GRASS imaging of knee hyaline cartilage: technique optimization and comparison with conventional MR imaging. AJR Am J Roentgenol 1994;163:887–892

17. Kramer J, Recht MP, Imof H, Stiglbauer R, Engel A. Postcontrast MR arthrography in assessment of cartilage lesions. J Comput Assist Tomogr 1994;18:218–224

18. Vande Berg BC, Lecouvet FE, Pollvache P, et al. Assessment of knee cartilage in cadavers with dual-detector spiral CT arthrography and MR imaging. Radiology 2002;222:430–436

19. Peterfy CG, van Dijke CF, Janzen DL, et al. Quantification of articular cartilage in the knee with pulsed saturation transfer subtraction and fat-suppressed MR imaging: optimization and validation. Radiology 1994;192:485–491

20. Pilch L, Stewart C, Gordon D, et al. Assessment of cartilage volume in the femorotibial joint with magnetic resonance imaging and 3D computer reconstruction. J Rheumatol 1994;21:2307–2321

21. Frank LR, Wong EC, Luh WM, Ahn JM, Resnick D. Articular cartilage in the knee: mapping of the physiologic parameters at MR imaging with a local gradient coil–preliminary results. Radiology 1999;210:241–246

22. Gray ML, Burstein D, Lesperance LM, Gehrke L. Magnetization transfer in cartilage and its constituent macromolecules. Magn Reson Med 1995;34:319–325

23. Brossmann J, Frank LR, Pauly JM, et al. Short echo time projection reconstruction MR imaging of cartilage: comparison with fat-suppressed spoiled GRASS and magnetization transfer contrast MR imaging. Radiology 1997;203:501–507

24. Gold GE, Thedens DR, Pauly JM, et al. MR imaging of articular cartilage of the knee: new methods using ultrashort TEs. AJR Am J Roentgenol 1998;170:1223–1226

25. Hargreaves BA, Gold GE, Lang PK, et al. MR imaging of articular cartilage using driven equilibrium. Magn Reson Med 1999;42:695–703

26. Burstein D, Gray ML, Hartman AL, Gipe R, Foy BD. Diffusion of small solutes in cartilage as measured by nuclear magnetic resonance (NMR) spectroscopy and imaging. J Orthop Res 1993;11:465–478

27. Bashir A, Gray ML, Boutin RD, Burstein D. Glycosaminoglycan in articular cartilage: in vivo assessment with delayed Gd(DTPA)(2-)-enhanced MR imaging. Radiology 1997;205:551–558

28. Insko EK, Reddy R, Leigh JS. High resolution, short echo time sodium imaging of articular cartilage. J Magn Reson Imaging 1997;7:1056–1059

29. Dardzinski BJ, Mosher TJ, Li S, Van Slyke MA, Smith MB: Spatial variation of T2 in human articular cartilage. Radiology 1997;205:546–550

30. Wagner M, Werner A, Grunder W. Visualization of collagenase-induced cartilage degradation using NMR microscopy. Invest Radiol 1999;34(10):607-614

31. Yoshioka H, Haishi T, Uematsu T, et al., MR microscopy of articular cartilage at 1.5 T: orientation and site of dependence of laminar structures. Skeletal Radiol 2002;31:505–510

32. Sanders TG, Mentzer KD, Miller MD, Morrison WB, Campbell SE, Penrod BJ. Autogenous osteochondral "plug" transfer for the treatment of focal chondral defects: postoperative MR appearance with clinical correlation. Skeletal Radiol 2001;30:570–578

33. Alparslan L, Minas T, Winalski CS. Magnetic resonance imaging of autologous chondrocyte implantation. Semin Ultrasound CT MR 2001;22(4):341–351

7

Classification of Articular Cartilage Injury and Repair

BERT R. MANDELBAUM, RALPH A. GAMBARDELLA, AND JASON M. SCOPP

The most important issue in the management of articular cartilage disorders is accurate and uniform characterization of the local, regional, systemic, and familial factors. Subjective and objective tools can be used to assess both the lesion and the disease process. These tools can also be used for therapeutic and prognostic indications.

The assessment tools and classification schemes must be accurate, reproducible, valid, cross-cultural, and unbiased by age, language, and demographic differences. In the contemporary milieu of digital databases and multimedia information sharing, uniformly accepted multidimensional tools of assessment is essential. This chapter presents the methods of subjective and objective assessment of articular cartilage disorders, including the spectrum of normal chondropenia and osteoarthritis, and identifies essential future directions.

■ Subjective Methods of Assessment

History

An accurate and thorough patient history is an essential first step in the evaluation of articular cartilage defects (ACDs). Important details include the patient's age, age at which the injury occurred, the defect etiology, mechanism of injury, and prior surgical interventions. Medical and family history of inflammatory arthritides such as lupus, rheumatoid arthritis, and human leukocyte antigen (HLA)-B27 associations are important factors to consider in treatment planning. Endocrine disorders including thyroid and diabetes, and collagen disorders such as Ehlers-Danlos and Marfan syndromes are known chondral modifiers and are important details in the patient's history.

Subjective Knee Scores

A subjective clinical survey outcome tool can be used to create a reliable, reproducible score. This score can then be used to stratify each patient along the continuum of articular cartilage disorders and provide insight into the specific and appropriate treatment profile. The continuum of articular cartilage disorders exists with normal cartilage on one end of the spectrum. As articular cartilage fails, *chondropenia* results. Chondropenia is defined as a loss of articular cartilage over time. Whereas *osteopenia* is a term used to describe the loss of bone form and function, *chondropenia* is an analogous term used to describe this process in articular cartilage. As cartilage loss continues, osteoarthritis results.

Various instruments have been used to stratify the subjective assessment ACDs and osteoarthritis. To date, there has been no effort to organize the subjective assessment tools to reflect the continuum that exists when describing articular cartilage disorders. As a consequence, patient population, age, and activity level are different. These differences are reflected in the scores. Therefore no consensus exists regarding an ideal scoring system.

The Cincinnati[1,2] **(Table 7–1),** International Knee Documentation Committee (IKDC), and International Cartilage Repair Society (ICRS) **(Fig. 7–1)** rating scales are excellent subjective and objective knee scores. They allow the patient and the clinician to rate symptoms quantitatively in relation to severity and functional level in a spectrum from sedentary life to return to sport.

TABLE 7–1   Cincinnati Knee Rating System (100 points)

This is an example of one of the modules of this system addressing a spectrum of function from strenuous sports (20 points) to minimal activity (0 points).

Function
Overall Activity Level
20_____No limitation. I have a normal knee and I am able to do everything including strenuous sports or heavy labor.
16_____I can partake in sports including strenuous ones but at a lower performance level. I must guard my knee and limit it to some heavy labor.
12_____Light recreational activities are possible with RARE symptoms. More strenuous activities cause problems. Active in non-strenuous sports.
8_____No sports or strenuous activities possible. Walking activities possible with RARE symptoms. I am limited to light work.
4_____Walking activities and daily living cause moderate problems. I frequently limit my activity.
0_____Walking activities and daily living cause severe problems and persistent symptoms.
_____I do not know what my real activity level is. I have not tested my knee.

The IKDC Subjective Knee Form is a reliable and valid measure of symptoms, function, and sports activity experienced by individuals with a variety of knee conditions including ligament and meniscal injury, patellofemoral problems, and osteoarthritis. A recent revision includes new demographic, subjective, and quality-of-life modules. The Subjective module includes 18 questions categorized by symptoms, pain, swelling, locking, giving way, sports activity, and function. In addition the knee history and surgical documentation forms have been developed with the ICRS and document articular cartilage, meniscal, and ligamentous status. The updated knee examination form includes documentation of effusion, passive motion deficit, ligament examination, compartment findings, harvest site pathology, radiographic findings, and functional tests.

Additionally, a quality of life survey like the Rand Short Form (SF)-36[3] is helpful to optimally define the impact of the problem and interventions on the patient's psychosocial and emotional lifestyle. Other accepted tools that have been utilized globally for assessment of articular cartilage lesions include the Hospital for Special Surgery Score, the Visual Analog Scale (VAS), the Lysholm, and the Tegener[4] scores. The major collective disadvantage of these tools is their lack of uniform and universal acceptance.

Several subjective outcome measurements have been developed to assess knee osteoarthritis (OA) disease severity at both baseline and after intervention. It is important to note, however, that patient perspective and physician perspective may differ. Therefore, symptom assessment tools used during treatment for OA should include a combination of patient and physician assessment. The VAS combined with either of two self-administered, algofunctional questionnaires can help to eliminate this potential bias. In North America, the Western Ontario McMaster Universities Osteoarthritis Index (WOMAC)[5] has achieved widespread acceptance as the gold standard for the assessment of OA-related symptoms, whereas in Europe the Lequesne Algofunctional Knee Index[6] has been preferred.

The WOMAC index is composed of pain, stiffness, and disability subscales.[5] Each subscale, and a variety of subscale combinations, has been validated for use with surgical and pharmaceutical intervention. The WOMAC bears excellent reproducibility as well as intra- and interobserver reliability. A modification of the WOMAC index, termed the Knee Injury and Osteoarthritis Outcome Score (KOOS) **(Table 7–2)** has been proposed by Roos et al.[7] for use in posttraumatic OA of the knee. The KOOS was developed as an instrument to assess patients' opinions about their knee and associated problems. The KOOS is intended to be used for knee injury that can result in posttraumatic OA, such as anterior cruciate ligament (ACL) injury, meniscus injury, and chondral injury. KOOS has high test-retest reproducibility. KOOS is meant to be used over short and long time intervals, and to assess changes from week to week induced by treatment (medication, operation, physical therapy) or over years due to the primary injury or posttraumatic OA. KOOS consists of five subscales: pain, other symptoms, function in daily living (activities of daily living, ADL), function in sport and recreation (Sport/Rec), and knee-related quality of life (QOL). KOOS is patient-administered, the format is user friendly, and it takes ~10 minutes to fill out. The KOOS system is self-explanatory and can be administered in the waiting room or used as a mailed survey. KOOS includes WOMAC Osteoarthritis Index LK 3.0 in its complete and original format, and WOMAC scores can be calculated. WOMAC is valid for elderly subjects with knee OA. KOOS construct validity has been determined in comparison with SF-36, and the

THE CARTILAGE STANDARD EVALUATION FORM/KNEE [1]

Patients Form

Name: _____ First Name: _____ Date of birth: _____

Street _____ Zip _____ Town _____ Country _____

Gender: ☐
Height: ☐ cm.   Examiner _____   Date of examination. _____   Med. Rec. No. ____
weight: ☐ Kg.

Localisation

      L   R

Knee involved: left: ☐   right: ☐   Opposite knee: normal ☐   injured ☐   Type of injury: _____

Etiology / Cause of injury

Date of injury: _____

Cause of injury: Activity of dailing living: ☐   Type of activity: _____

        Traffic ☐   Type of vehicle: _____   non-contact sport. ☐   Type of sport: _____

        Work ☐   Type of work: _____   contact sport ☐   Type of sport: _____

Onset of symptoms

Acute: ☐   Gradual: ☐   Date of symptom onset: _____

Which of the 3 faces fits to your basic mood

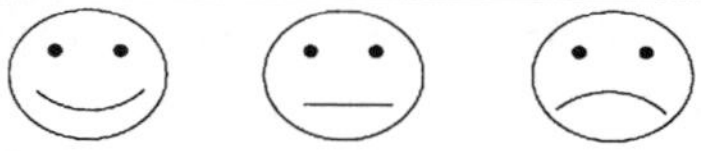

    ☺   😐   ☹

Previous surgery

Date: _____ Type: _____   Date: _____ Type: _____
Date: _____ Type: _____   Date: _____ Type: _____

Activity-Level

	Yes	No		Yes	No
I: Are You a high competitive sportsman/woman:	☐	☐	III : Sporting sometimes	☐	☐
II : Are You well-trained and frequently sporting	☐	☐	IV : Non sporting	☐	☐

Functional status

I : I can do everything that I want to do with my joint

II : I can do nearly everything that I want to do with my joint

III : I am restricted and a lot of things that I want to do with my joint are not possible

IV : I am very restricted and I can do almost nothing with my joint without severe pain and disability

	I	II	III	IV
Preinjury:	☐	☐	☐	☐
Activity level pretreatment:	☐	☐	☐	☐
Present activity level:	☐	☐	☐	☐

Eventual change related to the operative procedure: Yes ☐   No ☐

1. As compared to your healthy contralateral knee your injured knee is worth:

I	II	III	IV
90-100%	70-90%	40-70%	0-40%
☐	☐	☐	☐

2. On a scale mark the intensity of your knee pain

No Pain ▭▭▭▭▭▭▭▭▭▭ Severest Pain

0 1   3   6   10

  I   II   III   IV

© ICRS

FIGURE 7–1 International Cartilage Repair Society (ICRS) Patient's Subjective Rating System.

TABLE 7–2   Knee Injury and Osteoarthritis Outcome Score (KOOS)

Pain

P1 How often is your knee painful? ___ Never ___ Monthly ___ Weekly ___ Daily ___ Always

What degree of pain have you experienced the last week when...?

P2 Twisting/pivoting on your knee ___ None ___ Mild ___ Moderate ___ Severe ___ Extreme

P3 Straightening knee fully ___ None ___ Mild ___ Moderate ___ Severe ___ Extreme

P4 Bending knee fully ___ None ___ Mild ___ Moderate ___ Severe ___ Extreme

P5 Walking on flat surface ___ None ___ Mild ___ Moderate ___ Severe ___ Extreme

P6 Going up or down stairs ___ None ___ Mild ___ Moderate ___ Severe ___ Extreme

P7 At night while in bed ___ None ___ Mild ___ Moderate ___ Severe ___ Extreme

P8 Sitting or lying ___ None ___ Mild ___ Moderate ___ Severe ___ Extreme

P9 Standing upright ___ None ___ Mild ___ Moderate ___ Severe ___ Extreme

Symptoms

Sy1 How severe is your knee stiffness after first wakening in the morning?

___ None ___ Mild ___ Moderate ___ Severe ___ Extreme

Sy2 How severe is your knee stiffness after sitting, lying, or resting later in the day?

___ None ___ Mild ___ Moderate ___ Severe ___ Extreme

Sy3 Do you have swelling in your knee? ___ Never ___ Rarely ___ Sometimes ___ Often ___ Always

Sy4 Do you feel grinding, hear clicking or any other type of noise when your knee moves?

___ Never ___ Rarely ___ Sometimes ___ Often ___ Always

Sy5 Does your knee catch or hang up when moving?

___ Never ___ Rarely ___ Sometimes ___ Often ___ Always

Sy6 Can you straighten your knee fully? ___ Always ___ Often ___ Sometimes ___ Rarely ___ Never

Sy7 Can you bend your knee fully? ___ Always ___ Often ___ Sometimes ___ Rarely ___ Never

Activities of daily living

What difficulty have you experienced the last week...?

A1 Descending stairs ___ None ___ Mild ___ Moderate ___ Severe ___ Extreme

A2 Ascending stairs ___ None ___ Mild ___ Moderate ___ Severe ___ Extreme

A3 Rising from sitting ___ None ___ Mild ___ Moderate ___ Severe ___ Extreme

A4 Standing ___ None ___ Mild ___ Moderate ___ Severe ___ Extreme

A5 Bending to floor/pick up an object ___ None ___ Mild ___ Moderate ___ Severe ___ Extreme

A6 Walking on flat surface ___ None ___ Mild ___ Moderate ___ Severe ___ Extreme

A7 Getting in/out of car ___ None ___ Mild ___ Moderate ___ Severe ___ Extreme

A8 Going shopping ___ None ___ Mild ___ Moderate ___ Severe ___ Extreme

A9 Putting on socks/stockings ___ None ___ Mild ___ Moderate ___ Severe ___ Extreme

A10 Rising from bed ___ None ___ Mild ___ Moderate ___ Severe ___ Extreme

A11 Taking off socks/stockings ___ None ___ Mild ___ Moderate ___ Severe ___ Extreme

A12 Lying in bed (turning over, maintaining knee position) ___ None ___ Mild ___ Moderate ___ Severe ___ Extreme

A13 Getting in/out of bath ___ None ___ Mild ___ Moderate ___ Severe ___ Extreme

A14 Sitting ___ None ___ Mild ___ Moderate ___ Severe ___ Extreme

A15 Getting on/off toilet ___ None ___ Mild ___ Moderate ___ Severe ___ Extreme

A16 Heavy domestic duties (shoveling, scrubbing floors, etc. ___ None ___ Mild ___ Moderate ___ Severe ___ Extreme

A17 Light domestic duties (cooking, dusting, etc.) ___ None ___ Mild ___ Moderate ___ Severe ___ Extreme

(Continued)

TABLE 7–2 *(continued)*

Sport and recreation function

What difficulty have you experienced the last week...?

Sp1 Squatting ___ None ___ Mild ___ Moderate ___ Severe ___ Extreme

Sp2 Running ___ None ___ Mild ___ Moderate ___ Severe ___ Extreme

Sp3 Jumping ___ None ___ Mild ___ Moderate ___ Severe ___ Extreme

Sp4 Turning/twisting on your injured knee ___ None ___ Mild ___ Moderate ___ Severe ___ Extreme

Sp5 Kneeling ___ None ___ Mild ___ Moderate ___ Severe ___ Extreme

Knee-related quality of life

What difficulty have you experienced the last week...?

Q1 How often are you aware of your knee problems? ___ Never ___ Monthly ___ Weekly ___ Daily ___ Always

Q2 Have you modified your lifestyle to avoid potentially damaging activities to your knee? ___ Not at all ___ Mildly ___ Moderately ___ Severely ___ Totally

Q3 How troubled are you with lack of confidence in your knee? ___ Not at all ___ Mildly ___ Moderately ___ Severely ___ Totally

Q4 In general, how much difficulty do you have with your knee? ___ None ___ Mild ___ Moderate ___ Severe ___ Extreme

Scoring:

Each item is scored 0 to 4 and the raw score for each section is the sum of item scores.

Scores are then transformed to a 0 to 100 scale. A higher score indicates fewer problems.

Scale Raw score Transformed score MDC90

Scale	Raw score	MDC90
Pain /	36	12 points
Symptoms /	28	8 points
ADL /	68	10 points
Sport/Rec /	20	19 points
QOL /	16	

range score raw Possible

100 × score raw Actual Example: a pain raw score of 16 would be transformed as follows:

– 100

56

36

100) × (16 13 points

– 100

expected correlations were found. Moderate to high correlations were found when compared to the Lysholm knee scoring scale. The KOOS subscales Sport and Recreation Function and Quality of Life were more sensitive and discriminative than the WOMAC subscales Pain, Stiffness, and Function when studied in subjects meniscectomized 21 years ago and with definite radiographic signs of OA (mean age 57 years, range 38–76) compared with age- and gender-matched controls.

The KOOS's responsiveness has been determined in two separate studies. Significant improvement was found after reconstruction of the ACL, after physical therapy, and 3 months after arthroscopic partial meniscectomy. High effect sizes (mean score change/preoperative standard deviation, SD) were found, indicating fewer subjects needed to yield statistically significant differences. The subscales Sport and Recreation Function and Quality of Life were the most responsive, with effect sizes ranging from 1.16 to 1.65.

The addition of two subscales was found in an initial analysis of the KOOS to add significantly to the data generated by the WOMAC index when applied to patients who had undergone prior meniscectomy.[8] The two additional subscales are Sports and Recreation Function and Knee-Related Quality of Life. The clinometric properties of the KOOS have been found to be favorable in preliminary investigations.[7] Further, the KOOS reflects response to physical therapy and surgery, including ACL reconstruction. The use of this expanded form of the WOMAC instrument was specifically designed to measure several subsets of knee function and quality of life in response to meniscal injury. The KOOS provides excellent subjective information regarding the baseline and postintervention status of patients undergoing meniscal transplantation. Work on the validation KOOS is ongoing. The KOOS is currently being used in several clinical studies involving patients with meniscus injury, ACL injury, cartilage injury, or posttraumatic osteoarthritis. The KOOS is currently available in three languages: American English, Swedish, and Danish.

The Lequesne Index[6] also generates a score based on pain and functional limitations in response to various daily situations. To date, there have been few direct comparisons of the WOMAC and Lequesne instruments. Theiler et al[9] compared the WOMAC and Lequesne-Algofunctional Index in patients with osteoarthritis. This study suggests similar sensitivity to change in pain and quality of life after treatment. The WOMAC tends to display better performance in the pain subscale than the self-administered version of the Lequesne symptom sections.[10] Generally the data obtained from the two instruments is thought to be complementary, and the use of both scales may be advantageous.

Quality of life in osteoarthritis has been evaluated using the medical outcomes SF-36,[3] a well-documented health-related quality-of-life (HRQOL) instrument consisting of 36 questions compressed into eight scales and two primary dimensions: the physical and mental component scores. This questionnaire provides an assessment of HRQOL that is not specific to osteoarthritis, but it provides data complementary to the WOMAC instrument when applied to patients with osteoarthritis.[11]

■ Objective Methods of Assessment

Objective assessment of articular cartilage by both nonoperative and operative methods provides unbiased data regarding lesion size, depth, and location. Nonoperative tools include physical examination and imaging. Although this nonoperative assessment may provide vital information, the gold standard for lesion evaluation includes arthroscopy. Arthroscopic grading tools are presented in this section.

Physical Examination and Functional Assessment

Physical examination of the knee provides a functional assessment of articular cartilage status. Important elements include range of motion, effusion, and joint line tenderness. Additionally, varus or valgus malalignment and ligamentous integrity provide insight on the knee macroenvironment and possible forces transferred through an articular cartilage defect. The KT-1000 or -2000 Knee Ligament Arthrometer (Medmetric Corporation, San Diego, CA) allows measurements and side-to-side comparisons of anterior and posterior translation of the tibia on the femur. Isokinetic strength measurements are helpful to assess extremity and joint strength. Functional assessments such as the shuttle and the single leg hop define activity levels. Each of these physical examination tools is used to gather insight into the articular cartilage integrity and the lesion's effect on knee function.

Imaging Techniques

Radiography

Popular diagnostic techniques for the measurement of the structural integrity of cartilage of the knee include plain radiography and magnetic resonance imaging (MRI). Because cartilage is not visible on plain radiography, the joint space width seen on weight-bearing x-rays has been employed as a proxy for cartilage integrity. In addition, calculation of mechanical axis and patellofemoral alignment is essential in the pre- and postoperative assessment of alignment.

Plain radiographic systems have distinct advantages in cost and availability over MRI and arthroscopy. But standard radiographs are limited by magnification errors,[12] poor reproducibility,[13] and limited interobserver reliability.[14] The accuracy, reliability, and sensitivity to change of plain radiographs in patients with articular cartilage disorders of the knee can be optimized by correcting magnification errors, adhering to published protocols for radiographic technique, and using microfocal magnification and computerized interpretation of digitized radiographs.[15] Despite these protocols and techniques, radiographs remain unable to detect subtle changes in cartilage morphology associated with articular cartilage defects, chondropenia, and early OA.[16] In spite of these limitations, standardized enhanced plain radiographs remain the primary outcome measurements of choice for all studies of cartilage disorders of the knee. Standard radiologic projections include weight bearing anteroposterior (AP) projections, flexed 45-degree posteroanterior (PA), patella–femoral views, and lateral views. The most widely accepted quantitative radiographic assessment tool of articular cartilage disorders are the Kellgren-Lawrence and the Ahlbachk scoring systems.[17] These tools quantify the degree of mild, moderate, or severe joint space narrowing, subchondral sclerosis, osteophytes, and cysts.

Magnetic Resonance Imaging

Interest has centered on the ability of MRI to image articular cartilage. In the first report on the ability of MRI to assess articular cartilage, Yulish and colleagues[18] claimed that MRI could reliably diagnose early and late stages of osteoarthitis in the patella. These have been characterized by highly variable and generally not reproducible results. Nearly 13 years after the initial description of the use of MRI to assess articular cartilage, there remains a lack of consensus among investigators on what constitutes the normal MRI appearance of articular cartilage. Investigators have applied a wide variety of MRI pulse sequences toward the depiction of articular cartilage and have reached as many varied conclusions regarding its appearance as there have been published articles.[6,7] On high-resolution MRI, articular cartilage demonstrates a multilaminar appearance. However, there is lack of consensus on both the different numbers of layers in normal articular cartilage and on the histologic correlate of what these apparently different layers represent. Several investigators have suggested that the multilaminar appearance can be attributed to technical (truncation) and artifactual ("magic" angle) factors.[8,9]

Magnetic resonance imaging has improved dramatically in recent years and now has the potential to replace plain radiographs in assessing articular cartilage structural outcome.[13] The use of contrast enhancement through either direct or indirect injection increases the ability of MRI to detect articular cartilage lesions. A preliminary study demonstrated good correlation between an MRI-based quantification of cartilage damage and arthroscopic findings.[19] Other investigators have explored the statistical attributes of MRI-based measurements of cartilage thickness and volume[20] and the assessment of chondropenia and OA progression. Interobserver agreement, reproducibility, and accuracy remain significant problems for MRI-based evaluation of the severity of knee articular cartilage.[21] Moreover, optimal imaging protocols are evolving.[3] In the past, spin-echo (SE) sequences have shown poor sensitivity for detection of articular cartilage defects. Most recently the fat-suppressed T1-weighted 3D gradient echo, fast spin echo, or magnetic resonance (MR) arthrographic techniques with gadolinium have enhanced the sensitivity to over 85% in grade III and IV lesions. In addition, MR has been helpful as an adjunct in the assessment of articular cartilage repair in observing defect fill, continuity of surface, status of medullary bone, and definition of histology of repair tissues. Thus, the MRI as a diagnostic and outcome measurement tool for studies of articular cartilage disorders continues to evolve.

Arthroscopy

Arthroscopy provides direct visualization of articular cartilage and the knee macroenvironment. Articular cartilage defects can then be documented on operative reports, videos, photographs, and diagrams (grids and maps). These data can then be combined with subjective and objective findings obtained during history and physical examination. As a consequence, via arthroscopic lesion visualization, the clinician can define and classify the local, regional, and systemic factors that may influence lesion progression, joint degeneration, or defect regeneration. The following factors should be considered when visualizing articular cartilage defects:

1. Etiology: Is the defect acute or chronic? Was there a specific mechanism of injury or is the defect a consequence of chronic repetitive injury? This differentiation is often a difficult element to determine because there is typically a blend of acute and chronic etiologies.

2. Defect thickness: What is the thickness or depth of the defect? The most accepted method of depth classification is the Outerbridge Classification[22]). Recently, Brittberg and Winalski[23] modified the Outerbridge Classification (**Fig. 7–2**). Normal articular cartilage is grade 0, softening is grade I, fibrillation is grade II, fissuring is grade III, and full-thickness defect, with exposed subchondral bone, is grade IV. Grade I and II lesions are considered partial lesions, whereas grade III and IV lesions are full thickness. Tidemark penetration, avascular necrosis, bone bruises, or infarctions are also important factors to consider in the assessment of these defects.

3. Size: A probe can be used to accurately measure defect size. Defects less than 2 cm^2 are considered small, lesions between 2 cm^2 and 10 cm^2 are considered moderate, and lesions greater than 10 cm^2 are large.

4. Degree of containment: Lesion containment refers to the presence of an adequate margin of surrounding healthy articular cartilage. This margin can often be visualized on sagittal MRI images.

5. Location: What is the defect's location? Is it monopolar; bipolar, that is, a "kissing lesion" (medial femoral condyle and medial tibial plateau, for example); or multipolar? Each of these examples has different reparative and degenerative variables (**Fig. 7–2**).

6. Ligament integrity: Are the ACL and posterior cruciate ligament (PCL) intact? If there is ligamentous

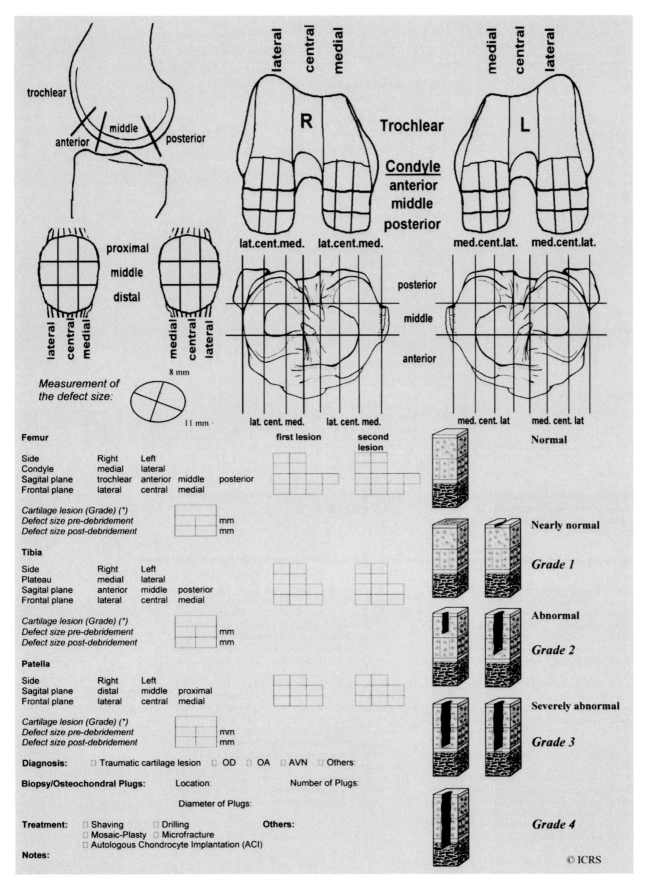

FIGURE 7–2 ICRS Classification Mapping Grid and Defect Thickness Assessment.

Cartilage Repair Assessment

Criteria	Points	
Degree of Defect Repair		
I Protocol A [1]	* In level with surrounding cartilage	4
	* 75% repair of defect depth	3
	* 50% repair of defect depth	2
	* 25% repair of defect depth	1
	* 0% repair of defect depth	0
I Protocol B [2]	* 100% survival of initially grafted surface	4
	* 75% survival of initially grafted surface	3
	* 50% survival of initially grafted surface	2
	* 25% survival of initially grafted surface	1
	* 0% (plugs are lost or broken)	0
II Integration to Border zone	* Complete integration with surrounding cartilage	4
	* Demarcating border <1mm	3
	* ¼ of graft integrated, ¼ with a notable border >1mm width	2
	* 1/2 of graft integrated with surrounding cartilage, 1/2 with a notable border >1mm	1
	* From no contact to ¼ of graft integrated with surrounding cartilage	0
III Macroscopic Appearance	* Intact smooth surface	4
	* Fibrillated surface	3
	* Small, scattered fissures or cracs	2
	* Several, small or few but large fissures	1
	* Total degeneration of grafted area	0

Overall Repair Assessment :				
	Grade I	normal	12	P
	Grade II	nearly normal	11-8	P
	Grade III	abnormal	7-4	P
	Grade IV	severely abnormal	3-1	P

An MRI and biomechanical evaluation form will be added to the cartilage repair assessment protocol in a near future

Cartilage Biopsy ☐ **Location** _____

(1) Protocol A : autologous chondrocyte implantation (ACI) ; periosteal or perichondrial transplantation ; subchondral drilling ; microfracturing ; carbon fibre implants ; others :

(2) Protocol B : mosaicplasty ; OAT ; osteochondral allografts ; others :

FOOTMARKS :

*[1] IKDC -Form extended by task force of ICRS

*[2] See patients subjective Assessment on the Patients form, point 1 and 2

*[3] DEFINITION OF ACTIVITY LEVELS: I: Jumping, pivoting, nard cutting, football, soccer; II: Heavy manual work, skiing, tennis;III: Light manual work, jogging, running; IV: Sedentary work (ADL)

*[4] Rate at the highest activity level, where the patient is confirming, that he would be able to function without symptoms, even if he is not actually practising activities on this level.

*[5] Use neutral-zero-method for documentation of the data of the passive range of motion. Write three figures for flexion / zero-point / hyperextension.
Examples:
150° flexion, 10° hyperextension =150/0/10
150° flexion, full extension = 150/0/0
150° flexion, 20° flexion contracture = 150/20/0

*[6] Write: M=manual, I=instrumented, R=x-ray.

*[7] Both endpoints must be firm, otherwise qualification <III> (abnormal).

*[8] Pivot shift is not rated in comparison to the opposite side, as a positive pivot shift is always pathologic and should not be confused with a physiologic reversed pivot shift.

*[9] Palpation of crepitus in the various compartments. The examination should be carried out during weightbearing flexion- and extension-movements. Crepitus is rated abnormal (III), if it is painful, and severely abnormal (IV), if it is not only palpable, but also audible.

*[10] X-rays should be taken as standing a.p.-x-rays in 30° flexion. They are rated normal, when there is no change. Nearly normal (II) should be marked, if there are minimal changes (e.g. small osteophytes, slight sclerosis or flattening of the femoral condyle), but the joint space is wider than 4 mm. For abnormal (III) and severely abnormal rating (IV) the absolute values of the joint (cartilage) space is determining.

*[11] As a functional test one leg hops are carried out on both legs. The percentage of hops on the injured side compared to the opposite side is noted.

© ICRS

FIGURE 7–3 ICRS Cartilage Repair Assessment.

disruption, is there a combined rotatory instability? If there has been ligamentous reconstruction, has joint stability been re-created?

7. Meniscus integrity: Are the menisci intact? If not, has partial, subtotal, or complete meniscectomy been performed? Has meniscal repair or allograft meniscal replacement been considered?

8. Previous management: Has there been prior debridement and chondroplasty, drilling, microfracture, bone graft, allograft, autologous chondrocyte implantation, or mosaicplasty?

9. Status of repair **(Fig. 7–3)**: If there has been previous management, repair tissue can be evaluated both biomechanically and histologically. An articular cartilage resilience and stiffness probe has been developed[24] to test arthroscopically the mechanical repair characteristics. Additionally, the ICRS visual histologic score[25] can be used to assess hyaline versus fibrocartilage repair.

10. Biochemical synovial markers: Synovial biopsy can be done during arthroscopy for evaluation of synovial disorders as well as joint microenvironment modifiers including stromelysin (matrix metalloproteinases MMP-1 and MMP-3) and other cytokines.

Arthroscopy remains the gold standard for the assessment of articular and meniscal cartilage lesions.[26] Arthroscopy also provides the only method for assessing the earliest superficial fibrillation of the surface of the articular cartilage,[16] which is undetectable by noninvasive means. Two damage assessment instruments have been proposed to translate the advantages of direct visualization of articulating surfaces to the quantification of cartilage damage. The French Society of Arthroscopy (SFA) scoring and grading systems[27,28] and the American College of Rheumatology Knee Arthroscopy Osteoarthritis Scale (ACR/KAOS)[29] include an overall assessment of cartilage damage in each compartment by VAS with a weighted estimate of the sum total of the lesions in a given compartment. The SFA system has superior intraobserver reliability and only the SFA has been assessed longitudinally for sensitivity to change.[27,28] However, the main advantage of the ACR/KAOS is its ease of use, because the SFA system may be limited by its complexity. Further, only the ACR/KAOS includes an assessment of the degree of synovitis present, which may have relevance to articular cartilage repair longevity. No data are available regarding the relevance of scores from these instruments to clinically relevant outcomes. The invasiveness of a second-look arthroscopy is a disadvantage that has limited the scores' emergence as routinely used outcome measures.

■ Conclusion

Despite the numerous theoretical advantages to MRI and arthroscopically based instruments, standardized

plain radiography remains the primary outcome measure of choice for all articular cartilage disorder-related research.[30] As such, trials of articular cartilage transplantation should utilize plain radiography as the primary outcome variable. Secondary outcome variables should include the same set of measures recommended for other articular cartilage clinical trials, including, the Cincinnati scale, WOMAC index[5] or its KOOS modification,[7] the Lequesne index,[6] the SF-36,[10] and global assessments by patient and physician by VAS. The emergence of MRI or arthroscopy as outcome measures could significantly decrease the required length of assessment or the required sample sizes by increasing sensitivity in the assessment of subtle chondropenia, osteoarthritis, or the articular cartilage defect's change over time. Overall, the need to create and utilize a universal multifaceted instrument that includes multiple subjective and objective data to assess disorders of articular cartilage has not yet been met. This ideal scoring system must be dynamic, global, Internet compatible, and accurate without bias for age, culture, and language. The clinical scientist must use an array of multimedia techniques to incorporate all comprehensive aspects of articular cartilage that may impact the intervention or the quality of life.

REFERENCES

1. Noyes FR, Mooar PA, Matthews DS,et al. The symptomatic anterior cruciate deficient knee. Part 1: The long-term functional disability in athletic active individuals. J Bone Joint Surg Am 1983;65:154–162

2. Noyes FR, Matthews DS, Mooar PA, et al. The symptomatic anterior cruciate deficient knee. Part 2: The results of rehabilitation, activity modification, and counseling on functional disability. J Bone Joint Surg Am 1983;65:163–174

3. Stewart A, Greenfield S, Hays R, et al. Functional status and well-being of patients with chronic conditions. JAMA 1989;262:907–913

4. Tegner Y, Lysholm J. Rating systems in the evaluation of knee ligament injuries. Clin Orthop 1985;198:43–49

5. Bellamy N. WOMAC Osteoarthritis Index—A User's Guide. London: London Health Science Centre, 1996

6. Lequesne M, Mery C, Samson M, Gerard P. Indexes of severity for osteoarthritis of the hip and knee. Validation-value in comparison with other assessment tests. Scand J Rheum 1987;85(suppl 65):85–89

7. Roos EM, Roos HP, Lohmander LS, Ekdahl C, Beynnon BD. Knee injury and osteoarthritis score (KOOS)—development of a self-administered outcome measure. J Orthop Sports Phys Ther 1998;28:88–96

8. Roos EM, Roos HP, Lohmander LS. WOMAC Osteoarthritis Index—additional dimensions for use in subjects with posttraumatic osteoarthritis of the knee. Western Ontario and MacMaster Universities.

9. Theiler R, Singha O, Schneren S, et al. Superior responsiveness of the pain and function sections of the Western Ontario and McMaster Universities Osteoarthritis Index (WOMAC) as compared to the Lequesne-Algofunctional Index in patients with osteoarthritis of the lower extremities. Osteoarthritis Cartilage 1999;7:515–519

10. Stucki G, Sangha O, Stucki S, et al. Comparison of the WOMAC (Western Ontario McMaster Universities) osteoarthritis index and a self-report format of the self-administered Lequesne-algofunctional index in patients with knee and hip osteoarthritis. Osteoarthritis Cartilage 1998;6:79–86

11. Bombardier C, Melfi CA, Paul J, et al. Comparison of a generic and a disease-specific measure of pain and physical function after knee replacement surgery. Med Care 1995;33(suppl 4): AS131–AS144

12. Mazzuca S. Plain radiography in the evaluation of knee osteoarthritis. Curr Opin Rheumatol 1997;9(3):263–267

13. Mazzuca SA, Brandt KD. Plain radiography as an outcome measure in clinical trials involving patients with knee osteoarthritis. Rheum Dis Clin North Am 1999;25(2):467–480

14. Rovati LC. Radiographic assessment. Introduction: existing methodology. Osteo Cart 1999;7(4):427–429

15. Dacre JE, Huskisson EC. The automatic assessment of knee radiographs in osteoarthritis using digital image analysis. Br J Rheumatol 1989;28(6):506–510

16. Loeuille D, Olivier P, Mainard D, et al. Magnetic resonance imaging of normal and osteoarthritic cartilage. Arthritis Rheum 1998;41:963–975

17. Petersson IF, Boegard T, Saxne T, et al. Radiographic osteoarthritis of the knee classified by the Ahlback and Kellgren-Lawrence systems for the tibiofemoral joint in people aged 35–54 years with chronic knee pain. Ann Rheum Dis 1997;56:493–496

18. Yulish BS, Montanez J, Goodfellow DB, Bryan PJ, Mulopulo GP, Modic MT. Chondromalacia patellae: assessment with MR imaging. Radiology 1987;164(3):763–766

19. Drape JL, Pessis E, Aulely GR, et al. Quantitative MR imaging evaluation of chondropathy in osteoarthritic knees. Radiology 1998;208:49–55

20. Eckstein F, Westhoff J, Sitteck H, et al. In vivo reproducibility of three dimensional cartilage volume and thickness measurements with MRI imaging. AJR Am J Roentgenol 1998;170:593–597

21. McNicholas MJ, Brooksbank AJ, Walker CM. Observer agreement analysis of MRI grading of knee osteoarthritis. J R Coll Surg Edinb 1999;44:31–33

22. Outerbridge RE. The etiology of chondromalacia patalloe. Clin Orthop Relat Res 2001; 389:5–8 Hochberg MC, Altman RD, Brandt KD, Moskowitez RW. Design and conduct of clinical trials in osteoarthritis: preliminary recommendations from a task force of the Osteoarthritis Research Society. J Rheumatol 1997;24(4): 792–794

23. Brittberg M, Winalski CS. Evaluation of cartilage injuries and repair. J Bone Joint Surg Am 2003;85-A(suppl 2):58–69

24. Lyyra T, Kiviranta I, Väätäinen U, et al. In vivo characterization of indentation stiffness of articular cartilage in the normal human knee. J Biomed Mater Res 1999;48:482–487

25. Mainil-Varlet P, Aigner T, et al. Histological Assessment of Cartilage Repair. J Bone Joint Surg Am 2003;85-A(suppl 2):45–57

26. Fife RS, Brandt KD, Braunstein EM, et al. Relationship between arthroscopic evidence of cartilage damage and radiographic evidence of joint space narrowing in early osteoarthritis of the knee. Arthritis Rheum 1991;34:377–382

27. Dougados M, Ayral X, Listrat V, et al. The SFA system for assessing articular cartilage lesions at arthroscopy of the knee. Arthroscopy 1994;10:69–77

28. Ayral X, Gueguen A, Listrat V, et al. Simplified arthroscopy scoring system for chondropathy of the knee (revised SFA score). Rev Rhum Engl Ed 1994;61:97–99

29. Ayral X, Gueguen A, Ike RW, et al. Inter-observer reliability of the arthroscopic quantification of chondropathy of the knee. Osteoarthritis Cartilage 1998; 6(3):160–166

■ SECTION THREE ■

Nonoperative Treatment

8

Analgesics and Antiinflammatory Medications

ORRIN M. TROUM

The presence of inflammation or comorbidities is the major determinant of which of the many available analgesic agents is most appropriate for controlling pain caused by cartilage injury in the athlete. However, agent selection requires careful assessment of patient preference as well. This assessment provides the opportunity to explain to the patient that analgesic agents may offer only modest and temporary benefit in managing the chronic pain that often results from cartilage damage. Moreover, because of side effects and lack or loss of efficacy, only a minority of osteoarthritis patients continues analgesic therapy for 1 year. Because of these limitations, patients must understand that pharmacotherapy is only one component of a comprehensive pain management program that may require considerable effort on their part.

In addition, determining the most appropriate analgesic therapy for long-term use in each patient may be more relevant to clinical practice than resolving the current debate regarding the first-line analgesic of choice for osteoarthritis pain. This approach may be particularly appropriate because patients often try several medications before seeking medical care and many combine acetaminophen and nonselective nonsteroidal antiinflammatory drugs (NSAIDs). Although acetaminophen has been preferred for long-term use in many patients with comorbidities, new studies regarding its hepatotoxic effects call this policy into question. However, these effects typically develop only in patients with underlying liver disease or in those using doses higher than recommended. Nonselective NSAIDs may be more effective than acetaminophen, particularly in patients with severe pain. Nevertheless, almost half of all patients surveyed have reported that acetaminophen is as effective as or more effective than NSAIDs. Determining which of these two first-line agents will be most effective for a given patient is further complicated by the absence of established clinical predictors of response.

Cyclooxygenase-2 (COX-2)-selective NSAIDs are as effective as, but no more effective than, nonselective NSAIDs and are generally reserved for patients at high risk of experiencing gastrointestinal bleeding. These patients can be easily identified on the basis of a history of similar bleeding or peptic ulcer, use of anticoagulants or glucocorticoids, cigarette smoking or ingestion of excessive amounts of alcohol, arthritis-related disability, or cardiovascular disease. However, because most athletes suffer gastrointestinal symptoms, and COX-2-selective therapy is less likely to exacerbate these symptoms than other agents, COX-2-selective NSAIDs may be particularly useful in athletes with pain related to cartilage degeneration.

Nevertheless, the gastrointestinal advantages of these agents must be balanced against their possible adverse cardiovascular effects. Because of their antiplatelet activity, nonselective NSAIDs may be associated with less cardiovascular morbidity than COX-2-selective NSAIDs. However, for many patients, any oral agent may be less appropriate than topical agents such as pharmacist-compounded NSAID creams and ointments or capsaicin cream. Such agents do not pose the risk of systemic side effects, may be as effective as oral agents, and are highly acceptable to patients.

For best results, any analgesic should be combined with nonpharmacologic treatments, which should form the main element of the treatment plan. Learning to pace athletic activity may be especially important. Weight reduction can help to control osteoarthritis pain and joint strain in active overweight or obese athletes. For example, a 10-pound weight loss was found to reduce the progression of osteoarthritis of the knee by 50% during a 10-year period, although data on the ability of weight loss to prevent the progression of hip osteoarthritis are not as clear. Assistive devices may also aid in pain management, particularly during the initial phase of treatment. For example, using a cane halves the amount of force placed on an osteoarthritic hip. Combining analgesic agents with wedged insoles, home exercise, physiotherapy, or self-care education have all been shown to provide pain reduction in addition to that provided by pharmacotherapy in controlled clinical trials. When combined with pharmacologic therapy, nonpharmacologic approaches may have synergistic effects that produce a degree of benefit greater than that obtainable when the effects of each approach used separately are totaled.

When nonpharmacologic therapies are added periodically, medication withdrawal or dosage reduction should be attempted to help prevent the side effects of chronic medication use. Simple advice that medication may no longer be required can enable many users to discontinue drug therapy without affecting symptoms, function, or quality of life. Incorporating these techniques in the treatment of younger patients may be especially crucial to prevent the adverse effects of chronic pharmacotherapy from accumulating over a life span.

■ Acetaminophen

Despite acetaminophen's lack of clinically significant antiinflammatory effects, its wide use as first-line therapy for mild to moderate osteoarthritis pain has been based on the opinion that it is as effective as NSAIDs but is less expensive and poses fewer side effects.

Mechanism of Action

The precise mechanisms of action by which acetaminophen (Tylenol) produces analgesia and exerts its weak antiinflammatory effects are unknown. However, it appears to act like salicylates by inhibiting the synthesis of prostaglandins, the precursors of prostanoids, which sensitize pain receptors both centrally and peripherally and increase blood flow to damaged tissue, thereby promoting edema and inflammation. By preventing the synthesis of prostanoids, acetaminophen prevents the pain

signals and edema they would otherwise produce. In addition, its central action may result from its ability to appreciably inhibit COX-3, a newly discovered cyclooxygenase enzyme expressed in human cerebral cortex, more than it inhibits either COX-1 or COX-2 at therapeutic dosages. This COX-3 selectivity may explain why acetaminophen selectively inhibits prostaglandin synthesis in brain tissue but not in platelets or gastric mucosa. Enhanced COX inhibition at low peroxide concentrations may also contribute to its tissue-specificity.

Dosage and Administration

The acetaminophen dose should not exceed 4000 mg/day initially and 3000 mg/day chronically because higher doses are associated with liver damage. Moreover, acetaminophen should be used cautiously in patients with hepatic dysfunction and in those who abuse alcohol, in whom risk of liver damage from acetaminophen use is increased. These patients are at particularly elevated risk of death due to liver failure from acetaminophen overdose. Because the only clinically significant interaction of acetaminophen with other drugs is that with high-dose warfarin, acetaminophen is particularly useful in treating patients who are taking several other drugs.

Efficacy

Because of its equivalent efficacy and superior safety compared with that of NSAIDs, acetaminophen has been recommended as the first-line therapy for osteoarthritic hip or knee pain in guidelines issued by the American College of Rheumatology (ACR). However, clinical trial evidence of the analgesic efficacy of acetaminophen is scanty. Only one small, 6-week, placebo-controlled study[1] found acetaminophen, 1000 mg/day, significantly reduced osteoarthritic knee pain at rest, but the report of that 1983 study did not indicate whether it incorporated the standard study methodology in use today. Other non–placebo-controlled older studies concluded that acetaminophen was as effective as an NSAID in treating osteoarthritic knee pain. However, acetaminophen produced a statistically significant response in only some of the variables evaluated, whereas the NSAID studied (either ibuprofen or naproxen) did so in all of them. A well-designed, placebo-controlled, 12-week trial whose results were reported in 2003 found that, whereas acetaminophen, 1000 mg, given four times daily, did not improve osteoarthritic hip or knee pain, diclofenac did.[2] These findings are consistent with those of an earlier study that found that diclofenac was more effective than acetaminophen for osteoarthritic knee or hip pain. However, because this earlier study was not placebo controlled, it did not establish the effectiveness of either treatment alone compared with placebo.

Adverse Effects and Safety

Because of its tissue-specific prostaglandin selectivity, acetaminophen does not promote bleeding in surgical patients or those with a bleeding diathesis and was not found to cause gastric injury in endoscopic studies. Moreover, no evidence exists to indicate that acetaminophen inhibits COX-1 in gastric mucosa even at high doses. However, results of recent studies indicate that acetaminophen may cause more adverse gastrointestinal events than previously believed. In a retrospective analysis of elderly patients, those taking high-dose acetaminophen (at least 2600 mg/day) had similar rates of adverse gastrointestinal events as those taking high-dose NSAIDs. However, after adjustment for gastrointestinal risk susceptibility, dyspepsia symptoms accounted for most of the gastrointestinal toxicity attributed to high-dose acetominophen.[3] In a similar study of a general patient population, high-dose acetaminophen (2000 mg/day or more) conferred the same risk for upper gastrointestinal complications as traditional NSAIDs did and increased the risk of adverse gastrointestinal events even after adjustment for age and other gastrointestinal risk factors. Moreover, in this study, high-dose acetaminophen increased the risk of serious gastrointestinal adverse events such as ulcer and its complications.[4] Nevertheless, the weight of clinical evidence indicates that the gastrointestinal risk conferred by acetaminophen therapy is less than that conferred by nonselective NSAID therapy, which was associated with more gastrointestinal side effects than acetaminophen in most direct comparisons.

As with gastrointestinal adverse events, acetaminophen may be more strongly associated with renal failure than previously believed. For example, heavy acetaminophen use (more than 365 doses annually) has been found to double the risk of end-stage renal disease.[5] Although this finding did not prevent the National Kidney Foundation Scientific Advisory Committee from recommending acetaminophen for analgesia in patients with impaired renal function, a later report supported the association between acetaminophen and chronic renal failure.[6]

Because acetaminophen does not affect platelet aggregation, it does not have the antifibrinolytic effects that may be advantageous in patients at elevated risk of thrombosis. Nevertheless, acetaminophen has not been associated with increased cardiovascular risk. Moreover, unlike NSAIDs, acetaminophen has not traditionally been associated with acute bronchospasm. Notwithstanding, one study reported an association between acetaminophen use and asthma. In that study, the odds ratio for asthma was 2.4 in daily users compared with those who never used acetaminophen.[7] Nevertheless, the causal link between acetaminophen use and asthma remains to be established in prospective studies. There are no data indicating that acetaminophen accelerates cartilage and bone degeneration, whereas some data indicate that NSAIDs such as indomethacin may do so.

■ Nonsteroidal Antiinflammatory Drugs

Because NSAIDs have both antiinflammatory and analgesic effects, they may be particularly useful for patients with detectable effusion indicating inflammatory osteoarthritis. Moreover, their analgesic effects are almost immediate, although their antiinflammatory effects require higher doses and 1 to 2 weeks of therapy.

Nonselective

Available Agents

In addition to the many different nonselective oral NSAIDs (**Table 8–1**), nonselective NSAIDs are also available in topical forms. These include methylsalicylate or capsaicin cream, which contains an extract from the

TABLE 8–1   Nonselective Nonsteroidal Antiinflammatory Drugs: Available Agents and Their Daily Dosages

Agent	Daily Dosage
Nonacetylated nonsalicylates	150–200 mg in 2–4 doses
Diclofenac	100–200 mg in 2–4 doses
Diclofenac plus misoprostol (Arthrotec)	100 mg in a single dose
Cataflam, Voltaren	
Voltaren XR	
Diflunisal (Dolobid)	500–1500 mg in 2 doses

(*Continued*)

TABLE 8–1 (continued)

Etodolac (Lodine)	800–1200 mg in 2–4 doses
Lodine XL	400–1000 mg in a single dose
Flurbiprofen (Ansaid)	200–300 mg in 2–4 doses
Ibuprofen	1200–3200 mg in 3–4 doses
Prescription (Motrin)	200–400 mg every 4–6 hours,
Nonprescription (Advil, Motrin IB, Nuprin)	not to exceed 1200 mg/day
Indomethacin (Indocin)	50–200 mg in 2–4 doses
Indocin SR	75 mg in a single dose or 150 mg in 2
Ketoprofen	200–225 mg in 3–4 doses
Prescription:	150–200 mg in a single dose
Orudis	12.5 mg every 4–6 hours as needed
Oruvail	
Nonprescription (Actron, Orudis KT)	
Ketorolac (Toradol)	20 mg followed by 10 mg every 4–6 hour not to exceed 40 mg/day[a]
Meclofenamate (Meclomen)	200–400 mg in 4 doses
Meloxicam (Mobic)	7.5–15 mg in a single dose
Nabumetone (Relafen)	1000 mg in 1–2 doses or 2000 mg in 2 doses
Naproxen	500–1500 mg in 2 doses
Naprosyn	750–1000 in a single dose
Naprelan	
Naproxen sodium	550–1650 in 2 doses
Prescription (Anaprox)	220 mg every 8–12 hours as needed
Nonprescription (Aleve)	
Oxaprozin (Daypro)	1200 or 1800 mg in a single dose
Piroxicam (Feldene)	20 mg in 1–2 doses
Sulindac (Clinoril)	300–400 mg in 2 doses
Tolmetin (Tolectin)	1200–1800 mg in 3 doses
Acetylated salicylates	2400–5400 mg in several doses
Aspirin (Anacin, Ascriptin, Bayer, Ecotrin)	
Nonacetylated salicylates	2000–3000 mg in 2–3 doses
Choline and magnesium salicylates	
(CMT, Tricosal, Trilisate)	
Choline salicylate (Arthropan liquid)	3480 mg or 20 mL in several doses
Magnesium salicylate	2600–4800 mg in 3–6 doses
Prescription (Magan, Mobidin, Mobogesic)	
Nonprescription	
(Arthritab, Bayer Select, Doan's Pills)	
Salsalate	1000–3000 mg in 2–3 doses
(Amigesic, Anaflex 750, Disalcid, Marthritic,	
Mono-Gesic, Salflex, Salsitab)	
Sodium salicylate (generic)	3600–5400 mg in several doses

[a]Oral ketorolac should only be used as continuation therapy after intramuscular ketorolac, and the maximum combined duration of use for both parenteral and oral ketorolac is 5 days.

chili pepper plant, or pharmacist-compounded NSAID creams such as diclofenac and ketoprofen. Topical agents are popular among patients and most useful in treating the knee or hand, to which they are more easily applied than they are to other areas. Moreover, they are particularly useful in patients who are unwilling or unable to take oral agents, and they are a valuable adjunct to oral agents as well.

In addition to being used alone, NSAIDS are frequently combined with acetaminophen. Concomitant use of acetaminophen may minimize NSAID side effects by allowing a lower dose of NSAIDs to be taken to achieve the same effect, and, in some surveys, up to 30% of patients taking NSAIDS also self-treated with acetaminophen. Although in general, NSAIDs should not be combined with one another, 81 to 325 mg/day of aspirin for cardioprotection may be combined with other NSAIDs, albeit at increased risk of gastrointestinal bleeding.

Mechanism of Action

Whether the pain relief provided by NSAIDs results primarily from their analgesic or from their antiinflammatory effects remains unclear. Although they reduce prostaglandin synthesis by inhibiting both COX-1 and COX-2, their main mechanism of antiinflammatory action is via COX-2 inhibition. Whereas COX-2 is induced at sites of inflammation to generate inflammation-mediating prostaglandins, COX-1 generates prostaglandins that protect the gastrointestinal mucosa and promote platelet function.

Efficacy

Nonselective NSAIDs have consistently been found superior to placebo and, in general, are similarly effective in treating osteoarthritic pain. For example, in meta-analyses of treatments for hip osteoarthritis,[8,9] differences in effectiveness between NSAIDs were rarely found. Nevertheless, indomethacin tended to be more effective as well as more toxic than other NSAIDs. Moreover, low doses of naproxen (less than 750 mg/day) and ibuprofen (less than 1600 mg/day) were less effective for hip osteoarthritis than were other NSAIDs. In contrast, meta-analyses of treatments for knee osteoarthritis provide little evidence regarding the superior effectiveness of one NSAID over another at equivalent recommended doses.[10,11] However, although NSAIDS are in general similarly effective, much variability in response to different NSAIDs has been shown both between patients and in the same patient at different times. Topical NSAIDs have proven to be as effective as oral NSAIDs in clinical trials. Meta-analysis has found them to be twice as beneficial as placebo,[12] and substituting a topical NSAID for its oral counterpart can allow dose reduction with equivalent pain control.

The NSAIDs may be more effective than acetaminophen in treating osteoarthritis pain. Meta-analyses have found that NSAID-treated patients with knee osteoarthritis had significantly greater improvement in both pain at rest and pain on motion than acetaminophen-treated patients.[13] However, absolute differences between the two treatments were slight, and no significant difference in walking time or quality of life was found.[13] Any superior effectiveness of NSAIDs relative to acetaminophen may result from the NSAIDs' antiinflammatory effects in patients whose osteoarthritis has a low-grade inflammatory component. The possible superior efficacy of NSAIDs compared with that of acetaminophen may be more pronounced in patients with severe pain. However, the results of one study indicating that NSAIDs were superior for treating osteoarthritis patients with severe pain were confounded by reanalysis, which indicated that severity of pain did not predict a better response to ibuprofen therapy when given in antiinflammatory doses.[14]

Results of two large surveys indicated that patients with rheumatoid complaints preferred NSAIDs to acetaminophen. However, in one survey, more osteoarthritis patients than rheumatoid arthritis or fibromyalgia patients preferred acetaminophen, and in another, therapy was more likely to be continued for more than 2 years in patients taking acetaminophen than in those taking NSAIDs. Improved compliance with acetaminophen appeared to be related to its superior side effect profile compared with that of NSAIDs.

Adverse Effects and Safety

Nonsalicylate NSAIDs result in adverse effects in 10 to 15% of patients. These effects are mainly related to the ability of these agents to inhibit platelet aggregation, which increases risk of bleeding. As a result, the ACR recommends that a complete blood count (CBC) be obtained before treatment with these agents is initiated, and that CBCs be repeated annually thereafter. More frequent reevaluation of hemoglobin/hematocrit may be prudent in patients at highest risk of gastrointestinal bleeding. Inhibition of prostaglandin synthesis by nonselective NSAIDs in the gastrointestinal mucosa can injure the lining of the stomach or intestines, which, when combined with the increased risk of bleeding posed by these agents, may result in perforated ulcer, gastrointestinal hemorrhage, and death. In a study from the United Kingdom, mortality related to the gastrointestinal complications of NSAIDs was found to be higher than that related to asthma, and an analysis in the United States found that as many as 16,500 NSAID-related deaths occur annually in arthritis patients.

The renal toxicity of these agents is also a concern. Although moderate intake of NSAIDs did not increase the risk of renal toxicity, after more than 5000 doses were taken the odds ratio for renal toxicity increased to 8.8.[5] Moreover, daily NSAID use has also been shown to increase the risk of chronic renal disease, although this risk was greatest in the elderly.[15] Nonselective NSAIDs are hepatotoxic as well as renotoxic. As a result, baseline measurements of creatinine and aspartate aminotransferase and alanine aminotransferase levels are recommended before NSAID therapy is initiated. Reevaluation after 1 month of therapy and as clinically indicated thereafter may be warranted in patients at higher risk of renotoxicity such as diabetic and/or hypertensive patients and patients with congestive heart failure.

Nonacetylated salicylates such as choline magnesium trisalicylate or salsalate do not have the antiplatelet effects of nonselective nonsalicylate NSAIDs or as significant a degree of renal toxicity as that associated with nonselective nonsalicylate NSAIDs. As a result, these salicylates may be more appropriate for patients with renal insufficiency or for those at high risk of gastrointestinal or other bleeding than other nonselective NSAIDs. However, at effective doses, these salicylates pose a risk of central nervous system toxicity and ototoxicity. In addition, some nonselective NSAIDs, such as etodolac and meloxicam, are more selective for COX-2 than other nonselective NSAIDs and therefore spare gastric prostaglandin synthesis somewhat. However, clinical evidence of reduced gastrointestinal damage with these agents is sketchier than that for more COX-2-selective agents.

Next to lack of efficacy, gastrointestinal side effects such as dyspepsia, nausea, and vomiting are the main reason patients discontinue or change NSAIDs. Because gastropathy induced by nonsalicylate NSAIDs is dose-dependent, the lowest effective dose should be used. In addition, screening for *Helicobacter pylori* infection before initiating NSAID therapy is important because such infection increases the risk of NSAID-related peptic ulcer. The association between NSAID use and peptic ulcer was well established by the results of a meta-analysis of current NSAID users, who were found to have a higher incidence of peptic ulcer than nonusers.[16] However, in another meta-analysis that controlled for the ulcer risk posed by *H. pylori* infection, the odds ratio for endoscopically determined ulcer related to NSAID use alone was 18, and when NSAID therapy was combined with *H. pylori* infection, it was 61. This controlled meta-analysis also found that, in patients with either NSAID use or *H. pylori* infection, the addition of either risk factor increased ulcer risk 3.5-fold.[17] *H. pylori* treatment has been found to reduce the risk of ulcer from 34% to 12% and the risk of complicated ulcer from 27% to 4% over 6 months in patients starting NSAID therapy.[18] Thus, if

infected, patients should be treated for *H. pylori* infection before NSAID therapy is initiated.

In patients at high risk of serious adverse gastrointestinal events, gastroprotective agents should be used even when low-dose nonselective NSAID therapy is prescribed. Although the most commonly used gastroprotective agent is misoprostol, 200 μg three or four times daily, it may cause diarrhea and flatulence when combined with an NSAID. Alternatives include histamine-2 receptor antagonists such as famotidine, which in the usual doses does not prevent gastric ulcers. Other possibilities include omeprazole, which, like high-dose famotidine, has been shown to prevent NSAID-related gastropathy in endoscopic studies. In patients with existing ulcers, omeprazole, 20 to 40 mg/day, is as effective as misoprostol, 200 μg twice daily, but better tolerated. In addition, lansoprazole (Prevacid), and esomeprazole (Nexium) are now Food and Drug Administration (FDA)-approved for the prevention of gastric ulcers in NSAID users at increased risk of developing gastrointestinal bleeding, perforations, or ulcers. Although proton-pump inhibitors are commonly used and have also been shown to prevent ulcer in patients taking NSAIDs, their cost may be limiting. Co-medication may also be required for NSAID-related constipation or diarrhea.

The NSAIDs may also promote fluid retention, edema, and hypertension. Therefore, when NSAIDs are combined with antihypertensive therapy in patients at high risk of these complications because of preexisting heart failure, hypertension, renal insufficiency, or impaired liver function, blood pressure should be monitored regularly. Even in patients who are not at high risk of hypertension, blood pressure should be checked a few weeks after NSAID therapy is initiated and two to three times annually thereafter. Because, like their gastrointestinal adverse effects, the hypertensive effects of NSAIDs are dose-dependent, these effects can be minimized by using the lowest effective dose.

Controversy exists as to whether the use of NSAIDs increases cardiovascular disease risk. Early findings regarding nonselective NSAIDs were inconclusive, suggesting either no effect or cardioprotection. However, a more recent study of more than 180,000 Medicaid patients found that use of various nonaspirin NSAIDs excluding COX-2-selective agents was not associated with altered risk of serious coronary heart disease or stroke compared with that found for controls.[19] Nevertheless, ibuprofen may impair the ability of aspirin to confer cardioprotection, as indicated by the effect of adding ibuprofen to aspirin on serum thromboxane formation and platelet aggregation in vitro. In contrast, like acetaminophen, diclofenac was not found to impair platelet disaggregation by aspirin.

Nonselective NSAIDs may induce bronchospasm by diverting arachidonic acid to the lipoxygenase pathway and increasing leukotriene synthesis. Thus, these agents should be avoided in patients with aspirin-sensitive asthma. In addition, some NSAIDs have been associated with worsening of degenerative joint disease. NSAIDs in vitro may retard, accelerate, or have no effect on osteoarthritis progression depending on the agent used. Indomethacin in particular may accelerate degeneration of cartilage and bone; piroxicam, diclofenac, and naproxen appear to have no such effect; and meloxicam may be chondroprotective. However, no clinical evidence exists to indicate that NSAIDs have favorable effects on cartilage. Moreover, although simple headache is a common side effect of NSAIDs, these agents may in rare cases produce aseptic meningitis. NSAIDs also interact with several drugs, which may pose problems for patients on multidrug regimens. The adverse effects of NSAID therapy can be avoided by the use of topical agents, which results in a nominal blood level of drug that limits systemic effects and enhances safety compared with that of oral NSAIDs. Meta-analysis has shown that topical NSAIDs are as safe as placebo,[12] and other studies have shown no association between topical agents and gastrointestinal bleeding.

COX-2 Selective

Available Agents and Mechanism of Action

Three COX-2-selective NSAIDs are available: celecoxib (Celebrex), rofecoxib (Vioxx), and valdecoxib (Bextra). In addition, although widely used in Europe and Mexico, the COX-2-selective NSAID etoricoxib (Arcoxia) was still under FDA review in the spring of 2005 for approval for U.S. use, as was parecoxib, an injectable prodrug of valdecoxib. At therapeutic doses, COX-2-selective NSAIDs exclusively inhibit prostaglandin synthesis through the COX-2 pathway, thereby sparing prostaglandin synthesis in the gastrointestinal mucosa.

Dosage and Indications

Effective dosages for osteoarthritis pain are celecoxib, 100 to 200 mg/day; rofecoxib, 12.5 to 25 mg/day; valdecoxib, 10 mg/day; etoricoxib, 60 to 90 mg/day; and parecoxib, 20 to 40 mg/dose. An acute pain indication also exists for rofecoxib, 50 mg/day, for up to 5 days, and for celecoxib, 400 mg, for the first dose, which may be followed by subsequent doses of 200 mg. However, no acute pain indication exists for valdecoxib. Parecoxib, which can be given either intravenously or intramuscularly, may be particularly useful for patients who need rapid control of moderate to severe pain or who are unable to take oral drugs because of surgical procedures or serious gastrointestinal distress.

The COX-2-selective NSAIDs can be useful for patients who have not responded adequately to nonpharmacologic treatments and maximum doses of acetaminophen or nonselective NSAIDs. However, greater efficacy of COX-2-selective NSAIDs compared with that of acetaminophen or nonselective NSAIDs has not been shown in these patients in clinical trials. COX-2-selective NSAIDs may also be used as initial therapy, particularly in patients with moderate to severe pain and inflammation. Because of their mechanism of action, COX-2-selective NSAIDs pose less risk of adverse gastrointestinal events than traditional NSAIDs but are similarly effective. As a result, guidelines recommend that COX-2-selective agents be reserved for use in patients at high risk of adverse gastrointestinal events. However, even in patients who are not at such high risk, the reduction in gastrointestinal side effects associated with COX-2-selective agents could be expected to result in better compliance and less need to change drugs, prescribe co-medications, or perform procedures. These advantages may thus support more widespread use of COX-2-selective NSAIDs.

Efficacy

Meta-analysis results have indicated that this class of agents appears to be as effective as nonselective NSAIDs.[20] However, no direct evidence indicates that one COX-2-selective agent is more effective than another.

Adverse Effects and Safety

Rofecoxib and celecoxib have an incidence of acute gastrointestinal injury and chronic ulceration that is half of that reported for nonselective NSAIDs. Use of COX-2-selective NSAIDs resulted in less risk of complicated and symptomatic ulcer after 6 to 9 months of therapy than use of nonselective NSAIDs in the Celecoxib Long-term Arthritis Safety Study (CLASS)[21] and the Vioxx Gastrointestinal Outcomes Research (VIGOR) study.[22] However, longer term study of celecoxib did not confirm this risk reduction after 12 or 16 months of therapy.[23] These negative results may have resulted from problems with study methodology and concomitant use of low-dose aspirin. For instance, in CLASS, celecoxib only reduced the rate of upper gastrointestinal complications in patients who were not taking aspirin concomitantly.[21] In contrast, the VIGOR study did not allow patients to take aspirin concomitantly. These studies thus indicate that COX-2-selective NSAIDs pose less risk of gastrointestinal side effects especially in patients who are not currently taking aspirin. However, other data suggest less gastrointestinal bleeding results from using a COX-2-selective NSAID with aspirin than from using a nonselective NSAID with aspirin. COX-2-selective NSAIDs may also be less likely to cause nuisance gastrointestinal side effects than nonselective NSAIDs. For example, celecoxib, 50 to 400 mg twice daily, appears slightly less likely to cause minor gastrointestinal symptoms, such as abdominal pain, dyspepsia, and nausea, than naproxen, 500 mg twice daily. Similarly, in the VIGOR study, rofecoxib was better tolerated than naproxen.

Unlike nonselective NSAIDs, COX-2-selective NSAIDs do not decrease platelet aggregation or increase bleeding time and thus may be used for surgical patients, patients with bleeding diathesis, and cautiously in those taking warfarin. Moreover, although all NSAIDs have been associated with hypertension, the cost of managing blood pressure destabilization was found to be significantly less for celecoxib than for higher-dose rofecoxib or nonspecific NSAIDs (diclofenac, ibuprofen, or naproxen). In addition, users of selective agents are more likely to concomitantly use other medications that may increase blood pressure than users of nonselective NSAIDs. Nevertheless, coprescribing antiplatelet agents with COX-2-selective NSAIDs appears prudent if there are no contraindications to combination therapy, particularly considering that combining 81 to 325 mg/day of aspirin with COX-2-specific NSAIDs has been found to pose a lower risk of endoscopically identified ulcers than combining aspirin with nonselective NSAIDs.

Although COX-2-selective NSAIDs were initially not expected to be renotoxic because of their selectivity, two separate investigative groups concluded that these agents may be so in certain patient populations. Thus, COX-2-selective agents should be used with caution in patients with mild to moderate renal impairment and avoided in patients with severe renal insufficiency. Similar precautions apply in patients with liver disease because, like nonselective NSAIDs, COX-2-selective agents may also be hepatotoxic. In addition, use of celecoxib and valdecoxib is contraindicated in patients who are allergic to sulfonamides because these COX-2-selective agents have a sulfonamide component. However, although some nonselective NSAIDs have been associated with the progression of osteoarthritis in in vitro studies, less is known about the effects of COX-2-selective NSAIDs in this regard. In addition, a few cases of aseptic meningitis related to rofecoxib use have been reported, as were several cases possibly related to celecoxib use.

Although the nonselective NSAID ketorolac is typically used in the emergency department and postoperatively for acute pain, it is associated with gastrointestinal ulceration and renal functional impairment. Moreover, because it predisposes patients to increased perioperative bleeding, it is contraindicated for preoperative use. In contrast, the COX-2-selective NSAID parecoxib does not impair platelet aggregation and produced no more gastrointestinal erosions or ulcers than placebo in healthy volunteers in a short-term trial. Moreover, parecoxib does not appear to have any significant drug interactions that may prevent its use in patients taking other drugs concurrently and appears equal to ketorolac and superior to morphine in controlling postsurgical pain in knee replacement patients. Therefore, once approved, parecoxib will probably replace ketorolac as the injectable NSAID of choice.

Addendum: While this manuscript was in press, rofecoxib was withdrawn worldwide on September 30, 2004, due to an increased risk of cardiovascular events seen in the Adenomatous Polyp Prevention on Vioxx (APPROVe) Trial.

The FDA Arthritis Advisory Committee and Drug Safety and Risk Management Advisory Committee subsequently met (February 16–18, 2005). Following public testimony and scientific presentations, the panel voted unanimously to advise the FDA that Vioxx, Bextra, and Celebrex can cause cardiovascular problems. In a separate vote a majority of the panel advised against removing these medications from the market.

The specific recommendations were:

Rofecoxib:

Initiate stronger black-box warning than celecoxib

Prohibit direct-to-consumer advertising

Add education materials

Cut dosing from 25 mg to 12.5 mg and virtually eliminate 50 mg

Commence patient informed consent (possibly)

Valdecoxib:

Initiate stronger black-box warning than celecoxib

Halt direct-to-consumer advertising

Add education materials

Contraindicated in cardiac surgery

Celecoxib:

Initiate black-box warning

Halt direct-to-consumer advertising

Add education materials

Call for lower 200 mg dose

A decision from the FDA is expected in the spring of 2005. In addition, the European Union has restricted the use of celecoxib (Celebrex), valdecoxib (Bextra), parecoxib (Dynastat), lumiracoxib (Prexige), and etoricoxib (Arcoxia) as of February 2005.

■ Opioids

Opioids are recommended for patients with severe pain who do not respond to or cannot tolerate COX-2 inhibitors, nonselective NSAIDs, or acetaminophen. They are particularly useful for patients with intense pain that cannot be adequately controlled by NSAIDs because, unlike NSAIDs, opioids do not have a dose level above which they can no longer exert analgesic effects. Nevertheless, although they are highly effective, opioids are considered third-line analgesics because they may cause tolerance, addiction, and respiratory depression. However, these limitations are less severe than previously believed. Thus, in most cases, when moderate or severe osteoarthritis pain cannot be controlled with nonopioid analgesics, a trial of opioid therapy is appropriate. Their use in competitive athletes may be limited due to the fact that these substances are banned by most athletic agencies.

Mechanism of Action

Opioids exert their analgesic effects by binding to one or more opioid receptors, which include μ, κ, and δ receptors. Each opioid binds to these receptors in different proportions and thus produces different effects in different patients. For example, oxycodone selectively binds to κ receptors and thus has a binding profile that may produce greater analgesia in women than in men. Because every patient has different alleles for opioid receptors and hence different mixtures of receptors, and because receptor populations vary with pain state, opioid treatment must be individualized, and achieving acceptable pain control often requires trying several different opioids in succession. However, little clinical trial evidence is available to indicate which agent should be tried first for a specific patient in a particular situation.

Nevertheless, some opioids act on other receptors in addition to those for opioids, and such dual action may make them particularly appropriate in specific situations. For example, the synthetic, centrally acting oral opioid tramadol (Ultram) also inhibits the reuptake of norepinephrine and serotonin by nerve cells, as may be the case for levorphanol. These two mechanisms synergistically combine the action of an opioid with that of an antidepressant to control pain. As a result, tramadol may be preferable to other less potent opioids such as codeine or propoxyphene, a centrally acting nonopiate narcotic structurally related to methadone, because tramadol produces fewer opioid-related adverse effects than these agents.

Agents, Dosage/Administration, and Indications

Available opioids with their equianalgesic doses for treating moderate to severe pain and their duration of action are listed in **Table 8–2.** More potent opioids such as morphine are reserved for the treatment of severe pain. Patients with moderate pain may be treated with low doses of a more potent opioid combined with a nonopioid, which allows lower opioid doses to be given. Examples of these combinations include acetamino-

phen and oxycodone (Percocet) or acetaminophen and pentazocine (Talacen). Although less potent opioids can be used alone, they are commonly combined with nonopioids in fixed-dose combinations for mild to moderate pain. An example of such a combination is acetaminophen and propoxyphene (Darvocet-N). In addition, because tramadol (Ultram) has a superior risk-benefit ratio to that of other less potent opioids, has minimal abuse potential, and is therefore an unscheduled opioid, it may be particularly appropriate for the long-term treatment of mild to moderate osteoarthritis pain when used either alone or in combination with acetaminophen (Ultracet). This combination has a faster onset of action than that of tramadol alone and provides better relief of pain than acetaminophen alone. Although Ultracet is presently approved for the treatment of acute pain, both of its components are also used for chronic pain, which indicates that it may be useful for chronic pain as well.

Treatment of severe pain in opiate-naive patients is usually initiated with an opioid with a short half-life and rapid clearance. These agents and their initial doses include codeine, 30 to 60 mg; hydromorphone, 2 to 4 mg; hydrocodone or oxycodone, 10 to 15 mg; or morphine, 15 to 30 mg. If patients in continuous pain respond well to initial treatment with short-acting agents and side effects can be managed, the short-acting agent can be discontinued and analgesic therapy with a long-acting, sustained-release agent can be initiated. The dose of the long-acting agent used should be equivalent to the average daily dose of the short-acting agent that controlled pain.

Long-acting agents include morphine (Kadian, MS Contin, Oramorph SR), transdermal fentanyl (Duragesic), and oxycodone (OxyContin). Although methadone and levorphanol have intrinsically long half-lives, they are generally considered second-line opioids because they are difficult to titrate and have delayed side effects. Like these agents, morphine also has relative disadvantages that limit its clinical utility. Because it induces its own metabolism, maintaining a steady serum level of morphine is difficult, and because it is relatively hydrophilic, its transport across the blood–brain barrier is delayed. In contrast, fentanyl is lipophilic and therefore faster acting, and because its potency is several hundred times greater than that of morphine, micrograms can provide pain relief for up to 3 days when administered transdermally. Like fentanyl, oxycodone is more potent than morphine, and its sustained release form has become the most popular opioid for the treatment of chronic nonmalignant pain in the United States. However, ~10% of patients have low levels of the cytochrome P-450 2D6 enzyme that converts oxycodone to its active metabolite, oxymorphone, and thus must take more than the usual dose to control pain.

TABLE 8–2 Opioid Analgesics: Equianalgesic Doses for Moderate to Severe Pain and Duration of Action

Agent	Dose	Duration (hours)
Less potent opioids:	200 mg (oral)	4
Codeine		
Dihydrocodeine	200 mg (oral)	4
Propoxyphene (Darvon, Dolene, SK65)	100 mg (oral)	4
Hydrocodone (Vicodin)	40 mg (oral)	4–6
Tramadol (Ultram)	100 mg (oral)	4–6
More potent opioids:	0.8 mg (sublingual),	6–9,
Buprenorphine (Subutex;	35 mg (transdermal)	72
Buprenorphine TDS)		
Fentanyl, transdermal (Duragesic)	25 μg/h (transdermal)[a]	48–72
Hydromorphone (Dilaudid)	7.5 mg (oral)	3–4
Levorphanol	4 mg (oral)	4–6
Meperidine (Demerol)	150–300 mg (oral)	3–4
Methadone (Methadose, Dolophine HCL)	10–20 mg (oral)	4–12
Morphine	30–60 mg (oral)	3–6
Continued release (MS Contin)		8–12
Sustained release (Kadian, Oramorph SR)		24
Oxycodone	20–30 mg (oral)	3–6
Immediate release		8–12
Continued release (OxyContin)		
Oxymorphone (Numorphan)	10 (rectal)	2–4
Pentazocine	100 mg (oral)	4

[a]25 μg/h is the lowest available dose of transdermal fentanyl and is equianalgesic to 45–135 mg/day of oral morphine.

In addition to these available long-acting opioids, a transdermal form of buprenorphine is being evaluated for U.S. use. Hydromorphone formulations that will allow once-daily dosing may be available in the United States by 2004· and several other sustained-release opioids are being tested. Such long-acting agents provide steady serum levels, which prevent mini-withdrawals or rebound reactions. In addition, long-acting agents have less abuse potential, are more convenient, and are associated with greater compliance, better quality of life, and more normal sleep patterns than short-acting agents. Moreover, if the dose of long-acting agents is carefully titrated, the intermittent sedation and related psychomotor impairment common during therapy with short-acting agents can be avoided.

However, most patients who are prescribed long-acting opioids should also be given fast-acting agents to treat breakthrough pain. For example, because it is rapidly absorbed bucally, the fast-acting fentanyl lozenge Actiq can be particularly useful for breakthrough pain. Such rescue medication can be given every 2 to 3 hours to enhance pain control. The usual dosage of rescue medication required is equivalent to 5 to 10% of the 24-hour dose of long-acting opioid, and the amount required indicates whether the dose of long-acting medication needs to be increased.

Pain levels sometimes increase after several weeks of acceptable control with opioid therapy because the patient's activity level increased after the pain was alleviated. In such cases, the opioid dose should be increased as well. Whether tolerance to the pain-relieving effects of opioids develops is unclear. Most studies of long-term opioid therapy in patients with chronic pain have found that the dose required for pain relief remains stable unless the underlying disease progresses. Nevertheless, patients receiving long-term opioid therapy typically experience withdrawal symptoms such as abdominal cramping, sweating, nausea, diarrhea, and irritability when therapy is abruptly ended or the dose is reduced considerably. Such symptoms are easily avoided by tapering the dose and can be relieved with clonidine or a benzodiazepine.

Efficacy

The efficacy of opioids in treating chronic pain is well established. For example, a retrospective study of long-term opioid use in 38 patients with chronic nonmalignant pain found that 63% obtained acceptable partial or full relief.[24] Moreover, a survey of 100 pain patients who received long-acting opioid therapy found that more than half had >50% reduction in pain and improved function.[25] However, about half of all patients typically discontinue opioid use within 1 year of initiation of therapy. Whether these discontinuations are related to loss of efficacy or to side effects is unclear. In many cases, lack of efficacy may result from the use of inappropriately low doses of opioids. For example, when given in the usual doses, less potent opioids alone do not appear to control chronic musculoskeletal pain better than nonopioids. Combining opioids with nonopioids also frequently results in inadequate pain control because of the inappropriately low dose of opioid contained in fixed-dose combinations. Nevertheless, codeine plus acetaminophen has been shown to control osteoarthritic hip pain significantly better than acetaminophen alone. However, a third of the patients discontinued therapy because of the side effects of this combination therapy. In contrast, propoxyphene plus acetaminophen was as effective as codeine plus acetaminophen for osteoarthritic hip or knee pain but significantly better tolerated.

Used alone, the less potent opioid tramadol was as effective as antiinflammatory doses of ibuprofen in patients with chronic hip and knee osteoarthritis studied in clinical trials and may offer greater analgesic potency than NSAIDs in selected patients. However, when tramadol was compared with diclofenac in patients with noninflammatory osteoarthritis of the hip or knee, the analgesia exerted by either agent was found to be highly individual. In addition, the effectiveness of one drug did not predict whether its alternate would be effective, and a considerable proportion of patients did not respond to either drug alone. Like other less potent opioids, tramadol can also be used in combination with nonopioids for mild to moderate pain. For example, in patients in whom the pain of osteoarthritis flares was not relieved by stable NSAID therapy, adding tramadol, 250 mg/day, for nearly 2 weeks resulted in significantly less pain at rest and less intense pain during movement. Like tramadol alone, tramadol combined with acetaminophen (Ultracet) can also be an effective add-on therapy for osteoarthritis pain flares in patients taking NSAIDs. Moreover, in patients at high risk of NSAID side effects, tramadol can also be used to reduce the dose of NSAIDs required to control pain. For instance, in patients with osteoarthritis of the knee who required 1000 mg/day of naproxen for pain relief, adding tramadol, 200 mg/day, allowed the naproxen dose to be reduced by three quarters without compromising pain control.

Adverse Effects and Safety

Because of reliance on outdated and biased study results, the addictive potential of opioid therapy for chronic pain has been exaggerated. A well-controlled study found that only four cases of addiction occurred in nearly 12,000 hospitalized patients who received opioids.[26] Thus, the risk of addiction appears low in patients with organic pain and no history of substance abuse, and such a history is not an absolute contraindication to opioid therapy if the patient is responsible and can be monitored carefully. Another excessively feared side effect of opioid therapy is respiratory depression, which can usually be prevented by carefully titrating the dose in response to pain. Careful dose titration is particularly important in patients with sleep apnea, in whom respiratory depression is especially dangerous.

Unlike NSAIDs, sustained-release opioids have not been shown to cause organ toxicity and therefore may be useful in treating patients with contraindications to NSAIDs such as renal insufficiency. Hydromorphone is particularly useful for patients with renal failure because none of its metabolites is active. However, morphine has several active metabolites whose levels vary with renal or hepatic function and its use is thus contraindicated in patients with renal or hepatic insufficiency. Unlike other opioids, the short-acting agent propoxyphene may result in cardiac toxicity owing to accumulation of one of its metabolites and thus should be avoided in patients at high risk of cardiovascular disease.

Opioids do not pose the risk of stomach ulcer, bleeding, or elevated blood pressure posed by NSAIDs. Thus, they can be particularly useful in treating patients with ulcer, bleeding diathesis, or hypertension. However, high doses of opioids may cause peripheral edema, which can be managed by a short course of diuretics. Opioids may also cause nausea, vomiting, constipation, cognitive impairment, dizziness, and drowsiness. The incidence of such side effects varies by agent. For example, although its analgesic effects are similar to those of morphine, hydromorphone, like oxycodone, has fewer side effects than morphine, which is more likely to cause nausea and pruritus than other opioids. Adverse effects tend to occur only upon initiation of therapy and decrease with increasing duration of treatment. They can usually be minimized with low initial doses and careful dose titration. Moreover, because opioid receptors also have a stimulatory function whose activation is responsible for many of the adverse effects of opioids, combining minuscule doses of opioid antagonists such as naltrexone and nalmefene with opioids can also minimize adverse effects.

If side effects remain but pain control is good, nausea can be controlled with prochlorperazine or promethazine given three to four times daily for a few days or, in some patients, with antihistamines such as hydroxyzine. Postprandial nausea, bloating, and early satiety can be controlled by metoclopramide, 10 to 20 mg three times daily. Although constipation may be persistent, it can be controlled with osmotic laxatives such as milk of magnesia, magnesium citrate, or lactulose, which are safer than bowel stimulants such as bisacodyl (Dulcolax). However, because opioid-related constipation results from lack of peristalsis, stool softeners alone are often ineffective. Compared with other sustained-release opioids, fentanyl causes less constipation because it does not enter the gastrointestinal tract.

Athletes who experience drowsiness during initiation of opioid therapy should be warned to limit activities while the dose is being titrated. Another approach is to reduce the dose by 25% until drowsiness resolves. If it persists, other sedating medications, such as antihistamines and antiemetics, may need to be eliminated or their doses decreased. In patients receiving long-term opioid therapy, sedation may indicate that osteoarthritis and its related pain are resolving and that the dose of pain medication should be tapered. Thus, assessing patients for sedation is particularly important after a new osteoarthritis therapy is added to the treatment regimen.

Other common side effects of opioid therapy include hives and itching. These adverse effects may result from the direct effect of opioids on mast cells, are more common with naturally occurring agents than synthetics, and can be controlled with nonsedating antihistamines. However, although tramadol may have less adverse impact on the immune system than other opioids, itchy rash appears to be a true hypersensitivity reaction and indicates that a patient is not a good candidate for continued therapy. Other adverse reactions to tramadol include pruritus, diarrhea, asthenia, and headache. Tramadol has also been associated with seizures, especially when taken with other opioids or selective serotonin reuptake inhibitors. However, its potential for drug interactions with highly protein-bound agents is minimal owing to its low degree of plasma protein binding.

Some patients receiving opioid therapy may experience myoclonus, which can be treated with clonazepam, a less sedating benzodiazepine than other drugs in its class. Opioids may also increase bladder sphincter tone and thereby cause urinary retention. Moreover, because opioids may also adversely affect the endocrine system and result in sexual dysfunction, patients should be warned that such dysfunction may occur and reassured that it is reversible.

REFERENCES

1. Amadio P, Cummings DM. Evaluation of acetaminophen in the management of osteoarthritis of the knee. Curr Ther Res 1983;34:59–66
2. Case JP, Baliunas AJ, Block JA. Lack of efficacy of acetaminophen in treating symptomatic knee osteoarthritis. Arch Intern Med 2003;163:169–178
3. Rahme E, Pettitt D, LeLorier J. Determinants and sequelae associated with utilization of acetaminophen versus traditional nonsteroidal antiinflammatory drugs in an elderly population. Arthritis Rheum 2002;46:3046–3054
4. Garcia Rodriguez LA, Hernandez-Diaz S. Risk of upper gastrointestinal complications among users of acetaminophen and nonsteroidal anti-inflammatory drugs. Epidemiology 2001;12:570–576
5. Perneger TV, Whelton PK, Klag MJ. Risk of kidney failure associated with the use of acetaminophen, aspirin, and nonsteroidal anti-inflammatory drugs. N Engl J Med 1994;331:1675–1679
6. Fored CM, Ejerblad E, Lindblad P, et al. Acetaminophen, aspirin and chronic renal failure. N Engl J Med 2001;345:1801–1809
7. Shaheen SO, Sterne JAC, Songhurst CE, Burney PG. Frequent paracetamol use and asthma in adults. Thorax 2000;55:266–270
8. Towheed T, Shea B, Wells G, Hochberg M. Analgesia and non-aspirin, non-steroidal anti-inflammatory drugs for osteoarthritis of the hip (Cochrane Review). In: The Cochrane Library, Issue 3. Oxford: Update Software, 2001
9. Towheed TE, Hochberg MC. A systematic review of randomized controlled trials of pharmacological therapy in osteoarthritis of the hip. J Rheumatol 1997;24:349–357
10. Towheed TE, Hochberg MC. A systematic review of randomized controlled trials of pharmacological therapy in osteoarthritis of the knee, with an emphasis on trial methodology. Semin Arthritis Rheum 1997;26:755–770
11. Watson MC, Brookes ST, Kirwan JR, Faulkner A. Non-aspirin, non-steroidal anti-inflammatory drugs for treating osteoarthritis of the knee (Cochrane Review). In: The Cochrane Library, Issue 3. Oxford: Update Software, 2001
12. Moore RA, Tramer MR, Carroll D, Wiffen PJ, McQuay HJ. Quantitative systematic review of topically applied non-steroidal anti-inflammatory drugs. BMJ 1998;316:333–338
13. Eccles M, Freemantle N, Mason J, for the North of England Non-Steroidal Anti-Inflammatory Drug Guideline Development Group. North of England evidence based guideline development project: summary guideline for non-steroidal anti-inflammatory drugs versus basic analgesia in treating the pain of degenerative arthritis. BMJ 1998;317:526–530
14. Bradley JD, Katz BP, Brandt KD. Severity of knee pain does not predict a better response to an antiinflammatory dose of ibuprofen than to analgesic therapy in patients with osteoarthritis. J Rheumatol 2001;28:1073–1076
15. Sandler DP, Burr R, Weinberg CR. Nonsteroidal anti-inflammatory drugs and the risk for chronic renal disease. Ann Intern Med 1991;115:165–172
16. Offman JJ, MacLean CH, Straus WL, et al. A metaanalysis of severe upper gastrointestinal complications of nonsteroidal antiinflammatory drugs. J Rheumatol 2002;29:804–812
17. Huang J-Q, Sridhar S, Hunt RH. Role of Helicobacter pylori infection and non-steroidal anti-inflammatory drugs in peptic ulcer disease: a meta analysis. Lancet 2002;359:14–22
18. Chan FK, To KF, Wu JC, et al. Eradication of Helicobacter pylori and risk of peptic ulcers in patients starting long-term treatment with non-steroidal anti-inflammatory drugs: a randomised trial. Lancet 2002;359:9–13
19. Ray WA, Stein CM, Hall K, Daugherty JR, Griffin MR. Non-steroidal anti-inflammatory drugs and risk of serious coronary heart disease: an observational cohort study. Lancet 2002;359:118–123
20. National Institute for Clinical Excellence Technology Appraisal Guidance No. 27. Guidance on the use of cyclo-oxygenase (COX) II selective inhibitors celecoxib, rofecoxib, meloxicam and etodolac for osteoarthritis and rheumatoid arthritis, 2001
21. Silverstein FE, Faich G, Goldstein JL, et al. Gastrointestinal toxicity with celecoxib versus nonsteroidal anti-inflammatory drugs for osteoarthritis and rheumatoid arthritis. JAMA 2000;284:1247–1255
22. Bombardier C, Laine L, Reicin A, et al. Comparison of upper gastrointestinal toxicity of rofecoxib and naproxen in patients with rheumatoid arthritis. N Engl J Med 2000;343:1520–1528

23. Hrachovec JB. Reporting of 6-month vs 12-month data in a clinical trial of celecoxib. JAMA 2001;286:2398, author reply 2399–2400
24. Portenoy RK, Foley KM. Chronic use of opioid analgesics in non-malignant pain: report of 38 cases. Pain 1986;25:171–186
25. Zenz M, Strumpf M, Tryba M. Long-term oral opioid therapy in patients with chronic non-malignant pain. J Pain Symptom Manage 1992;7:69–77
26. Porter J, Jick H. Addiction rare in patients treated with narcotics. N Engl J Med 1980;302:123

9

Glucosamine and Chondroitin Sulfate

RONALD A. NAVARRO

Osteoarthritis (OA) is an imbalance between the synthesis and degradation of cartilage that occurs in synovial joints.[1] It is characterized by disturbance in the smooth property of the cartilage, which results in the formation of subchondral cysts and marginal osteophytes.[2] Bone spurs may also form around the joint as the body's response. This process occurs until all layers of cartilage are lost, leaving only the bone layer.

Currently, the aim of OA treatment is to reduce pain and stiffness. Its management consists of pharmacologic and nonpharmacologic therapies. Pharmacologic treatment of OA begins with acetaminophen, adding a low-dose nonsteroidal antiinflammatory drug (NSAID), salicylate, selective cyclooxygenase-2 (COX-2) inhibitor, or topical capsaicin cream if needed. Analgesics or NSAIDs are the most common subscribed noninvasive treatment for reducing pain associated with early cases of OA. Pain reduction can also be achieved by nonpharmacologic treatment, for example, physical therapy and decreasing the load on the joint by changing the patient's lifestyle (e.g., weight loss and stress reduction). This can be challenging but of great benefit.[3] In more severe cases joint injections, irrigation, or arthroscopy may be beneficial. In patients who continue to have pain and limited function despite these measures, surgical intervention should be considered.[1] Although NSAIDs have definite effect in pain reduction, up to 2% of patients per year have severe gastrointestinal problems after prolonged intake.[4] Another important side effect is that with long-term usage of some of the NSAIDs, synthesis of cartilage matrix might be inhibited.[5]

The drawbacks of the long-term use of NSAIDs has inspired researchers to investigate agents that can help patients with OA with minimal or no side effects. A new class of agents termed symptomatic or disease modifying osteoarthritic drugs (S/DMOADs) is receiving wide publicity in the United States.[6] The results of 10+ years of investigation including 40 human clinical trials and over 300 studies overall in animals and in vitro can be summarized as follows: S/DMOADs demonstrate clinical efficacy in symptomatic relief of OA with little or no side effects, retard progression of arthritic lesions in animal models of OA, and in at least one clinical study show evidence of cartilage regeneration. Studies were conducted on nutraceuticals, such as chondroitin sulfate and glucosamine, to demonstrate their efficacy in the symptomatic treatment of OA. Meta-analyses reviewed clinical trials of the glucosamine and chondroitin, S/DMOADs, in the treatment of osteoarthritis. It was concluded that clinical trials of these two agents showed substantial benefit in the treatment of osteoarthritis, although they provided insufficient information about study design and conduct.[6–8]

■ Nutraceuticals and the Food and Drug Administration

The scientific community, nevertheless, expressed a high degree of skepticism toward nutraceuticals based on the concerns about the lack of quality control and of scientific testing of claims. The reason is that these substances are not Food and Drug Administration (FDA) regulated, and as a result, there is no requirement for rigorous scientific testing prior to marketing. The Dietary Supplement Health and Education Act (DSHEA) of 1994 established additional requirements for safety and made provisions for four categories of claims for nutritional support. However, because dietary supplements fall under the same general classification as "foods," there are no specific regulations to assure product quality. What is stated on the label may not reflect the actual composition or purity of the product inside.

The other important factor to consider is the lack of good manufacturing practices that should be in place to guarantee high quality and batch-to-batch consistency. Last and not least is the absence of a validated analytic method for the raw materials, which is the only way manufacturers can verify the purity of their products. Recent published reports of the analysis of randomly purchased dietary supplements have shown a wide deviation from label claim by the majority of products tested. The University of Maryland School of Pharmacy analysis of 32 products containing glucosamine and chondroitin sulfate reported that 84% of tested products did not meet the label claims, and 40% of the products contained less than 30% of the label claims, regardless of retail price. In light of this, when selecting a dietary supplement with reported efficacy in clinical trials, patients should be advised that "brand" does matter. The only way to expect a result from a supplement that is equivalent to that reported in a controlled clinical study is to use the same brand of supplement as used in the study.[9,10]

Therefore, it is not surprising to know that the Arthritis Foundation has recommended that "when a supplement has been studied with good results, find out which brand was used in the study, and buy that."[11]

■ Glucosamine

Glucosamine (GA) is an amino-monosaccharide. It is a precursor of the disaccharide unit of glycosaminoglycan (GAGs) and is reported to stimulate the production of proteoglycans, which is the ground substance of the articular cartilage.[12,13] Glucosamine also stimulates synovial production of hyaluronic acid (HA), which is responsible for the lubricating and shock-absorbing properties of synovial fluid.[14]

Improvement in the symptoms of OA associated with the use of GA has been observed in several clinical trials.[15–17] Reported short-term adverse effects include mild gastrointestinal problems, drowsiness, skin reactions, and headache. Houpt et al[18] conducted a double-blind study in Toronto, Canada investigating the efficacy of the hydrochloride salt of GA on pain and disability in knee OA. Although the primary end point was not met, a

positive trend was noted for the GA group. In addition, the secondary end points of cumulative pain reduction as noted by the patient in a daily diary and as assessed by knee examination were favorable, suggesting that glucosamine hydrochloride benefits some patients with knee OA.

■ Chondroitin Sulfate

Chondroitin sulfate (CS) is an important component of cartilage. Two types of CS exist: chondroitin-4-sulfate and chondroitin-6-sulfate. They vary in molecular weight and thus differ in their bioavailability and purity.[19] Chondroitin-4-sulfate is the most abundant GAG in growing mammalian hyaline cartilage. With age, chondrocytes secrete less chondroitin-4-sulfate and more amounts of the other GAGs. This change has been observed in the initiation and progression of the degenerative process within the cartilage in OA.[20]

Omata et al[21] injected bradykinin into the left knee articular cavities of rats three times a day for 2 days. Chondroitin sulfate was administered orally to rats for 14 days and was shown to inhibit the bradykinin-induced proteoglycan depletion of the articular cartilage in a dose-dependent manner. These results suggest that a reduction of the proteoglycan content of cartilage (similar to findings associated with osteoarthritis) can be inhibited by CS.

In another study, CS inhibited the aggrecanase enzyme in a dose-dependent manner, suggesting its protective effect. This is because aggrecanase has been believed to mediate aggrecans degradation in OA.[22] Several other studies reported similar inhibitory effect of CS on many degradative enzymes.[23]

Because of the large size of the CS, earlier reports voiced concerns about its bioavailability. However, radio-labeled CS given orally to humans was 70% absorbed. Its affinity for synovial fluid and articular cartilage has also been demonstrated.[24] In addition, many clinical trials have documented the clinical efficacy of CS in treating OA, showing significant symptomatic improvement and suggesting a structure modifying effect.[25,26]

■ Combined Therapy with Glucosamine and Chondroitin Sulfate

From the previous sections, it is evident that both CS and GA are effective. Over the years, the combined use of these nutraceuticals in OA treatment has become extremely popular.[3] This is because their use has much fewer side effects than do NSAIDs, and represents the only treatment suggested to prevent progression of the disease in preliminary reports.[25–27]

It is important to note that experimental studies have documented a synergistic effect when GA and CS are administered together. Lippiello et al[28] reported that the coadministration of TRH122(tm) (Nutramax Laboratories, Edgewood, Maryland) low molecular weight sodium chondroitin-4-sulfate and FCHG49(tm) (Nutramax Laboratories, Edgewood, Maryland) glucosamine hydrochloride resulted in a greater increase of GAGs production (96.6%) than for either agent alone (GA, 32%; CS, 32%). The same study showed that while CS inhibited interleukin-1, GA did not. Therefore, it is not a matter of which one is superior; they have two different mechanisms of action, so both of them should be given together to get a better result.

In another study, Woodward et al[29] investigated the efficacy of the same combination of nutraceuticals in modifying the cartilage in an OA model. Fifty percent of the rabbits were fed a regular diet whereas the rest were fed the studied combination in an amount equivalent to 2% of their body weight. At week 16 of the study, samples from the animals' medial condyles were evaluated histologically. The authors concluded that the studied combination has a significant structure-modifying effect in this OA model.

Two randomized, double-blind, placebo-controlled clinical trials investigated the efficacy of the same combination therapy in the management of OA. The first study was by Das et al,[30] who recruited 93 patients with knee OA. They found significant improvement in the treatment group of patients with mild or moderate knee OA at 4 and 6 months, compared with controls. The second 16-week crossover trial was conducted on 34 males from the U.S. Navy. It was also shown that the same combination therapy relieves symptoms of knee OA.[31]

■ Use of Glucosamine and Chondroitin Sulfate in Athletes

The use of S/DMOADs like GA and CS in sports injuries of athletes is a relatively new but promising application and a natural extension of their use in the treatment of osteoarthrosis.[32]

Although clinical trials examining this application have not been performed, a published clinical case study reported on improvement of an osteochondral impaction injury of the femoral head in a female collegiate basketball player. Resolution of pain and physical improvement evidenced by magnetic resonance imaging (MRI) was documented.[33] Other mostly anecdotal reports suggest a need for further controlled clinical investigation.

The direct effect of repetitive impact and torsional loading on articular cartilage especially in the presence of abnormal alignment, joint instability or muscle weakness, elevates the risk for subsequent joint degeneration.[2] Up to 87% of patients with meniscus and ligament injuries of the knee develop degenerative radiologic changes in a 10- to 20-year period.[34] Early OA in young sportsmen has been associated with severe anterolateral instability of the knee[35,36] but impact loading can also produce structural damage and osteoarthritic-like changes.[37] Indeed, a single contusion of cartilage often mimics lesions observed in patients with chondromalacia of the patella.[38]

Traumatic insults of sufficient magnitude may also release cartilage fragments or matrix products, which may engender a secondary inflammatory reaction.[39] Joint inflammation contributes to cartilage degeneration mediated by the action of proteases and inflammatory cytokines. Typically, elevated levels of interleukin-1, interleukin-6, and tumor necrosis factor found in synovial fluids indicate catabolism of articular cartilage associated with an inflamed joint. Hence, the therapeutic value of GA and CS in traumatic and inflammatory arthrosis relies on their ability to affect articular cartilage metabolism and minimize synovial tissue inflammation. In an editorial comment, the point is made that treatment of many young individuals with symptoms of damaged joints lies somewhere between arthroscopic debridement and total joint replacement.[40]

It is in this arena that the S/DMOADs may have the greatest application. For example, a study of 34 Navy Seals undergoing rigorous training was conducted at the Portsmouth Naval Medical Center. In a 16-week crossover trial, 34 males with chronic pain and radiographic degenerative joint disease (DJD) of the knee or low back used a combination of GA hydrochloride, CS, and manganese ascorbate (Cosamin® DS, Nutramax Laboratories, Edgewood, MD).[31] Assessment by summary of disease scores incorporating pain and functional questionnaires, and physical examination scores demonstrated significant improvement in summary disease scores (-16.3%; $p < .05$), patient assessment of treatment effect ($p < .02$), visual analog scale for pain recorded at clinic visits (-26.6%; $p \leq .05$) and physical examination score (-43.3%; $p < .01$). In addition, 93 patients with radiography-confirmed osteoarthritis of the knee participated in a 6-month, placebo-controlled clinical trial.[41] The intervention group received glucosamine hydrochloride, chondroitin sulfate with manganese ascorbate (CosaminDS). Patients were evaluated initially and at 2-month intervals for the course of the study. Primary outcome was assessed with the Lesquene Index of Severity of Osteoarthritis of the Knee (ISK). In the intervention group, patients with radiographically mild or moderate osteoarthritis ($N = 72$) showed significant improvement at 4 and 6 months ($p < .003$ and $p < .04$, respectively). The response rate to supplementation was 52% versus a response rate of 28% to placebo.

Although supporting evidence of efficacy in traumatic injuries to joints is not as extensive as in human OA, this application has the greatest potential for beneficial therapeutic intervention. Long-term, placebo-controlled clinical trials measuring change in tibiofemoral joint space radiographically have demonstrated that both GA and CS can effectively retard progressive narrowing of this joint in patients with mild to moderate osteoarthritis. A 3-year, randomized, placebo-controlled, double-blind study of 202 patients with knee OA reported that patients receiving 1500 mg of GA experienced minimal joint space narrowing while progressive joint space narrowing with placebo use was significantly greater.[42] A similarly controlled and measured 2-year study with CS was conducted with 300 knee OA patients. Both joint space width and joint space thickness decreased significantly in the placebo group; however, no change occurred in the CS group.[43] The difference between groups was significant. The only available evidence that S/DMOADs induce cartilage regeneration is a 3-year clinical trial of patients with OA. Radiographic evaluation indicated that GA administration had effectively increased joint space width.[44]

In animal studies, medication with polysulfated glycosaminoglycans (PSGAGs) enabled exercised carpal joints of equines to be flexed significantly further in an osteochondral defect model in ponies.[45] Intraarticular PSGAG in equines was chondroprotective in a chemically induced model of cartilage damage,[46] and a combination of GA and CS was effective in decreasing lameness in equines with degenerative joint disease.[47]

Scintigraphic evaluation of canines with induced acute synovitis showed that prior treatment with GA and CS had a protective effect on cartilage and reduced bone remodeling associated with the inflammation.[48] The significance of this study is that pretreatment with these agents minimized joint damage associated with inflammation. Additional support that prophylactic application of these agents is beneficial in maintaining joint function following trauma or inflammation was generated in a rat model of experimental immune arthritis. The histopathologic index in animals treated with GA and CS indicated a significant decrease in joint lesions.[49]

Joint instability induced by cruciate ligament transection mimics ligamentous instability associated with athletic trauma. In a canine model GA plus CS modulated cartilage metabolism minimizing degenerative activities.[50] Cruciate ligament transection coupled with partial meniscectomy is a standard instability model of osteoarthritis in rabbits.[51] Oral administration of GA plus CS inhibits the development of severe cartilage lesions in this model with anecdotal evidence of ligament regeneration.[28]

The mechanism of action whereby these agents exert their protective effect on joint tissues is related to their ability to stimulate synthetic activity in articular cartilage and to reduce inflammation (and symptoms associated with inflammation). Exposure of articular cartilage to physical or chemical stress, including mechanical, inflammatory, oxidative, and thermal entities, are possible factors initiating a series of events progressing to degenerative joint disease.[52–54] Under these circumstances, cartilage lesions ultimately develop because the stress-induced metabolic response of articular cartilage is dominated by a catabolic cascade and degradation of cartilage matrix.[55] Progressive degeneration of cartilage lesions is facilitated by a continual excessive or aberrant stress, such as joint instability. In fact, the latter may be the most prominent form of stress induced by athletic injury and the one most likely to lead to joint degeneration.

In more recent findings, chondroprotective agents like GA and CS were shown to enhance the ability of articular cartilage to respond to stress while minimizing inflammation.[56] In addition, preconditioning with a combination of GA and CS substantially improved restoration of joint function following induced synovitis.[49] Hence, therapeutic intervention and prophylactic treatment with these agents may significantly lessen the consequences of joint trauma and stress injury. What is the evidence that these agents function in this capacity? Much of the data are derived from in vitro studies.

■ In Vitro Studies of Glucosamine and Chondroitin Sulfate

In vitro, chondrocytes exposed to GA and CS were stimulated to synthesize new glycosaminoglycans. Further studies confirmed the anabolic activity on synovial tissue with findings of significant increases in the synthesis of proteoglycans and hyaluronic acid.[57,58] In addition to their ability to stimulate synthetic processes in joint cartilage and synovium, CS in particular has anticatabolic (inhibitory) activity on enzymes that degrade articular cartilage.[59] Hence the data generated by metabolic studies and confirmed at the molecular (messenger RNA, mRNA) level suggest that substantial increases in both anabolic and anticatabolic activity result from exposure of joint tissue to either or both agents.[60] In vitro studies also suggest that both GA and CS inhibit cytokine activity, responsible for generation of nitric oxide, proinflammatory prostaglandins, and metalloproteases, all agents that degrade cartilage matrix and elicit in part the clinical symptoms associated with OA.[52–54] It is clear that apoptosis (cell death) of chondrocytes follows exposure to inflammatory mediators[61] so that any reduction in this activity would be beneficial in preserving joint function.

In vitro and in vivo studies have also revealed two unique phenomena concerning the use of GA and CS on articular cartilage. Biosynthetic responses of young normal articular cartilage exposed to these agents are minimal, whereas aged or stressed tissues respond with greater intensity.[56] The increased responsiveness of stressed joint cartilage may reflect the natural increase in sensitivity of chondrocytes (or synoviocytes) previously activated by pathologic processes. Clinically, such activity may result in a greater capacity of articular cartilage to "repair" itself, that is, reconstitute matrix integrity. The second phenomenon is that synthetic processes in chondrocytes are stimulated with a combination of GA and CS to an extent greater than the additive value of each agent alone.[28,60] This synergy most likely results from the different mechanism of action of each agent. A controlled, in vivo animal study conducted in the United States provided evidence of a synergistic response to the combined use of GA and CS when compared with single ingredients and controls.[28] A significant decrease in the severity and number of cartilage lesions ($p < .05$) of the medial femoral condyles (measured by computerized quantitative histologic evaluation) followed the administration of a combination of GA and CS versus either component given alone or controls.[28] These data were verified by assessment of mRNA expression in tissues exposed to each agent alone and in combination.[60]

■ Conclusion

Although definitive clinical studies of the efficacy of S/DMOADs for management of sports-related cartilage injuries is lacking, sufficient controlled, clinical trials have demonstrated symptomatic relief in OA with no significant side effects. Animal models of joint stress have shown a slowing of degenerative change and lessening of inflammation. In addition, published in vitro work indicates that the agents GA and CS initiate an anabolic and anticatabolic effect on cartilage metabolism, which is significantly greater when they are used in combination. These benefits suggest a potential indication for use in professional as well as amateur athletes who have suffered joint trauma.[62]

REFERENCES

1. Rehman Q, Lane NE. Getting control of osteoarthritis pain. An update on treatment options. Postgrad Med 1999;106:127–134
2. Buckwalter JA, Lane NE. Athletics and osteoarthritis. Am J Sports Med 1997;25:873–881
3. Hungerford DS. Treating osteoarthritis with chondroprotective agents. Orthopedic Special Edition 1998;1:39–42
4. Schoenfeld P, Kimmey MB, Scheiman J, Bjorkman D, Laine L. Nonsteroidal anti inflammatory drug-associated gastrointestinal complications-guidelines for prevention and treatment. Aliment Pharmacol Ther 1999;13:1273–1285
5. Brandt K. Nonsteroidal anti-inflammatory drugs and articular cartilage. J Rheumatol 1987;14(suppl):132–133
6. Deal CL, Moskowitz RW. Nutraceuticals as therapeutic agents in osteoarthritis. The role of glucosamine, chondroitin sulfate, and collagen hydrolysate. Rheum Dis Clin North Am 1999;25:379–395
7. Barclay TS, Tsourounis C, McCart GM. Glucosamine. Ann Pharmacother 1998;32:574–579
8. McAlindon TE, LaValley MP, Gulin JP, Felson DT. Glucosamine and chondroitin treatment for osteoarthritis. A systematic quality assessment and meta-analysis. JAMA 2000;283:1469–1475
9. Adebowale A, Cox D, Liang Z, Eddington N. Analysis of glucosamine and chondroitin sulfate content in marketed products and the caco-2 permeability of chondroitin sulfate raw materials. JANA 2000;3:37–44
10. Russell AS, Aghazadeh-Habashi A, Jamali F. Active ingredient consistency of commercially available glucosamine sulfate products. J Rheumatol 2002;29:2407–2409
11. Horstman J. Arthritis Foundation's Guide to Alternative Therapies. Atlanta, GA: Arthritis Foundation, 1999.
12. Burkhardt D, Gosh P. Laboratory evaluation of antiarthritic drugs as potential chondroprotective agents. Semin Arthritis Rheum 1987;17:3–34
13. Piperno M, Reboul P, Hellio Le Graverand MP, et al. Glucosamine sulfate modulates dysregulated activities of human osteoarthritic chondrocytes in vitro. Osteoarthritis Cartilage 2000;8(3):207–212
14. McCarty MF. Enhanced synovial production of hyaluronic acid may explain rapid clinical response to high-dose glucosamine in osteoarthritis. Med Hypotheses 1998;50:507–510
15. Drovanti A, Bignamini AA, Rovati AL. Therapeutic activity of oral glucosamine sulfate in osteoarthritis: a placebo-controlled double-blind investigation. Clin Ther 1980;3:260–272
16. Reichelt A. Forster KK, Fischer M, Rovati LC, Setnikar I. Efficacy and safety of intramuscular glucosamine sulfate in osteoarthritis of the knee. Arzneimittelforschung 1994;44:75–80
17. Vaz AL. Double-blind clinical evaluation of the relative efficacy of ibuprofen and glucosamine sulphate in the management of osteoarthrosis of the knee in outpatient. Curr Med Res Opin 1982;8:145–149
18. Houpt JB, McMillan R, Wein C, Paget-Dellio SD. Effect of glucosamine hydrochloride in the treatment of pain of osteoarthritis of the knee. J Rheumatol 1999;26:2423–2430
19. Das A. Treatment of osteoarthritis with chondroprotective agents. Orthop Special Ed 1999;5:1–4
20. Ronca F, Palmieri L, Panicucci P, Ronca G. Anit-inflammatory activity of chondroitin sulfate. Osteoarthritis Cartilage 1998;6, suppl. A:14–21
21. Omata T, Segawa Y, Itokazu Y, Inoue N, Tanaka Y. Effects of chondroitin sulfate-C on bradykinin-induced proteoglycan depletion in rats. Arzneimittelforschung 1999;49:577–581
22. Sugimoto K, Takahashi M, Yamamoto Y, Shimada K, Tanzawa K. Identification of aggrecanase activity in medium of cartilage culture. J Biochem (Tokyo) 1999;126:449 455
23. Paroli E, Antonilli L, Biffoni M. Pharmacological approach to glycosaminoglycans. Drugs Exp Clin Res 1991;8:9–20

24. Conte A, Volpi N, Palmiera L, Bahous I, Ronca G. Biochemical and pharmacokinetic aspects of oral treatment with chondroitin sulfate. Drug Res 1995;45:918–925

25. Uebelhart D, Thonar EJ, Delmas PD, Chantraine A, Vignon E. Effects of oral chondroitin sulfate on the progression of knee osteoarthritis: a pilot study. Osteoarthritis Cartilage 1998;6(suppl A):39–46

26. Verbrugeen G, Goemaere S, Veys EM. Chondroitin sulfate S/DMOAD (structure/disease modifying antiosteoarthritis (OA) drug) in the treatment of finger joint OA. Osteoarthritis Cartilage 1998;6, suppl. A:37–38

27. Fillmore CM, Bartoli L, Bach R, Park Y. Nutrition and dietary supplements. Phys Med Rehabil Clin N Am 1999;10:673–703

28. Lippiello L, Woodward J, Karpman R, Hammad TA. In vivo chondroprotection and metabolic synergy of glucosamine and chondroitin sulfate. Clin Orthop Rel Res 2000;381:229–240

29. Woodward JK, Lippiello L, Karpman R. Beneficial effect of dietary chondroprotective agents in a rabbit instability model of osteoarthrosis. Proceedings of the 66th Annual Meeting of the American Academy of Orthopedic Surgeons, 1999, Anaheim, CA, paper No. 48

30. Das AK, Hammad T, Eitel J. Efficacy of a combination of glucosamine hydrochloride, sodium chondroitin sulfate and manganese ascorbate in the management of knee osteoarthritis: a randomized double-blind placebo-controlled clinical trial. Annual meeting of the American Association of Hip and Knee Surgeons, November 8, 1998

31. Leffler CT, Philippi AF, Leffler SG, Mosure JC, Kim PD. Glucosamine, chondroitin, and manganese ascorbate for degenerative joint disease of the knee or low back Mil Med 1999;164:85–91

32. Hungerford D, Navarro RA, Hammad T. Use of nutraceuticals in the management of osteoarthritis. JANA 2000;3:23–27

33. Schenck RC Jr, Clair DJ, Gilley JS, et al. Role of a glucosamine/chondroitin sulfate formula in treatment of an osteochondral impaction injury in a collegiate basketball player. Ortho Tech Rev 2000;2:12–15

34. Messner K. Current advances in sports-related cartilage research. Meniscus and ligament injuries are associated with increased risk of knee joint arthrosis. Lakartidningen 1998;95:4611–4612

35. Graham GP, Fairclough JA. Early osteoarthritis in young sportsmen with severe anterolateral instability of the knee. Injury 1988;19:247–248

36. Roos H. Are there long-term sequelae from soccer? Clin Sports Med 1998;17:819–831

37. Levin A, Burton-Wurster N, Chen CT, Lust G. Intercellular signaling as a cause of cell death in cyclically impacted cartilage explants. Osteoarthritis Cartilage 2001;9:702–711

38. Gedeon P, Mazieres B, Ficat P. A new model of experimental arthrosis: contusion of the cartilage. Experimental and clinical study. Rev Rhum Mal Osteoartic 1978;45:401–408

39. Howell DS, Pita JC, Woessner JF. Which comes first: Crystals, necrosis or inflammation. J Rheumatol 1983;10(suppl 9):59–61

40. Leach RE. Osteoarthritis—a sports medicine problem? Am J Sports Med 1999;27:1

41. Das AK, Hammad TA. Efficacy of a combination of FCHG49 glucosamine hydrochloride, TRHI22 low molecular weight sodium chondroitin sulfate and manganese ascorbate in the management of knee osteoarthritis. Osteoarthritis Cartilage 2000;8:343–350

42. Pavelka K, Gatterova J, Olejarova M, et al. Glucosamine sulfate use and delay of progression of knee osteoarthritis. A three year, randomized, placebo controlled double blind study. Arch Intern Med 2002;162:2113–2123

43. Michel B, Vignon E, Vathaire F, et al. Oral chondroitin sulfate in knee OA patients: radiographic outcomes of a two year prospective study. Trans Ortho Res Soc 2001;2:S68 (Abst)

44. Reginster JY, Deroisy R, Rovati LC, et al. Long-term effects of glucosamine sulphate on osteoarthritis progression: a randomized, placebo-controlled clinical trial. Lancet 2001;357:251–256

45. Todhunter RJ, Minor RR, Wootton JA, Krook L, Burton-Wurster N, Lust G. Effects of exercise and polysulfated glycosaminoglycan on repair of articular cartilage defects in the equine carpus. J Orthop Res 1993;11:782–795

46. Yovich JV, Trotter GW, McIlwraith CW, Norrdin RW. Effects of polysulfated glycosaminoglycan on chemical and physical defects in equine articular cartilage. Am J Vet Res 1987;48:1407–1414

47. Hanson RR, Smalley LR, Huff GK, White S, Hammad TA. Oral treatment with a glucosamine-chondroitin sulfate compound for degenerative joint disease in horses: 25 cases. Equine Practice 1997;19:16–20

48. Canapp SO, McLlaughlin RM, Hoskinson JJ, Roush JK, Butine MD. Scintigraphic evaluation of dogs with acute synovitis after treatment with glucosamine hydrochloride and chondroitin sulfate. Am J Vet Res 1999;60:1552–1557

49. Beren J, Hill SL, Diener-West M, Rose NR. Effect of pre-loading oral glucosamine HCL/chondroitin sulfate/manganese ascorbate combination on experimental arthritis in rats. Proc Exp Biol Med 2001;226:144–151

50. Johnson KA, Hulse DA, Hart RC, Kochevar D, Chu Q. Effects of an orally administered mixture of chondroitin sulfate, glucosamine HCL and manganese ascorbate on synovial fluid chondroitin sulfate 3B3 and 7D4 epitope in a canine cruciate ligament transection model of osteoarthritis. Osteoarthritis Cartilage 2001;9:14–21

51. Moskowitz RW, Davis W, Sammarco J. Experimentally induced degenerative joint lesions following partial meniscectomy in the rabbit. Arthritis Rheum 1973;16:397–405

52. Meyer GF, Ratcliffe BC, Mow VC. The effects of matrix compression on proteoglycan metabolism in articular cartilage explants. Osteoarthritis Cartilage 1994;2:91–101

53. Mazzetti I, Grigolo B, Pulsatelli L, et al. Differential roles of nitric oxide and oxygen radicals in chondrocytes affected by osteoarthritis and rheumatoid arthritis. Clin Sci 2001;101:593–599

54. Fernandes JC, Martel-Pelletier J, Pelletier JP. The role of cytokines in osteoarthritis pathophysiology. Biorheology 2002;39:237–246

55. Mankin HJ. The metabolism of articular cartilage in health and disease. In: Burleigh PMC, Poole AR, ed. Dynamics of Connective Tissue Macromolecules. Amsterdam, Holland: North Holland Publishers, 1975:189–215

56. Lippiello L. Articular cartilage response to the chondroprotective agents glucosamine and chondroitin sulfate under simulated conditions of joint stress (abstract). Annual meeting of the American Orthopaedics Society for Sports Medicine 2002, Orlando, FL

57. Bobacz K, Erlacher L, Graninger WB. The effect of chondrosulf (sodium chondroitin sulfate) on proteoglycan synthesis by human osteoarthritic and bovine juvenile articular cartilage chondrocytes—an in vitro study. Acta Med Austriaca 2002;29:20–25

58. McCarty MF, Russell AL, Seed MP. Sulfated glycosaminoglycans and glucosamine may synergize in promoting synovial hyaluronic acid synthesis. Medical Hypothesis 2000;54:798–802

59. Gouze JN, Bioanchi A, Dauca M, et al. Glucosamine modulates IL-1-induced activation of rat chondrocytes at a receptor level, and by inhibiting the NF-kappa B pathway. FEBS Lett 2002;510:166–170

60. Mims TT, O'Grady C, Marwin S, Grande DA. Effects of dietary supplements on cartilage metabolism and its potential role in osteoarthritis. Trans Ortho Res Soc (Abst.) 2000;25:240

61. Conrozier T. Death of articular chondrocytes. Mechanisms and protection. Presse Med 1998;27:1859–1861

62. Navarro RA. New concepts in the management of osteoarthritis. Orthopaedic Special Edition 2001;7:51–54

10

Hyaluronic Acid Injections: Viscosupplementation

RONALD A. NAVARRO AND JULIAN PAUL BALLESTEROS

With the rise in participation in both organized and recreational sports in the United States, the number of athletes with sports-related medical complaints has grown.[1] Acute injuries to joints and subacute or chronic joint pain are prevalent among athletes of all levels and are common reasons for visits to the general orthopaedist. Presently, a narrow spectrum of satisfactory nonoperative treatment regimens is available for such patients. The introduction of viscosupplementation via intraarticular injection of hyaluronic acids (HAs) offers an intriguing potential solution for many chondral pathologies in athletes.

■ Basic Science of Viscosupplementation

Numerous published reports have advocated the use of HA viscosupplementation in patients with symptomatic osteoarthritis, especially of the knee.[2–10] Understanding the mechanism of action of HAs is necessary to extrapolate the benefits of their use to patient-athletes. HAs are included in a class of molecules known as glycosaminoglycans (GAGs), and are composed of repeating polysaccharide units of glucuronic acid and *N*-acetylglucosamine. They are found in all human tissues, with the highest concentration in connective tissues and body fluids, especially synovial fluid.[11] In the extracellular matrix of articular cartilage, HAs provide intricate mechanical stability for both the chondrocytes that reside there and the type II collagen molecules that the cells manufacture.[12] The occurrence of HAs in synovial fluid is also

pivotal in the maintenance of articular cartilage. Because of the large molecular weight [up to 10×10^6 dalton (d)] of HAs, synovial fluid acts as a non-Newtonian solution. Therefore, it serves as a lubricant during normal movements of the joint (high viscosity/low elasticity) and as a shock absorber when more severe loading forces are withstood (low viscosity/high elasticity[3]). Much of the role HAs play in both articular cartilage and synovial fluid is understood because of research regarding osteoarthritis, a state in which it is known that HA concentration and molecular weight is significantly decreased.[13,14] These findings have also been noted in athletes and attributed to the cyclic loading impact sustained during athletic participation that can initiate or propagate such changes.[15,16] The lack of abundant, physiologically sound hyaluronan molecules deters the usual joint lubrication and protection, which leads to breakdown of cartilage matrix constitution, inflammatory changes, and the pain described by patients with degenerative joint disease.

■ Types of Commercially Available Hyaluronic Acids

There are currently three preparations of hyaluronan that are approved in the United States for intraarticular therapy in patients with arthritis pain of the knee. Sodium hyaluronate (Hyalgan®, Sanofi-Synthelabo, New York, NY) and hylan G-F 20 (Synvisc®, Wyeth Pharmaceuticals, Madison, NJ) were approved by the Food and Drug Administration in 1997; sodium hyaluronate

(Supartz®, Smith and Nephew, Memphis, TN) was approved in 2001.[17–19] All three are extracted from rooster combs but purified differently by each manufacturer. Other HA therapies are available overseas or are still in development. The main differences in the forms available in the United States are based on preparation, molecular weight, dose, and frequency of administration as intraarticular injections for patients with osteoarthritis of the knee. Synvisc is a much larger molecule than the other two, averaging more than 6000 kd (compared with average molecular weights of 500–730 kd and 620–1170 kd for Hyalgan and Supartz, respectively) by virtue of the cross-linking of hyaluronan molecules.

The importance of molecular weight differences is debatable. It was initially thought that viscosupplementation should consist of hyaluronan molecules of higher molecular weight than those naturally occurring to restore synovial fluid viscosity by resisting breakdown and catabolism. On the other hand, smaller HA molecules should theoretically have the ability to more effectively penetrate articular cartilage to restore the matrix and chondrocyte support lost in arthritic tissue. In fact, there are data to support some therapeutic benefit of small, moderate, and large preparations of HAs.[5,6,20–23] Furthermore, despite evidence demonstrating that actual intraarticular duration of exogenous HAs is between one and a few days, clinical pain relief has been shown to persist for months, suggesting an in vivo biologic modification of joint architecture.[2,7,24–26] A more viscous and elastic HA is seen in the synovial fluid.[14] HAs have been seen to promote endogenous HA synthesis and inhibit induction of degradative enzymes.[21] Additional benefits of antiinflammatory activity by inhibition of induction of proinflammatory signals[27] as well as a direct analgesic effect via nociceptors have also been documented.[28] Most of the commercial preparations call for between three and five injections, given once per week over 3 to 5 weeks.[29]

■ Adverse Effects of Hyaluronic Acids

To date, the most common adverse effect of intraarticular viscosupplementation with HA has been acute local inflammatory reactions, which is reflected in the prescribing information of all three commercially available preparations.[17–19] It is difficult to determine the rate with which these reactions occur or the magnitude of their severity due to the different incidences published in the literature; however, in general HA injections have been well tolerated.[9,30] Characterized by pain, effusions, and warmth with difficulty ambulating, most of these episodes were mild and lasted no more than a few days.[31] Although under investigation, the mechanism of these reactions remains unclear. Serum antibodies to chicken serum proteins were found in one patient, suggesting the reactions could be due to allergic response to HA injection components.[31] Another possibility for such reactions may be extraarticular soft tissue injections, as was demonstrated by a study determining that intraarticular needle placement accuracy may be as low as 71% depending on the experience of the administrator and which approach is used.[32]

Additionally, no known contraindications due to drug interactions have been reported thus far, and HAs have not been associated with abnormalities in liver or renal laboratory values.[32] Continued monitoring for and reporting of adverse effects of HA use is warranted.

■ Hyaluronic Acid and Osteoarthritis

Forster and Straw[33] recently studied 38 patients with symptomatic knee arthritis without mechanical symptoms and randomized them to HA injections versus arthroscopic washout. Pre- and postintervention assessments with a visual analog scale (VAS) for pain, Knee Society function score, and the Lequesne Index revealed no difference between the groups at all data collection points up to 1 year. The authors concluded that HA therapy can be considered an alternative to arthroscopy in this patient group, but results can be strengthened with longer follow-up.

Jubb et al[34] compared HA therapy with saline placebo and investigated the structural changes, as measured by joint space narrowing (JSN) within the medial knee. Patients received either three weekly injections of commercially available HA or a placebo vehicle of saline. The course was repeated twice more at four monthly intervals and concomitant treatment with analgesics or NSAIDs was allowed. At 52 weeks 319 out of 408 total had completed the study (HA: $n = 160$, saline: $n = 159$). Only 273 were included in the primary analysis and there was no statistically significant difference between the groups. When assessing for baseline JSN, a difference was measured. In those with radiologically milder disease at baseline and receiving HA, the JSN was significantly reduced compared with placebo ($p = .02$). This assessment is supported by the belief that HA can work better if there is cartilaginous substrate it can work with. Patients with milder disease have less wear of native articular cartilage and therefore have a cartilaginous substrate where the exogenous HA can have an effect.

In a recent prospective, randomized trial of 100 patients, corticosteroid and hyaluronic acid injections were studied for treatment of knee osteoarthritis.[35] The authors tested the hypothesis that there was no difference between Hylan GF-20 and the corticosteroid betamethasone sodium phosphate-betamethasone acetate in terms of pain relief or improved function. All patients given HA received three weekly injections, whereas the steroid injection group received one and could receive another during the 6-month course of the study. A blinded evaluator assessed the patients with the Western Ontario and McMaster University Osteoarthritis Index (WOMAC), a modification of the Knee Society rating system, and the VAS for pain. In the aggregate, no significant differences between the two treatment groups were found with respect to the WOMAC, Knee Society system, or VAS results. However, women demonstrated a significant improvement in only one of the six possible outcome-treatment combinations (the WOMAC scale), whereas men demonstrated significant improvements in five of the six outcomes (all measures except the Knee Society rating system). Because women demonstrated significantly less response to treatment than men did for both treatments on all three outcome scales, the authors believe such significant gender-related differences warrant further investigation.

In another study comparing HA and corticosteroid injections specifically in female patients with knee osteoarthritis,[36] 60 female patients were randomized to three weekly intraarticular injections of 30 mg sodium hyaluronate (Na HA) with a high molecular weight (1.0 to 2.9 million d) or 40 mg 6-methylprednisolone acetate (6-MPA). The clinical assessments included pain at rest, at weight bearing, and on walking; the Lequesne Index; and active range of knee flexion. Assessments were done at baseline, at week 4, and at months 3 and 6. A significant decrease in VAS scores for pain at rest, at weight bearing and pain on walking, and in the Lequesne Index was found in both groups at week 4 when compared with baseline, and there was no significant differences between the two groups. However at month 3, improvement in all pain scores and the Lequesne Index was found in favor of hyaluronic acid. At the month 6 time period, no significant difference was found between the treatment groups. Improvement in pain was accompanied by an increase in joint flexion at week 4 and at month 3 in both groups. Both treatments were well tolerated. The authors believed that the results showed that both intraarticular HA and 6-MPA treatments provide clinically significant improvement, and demonstrated that Na HA has a long-term beneficial effect in patients with knee osteoarthritis.

In a study aimed at assessing the efficacy of repeat treatment cycles of intraarticular HA,[37] 49 of 108 patients had a repeat course administered (the other 59 patients had only a single treatment cycle) because they continued to fulfill the inclusion criteria, but the repeat was done no earlier than month 4 after the first cycle of five injections. The primary efficacy parameter was pain on movement measured by VAS. Secondary parameters were pain on movement and pain at rest (5-point Likert ordinal rating scale), pain at rest (VAS), knee joint function (Larson scale), walking time, and global assessment of efficacy. There were significant improvements in all efficacy parameters compared with the baseline values starting from 1 week after the last injection until month 12 for the 59 completed patients and for all 108 enrolled patients. Safety and tolerability of HA were good or very good in more than 90% of patients. Of four patients who withdrew because of adverse events, only one event (knee joint effusion) was judged as possibly drug related. Two other adverse events judged to be drug related (generalized skin eruption; pruritus and knee joint effusion) resolved and did not lead to study withdrawal. The authors believed that the results of this observational study suggest that HA, administered either as a single or repeat course, is an effective and well-tolerated therapy for the long-term treatment of the pain of OA.

A well done study looked at the long-term efficacy on intraarticular HA in moderate to severe osteoarthritis.[38] The author studied a regimen of five weekly intraarticular injections of sodium hyaluronate in 76 patients (92 knees) with moderate to severe osteoarthritis of the knee in which the pain was not controlled by conventional measures. Thirteen patients had a repeat treatment course. A total of 72% of patients achieved >50% improvement (defined by physical examination and assessment of pain using a VAS) for 1 year or longer; 9% of patients failed to achieve >50% improvement for any period of time. The duration of response exceeded 2 years in some patients. Total knee replacement surgery was avoided or significantly delayed in 15 of 19 patients who were considering surgery prior to the injections. Ten of 15 (67%) knees improved after a repeat treatment course. Local adverse events were minor and infrequent. In this setting, the authors believed intraarticular sodium hyaluronate was an effective and safe treatment for pain in difficult-to-treat patients with moderate to severe OA of the knee.

■ Potential Application of Hyaluronic Acid to High-Endurance Athletes

The proposed augmentation of both synovial fluid viscosity and articular cartilage constitution could theoretically be of benefit to high-endurance athletes such as marathoners. Published data extolling the resulting clinical syndrome of osteoarthritis from repeated loading forces upon joints are prevalent in the orthopaedic literature.[13,15,16,39] Although a role in articular cartilage protection has yet to be advocated, animal meniscectomy models of osteoarthritis have indicated that a diminished degree of degeneration in joints treated with intraarticular HAs is witnessed when compared with controls.[23,40] If further research continues to bear out a safeguarding effect against arthritis, HAs may one day be in great demand by high-endurance athletes as are current products such as shoes, inserts, and orthotic braces that assert enhanced cushioning and shock absorption.

Older runners who experience limitation of desired distance or frequency secondary to knee pain from osteoarthritis would be the most obvious beneficiaries of the purported augmentation offered by HAs, but patients suffering from additional joint pain may also be interested in viscosupplementation. Although not yet approved for use in joints other than the knee, a study has already shown improvement of pain and mobility in degenerative hip joints injected with HAs.[41] Younger athletes with early degenerative joint disease from previous trauma may also benefit from visocosupplementation as their use has been proposed in the shoulder and ankle.

■ Application of Hyaluronic Acid to Acutely Injured Athletes

The acutely injured athlete or elite level athlete may also regard HA with interest as the incidence or recognition of injuries to articular cartilage becomes more frequent. A recent study of magnetic resonance imaging (MRI) scans obtained from 34 presumably asymptomatic knees of Division I college basketball players revealed that 41% had bone marrow edema and 41% had abnormal cartilage signal or focal abnormality.[42] It is likely that many players are not entirely forthright about their symptomatology, as playing time is often at stake for players who report having pain; therefore, it is impossible to determine how many of these players were in fact asymptomatic. In any event, it is reasonable to predict that a significant percentage of these players, whether or not they experience knee pain (or are honest about such pain), could potentially suffer from early-onset osteoarthritis, as the correlation has been made that bone marrow edema can predict for this.[43]

As MRI becomes more economical and prevalent, the indications for its utilization earlier in the protocol for evaluation of injured amateur athletes will likely expand as has occurred in the ranks of professional athletes. Breathless reports in newspapers recounting official statements from teams that an MRI will be done to determine the extent of the injury to the star player are frequently followed by news that the MRI revealed only a "bone bruise" and no ligament damage. It is unclear how significant such injuries are for athletes and how much subsequent time is lost to associated rest and rehabilita-

tion. If it is found that a correlation exists between traumatic bone bruising and significant time away from athletic participation, then viscosupplementation may play a role in athletes with documented bone bruises to decrease healing time and return the athlete to competition more rapidly. In addition, although surgical techniques have become more and more successful in athletes with chondral injuries,[10,44] less conservative interventions are presently unavailable. HAs do not currently play a prominent role in the treatment regimen, but may be useful either as first-line agents or in addition to surgical intervention. For instance, supplementing the osteochondral autograft transfer (OAT) procedures, microfracture, meniscal repair/debridement, or anterior cruciate ligament (ACL) reconstruction with HA therapy perioperatively may be of some benefit to patients.

■ Conclusion

Viscosupplementation with intraarticular injections of hyaluronic acid is a potential boon for orthopaedic surgeons who treat a substantial number of athletes with joint pain. It is becoming a more widely accepted answer to the demand of patients with osteoarthritis of the knee who are not yet candidates for total joint replacement.[45] Although not yet currently used for athletes by a majority of orthopaedists, HAs offer potential therapeutic impact both for prophylaxis from degenerative chondral changes in high-endurance or elite-level athletes as well as in the setting of acutely injured athletes with ligamentous, meniscal, or cartilaginous defects. As research into these indications continues, the actual value of viscosupplementation will soon be realized.

REFERENCES

1. From the Centers for Disease Control and Prevention. Nonfatal sports- and recreation-related injuries treated in emergency departments—United States, July 2000–June 2001. JAMA 2002;288: 1977–1979
2. Balazs EA, Denlinger JL. Viscosupplementation: a new concept in the treatment of osteoarthritis. J Rheumatol 1993;20:3–9
3. Kirwan J. Is there a place for intra-articular hyaluronate in osteoarthritis of the knee? Knee 2001;8:93–100
4. Simon LS. Viscosupplementation therapy with intra-articular hyaluronic acid. Osteoarthritis 1999;25:345–357
5. Marshall KW. Intra-articular hyaluronan therapy. Curr Opin Rheumatol 2000;12:468–474
6. Asari A, Miyauchi S, Matsuzaka S, Ito T, Kominami E, Uchiyama Y. Molecular weight dependent effects of hyaluronate on the arthritic synovium. Arch Histol Cytol 1998;61:125–135
7. Listrat V, Ayral X, Patarnello F. Arthroscopic evaluation of potential structure modifying activity of hyaluronan (Hyalgan(r)) in osteoarthritis of the knee. Osteoarthritis Cartilage 1997;5:153–160
8. Adams ME, Lussier AJ, Peyron JG. A risk-benefit assessment of injections of hyaluronan and its derivatives in the treatment of osteoarthritis of the knee. Drug Saf 2000;23:115–130

9. Lussier A, Cividino AA, McFarlane CA, Olszynski WP, Potashner WJ, De Medicis R. Viscosupplementation with hylan for the treatment of osteoarthritis: findings from clinical practice in Canada. J Rheumatol 1996;23:1579–1584

10. Blevins FT, Steadman JR, Rodrigo JJ, Silliman J. Treatment of articular cartilage defects in athletes: an analysis of functional outcome and lesion appearance. Orthopedics 1998;21:761–767

11. Fraser JR, Laurent TC, Laurent UB. Hyaluronan: its nature, distribution, functions and turnover. J Intern Med 1997;242:27–33

12. Buckwalter JA, Mankin HJ. Articular cartilage. Part I: tissue design and chondrocyte-matrix interactions. J Bone Joint Surg 1997;79A:600–611

13. Athanasiou KA, Shah AR, Hernandez RJ, LeBaron RG. Basic science of articular cartilage repair. Clin Sports Med 2001;20:223–247

14. Balazs EA, Watson D, Duff IF. Hyaluronic acid in synovial fluid. I: molecular parameters of hyaluronic acid in normal and arthritic human fluids. Arthritis Rheum 1967;10:357–375

15. Arokoski JP, Jurvelin JS, Vaatainen U, Helminen HJ. Normal and pathological adaptations of articular cartilage to joint loading. Scand J Med Sci Sports 2000;10:183–185

16. Buckwalter JA, Lane NE. Athletics and osteoarthritis. Am J Sports Med 1997;25:873–881

17. Hyalgan® (sodium hyaluronate) prescribing information, Sanofi-Synthelabo Inc., New York, NY

18 Synvisc® (hylan G-F 20) prescribing information, Wyeth Pharmaceuticals, Madison, NJ

19. Supartz® (sodum hyaluronate) prescribing information, Seikagaku Corporation, Tokyo, Japan

20. Wobig M, Dickhut A, Maier R, Vetter G. Viscosupplementation with hylan G-F 20: a 25-week controlled trial of efficacy and safety in the osteoarthritic knee. Clin Ther 1998;20:410–423

21. Smith MM, Ghosh P. The synthesis of hyaluronic acid by human synovial fibroblasts is influenced by the nature of the hyaluronate in the extracellular environment. Rheumatol Int 1987;7:113–122

22. Aviad AD, Houpt JB. The molecular weight of therapeutic hyaluronan (sodium hyaluronate): how significant is it? J Rheumatol 1994;21:297–301

23. Kikuchi T, Yamada H, Shimmei M. Effect of high molecular weight hyaluronan on cartilage degeneration in a rabbit model of osteoarthritis. Osteoarthritis Cartilage 1996;4:99–110

24. Jubb RW, Plva S, Beinat L, Dacre J, Gishen P. A one-year, randomized, placebo (saline) controlled trial of 500–730 kDa sodium hyaluronate (Hyalgan) on the radiological change in osteoarthritis of the knee. Int J Clin Pract 2003;57(6):467–474

25. Schiavinato A, Lini E, Guidolin D. Intra-articular sodium hyaluronan injections in the Pond Nuki experimental model of osteoarthritis in dogs. II. Morphological findings. Clin Orthop 1989;241:286–299

26. Frizziero L, Govoni E, Bacchini P. Intra-articular hyaluronic acid in the treatment of osteoarthritis of the knee: clinical and morphological study. Clin Exp Rheumatol 1998;16:441–449

27. Tobetto K, Yasui T, Ando T, et al. Inhibitory effects of hyaluronan on arachidonic acid release from labeled human synovial fibroblasts. Jpn J Pharmacol 1992;60:79–84

28. Gotoh S, Miyazaki K, Onaya J, Sakamoto T, Tokuyasu K, Mamiki O. Experimental knee pain model in rats and analgesic effects of sodium hyaluronate. Nippon Yakurigaku Zasshi 1998;92:17–27

29. Navarro RA, Soifer TB. Treating the pain of osteoarthritis. Orthopedic Technology Review 2002;4:18–22

30. Evanich JD, Evanich CJ, Wright MB, Rydlewicz JA. Efficacy of intra-articular hyaluronic acid injections in knee osteoarthritis. Clin Orthop 2001;390:173–181

31. Puttick MP, Wade JP, Chalmers A, Connell DG, Rangno KK. Acute local reactions after intra-articular hylan for osteoarthritis of the knee. J Rheumatol 1995;22:1311–1314

32. Jackson DW, Evans NA, Thomas BM. Accuracy of needle placement into the intra-articular space of the knee. J Bone Joint Surg 2002;84-A:1522–1527

33. Forster MC, Straw R. A prospective randomized trial comparing intra-articular Hyalgan injection and arthroscopic washout for knee osteoarthritis. Knee 2003;10:291–293

34. Jubb RW, Piva S, Beinat L, Dacre J, Gishen P. A one year, randomized, placebo (saline) controlled clinical trial of 500–730 kDa sodium hyaluronate (Hyalgan) on the radiological change in osteoarthritis of the knee. Int J Clin Pract 2003;57:467–474

35. Leopold SS, Redd BB, Warme WJ, Wehrle PA, Pettis PD, Shott S. Corticosteroid compared with hyaluronic acid injections for the treatment of osteoarthritis of the knee. A prospective, randomized trial. J Bone Joint Surg Am 2003;85-A:1197–1203

36. Tasciotaoglu F, Oner C. Efficacy of intra-articular sodium hyaluronate in the treatment of knee osteoarthritis. Clin Rheumatol 2003;22:112–117

37. Kolarz G, Kotz R, Hochmayer I. Long-term benefits and repeated treatment cycles of intra-articular sodium hyaluronate (Hyalgan) in patients with osteoarthritis of the knee. Semin Arthritis Rheum 2003;32:310–319

38. Neustadt DH. Long-term efficacy and safety of intra-articular sodium hyaluronate (Hyalgan) in patients with osteoarthritis of the knee. Clin Exp Rheumatol 2003;21:307–311

39. Saxon L, Finch C, Bass S. Sports participation, sports injuries and osteoarthritis: implications for prevention. Sports Med 1999;28:123–135

40. Armstrong S, Read R, Ghosh P. The effects of intra-articular hyaluronan on cartilage and subchondral bone changes in an ovine model of early osteoarthritis. J Rheumatol 1994;21:680–688

41. Bragantini A, Molinaroli F. A pilot clinical evaluation of the treatment of hip osteoarthritis with hyaluronic acid. Curr Ther Res 1994;55:319–330

42. Major NM, Helms CA. MR imaging of the knee: findings in asymptomatic collegiate basketball players. AJR 2002;179:641–644

43. Zanetti M, Bruder E, Romero J, Hodler J. Bone marrow edema pattern in osteoarthritic knees: correlation between MR imaging and histologic findings. Radiology 2000;215:835–840

44. Levy AS, Lohnes J, Sculley S, LeCroy M, Garrett W. Chondral delamination of the knee in soccer players. Am J Sports Med 1996;24:634–639

45. Navarro RA. New concepts in the management of osteoarthritis. Orthopaedic Special Edition. 2001;7:51–54

■ SECTION FOUR ■

Operative Treatment

11

Arthroscopic Management of the Early Arthritic Joint

STEVEN S. GOLDBERG, RAFFY MIRZAYAN, AND C. THOMAS VANGSNESS, JR.

The first known use of arthroscopy to treat osteoarthritis of the knee was reported in 1934 by Burman et al[1] in their group of 11 patients. They remarked, "It was in a group of arthritic cases that we had the pleasant surprise of seeing a marked improvement in the joint following arthroscopy." Haggart[2] and Magnuson,[3] a decade later, pioneered joint debridement of osteoarthritis using open arthrotomy. Haggart improved symptoms in 19 of 20 patients, whereas Magnuson touted "complete recovery" in 60 of 62. Both of these studies attribute improvement in symptoms to the removal of rough and irritating material. In 1950, Isserlin[4] claimed success in 23 of 35 debridement arthrotomies, greatly reducing pain and achieving motion from nearly full extension to 90 degrees.

With the advancement of arthroscopy during the 1970s, surgeons realized its diagnostic and therapeutic value without the morbidity associated with arthrotomy. Jackson and Abe[5] demonstrated pain relief with debridement and also recognized the therapeutic value of irrigation. At the same time, O'Connor[6] relieved symptoms of crystal-induced synovitis with arthroscopic lavage. Since that time, multiple studies have reported symptomatic relief in the arthritic patient following lavage and/or debridement of the knee.[7-20] The procedure gained popularity because it is a relatively safe, palliative form of therapy, and according to Schonholtz,[21] "no bridges are burned with arthroscopic surgery, [and] more extensive surgery can be carried out later." This is of particular importance for the athlete, in whom a major reconstructive procedure may be the end of a favorite activity or even a career. The increasing awareness by the public of a presumed safe, rapid source of relief with minimal recovery period has driven demand for use of arthroscopy for this purpose.

Although the literature on this subject is abundant, only a minority of studies is prospective or controlled.[22-26] Other studies have been less enthusiastic, criticizing the study designs and the paucity of evidence demonstrating change in the course of disease.[27-29] A recent randomized, prospective, placebo-control study[30] has renewed orthopaedists' and the public's interest in closely examining this procedure from both a medical and an economic standpoint. This chapter defines the various modalities of arthroscopic debridement, describes the physiologic changes, and reviews the literature of outcomes for these procedures.

■ Indications

As with any procedure, appropriate patient selection is important to a successful outcome. Generally, the indications for arthroscopic debridement in athletes are patients who have failed previous nonoperative management including rest, physical therapy, nonsteroidal antiinflammatory medications, and steroid injections. No standard algorithm exists for the timing of surgery, and the optimal age groups varies in reported studies.[31,32] To our knowledge, no study reports on the success of this operation in the isolated athletic patient group.

Age alone is not a reliable predictor of successful treatment.[33] Jackson and Rouse[34] reported on 68 patients over 40 years of age treated with partial arthroscopic meniscectomy and found that age did not effect the outcome. Lotke et al[10] concluded that traumatic meniscal tears treated with debridement might do well regardless of the patient's age.

In Insall's[33] review of the Pridie resurfacing technique, he stressed that the ideal patient was middle-aged and active, rather than the elderly who may be incapable of postoperative rehabilitation. This contradicts Burks's[35] review of the arthroscopy literature, which showed that the elderly benefit most from lavage, probably due to their lower level of activity.

The duration of symptoms is an indicator of how much the patients will improve following arthroscopic debridement. Baumgaertner et al[8] stated that symptoms of less than 12 months' duration significantly predicted better outcome, as did Lotke.[10] Wouters[36] showed that pain of less than 3 months' duration, a history of twisting injury, or locking was a significant predictor of a better postoperative outcome.

Malalignment is repeatedly blamed for poor results following arthroscopy.[8,36] Harwin[37] showed that patients with malalignment greater than 5 degrees had only 26% satisfactory results by subjective measurements compared with 84% of patient with normal alignment. Salisbury et al[38] concluded that patients with malalignment "should be excluded from consideration for arthroscopic debridement." Younger patients with varus knees are better served by undergoing high tibial osteotomy.[38,39] Arthroscopy is not a substitute for a definitive reconstructive procedure in a young athlete with varus deformity.[28] Patients who have laxity due to ligamentous insufficiency also do poorly.

Radiographic findings such as large osteophytes and loose bodies indicate that the patient will not see much improvement. Severity of arthritis is a prognostic indicator for the success of arthroscopic debridement.[8,36,40] A complete loss of joint space, as opposed to minor narrowing, is a poor prognostic indicator. Aichroth[7] showed significantly better results in patients with Outerbridge[41] stage I and II knees versus stage III and IV. Looking at preoperative radiographs, Lotke[10] found that patients with normal radiographs had a 90% chance of good to excellent symptom relief following a medial meniscectomy versus only a 21% chance of similar results if the patient showed moderate to marked arthritic changes. In Baumgaertner et al's[8] study, 77% of patients with mild or moderate changes on x-rays had a good to excellent result, according to a grading system of pain, function, and patient enthusiasm, versus 33% with severe changes.

TABLE 11–1   Prognostic Indicators for Arthroscopic Debridement

Positive	Negative
Normal alignment	Malalignment >5 degrees
Minimal radiographic changes	Radiographic signs of osteoarthritis
Symptoms <3 months	Symptoms >1 year
Mechanical symptoms	Pending litigation
Flap tears	Degenerative tears
Isolated medial femoral condyle lesions	Diffuse chondromalacia

Patients who are filing workman's compensation claims or are in the process of litigation also tend to do poorly.

Novak and Bach[39] summarized the factors predicting a better outcome in their study. These factors included normal alignment, a history of mechanical symptoms, minimal roentgenographic degeneration, and a short duration of symptoms. **Table 11–1** lists predictors of outcome summarized from several studies on arthroscopic debridement.

■ Overview of Orthoscopic Choices

Arthroscopic debridement can generally be divided into three categories, in order of increasing alteration of the native tissue: (1) lavage, (2) debridement, and (3) abrasion arthroplasty.

Arthroscopic lavage involves washing the knee with fluid, usually lactated Ringer's solution or saline. The mechanism of benefit of lavage is thought to be the removal of prostaglandins,[42] enzymes,[43] crystals,[6] and cartilaginous debris,[44] mechanically loosened from the surfaces.

Debridement includes removal of loose bodies, osteophytes, and fibrillated chondral flaps of roughened articular and meniscal cartilage to create smooth cartilage surfaces using a motorized shaver. The irritants that stimulate the synovial lining of the joint are reduced, which in turn decreases joint effusions, and proteolytic enzymes.

Abrasion arthroplasty involves scraping the articular surface 1 to 2 mm until bleeding bone is encountered.[45] Techniques that penetrate the subchondral bone are not considered arthroscopic debridement and are discussed in other chapters.

■ Surgical Debridement Technique

Arthroscopy is performed through the standard antero-medial and anterolateral portals and occasionally a third, superomedial portal. A systematic diagnostic examination of the joint is performed, including inspection for loose bodies in the suprapatellar pouch, medial and lateral gutters, and the popliteus hiatus. The Gillquist views are used to evaluate the posterior joint for loose bodies.[46] The posteromedial compartment can be visualized by placing the arthroscope between the posterior cruciate ligament and medial femoral condyle from the lateral portal. The posterolateral compartment can be visualized by placing the arthroscope between the anterior cruciate ligament and the lateral femoral condyle from the anteromedial portal.

The cartilaginous surfaces of the joint are graded based on the Outerbridge[41] classification. A probe is inserted and the cartilaginous surfaces are palpated. Loose flaps of cartilage are elevated and the extent of delamination is evaluated. The menisci are evaluated as well with a probe and their stability is assessed. A motorized shaver can be used to debride loose flaps of cartilage with variable results. For example, when the cartilage is softened and has a "crab meat" appearance (**Fig. 11–1**), the shaver can be used to remove the abnormal cartilage and smooth down the articular surface. This is much easier to accomplish if the shaver is used in the "fast forward" mode instead of the "oscillate" mode. Degenerated menisci with flap tears are first debrided with an arthroscopic basket or shaver, and then smoothed to provide a smooth transition with the remaining horns of the meniscus. Radiofrequency devices on the articular cartilage are not recommended. The knee is then thoroughly irrigated and massaged to remove any remaining loose debris. Once the wounds are closed, a soft

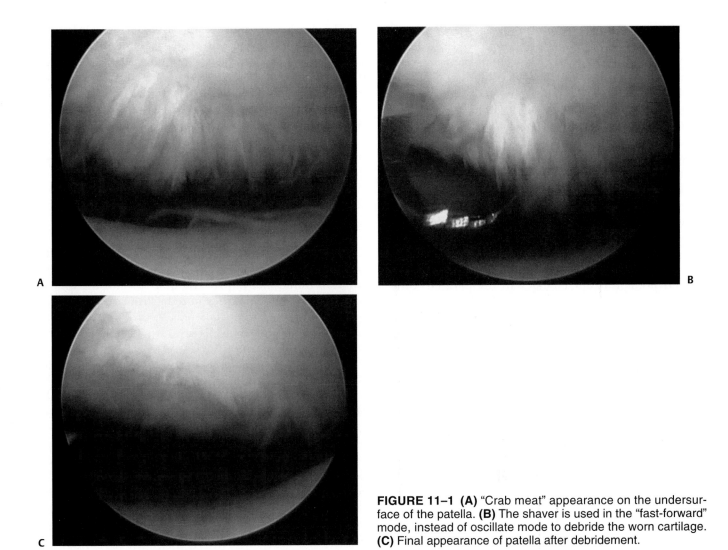

FIGURE 11–1 (A) "Crab meat" appearance on the undersurface of the patella. **(B)** The shaver is used in the "fast-forward" mode, instead of oscillate mode to debride the worn cartilage. **(C)** Final appearance of patella after debridement.

compressive dressing is applied. Patients are permitted to bear weight as tolerated but activities are limited until the sutures are removed 7 to 10 days later. Athletes usually return to sports when pain and swelling is controlled, and when muscle strength is equal to the contralateral limb.

■ Published Results

Lavage

Arthroscopic lavage has been proposed as a treatment for osteoarthritis since Burman[1] published his first results in 1934. Since that time, several authors have supported the use of lavage.[47,48,49] Livesley et al[23] prospectively compared patients with physiotherapy to patients with arthroscopic lavage plus physiotherapy. They found that the lavage patients had a significant overall relief of pain for up to 1 year and that signs of inflammation were significantly better for up to 3 months when looking at joint tenderness, warmth, morning stiffness, swelling, and disturbance in the patient's sleep pattern. Edelson et al[47] retrospectively reported that knee washout resulted in good or excellent pain relief and functional improvement in 86% of patients at 1 year and 81% of patients at 2 years. This study did not have a control group, and the author stated in the discussion "it is possible that some placebo effect may have contributed to the perceived benefit." Eriksson and Haggmark[48] reported on 10 runners who improved with arthroscopy and continued to be able to run with repeat needle lavage every 4 to 12 months.

Other studies have not been as supportive of the benefits. Bird and Ring's[50] percentage of patients with improvement dropped from 93% to 50% between postoperative week 1 and week 4. Using infrared thermography, a quantifiable measurement of inflammation showed no significant changes in unoperated knees. Lindsay et al's[22] prospective, double-blind controlled study found no additional benefit to synovial irrigation when compared with needle aspiration.

Arthroscopic Debridement

Haggart[2] and Magnusson[3] first reported debridements of arthritic knees with arthrotomy in 1940 and 1941, and in the 1970s, Jackson and Abe[5] advanced the technique by employing the arthroscope for the same procedure. Sprague[51] published an early report of arthroscopic debridement of a degenerative knee. In his study, 62 patients were followed for an average of 13 months and 74% had good results, as determined by a patient's subjective assessment of improvement compared with before surgery. Because of the limited morbidity and good results, Sprague stated, "arthroscopic debridement of the knee joint is recommended as a useful therapeutic modality in many patients with degenerative arthritis of the knee." Since that time there have been multiple reports of the beneficial effects of arthroscopic debridement for osteoarthritis.[20]

Despite good initial results only a small number of studies have evaluated the beneficial effects over time. Jackson[19] achieved symptom improvement in 68% of patients at 3 years, Timoney et al[17] in 63% at 4 years, and Bert and Maschka[16] in 66% at a minimum of 5 years. But in Baumgaertner et al's[8] retrospective study of patients over 50 years of age, only 40% of patients maintained good or excellent results through the 33-month follow-up.

McLaren et al[15] retrospectively reviewed 171 patients ranging in age from 23 to 82 years undergoing arthroscopic debridement, and although 65% of the patients felt their symptoms were improved, there was no identifiable trend with respect to age, severity of disease preoperatively or witnessed during surgery, alignment, or presence of osteophytes. The authors noted that improvement in symptoms is "marked, but unpredictable."

In England, Aichroth et al[7] reported on 254 patients undergoing arthroscopic debridement, ranging in age from 28 to 82 years, half of which were under 50. At an average follow-up of 44 months, 75% had minimal discomfort and improved function. They also noted that only 14% of the patients required subsequent surgery at an average of 4 years postoperatively. They stratified the results according to several categories and found that statistical predictors of good results were age under 60 years, Outerbridge grade I and II, and Ahlback[52] radiographic grade of 0 or 1. They noted, however, that the percentage of satisfactory results deteriorated with time. However, the information gained during the diagnostic portion of the procedure was helpful in planning future reconstructive surgery.[7]

Gross et al[14] retrospectively reviewed 40 patients with an average age of 54 years and noted 72% with subjective and functional improvement at 24 months follow-up. In their discussion they noted, "Procedures in these patients were not undertaken as a cure, but rather for palliation of their symptoms until a more extensive procedure might be needed."

Other studies specifically looked at the results of debridement compared with simple lavage of the knee. In a prospective, randomized study performed in England, Hubbard[25] found a significant difference between the two groups at 1 year. Eighty percent of the debridement patients had relief of pain, whereas only 20% with lavage continued to have relief. At 5-year follow-up, 59% of the debridement patients continued to have pain relief compared with only 10% of the lavage group. The patients in this study were limited to only lesions of the medial femoral condyle, and all patients had full range of motion and normal alignment preoperatively.

A recent report by Moseley and O'Malley[30] prospectively and randomly assigned 180 patients to receive arthroscopic debridement, arthroscopic lavage, or a "placebo" surgery consisting of anesthesia and incisions, but no insertion of instruments. This was an expansion of a pilot study first reported in 1996.[53] Both patients and reviewers were blinded to the treatment. The patients were graded over a 24-month period with regard to pain and function. In this study, there was no difference with regard to pain or function level among any of the groups at any time in the 2-year follow-up period. Critics of Moseley and O'Malley's study pointed out that (1) nearly all the participants were men despite the fact that osteoarthritis is more common in women; (2) patients were not stratified for body weight, malalignment and mechanical symptoms, and severity of disease; (3) coexisting meniscal pathology was not accounted for; and (4) there was potential selection bias caused by the number of patients who decided not to participate. This article was widely reported in the press and has generated controversy within the orthopaedic community. It has also renewed the interest in this controversial subject, both among physicians and the general public.

To make informed decisions regarding when and how to operatively treat patients with cartilage injury, the physician must understand the physiologic changes occurring in response to the treatments proposed. Schmid and Schmid[54] examined samples taken from knees in patients 18 to 42 years with posttraumatic arthritis and found "architecture of fibers and the chondrocytes show significantly more pathologic alterations after cartilage shaving of traumatically injured cartilage than after no surgical therapy" including increased cell necrosis and disorientation of collagen. Kim et al,[55] using a rabbit model, simulated debridement by partial-thickness shaving of patellar articular cartilage, and found no histologic evidence of regeneration of tissue. They noted that underlying tissue may even degenerate further. Gibson et al[56] compared arthroscopic debridement to lavage by measuring quadriceps strength before and after surgery. At 6 and 12 weeks postoperatively, the lavage group showed an increase in quadriceps isokinetic torque. The debridement group failed to show a similar improvement, although on biopsy the diameter of type II muscle fibers did increase.

Concerns about the amount of trauma to the healthy cartilage and the desire for a more precise method of ablating unstable tissue led to the development of laser and radiofrequency ablation techniques for chondroplasty. Laser ablation has the advantage of controlling the depth of penetration of emitted photons.[57] Despite initial interest, studies showed laser ablation can lead to thermal damage and osteonecrosis in normal tissue.[58] Radiofrequency ablation is another, less expensive method of delivering thermal energy to destroy abnormal tissue.

The depth of energy penetration in vivo is still debated.[59,60] Techniques and outcomes of this method are discussed in other chapters.

Abrasion Arthroplasty

Debridement of knee arthritis was advanced in 1959 when Pridie[61] published a method of resurfacing osteoarthritic knee joints by drilling through eburnated bone. He believed articular surfaces could be restored by bleeding to induce growth of fibrocartilage. Salter et al[62] demonstrated hyaline cartilage growth in animals after drilling 2-mm holes in the cancellous bone followed by continuous passive motion. Johnson[63] advanced the current techniques of abrasion arthroplasty and advocated this procedure for patients with good alignment, good motion, and low demand. He stressed that the depth of abrasion be limited to 1 to 2 mm and that deeper abrasion would hinder good results. Friedman et al[64] showed encouraging results with abrasion arthroplasty with an early short-term follow-up of 1 year. Looking specifically at younger patients, those under 40 years of age had an 86% rate of symptom improvement following abrasion arthroplasty.

Other results were not as encouraging. Bert and Maschka[16] reported in a study comparing patients undergoing arthroscopic debridement compared with arthroscopic debridement plus abrasion arthroplasty that the results were "totally unpredictable" and were "unrelated to any identifiable patient characteristics." They noted arthroscopic debridement alone resulted in higher Hospital for Special Surgery knee scores[65] than abrasion arthroplasty. Rand[20] came to a similar conclusion that abrasion arthroplasty offered no benefit over arthroscopic debridement alone. Although this was an older age group averaging 63 years, it was noted that 50% of the patients in the abrasion arthroplasty group underwent total knee arthroplasty within 3 years of their abrasion arthroplasty procedure. Mankin[66] demonstrated that fibrocartilage created by abrasion arthroplasty had wear characteristics inferior to native articular cartilage.

Abrasion arthroplasty has failed to clearly show significant improvement over arthroscopic debridement alone and, therefore, it is generally not regarded as a primary treatment for the athlete with early degenerative arthritis.[67]

Isolated Patellofemoral Debridement

As an isolated procedure, debridement of the patellofemoral joint has had generally good results. Friedman et al's[64] early study of abrasion arthroplasty noted that 82% of their patients with patellofemoral compartment abrasion alone reported improvement in function compared with only 56% and 50% in the medial and lateral compartment groups, respectively. Federico and Reider[68] reviewed the results of patellofemoral debridement in 36 patients with patellofemoral pain. Eighty-nine percent of the patients reported subjective improvement following this procedure, despite the fact that only 58% of the patients with traumatic chondromalacia patella have good or excellent results and only 41% of patients with atraumatic chondromalacia had good or excellent results, as determined by their functional limitations. With regard specifically to sporting activities, 27 of 29 patients who were active in sports prior to the onset of their symptoms were able to return to active sporting activities, including one at the elite level and two at the competitive level. The authors concluded that patients with normal patellar alignment and who have failed nonoperative care might benefit from this procedure, although it is unclear why some patients improve more than others.

Other Joints

Arthroscopic debridement has been advocated for joints besides the knee. Weinstein et al[69] reported 80% good to excellent results in 25 patients averaging 46 years of age who underwent arthroscopic debridement of the shoulder. The operative procedure consisted of glenohumeral joint lavage, debridement of chondral lesions and labral tears, loose body removal as well as partial synovectomy and subacromial bursectomy. The authors recommended that this procedure be reserved for patients with a concentric humeral head and the presence of visible joint space on the axillary radiograph. It is not recommended for joint incongruity or large osteophytes. They also noted that 10 of 12 patients with preoperative stiffness had a postoperative improvement in range of motion, most markedly with external rotation, and that 7 of 13 patients in the study who had restricted sports preoperatively returned to their activity. A smaller study by Johnson[70] also showed good results following arthroscopic lavage and debridement of the shoulder, whereas Cofield[71] noted its value in staging arthritic diseases.

Ogilvie-Harris et al[11,72,73,74] have reported successful results of arthroscopic debridement for the shoulder,[72] elbow,[73] ankle,[74] as well as the knee.[11] In their review of arthroscopic ankle debridement, 17 of 27 patients showed improvement, although only two ankles restored normal function. In this young group averaging 40 years of age, 18 patients preoperatively limited their sporting activities compared with only 6 patients postoperatively with similar limitations. Two complications were reported, relating to numbness at the anterolateral portal that resolved over 6 months in both cases. The same authors reported on 21 patients followed for nearly 3 years following arthroscopic treatment of degenerative arthritis of the elbow. In this group, all patients had excellent or good results postoperatively with statistically significant improvements in pain, strength, motion, stability, and function of the elbow.[73]

■ Complications

The most common complication with these procedures is worsening of the patient's original symptoms, caused by excessive debridement of the patient's cartilage surfaces. Abrasion arthroplasty has the highest potential for this problem, and is primarily why this technique has fallen out of favor. In Rand's[20] study, 9 of 28 patients became worse subsequent to abrasion arthroplasty. In Bert and Maschka's[16] series, 10 of 59 became worse. Other complications, albeit rare, are similar to other arthroscopic procedures. Even though the majority of studies do not even report complications, such as infection, instrument breakage, hemarthrosis, stiffness, tourniquet problems, and peripheral nerve injury, the incidence is as high as 7% to 31% in some series.[75]

■ Evidence-Based Medicine

Although numerous studies have been published on this topic, only a few studies are prospective, with even fewer having a control group or blinded evaluations. In an era of increasing cost awareness and scrutiny by patients and third-party payers, more emphasis is placed on the practice of evidence-based medicine. These studies, although dramatically fewer in number, are relied on far more in determining the standard of care and forming public health policy decisions. The cost and time needed to carry out these investigations far exceeds the work required to write a historical review. The pertinent evidence-based medicine studies regarding arthroscopic debridement are summarized in **Table 11–2.**

■ Controversy

Although the orthopaedic community generally believed arthroscopic debridement was a beneficial palliative treatment of arthritis, some authors voiced reservations. As early as 1990, S. Ward Casscells,[28] editor-in-chief of *Arthroscopy: The Journal of Arthroscopic and Related Surgery,* questioned the cost-effectiveness and scrutinized the overall lack of selection criteria. He stated, "There is no evidence thus far that irrigation, debridement, and/or abrasion arthroplasty produce relief for more

TABLE 11–2 Select Evidence-Based Medicine Studies of Arthroscopic Debridement

Author	Lindsay et al.[22]	Livesley et al.[23]	Chang et al.[24]	Moseley et al.[53]	Hubbard[25]	Bradley et al.[26]	Moseley and O'Malley[30]
Year	1971	1991	1993	1996	1996	2002	2002
Participants	24	61	32	10	76	177	165
Method	Compare closed needle irrigation to closed needle aspiration	Compare arthroscopic lavage plus physiotherapy to physiotherapy alone	Compare arthroscopic debridement to closed needle lavage	Compare arthroscopic debridement to arthroscopic lavage to "placebo" surgery	Compare arthroscopic debridement to arthroscopic washout	Compare needle irrigation to "sham" lavage	Compare arthroscopic debridement to arthroscopic lavage to "placebo" surgery
Design	Prospective, randomized, double blind	Prospective, nonrandomized, nonblinded	Prospective, randomized, blinded independent examiner	Prospective, randomized, double-blind, placebo controlled	Prospective, randomized, nonblinded	Prospective, randomized, double-blind, placebo controlled	Prospective, randomized, double-blind, placebo controlled
Duration of follow-up	47 days	12 months	12 months	6 months	12 months	12 months	24 months
Conclusion	Subjective, objective and synovial fluid analyses all similar	Less pain for 1 year, fewer signs of inflammation for 6 months	Subjective evaluations, physical evaluations, and utilization of medical services similar	Subjective, objective, patient satisfaction measurements similar	Percentage of patients pain free: 80% with debridement, 20% with washout ($p = .05$)	Subjective, objective, measurements similar	Subjective, objective, patient satisfaction measurements similar

than a few months or, at most, several years." He noted that most studies did not preoperatively select patients with regard to age, degree of disease, or, what he felt was most important, alignment. He further stated, "Enthusiasm for arthroscopic procedures appears to know no limits at the present time," and urged a more scientific approach to the problem. Noting the intense scrutiny by the government, insurance and public health institutions, he warned orthopaedic surgeons to be more selective with this procedure or "it will be done for us regardless of our wishes."

An editorial by Dandy[27] expressed concern that using arthroscopy as first-line treatment of osteoarthritic knees would pose a strain on available health care resources. In his opinion, arthroscopic debridement is not a substitute for conservative management, osteotomy or joint replacement, and he hopes "it does not become a vehicle for misplaced optimism."

Sharkey[29] raised three fundamental questions: (1) Does arthroscopy for osteoarthritis change the natural history of the disease? (2) How can any improvement from arthroscopic debridement be explained on a cellular or biologic level? (3) Is the outcome of arthroscopic debridement related to a placebo effect.[29,75] Moseley and O'Malley's[30] attempt to answer the final question has recently become a major topic of debate among orthopaedists and the health care community. The study generated significant media attention both for its conclusions and because patients were anesthetized without undergoing actual surgery ("sham surgery").

The next question that then arises is how to treat the patient who has both arthritis and a meniscal tear. Bhattacharyya and Gale[76] performed magnetic resonance imaging (MRI) and plain radiography on 154 symptomatic osteoarthritic patients and 49 age-matched controls, and found the prevalence of meniscal tears was 91% in symptomatic patients, but more surprisingly 76% prevalence in asymptomatic controls. Among patients with osteoarthritis, those with a meniscal tear were not more painful than those without a tear, and the authors concluded that meniscal tears do not affect functional status in this population. However, a prospective study[77] assessing the impact of arthroscopic debridement on health-related quality of life, as determined by the Western Ontario and McMaster Universities Osteoarthritis Index (WOMAC)[78] and Short Form-36 (SF-36)[79] scores, concluded that an unstable meniscus tear at arthroscopy was one of only three statistically significant ($p = .01$) predictors of patient satisfaction. The other two predictors were medial joint line tenderness ($p = .04$) and a positive Steinman test ($p = .01$), the presence of pain referred to the joint line during internal and external rotation in a knee flexed to 90 degrees. Forty-four percent of patients in that study had clinically important reductions in pain with debridement at 2-year follow-up as determined by the WOMAC score. Garret's[80] editorial regarding these two seemingly conflicting reports, published in the same issue of the *Journal of Bone and Joint Surgery*, effectively stated that orthopaedists must attempt to distinguish if patient symptoms are attributable to a meniscal tear, arthritis alone, or both. "It remains to be determined in future studies whether arthroscopic surgery can benefit patients who have mechanical symptoms primarily and symptoms of osteoarthritis secondarily."

■ Conclusion

The use of arthroscopic debridement for treatment of arthritis and cartilage injury in the athlete remains controversial, and no clear indications regarding when or exactly how to treat these patients is established. From extensive historical literature, patients with mild arthritic changes, a short duration of symptoms, and good mechanical alignment frequently show symptomatic relief from this procedure. In general, most younger, athletic patients fit those criteria. However, the degree and duration of benefit is often unpredictable. Though much fewer in number, most evidence-based medicine studies are not as encouraging and point to a significant placebo effect of arthroscopic debridement. What can be concluded is that patients with severe arthritis generally will not improve. Although the morbidity associated with performing these procedures is low, athletes with obvious malalignment would be better served with procedures such as tibial osteotomy. The belief that debridement can delay future reconstruction is speculative. Future evidence-based studies will demonstrate the more appropriate indications and the exact role of arthroscopic debridement as a treatment of arthritis in the athlete and as well as the general population.

REFERENCES

1. Burman MS, Finklestein H, Mayer L. Arthroscopy of the knee joint. J Bone J Surg 1934;16-A:255–268
2. Haggart GE. Surgical treatment of degenerative arthritis of the knee joint. J Bone J Surg 1940;22-B:717–729
3. Magnuson PB. Joint debridement: surgical treatment of degenerative arthritis. Surg Gynecol Obstet 1941;73:1–9
4. Isserlin B. Joint debridement for osteoarthritis of the knee. J Bone J Surg 1950;32-B:302–306
5. Jackson RW, Abe I. The role of arthroscopy in the management of disorders of the knee: an analysis of 200 consecutive cases. J Bone J Surg 1972;54-B:310–322
6. O'Connor RL. The arthroscope in the management of crystal-induced synovitis of the knee. J Bone J Surg 1973;55-A:1443–1449
7. Aichroth PM, Patel DV, Moyes ST. A prospective review of arthroscopic debridement for degenerative joint disease of the knee. Int Orthop 1991;15:351–355

8. Baumgaertner MR, Cannon WD, Vittori JM, Schmidt ES, Maurer RC. Arthroscopic debridement of the arthritic knee. Clin Orthop 1990;253:197–202

9. Shahriaree H. Arthroscopic debridement. In: Shahriaree H, ed. O'Connor's Textbook of Arthroscopic Surgery, 2nd ed. Philadelphia: JB Lippincott, 1992:433–436

10. Lotke PA, Lefkoe RT, Ecker ML. Late results following medial meniscectomy in an older population. J Bone J Surg 1981;63-A: 115–119

11. Ogilve-Harris DJ, Fitsialos DP. Arthroscopic management of the degenerative knee. Arthroscopy 1991;7:151–157

12. Hubbard MJS. Articular debridement versus washout for degeneration of the medial femoral condyle: a five year study. J Bone J Surg 1996;78-B:217–219

13. Shannon FJ, Devitt AT, Poynton AR, Fitzpatrick P, Walsh MG. Short-term benefit of arthroscopic washout in degenerative arthritis of the knee. Int Orthop 2001;25:242–245

14. Gross DE, Brenner SL, Esformes I, Gross ML. Arthroscopic treatment of degenerative joint disease of the knee. Orthopedics 1991;14:1317–1321

15. McLaren AC, Blokker CP, Fowler PJ, Roth JN, Rock MG. Arthroscopic debridement of the knee for osteoarthrosis. Can J Surg 1991;34:595–598

16. Bert JM, Maschka K. The arthroscopic treatment of unicompartmental gonarthrosis: a five-year follow-up study of abrasion arthroplasty plus arthroscopic debridement and arthroscopic debridement alone. Arthroscopy 1989;5:25–32

17. Timoney JM, Kneisl JS, Barrack RL, Alexander AH. Arthroscopy in the osteoarthritic knee: long-term follow-up. Orthop Rev 1990;19:371–379

18. McGinley BJ, Cushner FD, Scott WN. Debridement arthroscopy: 10-year follow-up. Clin Orthop 1999;367:190–194

19. Jackson RW, Silver R, Marans H. Arthroscopic treatment of degenerative joint disease. Arthroscopy 1986;2:114

20. Rand JA. Role of arthroscopy in osteoarthritis of the knee. Arthroscopy 1991;7:358–363

21. Schonholtz GJ. Arthroscopic debridement of the knee joint. Orthop Clin North Am 1989;20:257–263

22. Lindsay DJ, Ring EF, Coorey PF, Jaysan MIU. Synovial irrigation in rheumatoid arthritis. Acta Rheumatol Scand 1971;17:169–174

23. Livesley PJ, Doherty M, Needoff M, Moulton A. Arthroscopic lavage of osteoarthritic knees. J Bone J Surg 1991;73-B: 922–926

24. Chang RW, Falconer J, Stulberg SD, Arnold WJ, Manheim LM, Dyer AR. A randomized, controlled trial of arthroscopic surgery versus closed-needle joint lavage for patients with osteoarthritis of the knee. Arthritis Rheum 1993;36:289–296

25. Hubbard MJS. Articular debridement versus washout for degeneration of the medial femoral condyle: a five year study. J Bone J Surg 1996;78-B:217–219

26. Bradley JD, Heilman DK, Katz PB, G'Sell P, Wallick JE, Brandt KD. Tidal irrigation as treatment for knee osteoarthritis: a sham-controlled, randomized, double-blinded evaluation. Arthritis Rheum 2002;46:100–108

27. Dandy DJ. Arthroscopic debridement of the knee for osteoarthritis. J Bone J Surg 1991;73-B:877–878

28. Casscells SW. What, if any, are the indications for arthroscopic debridement of the osteoarthritic knee. Arthroscopy 1990;6:169–170

29. Sharkey PF. The case against arthroscopic debridement. J Arthroplasty 1997;12:467–469

30. Moseley JB, O'Malley K, Petersen NJ, et al. A controlled trial of arthroscopic surgery for osteoarthritis of the knee. N Engl J Med 2002;347:81–88

31. Gambardella RA. Arthroscopic treatment of degenerative joint disease. In: Fu FH, Harner CD, Vince KG, eds. Knee Surgery. Baltimore: Williams and Wilkins, 1994:1113–1120

32. Hunt SA, Jazrawi LM, Sherman OH. Arthroscopic management of osteorthritis of the knee. J Am Acad Orthop Surg 2002;10: 356–363

33. Insall J. The Pridie debridement operation for osteoarthritis of the knee. Clin Orthop 1974;101:61–67

34. Jackson RW, Rouse DW. The results of partial arthroscopic meniscectomy in patients in patients over 40 years of age. J Bone J Surg 1982;64-B:481–485

35. Burks RT. Arthroscopy and degenerative arthritis of the knee: a review of the literature. Arthroscopy 1990;6:43–47

36. Wouters E, Bassett FH, Hardaker WT, Garrett WE. An algorithm for arthroscopy in the over-50 age group. Am J Sports Med 1992; 20:141–145

37. Harwin SF. Arthroscopic debridement for osteoarthritis of the knee: predictors of patient satisfaction. Arthroscopy 1999;15:142–146

38. Salisbury RB, Nottage WN, Gardner V. The effect of alignment on results in arthroscopic debridement in the degenerative knee. Clin Orthop 1985;198:268–272

39. Novak PJ, Bach BR. Selection criteria for knee arthroscopy in the osteoarthritic patient. Orthop Rev 1993;22:796–804

40. Ogilve-Harris DJ, Fitsialos DP. Arthroscopic management of the degenerative knee. Arthroscopy 1991;7:151–157

41. Outerbridge RE. The etiology of chondromalacia patellae. J Bone J Surg 1961;43-B:752–757

42. Ogilve-Harris DJ, Bauer M, Corey P. Prostaglandin inhibition after arthroscopy. J Bone J Surg 1985;67-B:567–571

43. Evans CH, Mazzocchi RA, Nelson DD, Rubash HE. Experimental arthritis induced by intraarticular injection of allogenic cartilagious particles into rabbit knees. Arthritis Rheum 1984;27:200–207

44. Chrisman OD, Fessel JM, Southwick WO. Experimental production of synovitis and marginal articular exostoses in the knee joints of dogs. Yale J Biol Med 1965;37:409–412

45. Insall J. The Pridie debridement operation for osteoarthritis of the knee. Clin Orthop 1974;101:61–67

46. Gillquist J, Hagberg G, Oretorp N. Arthroscopic examination of the posteromedial compartment of the knee joint. Int Orthop 1979;3:13–18

47. Edelson R, Burks RT, Bloebaum RD. Short-term effects of knee washout for osteoarthritis. Am J Sports Med 1995;23:345–349

48. Eriksson E, Haggmark T. Knee pain in the middle-aged runner. In: Symposium on the Foot and Leg in Running Sports. Park Ridge, IL: American Academy of Orthopaedic Surgeons, 1980:106–108

49. Jayson MIV, Dixon AStJ. Arthroscopy of the knee in rheumatic diseases. Ann Rheum Dis 1968;27:503–511

50. Bird HA, Ring EF. Therapeutic value of arthroscopy. Ann Rheum Dis 1978;37:78–79

51. Sprague NF III. Arthroscopic debridement for degenerative knee joint disease. Clin Orthop 1981;160:118–123

52. Ahlback S. Osteoarthritis of the knee: a radiographic investigation. Acta Radiol Diagn (Stockh) 1968;(suppl 277):7–72

53. Moseley JB, Wray NP, Kuykendall D, Willis K, Landon G. Arthroscopic treatment of osteoarthritis of the knee: a prospective, randomized, placebo-controlled trial. Results of a pilot study. Am J Sports Med 1996;24:28–34

54. Schmid A, Schmid F. Results after cartilage shaving studied by electron microscopy. Am J Sports Med 1987;15:386–387

55. Kim HKW, Moran ME, Salter RB. The potential for regeneration of articular cartilage in defects created by chondral shaving and subchondral abrasion: an experimental investigation in rabbits. J Bone J Surg 1991;73-A:1301–1315

56. Gibson JNA, White MD, Chapman VM, Strachan RK. Arthroscopic lavage and debridement for osteoarthritis of the knee. J Bone J Surg 1992;74-B:534–537

57. Raunest J, Lohnert J. Arthroscopic cartilage debridement by excimer laser in chondromalacia of the knee joint. Arch Orthop Trauma Surg 1990;109:155–159

58. Garino JP, Lotke PA, Sapega AA, Reilly PJ, Esterhai JL. Osteonecrosis of the knee following laser assisted arthroscopic surgery: a report of six cases. Arthroscopy 1995;11:467–474

59. Turner AS, Tippett JW, Powers BE, Dewell RD, Mallinckrodt CH. Radiofrequency (electrosurgical) ablation of articular cartilage: a study in sheep. Arthroscopy 1998;14:585–591

60. Lu Y, Hayashi K, Hecht P, et al. The effect of monopolar radiofrequency energy on partial-thickness defects of articular cartilage. Arthroscopy 2000;16:527–536

61. Pridie KH. A method of resurfacing osteoarthritic knee joints. J Bone J Surg 1959;41-B:618–619

62. Salter RB, Simmonds DF, Malcomb BW, Rumble EJ, MacMichael D, Clements ND. The biologic effects of continuous passive motion on the healing of full thickness defects in articular cartilage. J Bone J Surg 1980;62-A:1232–1251

63. Johnson LL. Arthroscopic abrasion arthroplasty: historical and pathologic perspective: present status. Arthroscopy 1986;2:54–69

64. Friedman MJ, Berasi CC, Fox JM, Del Pizzo W, Snyder SJ, Ferkel R. Preliminary results with abrasion arthroplasty in the osteoarthritic knee. Clin Orthop 1984;182:200–205

65. Insall J, Ranawat CS, Aglietti P, Shine J. A comparison of four models of total knee replacement prosthesis. J Bone J Surg 1976;58-A:754–758

66. Mankin HJ. The response of articular cartilage to mechanical injury. J Bone J Surg 1982;64-A:460–466

67. Goldman RT, Scuderi GR, Kelly MA. Arthroscopic treatment of the degenerative knee in older athletes. Clin Sports Med 1997; 16:51–68

68. Federico DJ, Reider B. Results of isolated patellar debridement for patellofemoral pain in patients with normal patellar alignment. Am J Sports Med 1997;25:663–669

69. Weinstein DM, Bucchieri JS, Pollock RG, Flatow EL, Bigliani LU. Arthroscopic debridement of the shoulder for osteoarthritis. Arthroscopy 2000;16:471–476

70. Johnson LL. The shoulder joint: an arthroscopist's perspective of anatomy and physiology. Clin Orthop 1987;223:113–125

71. Cofield RH. Arthroscopy of the shoulder. Mayo Clin Proc 1983;58:501–508

72. Ogilve-Harris DJ, Wiley AM. Arthroscopic surgery of the shoulder: a general appraisal. J Bone J Surg 1986;68-B:201–207

73. Ogilve-Harris DJ, Gordon R, MacKay M. Arthroscopic treatment for posterior impingement in degenerative arthritis of the elbow. Arthroscopy 1995;11:437–443

74. Ogilve-Harris DJ, Sekyi-Otu A. Arthroscopic debridement for the osteoarthritic ankle. Arthroscopy 1995;11:433–436

75. Stuart MJ. Arthroscopic management for degenerative arthritis of the knee. In: Zuckerman JD, ed. Instructional Course Lectures, vol 48. Rosemont, IL: American Academy of Orthopaedic Surgeons, 1999:135–141

76. Bhattacharyya T, Gale D, Dewire P, et al. The clinical importance of meniscal tears demonstrated by magnetic resonance imaging in osteoarthritis of the knee. J Bone J Surg 2003;85-A:4–9

77. Dervin GF, Stiell IG, Rody K, Grabowski J. Effect of arthroscopic debridement for osteoarthritis of the knee on health-related quality of life. J Bone J Surg 2003;85-A:10–19

78. Bellamy N, Buchanan WW, Goldsmith CH, Campbell J, Stitt LW. Validation study of WOMAC: a health status instrument for measuring clinically important patient-relevant outcomes following total hip or knee arthroplasty in osteoarthritis. J Rheumatol 1988;1:95–108

79. Ware JE Jr, Sherbourne CD. The MOS 36-item short-form health survey (SF-36): conceptual framework and item selection. Med Care 1992;30:473–483

80. Garrett W. The orthopaedic forum: evaluation and treatment of the arthritic knee. J Bone J Surg 2003;85-A:156–157

12

Electrothermal Chondroplasty

AMIR M. KHAN AND GARY S. FANTON

Few effective options are available to the orthopedic surgeon in the treatment of advanced chondromalacia and arthritis following failure of medical management. Currently, lavage[1-3] and debridement,[4-6] repair stimulation techniques,[7,8] cell and tissue transplantation,[9-11] osteochondral plugs,[12-15] and biologic and synthetic matrices[16] are options in the treatment of arthritis. Cartilaginous defects that do not penetrate through to the subchondral bone show little or no reparative response.[17,18] It is believed that grade I, II, and III lesions propagate through a process of delamination, fragmentation, or fibrillation.[19] This degradative process can be slowed in grade II, III, and IV lesions with debridement of the loose cartilage to a stable rim. Generally, this is accomplished by the use of mechanical instruments such as rotary shavers, hand instruments, or thermal devices such as lasers and more recently the use of radiofrequency energy (RFE) probes.

Mechanical debridement with shavers and probes has been the mainstay of cartilage debridement and regeneration but it is not without deleterious effects.[20,21] It results in fine surface fibrillation as well as iatrogenic defects involving normal cartilage of various sizes. Cartilage regeneration can be accomplished by abrading the subchondral bone, which results in subchondral bleeding and formation of fibrocartilage, which is not as functional as normal hyaline cartilage.[22]

Thermal energy used to debride cartilage was initially attempted with laser, and it showed some early promise.[23,24] However, the depth of thermal damage and healing response following application of lasers has been a concern.[25] Histologic and biochemical studies on rabbit articular cartilage after laser treatment confirmed extensive damage reducing cell viability and expression of proteoglycans.[26] Another study of acute and chronic response of articular cartilage to holmium:yttrium-aluminum-garnet (Ho:YAG) laser treatment confirmed no healing of full- or partial-thickness defects in hyaline cartilage.[27] At present the healing of articular cartilage following laser energy application remains controversial.

Thermal chondroplasty with RFE has become tremendously popular over the past few years. It is believed that up to 10,000 procedures are being performed monthly. RFE chondroplasty has gained popularity based on anecdotal reports of clinical success and lack of peer reviewed prospective clinical studies.

Several basic science studies have shown the effect of bipolar (bRFE) and monopolar (mRFE) radiofrequency energy on animal and human cartilage models.[21,28-38] Chondrocyte death has been observed following RFE chondroplasty and remains a concern in the clinical setting.[29-31,35-38] It is believed that thermal chondroplasty alters the mechanical and or structural properties of the superficial layer of the articular cartilage that slows or possibly stops the degenerative cycle.[21] Some hypothesize that RFE may also reduce the release of collagen and proteoglycan epitopes into the synovial fluid, thus reducing the cycle of cartilage degradation, synovial inflammation, and further articular degeneration.[30] Radiofrequency energy is an inexpensive tool that is easy to use for the surgeon and operative personnel, and it can be delivered arthroscopically with a wide variety of probes that offer extended flexibility to the surgeon. In addition, mRFE has the advantage of providing temperature-controlled application, thus potentially widening the margin of safety when treating intraarticular structures.[30,35-38] Nevertheless, application of RFE for chondroplasty in the clinical setting should proceed with caution until more basic and clinical studies can confirm the efficacy and safety of these devices.

■ Radiofrequency Energy

There are two basic types of radiofrequency (RF) circuitry for use in orthopedic applications: monopolar and bipolar. The tissue temperature profiles for these two systems are vastly different. The RFE oscillates the electrolytes in the intracellular and extracellular solutions producing molecular friction.

In the monopolar setting, the current flows from the current generator **(Fig. 12–1),** which takes power from a line source such as 110 V at 60 Hz, boosts the power to as high as 600 V or even greater, and transforms it into an alternating current at 460 kHz by oscillating a crystal tuned to 460,000 on/off per second. The current passes from the box through the connecting cable, through the probe (active electrode) into the patient, through the patient to the return electrode (indifferent electrode or ground pad), and back to a return within the box. Because the patient's tissue has a higher resistance than the rest of the circuit, heat is produced at the point where there is a step-up in the resistance. During chondroplasty, the RFE may choose to pass from the probe through the cartilage surface and subchondral bone to the grounding plate on the skin, or from the probe through the irrigation solution to the joint capsule and then to the grounding plate. The path selected is most likely determined by the impedance encountered as it passes along the cartilage surface and may be influenced by the cartilage thickness, water content, proteoglycan concentration, collagen content,

subchondral bone thickness, and the conductive characteristics of the irrigation solution selected.[30] Primary heating occurs in the upper layers of the tissue, which then heats the deeper layers of tissue.[39] The temperature is monitored 50 times per second, providing a constant feedback to the RF generator that automatically adjusts power output accordingly, much like the thermostat in a room. The gradient of thermal effect seen with monopolar RF arthroscopy is capable of achieving a deeper tissue response if necessary.[40]

This is in distinction to laser energy, which produces heat through direct photostimulation of cellular ions, and bipolar RF, which creates a conduction path through the arthroscopy fluid rather than through the treated tissue. The current produced by bipolar RF follows a path of least resistance from the probe tip, through the conductive irrigating solution, and back to another conductive electrode a very short distance away. High temperatures between bipolar probe electrodes are reached as the current "arcs" between them heating the surrounding solution. The heated solution provides high surface temperatures with limited ability to penetrate deeper tissue. Less current is required with a bipolar device to achieve the same effect, because the current passes through a much smaller volume of tissue. The thermal effect of RFE is determined by the level of energy used, duration of treatment, type of tissue treated, and type of electrode used. In addition, the extent of thermal modification is operator dependent and due to the lack of tactile response in the no contact approach, it relies on visual observation of the tissue response.

■ Basic Science of Thermal Chondroplasty

The Ho:YAG laser has been used to treat chondromalacia,[21] but concerns of avascular necrosis in the clinical setting and large zone of thermal injury in animal studies[22] has resulted in limited use of this approach. Lane et al[26] performed matrix assessment in a rabbit model following Ho:YAG laser treatment of articular cartilage and found that extensive articular cartilage damage is caused by the laser. Biochemically, the amount of glycosaminoglycan in the treated cartilage, and the amount of sulfate incorporation into proteoglycans was significantly less in laser-treated articular cartilage than controls. In addition, subchondral changes including bony architectural damage, blood vessel membrane damage, and lack of osteocytes in lacunae was also observed. They postulated that cell viability was greatly reduced, and the subchondral changes could possibly explain the clinical avascular necrosis observed in some cases.

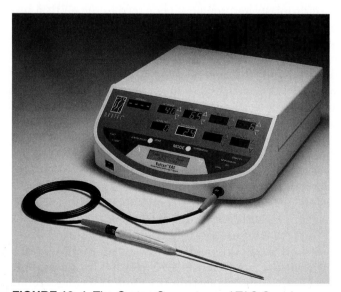

FIGURE 12–1 The Oratec Generator and TAC C probe.

Another study of acute and chronic response of articular cartilage to Ho:YAG laser treatment confirmed no healing of full- or partial-thickness defects in hyaline cartilage.[27]

Several in vitro and in vivo studies have demonstrated the ultrastructural and histologic changes that occur after mRFE treatment of capsular tissue.[39–45] However, studies on RFE chondroplasty are limited. Peer-reviewed prospective clinical outcome studies have not been published, but basic science studies of the effect of RFE on human and animal cartilage models have been published.[21,28–38]

A study compared rotary shaver debridement of articular cartilage with that of a bipolar RF probe on distal femur of sheep. A modification of Mankin's scoring system using six histologic variables was evaluated in terms of favorable and unfavorable response to treatment. The outcome was superior for the bipolar probe, and in addition, viability of remaining cartilage with less destruction of normal architecture was noted.[21] However, this study did not report on the power settings and energy delivery and did not use the currently accepted methods for evaluating cell viability. In addition, a major shortcoming of this study was that the cartilage defects did not represent degenerative chondromalacia changes. Instead, the investigators created a fracture in healthy cartilage and used this to simulate the changes seen with grade II and grade III chondromalacia.

To address this concern, Kaplan et al[33] evaluated the effects of RF ablation on freshly acquired human knee cartilage from patients undergoing total knee arthroplasty. Although cartilage smoothing was obtained, the authors discovered no increased incidence of chondrocyte death in the adjacent areas after the debridement. They concluded that the probe did not cause any significant injury to the surrounding tissue. The shortcomings of this study include the use of insensitive techniques of light microscopy with hematoxylin and eosin and periodic acid-Schiff staining to determine cell viability. In addition, the authors recognized that their study examined the changes at time zero, and that the need for additional evaluation of this technique to determine long-term chondrocyte survival and function was necessary. A case report of a second-look arthroscopy 1 year following bipolar chondroplasty revealed a scalloped cavity with appreciable thinning of the articular surface in the treated region.[46] This raises concern about the delayed appearance of injury to the chondrocytes with subsequent formation of a depression in the articulating surface. The authors of this chapter have also encountered similar isolated cases.

Lu et al[35] evaluated in vitro chondrocyte viability and surface contouring of human articular cartilage using confocal laser microscopy (CLM) and scanning electron microscopy (SEM) after treatment with different time intervals of RFE and bRFE. Monopolar RFE probe was applied in light contact without flow and the bRFE probe was applied noncontact with flow as per manufacturers recommendations. The authors found that bRFE caused significantly greater chondrocyte death than did mRFE at identical treatment time intervals. The SEM results showed that mRFE created a smoother surface than bRFE at 5-second application, but no significant differences were seen at longer application intervals. At a 15-second interval the cartilage met the authors' definition of optimal contouring based on SEM grading system. The authors feel that arthroscopy may overestimate the degree of smoothing given its low magnification, but it remains unclear if SEM grading correlates with clinical outcome. In a previous study, Lu et al[30] compared two bipolar and one monopolar RFE probes. Each probe type was applied to the cartilage using a controlled mechanical jig, noncontact mode, and paintbrush pattern. A higher chondrocyte death in the two bipolar probe types was confirmed. In addition, the bipolar systems penetrated to the level of subchondral bone in all osteochondral sections during arthroscopically guided paintbrush pattern treatment. Monopolar probes did not penetrate the subchondral bone in the three modes of application studied. In summary, the researchers concluded that RFE should be used cautiously for thermal chondroplasty until viability of chondrocytes could be improved. In addition, a recent study reported that the lavage solution temperature may have significant influence on chondrocyte viability when thermal chondroplasty is being conducted.[38] Further in vivo studies investigating the long-term effects of lavage solution temperature are needed.

■ Clinical Considerations for Thermal Chondroplasty

The term *chondroplasty* implies a surgical procedure, which promotes or facilitates the development or regeneration of normal articular cartilage. Traditionally cold cutting instruments such as drills and mechanical burrs or curettes have been used to perform these procedures. The nature of these procedures involves debriding eburnated bone to stimulate a bleeding response and allow migration of marrow cells with high potential for repair. Under appropriate biomechanical conditions, the ensuing blood clot becomes fibrous tissue, which subsequently undergoes metaplasia to fibrocartilage and, it is hoped, hyaline-like articular material. The use of thermal energy, such as RFE or laser energy, in the performing of "chondroplasty" really represents a surgical debridement of damaged articular surfaces. The primary goal is not to stimulate repair but debride unstable fragments and prevent further mechanical disruption of remaining cartilage layers. Although, some studies have suggested that repair is stimulated in laser-treated articular cartilage.[23,24]

The Ho:YAG laser when properly used is tangentially applied parallel to the articular surface to avoid iatrogenic damage to underlying normal chondrocytes. Grade II and III chondromalacia represent the best indications for this thermal coagulation of damaged articular surfaces. Many second-look arthroscopies have noted the sealing of articular cartilage fissures to be mechanically stable without further expansion of the degenerative areas previously treated.[47]

Great confusion currently exists over the indications and contraindications for RFE-assisted chondroplasty. Earlier RF chondroplasty studies were done on animal models; however, more recent in vitro human cartilage studies have allowed potential extrapolation of data to clinical situations. Despite an abundance of basic science studies, there is a lack of well-designed clinical studies, which can truly assess the benefits of RFE chondroplasty. Anecdotal reports of successful mRFE chondroplasty as assessed by second-look arthroscopies and high-field magnetic resonance imaging (MRI) have been published.[47] Khan et al[48] performed a retrospective study of 12 patients with grade III chondromalacia of the patella who were treated with mRFE chondroplasty. All patients had chronically symptomatic patellofemoral pain with clinical findings indicative of chondromalacia, and all patients had failed a conservative program of physical therapy and patellar taping for at least 3 months. All patients underwent preoperative MRI evaluation including T1, T2, and fast spin echo short-time inversion recovery (STIR) sequences of patellofemoral joint in sagittal, coronal, and axial planes. Special attention was paid to the evaluation of the subchondral bone for osseous edema. All patients underwent low power temperature regulated arthroscopic monopolar thermal chondroplasty of the patella. Postoperatively, three patients had the MRI evaluation at 3 months, six at 6 months, and three at 1 year. All pre- and postoperative MRIs were assessed by a board-certified radiologist. None of the 12 patients had any discernible signal changes on postoperative MRI scans of the underlying bone on T1, T2, and STIR sequences to suggest avascular necrosis. Eleven of 12 patients reported improvement in clinical symptoms at 1 year, and one patient was symptomatically unchanged compared with preoperatively.

Similar clinical successes have been presented following RFE chondroplasty.[49–52] Baker et al[53] noted excellent functional results along with favorable MRI findings following ablative chondroplasty. Owens et al[50] reported superior clinical outcomes with bRFE debridement of patellar grade II and III chondral lesions when compared with mechanical devices. However, Stein et al,[51] in a prospective study of 146 patients who were randomly placed in either a control group (chondroplasty alone) or a treatment group (chondroplasty and electrocautery), showed that electrocautery as an adjunct to chondroplasty offered little benefit in the treatment of chondromalacic lesions and in fact may limit successful outcome. Several multicenter trials are ongoing and early reports suggest RFE to be promising in the treatment of chondromalacia.[52] Nevertheless the effect of RFE on articular cartilage confirms that chondrocytes are temperature sensitive, and temperatures greater than 45°C can cause excessive chondrocyte death and may promote further degeneration of the articular cartilage.[28] Great care is emphasized in the selection of operative parameters regarding the RFE chondroplasty until safety and efficacy are confirmed via well-designed prospective randomized clinical studies.

■ Surgical Technique

Current options for thermal chondroplasty include the use of laser, bRFE **(Fig. 12–2)**, or mRFE **(Fig. 12–3)**. In our institution mRFE treatment of the articular surface is performed with a specially designed TAC-C probe (Oratec Interventions, Menlo Park, CA). Our selection of this probe is based on basic science studies that confirm mRFE to have the safest profile in regard to depth of chondrocyte death. Operative parameters for performing thermal chondroplasty should not exceed 50°C and 30 W of power. The current Oratec system automat-

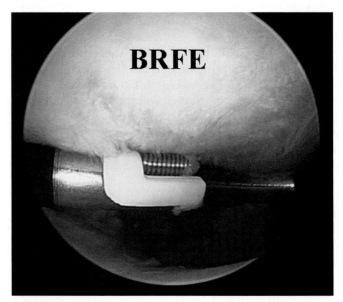

FIGURE 12–2 Bipolar Mitek Vapor probe device being used to treat the cartilage.

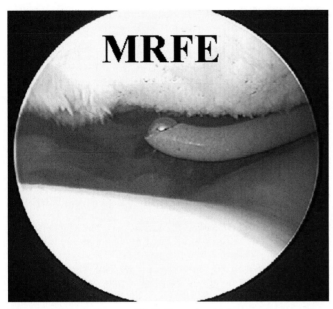

FIGURE 12–3 Oratec TAC C probe being used in a "near contact" or gentle contact method to treat the cartilage.

ically senses the probe being attached and defaults to the set parameters. In practice, the lowest possible temperature and power settings are used to achieve the desired visual thermal effect. At this time, the lavage solution is kept at room temperature but further studies are being conducted to identify the optimal lavage solution temperature for mRFE chondroplasty.

Initially, loose and fibrillated cartilage is mechanically shaved. This is done to even out the cartilage fibril length and remove larger unstable flaps allowing a more effective thermal depth of penetration and contouring. A no-contact application by bipolar probes can produce smoothing of the articular cartilage and application longer than 2 to 3 seconds is discouraged. However, a no-contact application of the monopolar probe does not produce any smoothing of the articular cartilage.[30] Therefore, a "near contact" or gentle contact method is used, lightly brushing the damaged cartilage surface as it congeals and shrinks the fibrils like the end of a nylon rope. Avoid prolonged application of RFE to one place and avoid pushing the probe deep into the lesion. In vitro studies have suggested application times of up to 15 seconds for optimal contouring. However, we rely on visual assessment of smoothing and do not apply the probe for more than a few seconds to one area. At this time, the concern of causing chondrocyte death supersedes optimal contouring. In cases of grade IV lesions, the edges of the defect should be carefully smoothed to minimize step-off against areas of normal cartilage. Avoid direct application of RFE to the subchondral bone as irreversible damage may occur. The safety of this procedure lies in the surgeon's understanding of the potential deleterious effect of temperature on chondrocyte viability

and the potential of full-thickness loss of articular cartilage secondary to inappropriately high power settings. We have encountered a few cases of cartilage damage of the femoral condyles referred to us following treatment with bRFE chondroplasty. Other reports of cartilage damage following bRFE have also been published.[46]

Postoperatively, rehabilitation is begun with no specific restrictions other than patient comfort. Generally, this occurs a few days after surgery and emphasizes range-of-motion and progressive closed kinetic chain exercises. Although we have not had any cases of avascular necrosis of the subchondral bone following monopolar RF chondroplasty, the presence of continued pain postoperatively may warrant a workup for avascular necrosis.

■ Conclusion

Radiofrequency energy is currently being used in the treatment of grade II, III, and IV chondromalacia. Basic science studies have confirmed that RFE can mechanically debride the articular surface by smoothing, thus potentially reducing further delamination. However, a zone of thermal injury in the areas of treatment has been observed with loss of chondrocyte viability. bRFE appears to create a larger zone of cartilage injury than does mRFE, but other factors such as application technique, duration of application, and lavage solution temperature may also effect the viability of chondrocytes. Therefore, further use of this procedure lies in the surgeon's understanding of the limitations of alternate treatment options and the risks and benefits of RFE chondroplasty on chondrocyte viability. At this time, we prefer mRFE, although bRFE remains a potential alternative. Great care should be taken in the selection of operative parameters by individual clinicians when using RFE chondroplasty until more clinical and basic science studies can define appropriate safety and efficacy protocols.

REFERENCES

1. Jackson RW. Arthroscopic treatment of degenerative arthritis. In: McGinty JB, Caspari RB, Jackson RW, Poehling GG, eds. Operative Arthroscopy. New York: Raven Press, 1991:319–323
2. Livesley PJ, Doherty M, Needoff M, Moulton A. Arthroscopic lavage of osteoarthritic knees. J Bone Joint Surg Br 1991;73:922–926
3. Gibson JN, White MD, Chapman VM, Strachan RK. Arthroscopic lavage and debridement for osteoarthritis of the knee. J Bone Joint Surg Br 1992;74:534–537
4. Baumgaertner MR, Cannon WD Jr, Vittori JM, Schmidt ES, Maurer RC. Arthroscopic debridement of the arthritic knee. Clin Orthop 1990;253:197–202
5. Sprague NK III. Arthroscopic debridement for degenerative knee joint disease. Clin Orthop 1990;253:197–202
6. Hubbard MJ. Articular debridement versus washout for degeneration of the femoral condyle: a five year study. J Bone Joint Surg Br 1996;78:217–219

7. Buckwalter JA, Mankin HJ. Articular cartilage: tissue design and chondrocyte-matrix interactions. Instr Course Lect 1998;47: 477–486

8. Steadman JR, Rodkey WG, Singleton SB, Briggs KK. Microfracture technique for full-thickness chondral defects: technique and clinical results. Op Tech Orthop 1997;7:300–304

9. Grande DA, Pitman MI, Peterson L, Menche D, Klein M. The repair of experimentally produced defects in rabbit articular cartilage by autologous chondrocyte transplantation. J Orthop Res 1989;7:208–218

10. Brittenberg M, Nilsson A, Lindahl A, Ohlsson C, Peterson L. Rabbit articular cartilage defects treated with autologous cultured chondrocytes. Clin Orthop 1996;326:270–283

11. Peterson L, Minas T, Brittberg M, Nilsson A, Sjogren-Jansson E, Lindahl A. A two year to 9-year outcome after autologous chondrocyte transplantation of the knee. Clin Orthop 2000;374: 212–234

12. Hangody L, Kish G, Karpati Z, Udvarhelyi I, Szigeti I, Bely M. Mosaicplasty for the treatment of articular cartilage defects: application in clinical practice. Orthopedics 1998;21:751–756

13. Garrett JC. Osteochondral allografts for reconstruction of articular defects of the knee. Instr Course Lect 1998;47:517–522

14. Czitrom AA, Keating S, Gross AE. The viability of articular cartilage in fresh osteochondral allografts after clinical transplantation. J Bone Joint Surg Am 1990;72:574–581

15. Garrett JC. Osteochondritis dissecans. Clin Sports Med 1991;10:569–593

16. Jackson DW, Felt JC, Song Y, Van Sickle DC, Simon TM. Restoration of large femoral trochlear sulcus articular cartilage lesions using a flowable polymer: an experimental study in sheep. Trans Orthop Res Soc 2000;25:670

17. Mankin HJ. Responses of articular cartilage to mechanical injury. J Bone Joint Surg Am 1982;54:460–466

18. Goldberg VM, Caplan AI. Biologic restoration of articular surfaces. Instr Course Lect 1999;12:474–484

19. Kevin AJ, Coleman A, Wisnom MR, et al. Propagation of surface fissures in articular cartilage subjected to cyclic loading. Orthopedic Research Society 1998, New Orleans

20. Grigka J, Boenke S, Schreiner C, Lohnert J. Significance of laser treatment in arthroscopic therapy of degenerative gonarthritis. Knee Surg Sports Traumatol Arthrosc 1994;2:88–93

21. Turner AS, Tippett JW, Powers BE, Dewell RD, Hallinckrodt CH. Radiofrequency (electrosurgical) ablation of articular cartilage: a study in sheep. Arthroscopy 1998;14:585–591

22. Wirth CJ, Ruddert M. Techniques of cartilage growth enhancement: a review of the literature. Arthroscopy 1996;12:300–308

23. Collier MA, Haugland LM, Bellamy J, et al. Effects of holmium:YAG laser on equine articular cartilage and subchondral bone adjacent to traumatic lesions: a histopathological assessment. Arthroscopy 1993;9:536–545

24. Miller DV, O'Brien SJ, Arnoczky SS, Kelly A, Fealy SV, Warren RF. The use of the contact Nd:YAG laser in arthroscopic surgery: effects on articular cartilage and meniscal tissue. Arthroscopy 1989;5:245–253

25. Fink B, Schneider T, Braunstein S, et al. Holmium:YAG laser-induced aseptic bone necroses of the femoral condyle. Arthroscopy 1996;12:217–223

26. Lane JG, Amiel ME, Monosov AS, Ameil D. Matrix assessment of the articular cartilage surface after chondroplasty with the holmium:YAG laser. Am J Sports Med 1997;25:560–569

27. Trauner KB, Nikoshita NS, Flotte T, Patel D. Acute and chronic response of articular cartilage to holmium:YAG laser irradiation. Clin Orthop 1995;310:52–57

28. Lu Y, Hayashi K, Hecht P, et al. The effect of monopolar radiofrequency energy on partial-thickness defects of articular cartilage. Arthroscopy 2000;16:527–536

29. Edwards RB III, Markel MD. Radiofrequency energy treatment effects on articular cartilage Op Tech Sports Med 2001;11: 96–104

30. Lu Y, Edwards RB III, Cole BJ, Markel MD. Thermal chondroplasty with radiofrequency energy, an in vitro comparison of bipolar and monopolar radiofrequency devices. Am J Sports Med 2001;29:42–49

31. Lu Y. MD, Edwards RB III, Kalscheur VL, Nino S, Cole BJ, Markel MD. Effect of bipolar radiofrequency energy on human articular cartilage: comparison of confocal laser microscopy and light microscopy. Arthroscopy 2001;17:117–123

32. Krenzel BA, Mann CH, Kayes AV, Speer KP. The effects of radiofrequency ablation on articular cartilage: a time dependent analysis. Presented at the 67th Annual Meeting of the American Academy of Orthopaedic Surgeons 2000, March 15–19, Orlando FL

33. Kaplan L, Uribe JW, Sasken H, Markarian G. The acute effects of radiofrequency energy in articular cartilage: an in vitro study. Arthroscopy 2000;16:2–5

34. Gundel J, Saskin H, Popovitz L, et al. The effect of bipolar radiofrequency energy on partial-thickness defects in a sheep model. Arthroscopy Association of North America 20th Annual Meeting, April 19–22, 2001, Seattle

35. Lu Y, Edwards RB, Nho S, Heiner JP, Cole BJ, Markel MD. Thermal chondroplasty with bipolar and monopolar radiofrequency energy: effect of treatment time on chondrocyte death and surface contouring. Arthroscopy 2002;18:779–788

36. Edwards RB, Lu Y, Nho S, Heiner JP, Cole BJ, Markel MD. Thermal chondroplasty of chondromalaic human cartilage. Am J Sp Med 2002;30:90–97

37. Edwards RB, Lu Y, Nho S, Rodriguez E, Markel MD. Thermometric determination of cartilage matrix temperatures during thermal chondroplasty: comparison of bipolar and monopolar radiofrequency devices. Arthroscopy 2002;18:779–788

38. Lu Y, Edwards RB, Nho S, Heiner JP, Cole BJ, Markel MD. Lavage solution temperature influences depth of chondrocyte death and surface contouring during thermal chondroplasty with temperature-controlled monopolar radiofrequency energy. Am J Sp Med 2002;30:667–673

39. Hayashi K, Markel MD. Thermal modification of joint capsule and ligamentous tissues. Op Tech in Sports Med 1998;6:120–125

40. Hecht P, Hayashi K, Cooley AJ, et al. The thermal effect of monopolar radiofrequency energy on the properties of joint capsule. An in vivo histologic study using a sheep model. Am J Sports Med 1998;26:808–814

41. Lopez MJ, Hayashi K, Fanton GS, Thabit G III, Markel MD. The effect of radiofrequency on the ultrastructure of joint capsule collagen. Arthroscopy 1998;14:495–501

42. Hecht P, Hayashi K, Lu Y, et al. Monopolar radiofrequency energy effects on joint capsule tissue: potential treatment for joint stability. An in vivo mechanical, morphological, and biochemical study using an ovine model. Am J Sports Med 1999;27:761–771

43. Lopez MJ, Hayashi K, Vanderby R, Thabit G III, Fanton GS, Markel MD. Effects of monopolar radiofrequency energy on ovine joint capsular mechanical properties. Clin Orthop Rel Res 2000;374:286–297

44. Hayashi K, Thabit G, Massa KL, et al. The effect of thermal heating on the length and histologic properties of the glenohumeral joint capsule. Am J Sports Med 1997;25:107–112

45. Naseef GS, Foster TE, Trauner K, Solhpour S, Anderson RR, Zarins B. The thermal properties of bovine joint capsule. The basic science of laser and radiofrequency induced capsular shrinkage. Am J Sports Med 1997;25:670–674

46. Hogan CJ, Diduch DR. Progressive articular cartilage loss following radiofrequency treatment of a partial-thickness lesion. A case report. Arthroscopy 2001;17:E24

47. Dillingham MF. Arthroscopic electrothermal surgery of the knee. Op Tech Sports Med 1998;6:154–156

48. Khan AM, Bonzon CJ, Indelli PF, Fanton GS. Magnetic resonance imaging of the patella following arthroscopic monopolar radiofrequency chondroplasty. Presented at the Arthroscopy Association of North America 20th Annual Meeting, April 19–22, 2001, Seattle

49. Antounian F. Nonrandomized study of coblation treatment in articular cartilage surgery: interim findings. Presented at the Arthrocare-sponsored symposium during the 67th Annual Meeting of the American Academy of Orthopaedic Surgeons, March 15–19, 2000, Orlando, FL

50. Owens BD, Stickles BJ, Balikian P, Busconi BD. Arthroscopy. Prospective analysis of radiofrequency versus mechanical debridement of isolated patellar chondral lesions. Arthroscopy 2002;18:151–155

51. Stein DT, Ricciardi CA, Viehe T. The effectiveness of the use of electrocautery with chondroplasty in treating chondromalacic lesions: A randomized prospective study. Arthroscopy 2002;18: 190–193

52. Tasto J. Radiofrequency and articular cartilage debate. Presented at the Arthroscopy Association of North America 21st Fall Course, November 17–20, 2002, Palm Desert, CA

53. Baker MD, Branche MD. Megnetic resonance imaging evaluation of ablative chondroplasty. Presented at the Arthroscopy Association of North America 21st Fall Course, November 17–20, 2002, Palm Desert, California

13

Microfracture Technique

PAUL SETHI, RAFFY MIRZAYAN, AND F. DANIEL KHARRAZI

Chondral defects of the knee are frequently associated with ligamentous, meniscal and combined injuries of the athlete's knee.[1] Alone, or in conjunction with other associated intrinsic knee injuries, chondral and osteochondral defects can be responsible for pain, effusion, mechanical symptoms, and significant limitation of the athlete. Rarely do these lesions heal spontaneously, and with time most patients develop degenerative changes associated with these defects.[2–4] A variety of treatment options including arthroscopic lavage, marrow stimulating or microfracture techniques, autologous chondrocyte implantation, and osteochondral implantation, allogenic and autograft, have been described with variable success.[1] Unlike ligament disruption, there are no reconstructive or restorative techniques at present that restore the chondral defect to normal hyaline articular cartilage. This chapter describes the indications, patient selection, surgical technique, postoperative care, and complications associated with the microfracture technique.

■ Evaluation

Evaluation of the patient with an articular cartilage lesion is best accomplished with a methodical approach. There are numerous published treatment algorithms,[1] but understanding how best to navigate the algorithm is probably of greater importance. In 1998, the International Cartilage Repair Society made recommendations on an approach to include specific variables so that comprehensive understanding of the injury was elucidated.

A thorough history should elucidate the onset and chronicity of symptoms, describe and assess the symptoms, and determine their traumatic or spontaneous origin. A history of systemic medical problems including collagen disorders or human leukocyte antigen (HLA)-B27 associations is also essential. Previous treatment for the problem is also instrumental in the management and decision-making process.

Despite a complete physical examination, the most likely clinical presentation of full-thickness cartilage injuries are mechanical complaints consistent with a loose body or simply pain that is localizable to a specific compartment. Patients frequently have recurrent effusions, but joint line pain or a palpable point of tenderness is not always present. Ligamentous examination and assessment of overall alignment are essential.

Radiographic assessment is discussed in greater detail in earlier chapters. Standard radiographs [standing full length anteroposterior (AP), lateral, and 45-degree posteroanterior (PA) views] are used to evaluate the presence of a lesion, arthritic changes, and axial alignment. Magnetic resonance imaging (MRI) is also used to delineate the location, size, and depth of the lesion, as well as to help define associated subchondral bone bruising and meniscal and ligamentous injury. The use of radionucleotide bone scan is not as well defined, but we believe it can be a useful tool, especially in determining bony activity in previously operated knees.

■ Indications

The general indication for microfracture is a full-thickness articular cartilage defect on the weight-bearing aspect of the tibia, femur, trochlear groove, or patella. Microfracture has also been used on chondral defects in the humerus, glenoid, talus, and capitellum. It is difficult to apply an age threshold; however, usually young patients with a small, contained defect are likely to improve. Microfracture is not our recommended treatment for osteoarthritis. The ideal condition for a microfracture is a symptomatic, contained, femoral condylar lesion that is less than 2 cm^2 in size. We do not routinely prophylactically treat asymptomatic defects, nor do we convert partial-thickness lesions into full-thickness lesions.

We are very hesitant to perform microfracture or any articular cartilage preservation procedure in patients with axial malalignment. Sharma et al[5] reported that a varus malalignment of greater than 5 degrees increases the risk of medial compartment osteoarthritis fourfold, and that valgus alignment increases the risk of lateral compartment osteoarthritis fivefold. These patients are often candidates for tibial or femoral osteotomy in a staged or sometimes simultaneous fashion. Patients with systemic diseases and inflammatory arthritides, such rheumatoid arthritis and systemic lupus erythematous, are not candidates for microfracture.

■ Surgical Technique

The goal of this procedure is to penetrate the calcified cartilage layer, leave the subchondral plate intact, and penetrate the subchondral bone to create an access channel for mesenchymal stem cells to differentiate into a stable repair tissue, that is, fibrocartilage.

Standard arthroscopic portals are made anterolateally and anteromedially. A suprapatellar portal can also be added at the individual surgeon's preference. We find it useful when there is copious joint debris. After completing diagnostic arthroscopy, we perform all intraarticular work including debridement, removal of any loose chondral fragments, and then microfracture. In conjunction with anterior cruciate ligament (ACL) reconstruction, we perform the microfracture first so as not to put additional stress on the new graft.

In preparation for microfracture, the lesion is identified and all loose or delaminated fragments are removed to create stable edges of articular cartilage. We do not routinely use thermal or radiofrequency energy to treat the cartilage defects. If a sclerotic base is present, abrasion chondroplasty is used in conjunction with a microfracture to create a bleeding base.

Small partial-thickness lesions are debrided of unstable fragments, and no further procedure is undertaken. Spuriously diagnosed lesions that are smaller than 2 cm^2 and asymptomatic are debrided of any unstable edges and left alone. Partial-thickness lesions should not be debrided into full-thickness lesions.

The contained lesion is debrided down to exposed bone using an arthroscopic shaver. A stable rim of cartilage now surrounds the lesion **(Fig. 13–1)**. Steadman et al[4] point out that it is essential to remove the layer of

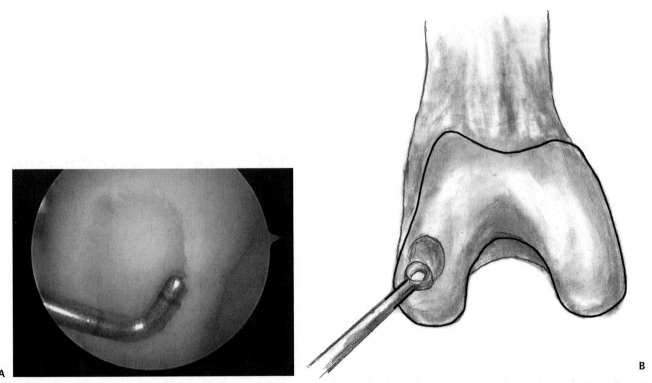

A   B

FIGURE 13–1 (A) The lesion has been debrided of loose and worn cartilage. Care is taken to remove the calcified cartilage layer and to leave a stable rim of healthy cartilage around the lesion. **(B)** A ring curette may be used to remove the calcified cartilage layer.

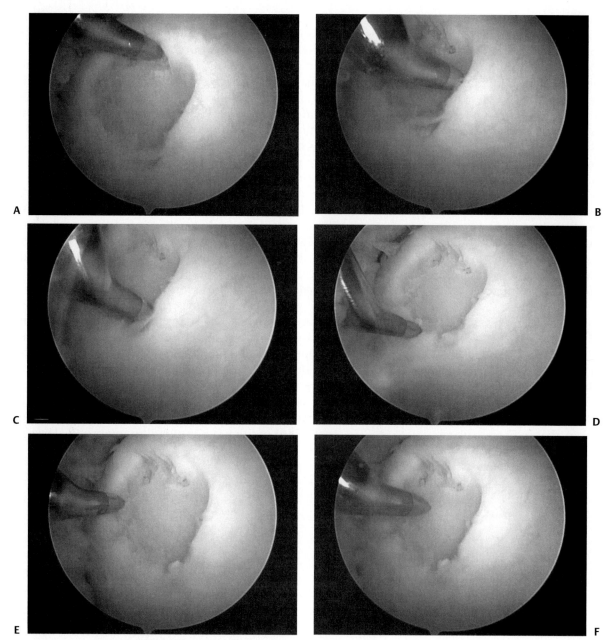

FIGURE 13–2 (A) Microfracture is performed systematically at the periphery of the lesion starting at the 12 o'clock position. **(B-E)** The microfracture is then carried around like the face of a clock until the 12 o'clock position is reached again. **(F)** Once the periphery has been microfractured, then the central portion of the lesion is addressed.

calcified cartilage. This is performed with a curette, or with the shaver used in the high-speed forward mode, but not with a high-speed burr. Although it is important to create a roughened surface for a clot to adhere to, it is equally important not to remove so much subchondral bone as to compromise the structural integrity of the bone.

Starting peripherally in the lesion, an awl is penetrated ~4 mm into the bone, such that the subchondral bone is penetrated and either fat or blood is seen com-

ing from the hole **(Fig. 13–2).** Penetration of the bone is ideally accomplished perpendicular to the articular surface. This is done with various angled awls, or more simply at different knee flexion angles. The procedure is continued around the periphery, using the awl to penetrate subchondral bone, leaving 2-mm bridges between the punctures, without causing adjacent holes to become confluent with one another. This is continued, working centrally until the defect is filled **(Fig. 13–3).** Satisfactory penetration of the subchondral bone may

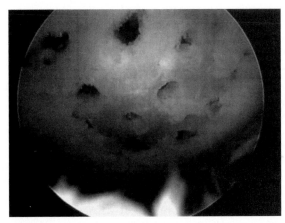

FIGURE 13–3 The defect is then completely filled, taking care not to allow the channels to coalesce, which would lead to breakdown of subchondral bone.

be assessed by visualization of bleeding bone or fat droplets, which is most easily obtained by creating a negative pressure (inflow off, suction on) at the end of the microfracture procedure **(Fig. 13–4).**

The high cost of awls has been criticized, and the less expensive use of Kirschner wires (K-wires) has been advocated. However, K-wires, when drilled into hard subchondral bone, can generate heat and subsequent thermal necrosis of the same tissue that is being stimulated to fill the chondral defect. The theoretical advantage of arthroscopic awls versus the risk of thermal necrosis with drilling technique is not proven, and we recommend using whichever technique surgeons are most comfortable with. Drilling with K-wires can also theoretically leave smooth channels, which "super-clot" will not adhere to, but again this has not been proven. Retrograde drilling, using the ACL guide to pinpoint

the area of osteonecrosis can assist in difficult to reach areas of necrosis.

The patellofemoral joint warrants special mention. It is paramount to keep in mind that chondromalacia patella frequently exists in the asymptomatic state, and responds to a wide number of treatments that do not address the articular surface.[6] Similarly, trochlear lesions are usually well shouldered and nonprogressive. Trochlear defects are usually long and narrow. If the lesion is large enough to engage the patella and allow the patella to articulate on bare bone, the area is treated. It may be that the patellofemoral lesions are less likely to be pain sources and more likely to be particle generators. Looking for the exact etiology of the anterior knee pain can be challenging. Only when the more probable cause of anterior knee pain, such as malalignment and instability, are ruled out or treated should patellofemoral microfracture be undertaken. This is not to suggest that microfracture is not a viable option in this anatomic location; rather, we are suggesting that the surgeon proceed systematically.

■ Postoperative Protocol

The correct rehabilitation of any surgical procedure can often be one of the most critical aspects of successful outcomes. The same principle holds true for microfracture techniques, as the proper physical environment for mesenchymal cell differentiation into stable repair tissue can be modulated by therapy.

We believe that motion after microfracture treatment is critical. The motion may simply encourage nourishment for the differentiating mesenchymal cells. It has been suggested that the motion may mediate a cellular

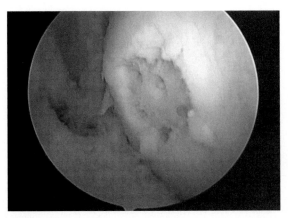

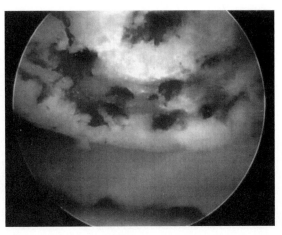

A   B

FIGURE 13–4 (A) Fat droplets (at the 4 o'clock and 5 o'clock positions). **(B)** Blood may be seen to extravasate from the channels.

signal for the mesenchymal cells to differentiate in articular cartilage-like cells.[3] Accordingly, we are firm proponents of immediate motion. We use a continuous passive motion (CPM) device initially; however, it is discontinued as soon as uninhibited pain-free range of motion is achieved. This is routinely assessed at the first postoperative visit, 7 days after surgery. We recommend stationary cycling as an integral part of the daily postoperative protocol. Steadman et al[4] are strong proponents of CPM for 8 hours per day for more than 8 weeks. This is often too cumbersome and impractical for our patient population.

In general, patients are encouraged to walk with crutches, initially non-weight bearing, and to be as mobile as possible to help limit the risk of venous thromboembolism. We do not use any pharmacologic agents to specifically decrease this risk. Treatment with ice or a cold therapy system is very important to help control postoperative swelling. We recommend ice for 20 minutes three to four times a day until swelling is essentially absent. We do not routinely use postoperative bracing, unless a ligamentous procedure has been performed. In isolated lesions, we ideally keep the patient touch-down weight bearing (the weight of the patients leg may rest comfortably on the ground) for 4 to 6 weeks.

Early range-of-motion exercises are important to emphasize. Equally important are immediate initiation of isometric quadriceps exercises and straight leg raises with ankle weights. Two weeks postoperation, aquatic exercises and swimming are encouraged. Gait retraining and strength training are initiated at 8 weeks, and return to sports is permitted when effusion is minimal or absent after exercise, and strength testing reveals 85% of the contralateral leg strength. This is usually at 4 to 6 months, depending on the size of the lesion. Maximal improvement is commonly observed as late as 2 years after the index procedure.[7]

■ Complications

The most common complications of microfracture are more specific to knee arthroscopy rather than to the microfracture technique. Certainly wound infection, pain, and persistent effusions are possible, and all are treated with conventional means. Deep venous thrombosis is an uncommon event and should be treated accordingly.

A failed microfracture, whether defined as persistent focal pain, recurrence of preoperative symptoms, or development of mechanical catching symptoms, is a recognized complication. Occasionally, repeat arthroscopy reveals a hypertrophic scar, which can be debrided to a more congruent bed. This is frequently successful. Treatment of failed microfracture lesions requires further workup and depends on the size and location. Rarely will we treat a lesion that has failed microfracture with a second microfracture procedure; rather, we consider autologous chondrocyte implantation or osteochondral auto/allografting, depending on the size of the residual defect.

■ Healing

Similar to the other marrow stimulating techniques, the basic premise of microfracture is to penetrate the subchondral bone, leaving the bony architecture intact, and create an access channel to the pluripotential mesenchymal stem cells that reside within the bone marrow. The healing response of articular cartilage is well described in an earlier chapter. Simplified, marrow-stimulating techniques generate reparative tissue that is fibrocartilage **(Fig. 13–5)**. Instead of principally type II collagen (along with types VI and IX) normally found in articular cartilage, the repair tissue is predominantly type

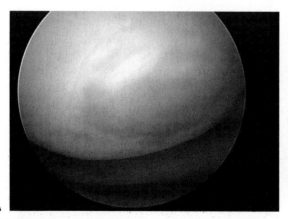
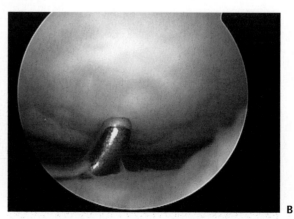

A   B

FIGURE 13–5 (A) Lesion 6 months after microfracture filled with fibrocartilage. **(B)** Note that the repair tissue is soft and is "dimpled" with a probe.

I collagen. It is likely that the composition difference accounts for the wear characteristics and longevity of the repair.[2–4]

■ Results

Left untreated, cartilage defects rarely heal spontaneously. Messner and Maletius[8] reported on the natural history of traumatically acquired full-thickness cartilage injuries in 28 athletes treated conservatively. Good or excellent results were reported in 22 of 28 patients at 14 years when left untreated. However, radiographic evidence of joint space narrowing was observed in 43% of patients, and these authors concluded that this rate of radiographic change was "twice as high as in patients with partial meniscectomy with intact cartilage at similar follow-up time." It is important to recognize that not all chondral defects are symptomatic, and prophylactic treatment of asymptomatic lesions is at best controversial. However, patients who have symptoms that are consistent with their articular cartilage lesions probably will have the best outcome when they are treated.

To best understand the benefits of microfracture it is useful to evaluate the benefits of arthroscopic lavage and debridement. The treatment of athletes poses greater therapeutic challenges than treating a lower demand patient, who may not have the same time constraints to return to practice. As such, there may be a role for lavage. Although they have been recently criticized in the literature for the treatment of degenerative cartilage changes,[9] lavage and debridement may have a role in the athlete who has symptoms from free cartilage fragments. In fact, lavage alone may have some therapeutic role. Certainly any free-floating fragments should be removed, as they may contribute to recurrent effusions or synovitis. Loose edges of articular cartilage may cause mechanical symptoms and be a source for debris. Fu et al[10] examined the results of debridement for full-thickness defects and demonstrated a 55% improvement at 3-year follow-up. Hubbard's[11] results demonstrated a 59% improvement for debridement of the medial femoral condyle at 5-year follow-up, versus only 12% for patients with similar lesions treated with lavage alone. Levy et al[12] independently corroborated these results with reported improvement and return to play in soccer players with lavage and debridement alone.

When a symptomatic focal chondral lesion is identified, lavage alone may be insufficient, and a marrow stimulating technique may be useful. The concept of mesenchymal stem cell stimulation was initiated over 50 years ago. In 1959, Pridie reported on open arthrotomy and drilling to treat cartilage defects.[13] In 1979, Ficat et al[14] introduced spongialization, in which the

subchondral bone was debrided to stimulate a healing response. Sprague[15] first introduced arthroscopic treatment in 1981, Jackson[16] introduced abrasion arthroplasty in 1984, and Steadman and Rodrigo's group[17] introduced "ice-pick" microfracture in 1994. It is important to differentiate microfracture from the more invasive abrasion arthroplasty, where the subchondral plate is disrupted. With the exception of the "ice-pick" microfracture, most of these treatments offered the patient initial relief, but it was all short-term, as the clinical results deteriorate over time and may not be significantly different from those of debridement.[1]

Steadman et al[18] reported on microfracture results at 3- to 5-year follow-up, and they found 75% of patients were improved, 20% unchanged, and 5% were worse. Activities of daily living (ADL) could be performed by 67% of patients. The ability to do strenuous work also improved. The specific negative predictive factors included advanced age, preoperative joint space narrowing, and isolated chondral defects. It is important to recognize that the histology of these repairs was a hybrid mixture of hyaline and fibrocartilage, and that the durability of this tissue still remains to be fully elucidated.

In a second study, Steadman and Rodrigo's group[17] reported improvement in the appearance of the articular surface following microfracture. Patients who received CPM for 6 to 8 hours a day for more than 6 weeks had better results. Furthermore, at follow-up, patients who did not receive CPM had a threefold chance of having exposed subchondral bone after microfracture.

Williams et al[19] examined 34 patients, most with isolated Outerbridge grade IV lesions, who were treated with microfracture. The mean interval to follow-up was 21.1 months. They reported that the mean ADL score increased, the mean Short Form (SF-36) physical component score increased, the mean SF-36 mental component score decreased, and that none of the 34 patients required further surgery of the affected limb. The authors concluded that patients with chondral and osteochondral lesions who undergo the microfracture abrasion technique experience significant clinical improvement at an approximate 2-year follow-up interval.

The routine use of microfracture in older patients, with focal degenerative changes has previously not been recommended. However, Steadman et al[20] examined the results of microfracture technique in patients 40 years of age or over (range: 40–70 years) with Outerbridge grade IV degenerative lesions and no evidence of concomitant ligament or meniscus injury or varus/valgus malalignment. At an average of 2.5 years follow-up, all subjective parameters measured (pain, swelling, limping, walking, stair climbing, level of sport, and ADL) demonstrated significant improvement over preoperative status. Similarly, functional outcome scores demonstrated significant improvement: mean Lysholm score and mean Tegner Activity Scale score improved. Thirteen patients (15.5%) required repeat arthroscopy within 5 years of the initial microfracture procedure for lysis of adhesions. The authors concluded that the microfracture technique is an efficacious surgical option for the treatment of degenerative chondral lesions of the knee. This solitary report does not justify microfracture techniques as an option for arthritis, but perhaps pushes the indication envelope further back.

There are limited data comparing microfracture to alternative treatments. The largest prospective randomized study[21] comparing autologous chondrocyte implantation (ACI) and microfracture examined 80 patients; 40 patients were treated with ACI and 40 with microfracture. The patients had symptomatic single defects on the femoral condyle between 2 and 10 cm^2. They all had stable knees with no osteoarthritis. The two groups followed identical rehabilitation protocol after surgery. Follow-up examination by an independent observer was done after 12 and 24 months. There were four failures in the ACI group, defined as reoperation because of nonhealing of the primary treated defect, and two in the microfracture group. Reoperations due to trimming and debridement were done in 10 patients in the ACI group and four in the microfracture group. After 1 year, both groups had significant clinical improvement (Lysholm and visual analog scale pain score). The outcome was slightly, but not significantly, better in the microfracture group than in the ACI group after 1 year. Histologic evaluation of 67 patients was performed and graded as hyaline-like (versus hyaline-fibrocartilage or fibrous) in 71% of ACI patients as compared with only 40% of the microfracture patients. Histology was graded as fibrous in 31% of the microfracture patients, compared with 3.1% in the ACI group. This important study suggested that there was no significant clinical benefit of one treatment versus the other. The ACI group had a higher likelihood of requiring a second surgery; however, the histology in the ACI group was more like hyaline cartilage. The clinical importance of this is still yet to be determined, although we speculate that the longevity will be important for long-term outcome

Preliminary reports from a multicenter, prospective study[7] also compared patient reported outcomes between patients treated with ACI and those treated with marrow stimulation techniques (MSTs) at a minimum of 3 years. They did not include patellar or tibial defects. At follow-up, ACI patients reported greater improvement in their overall Cincinnati Knee Rating Scale Score, pain scores, and swelling when compared with MST patients. Although ACI patients were characterized at the preoperative baseline by lower overall modified Cincinnati Knee Rating Scale scores, they were more likely to have had at least one prior surgery and to be receiving worker's compensation. ACI patients reported greater functional improvements and significantly reduced symptoms at 3 to 5 years than did MST patients. The results from this prospective comparative study demonstrate that ACI may be more effective than MST for certain patients.

It has been repeatedly demonstrated that the collagen makeup of cartilage repairs does not match that of native cartilage. As such, efforts to improve the histologic characteristics of the regenerated cartilage include hybridization of microfracture and autologous chondrocytes or microfracture and a collagen matrix. Nehrer et al[22] reported the results of microfracture with a collagen matrix added and ACI with a collagen matrix added. The animals treated with collagen implants showed better filling of the defects than did the untreated or only microfractured knees. Histologic analysis revealed the biggest amount of hyaline-like tissue was in the matrix augmented treatment group. Reparative tissue was predominantly fibrocartilage in the other groups. Although very preliminary, this is the only report of combined therapy in single defects, and suggests that there are potential methods to modulate the collagen expression in reparative tissues. This report may offer a glimpse into future treatment options.

■ Conclusion

The future direction of articular cartilage repair will certainly involve a more complete understanding of the molecular biology of cartilage repair and development. Eventually the local delivery of the appropriate growth factors and signal molecules for the body to regenerate articular cartilage will become a reality, in contrast to fibrocartilage that we currently stimulate. Until that time, we will continue to utilize and improve upon the techniques discussed here. Microfracture should continue to play an appropriate role in the treatment of chondral injuries until better treatment options are elucidated.

REFERENCES

1. Mandelbaum B, Browne J, F, et al. Articular cartilage lesions of the knee. Am J Sports Med 1998;26:853–861
2. Buckwalter JS. Articular cartilage: injuries and potential for healing. J Orthop Sports Phys Ther 1998;28:192–202
3. Cohen NP, Foster RJ, Mow VC. Composition and dynamics of articular cartilage: Structure, function and maintaining healthy state. J Orthop Sports Phys Ther 1998;28:203–215
4. Steadman J, Rodkey W, Rodrigo J. Microfracture: surgical technique and rehabilitation to treat chondral defects. Clin Orthop Rel Res 2001;391:s362–s369
5. Sharma L, Song J, Felson D, et al. The role of knee alignment in disease progression and functional decline in knee osteoarthritis. JAMA 2001;286:188–195

6. Unverferth K, Minas T. Surgical management of isolated chondral defects. Current Opinions in Orthopedics 2002;13:1–8

7. Erggelet C, Anderson A, Arciero R et al. Marrow stimulation techniques versus autologous chondrocyte implantation for treatment of full-thickness chondral defects of the knee. Comparison of patient outcomes at 3–5 years. Proceedings of the 4th International Symposium on Cartilage Repair. June 2002, Toronto, Canada

8. Messner K, Maletius W. The long term prognosis for severe damage to weight bearing cartilage in the knee. Acta Orthop Scand 1996;67:165–168

9. Mosely J, O'Malley K, Petersen NJ, et al. A controlled trial of arthroscopic surgery for osteoarthritis of the knee. N Engl J Med 2002;347:81–88

10. Fu F, Browne JE, Errgelet C, et al. A controlled study of autologous chondrocyte implantation versus debridement for full thickness articular cartilage lesions of the femur: results at three years. AAOS 68th Meeting Proceedings 2001, Poster No. PE 035, pp. 377-378

11. Hubbard J. Arthroscopic surgery for chondral flaps in the knee. J Bone Joint Surg Am 1987;69:794–796

12. Levy AS, Lohnes J, Sculley S. Chondral delamination of the knee in soccer players. Am J Sports Med 1996;67:165–168

13. Insall J. Intra-articular surgery for degenerative arthritis of the knee. A report of the work of the late K. H. Pridie. J Bone Joint Surg Br 1967;49:211–228

14. Ficat RP, Ficat C, Gedeon P, Toussaint JB. Spongialization: a new treatment for diseased patellae. Clin Orthop 1979;144:74–83

15. Sprague NF. Arthroscopic debridement for degenerative knee joint disease. Clin Orthop 1981;160:118–123

16. Jackson RW. Arthroscopic surgery. J Bone Joint Surg Am 1983;65:416–420

17. Rodrigo JS, Steadman JR, Sillman JF, et al. Improvement of full thickness chondral defect in the human knee after debridement and microfracture using continuous passive motion. Am J Knee Surg 1994;7:109–116

18. Steadman JR, Rodkey WG, Singleton SB, et al. Microfracture technique for full thickness chondral defects. Technique and clinical results. Oper Tech Orthop 1997;7:300

19. Williams R, Marx R, Jones E, et al. A prospective outcome analysis of patients treated with microfracture abrasion for chondral lesions of the knee: a preliminary review. Proceedings of the 4th International Symposium on Cartilage Repair, June 2002, Toronto, Canada

20. Steadman MD Jr, Miller B, Briggs K, et al. Patient satisfaction and functional outcome after microfracture of the degenerative knee. Proceedings of the 4th International Symposium on Cartilage Repair, June 2002, Toronto, Canada

21. Knutsen G, Lars Engebretsen L, Ludvigsen T, et al. Autologous chondrocyte implantation versus microfracture. A prospective randomized Norwegian multicenter-trial. Proceedings of the 4th International Symposium on Cartilage Repair, June 2002, Toronto, Canada

22. Nehrer S, Dorotka R, Bindreiter U, et al. Repair in articular cartilage defects in a sheep model treated by microfracture and a collagen trilayer matrix. Proceedings of the 4th International Symposium on Cartilage Repair, June 2002, Toronto, Canada

14

Osteochondral Autograft Transfer (OATS/Mosaicplasty)

JASON L. KOH, LÁSZLÓ HANGODY, AND GABOR KRISTOF RÁTHONYI

Osteochondral autografts were originally described by several authors.[1,2] These early reports described the use of a single osteochondral autograft, with success at follow-up ranging from 6 months to 10 years.[1,3,4] Matsusue et al[5] reported excellent results 3 years after arthroscopic transplantation of multiple osteochondral fragments, harvested from the same knee, to a chondral lesion in a patient with anterior cruciate ligament (ACL) deficiency. This was one of the first reports of the use of multiple fragments. Outerbridge,[3] in 1995, published the results of transplantation of osteochondral fragments of the patella to the femoral condyle, with relief of symptoms and survival of hyaline cartilage up to 9 years. Together, these results suggested that osteochondral autografts could provide a durable repair of articular cartilage lesions.

Independently, Hangody et al[6] and Bobic[7] published their results with the use of standardized tubular instruments for the harvesting of cylindrical osteochondral autografts from relatively non-weight-bearing areas of the knee. Their early promising results have been duplicated by other groups working in North America and Europe,[8–10] and indications have been expanded to other areas of the body as well.[11]

■ Description of Osteochondral Autografting

Osteochondral autograft transfer (OATS), or "mosaicplasty," involves the harvesting of cylindrical osteochondral plugs from relatively non-weight-bearing areas of the knee (such as the intercondylar notch or the femoral periphery of the patellofemoral joint) to areas of symptomatic full-thickness cartilage or osteochondral injury **(Figs. 14–1, 14–2, 14–3, 14–4,** and **14–5).** These plugs are placed to fill in the majority (60–80%) of the defect with intact osteochondral tissue, with the remaining defect to be eventually filled in with fibrocartilaginous repair tissue.[12] Variations exist in the size of plugs used (both in diameter and depth), methods of harvest, methods of graft site preparation, and density of plugs used to fill an area.[6,7] One of the authors (J.L.K.) prefers to use fewer, larger (6–9 mm) plugs to completely fill a defect,[13] whereas another (L.H.) prefers multiple, smaller plugs.[14] Harvesting and grafting may be conducted either through a small arthrotomy or arthroscopically, although it is strongly recommended that such grafting be done through an incision early in the learning curve or for large lesions. It is of vital importance that both harvesting and implantation of plugs be conducted at 90 degrees to the articular cartilage to ensure maximum surface congruity, and this remains one of the most technically demanding aspects of the procedure.[15]

■ Indications and Patient Selection

We emphasize that this technique is limited to patients with a relatively well-defined articular cartilage or osteochondral lesion, without significant degeneration of the joint. The maximum lesion size typically recommended is up to 2 cm in diameter (J.L.K.) or 4 cm

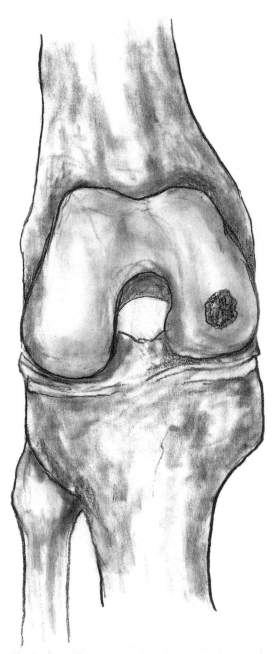

FIGURE 14–1 The initial assessment of the lesion is done arthroscopically and the size of the lesion is measured.

(L.H.), although in certain salvage situations lesions up to 9 cm² have been grafted. The patient must be willing to limit weight bearing for a period of 3 to 6 weeks, because early weight bearing has been associated with subsidence in some animal models[12] and case reports.[15,16] Patients older than 50 years or with thin cartilage are also contraindicated. Any malalignment or instability should be corrected prior to or concurrently with the grafting procedure to create the most favorable biomechanical environment.

■ Preoperative Evaluation

A careful history and physical examination often identify the activities that trigger discomfort. Areas of articular cartilage damage on the distal femoral condyles may be tender on physical examination, especially when the knee is flexed. Patellofemoral pathology and symptoms may be reproducibly elicited at a specific angle of knee flexion, suggesting a particular area of trochlear damage. Full-length standing (hip to ankle) films of the lower extremity are obtained to evaluate for

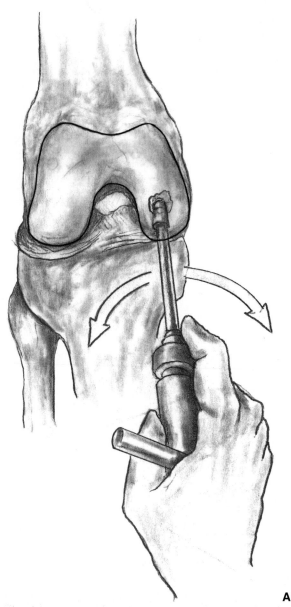

A

FIGURE 14–2 (A) Once the appropriate site is determined, the recipient harvester is introduced at a 90-degree angle with the joint surface.

(Continued)

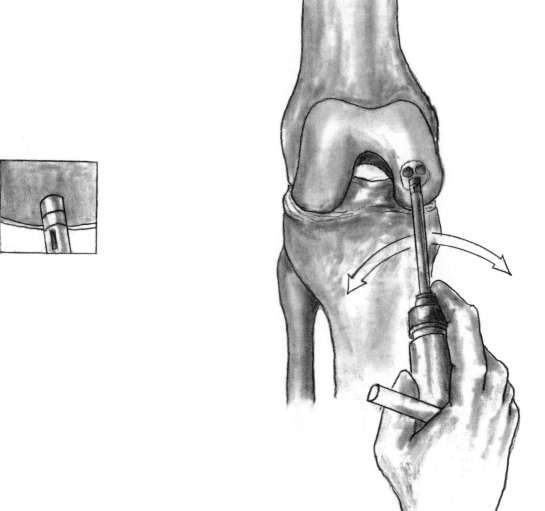

FIGURE 14–2 (*Continued*) **(B)** Bone plugs are removed.

malalignment. Magnetic resonance imaging (MRI) or previous arthroscopy photos, if available, are reviewed to help determine the size and location of the lesion, and assess for concurrent pathology.

■ Patient Positioning

Patient and portal positioning are critical using this technique. Preoperative evaluation of the location of the defect allows for appropriate portal position. If the defect is located on the posterior aspect of the femoral condyle, a significant amount of knee flexion (up to 120 degrees) may be necessary to achieve perpendicular positioning of the instrumentation. An assistant or leg holder may be useful to stabilize the hyperflexed knee.

■ Arthroscopic Technique

Portal Placement

Perpendicular access to the lesion and harvest sites is critical for proper insertion of the grafts. Viewing and working portals should be carefully positioned. An 18-gauge spinal needle or 1.2-mm Kirschner wire (K-wire) is initially used to determine the appropriate portal sites. Moving the standard portals centrally closer to the patellar tendon allows a more perpendicular path to the inward curve of the femoral condyles. Note that in certain cases a transligamentous portal may be necessary.

Defect Preparation and Templating

The defect site is measured and templated for grafting. Using various circular sizers of known diameters, the

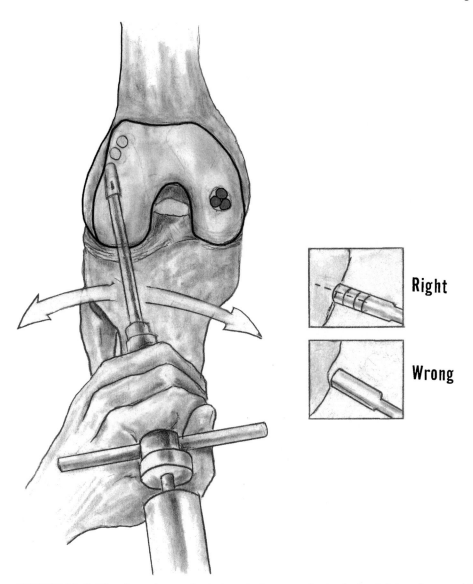

Right

Wrong

FIGURE 14–3 The donor harvester is inserted perpendicular to the joint surface and the osteochondral plugs are extracted.

appropriate number and location of plugs for a particular defect can be determined. Delaminated or unstable articular cartilage can be sharply removed at a right angle with a full radius resector, a sharp curette, or an arthroscopic scalpel. During this stage, the ability to achieve appropriate perpendicular graft orientation should also be verified. If the defect cannot be filled completely with a plug, preparation of the defect bed is conducted to promote fibrocartilage grouting of the defect site. The base of the lesion is lightly abraded to remove the calcified cartilage layer, and the uncovered area can be treated with microfracture.

It can be difficult to appropriately visualize the orientation of the grafting/harvesting tools, particularly in the anterior aspect of the knee when flexion pulls the fat pad against the condyles. Nevertheless, the 180-degree visualization of circumferential marks on the in-

strumentation can and must be achieved to ensure perpendicular harvesting of the graft. Equal laser marks on the tubular harvesting chisel at the 12, 6, and 9 or 3 o'clock positions indicate a nearly perpendicular graft. Visualization can be aided by the partial resection of the fat pad, the use of traction sutures or a fat pad retractor, retraction with small probes or spinal needles, or threaded/lipped clear cannulas. "Past-pointing" of instruments tends to also retract the capsular soft tissue when pulled back to the appropriate position.

Defects up to 9 mm in diameter can often be filled using a single plug. Larger defects can be filled with multiple plugs, achieving a 70 to 80% fill rate with identical sized plugs. The use of variable size plugs can increase the fill rate from 90 to 100%. Marking the base of the defect with the sharp-edged guide helps to optimize coverage and determine the number and the sizes of grafts

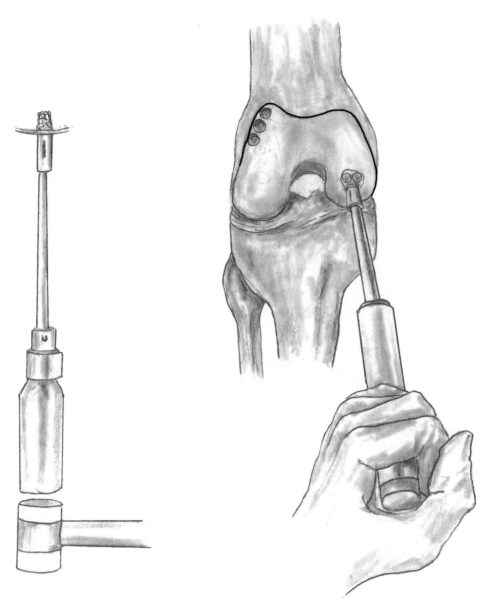

FIGURE 14–4 The plugs are then transferred to the recipient site and are introduced through a tube with a mallet.

needed. Finally, the depth of the defect should be measured with the dilator.

Graft Harvest

Several locations have been recommended for graft harvest. Arthroscopically accessible harvest sites include the periphery of the medial and lateral femoral condyles at the level of the patellofemoral joint above the sulcus terminalis, and the notch area. Notch area grafts can have less desirable features, such as concave surfaces and underlying bone, which is less elastic. Note that it is easier to access the medial patellofemoral periphery than the lateral technically.

Optimal view for graft harvest is obtained by introducing the arthroscope through the standard contralateral portal. With the knee in extension, the standard ipsilateral portal can be used to provide perpendicular access to the donor site. Knee extension eases access to the most superior donor plug. Additional portals should be made if the desired perpendicular access cannot be achieved from the existing one. A spinal needle or a K-wire can be used to determine the location of the additional harvesting portals. Gradual knee flexion allows sequential graft harvesting extending from the upper to the lower portions of the periphery of the femoral condyle.

After the necessary portals have been established, the proper size tube chisel, with the appropriate harvesting

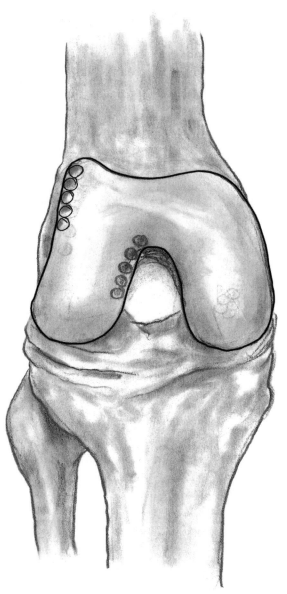

FIGURE 14–5 Acceptable donor sites include the lateral edge of the lateral femoral condyle, and the medial edge of lateral femoral condyle by the trochlea.

tamp, is introduced. Once the harvest site is clearly identified the chisel is placed perpendicular to the articular surface and is hammered to the appropriate depth. Laser markings on the harvesting chisels guide this step. Various systems have varying depth of cores, but the minimum length should be enough to ensure sufficient stability. In treating osteochondral defects where little surrounding bone is available, longer plugs are needed. Increasing flexion of the knee allows the use of inferior harvesting sites. In some systems, the graft is removed from the harvesting tube and placed in a saline-soaked sponge; in others the graft remains in the chisel until implanted. The length of the plug and the articular surface height of the graft at the 12, 3, 6, and 9 o'clock po-

sitions are determined and recorded. The donor tunnels typically fill with cancellous bone in 4 weeks and the surface fibrocartilage is formed after 8 to 10 weeks.

In case of technical difficulties or during the learning curve, the grafts can also be harvested through a mini-arthrotomy, 1.5 to 2 cm long.

Implantation of the Grafts

Knee flexion allows perpendicular access to the recipient site, and appropriate distention of the joint establishes enough space for the implantation. The recipient site can be drilled, or recipient site plugs can be harvested for implantation into the donor site. Again, it is critical to establish that the socket orientation is perpendicular to the articular surface. This can be confirmed by viewing from different angles with the arthroscope. The socket is then dilated appropriately to the measured depth of the harvested donor site plug. If there are small differences in depth at the edges of the socket, the graft should be appropriately oriented to minimize step-offs with the surrounding cartilage.

The graft is then delivered into the prepared socket, by the use of either a tamp or a screw applying pressure. Typically, the graft is allowed to protrude slightly from the surrounding cartilaginous articular surface, and final adjustments are made with a slightly oversize tamp to ensure that the graft is flush with the surface. Several studies[15,17,18] indicate that it is preferable for the graft to be slightly countersunk rather than proud. The same steps are repeated in the subsequent implantations. To achieve a good fill rate, the subsequent grafts should be inserted immediately adjacent to the previously placed grafts. Step-by-step graft implantation has several advantages. Although dilation of the actual recipient hole allows easier graft insertion, by lowering the insertion force on the hyaline cartilage cap, dilation of the adjacent hole impacts the surrounding bone back against the previously implanted grafts, resulting in a very safe press fit fixation.

When the entire recipient site is covered, a functional test is performed to check the congruency of the implanted area. Grafts that are implanted in a contact manner produce a convex, smooth articular surface, which allows the initiation of an accelerated rehabilitation protocol. During portal closure, a suction drain may be inserted into the joint. An elastic bandage lessens postoperative bleeding from the donor sites.

■ Open Mosaicplasty

Mini-arthrotomy using a 3- to 4-cm-long medial or lateral parapatellar sagittal incision may be necessary if an arthroscopic approach is not possible **(Figs. 14–6 and 14–7)**. The extended anteromedial approach may be required for reconstruction of trochlear, patellar, and

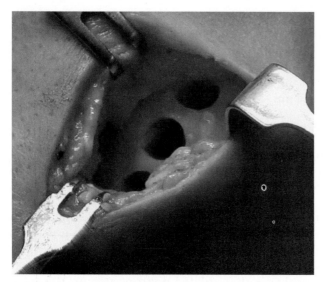

FIGURE 14–6 Mini-parapatellar arthrotomy may be used.

tibial defects. The implantation technique is identical to the arthroscopic procedure described above. Mosaicplasty in other sites (talus, femoral or humeral head, humeral capitellum) requires special open approaches and arthroscopic graft harvesting from the knee.

■ Postoperative Protocol

The osteochondral plug graft should be viewed as a fracture site and appropriate union should be achieved prior to excessive load. One of us (J.L.K.) recommends

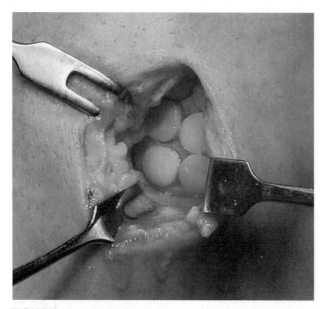

FIGURE 14–7 Multiple plugs have been used to fill a defect.

touch-down weight bearing only for 6 weeks for lesions on the weight-bearing surface of the femoral condyles, unless the lesion is small and the surrounding surface is supportive. The other senior author (L.H.) recommends 2 to 3 weeks non-weight bearing and 2 to 3 weeks of partial loading (30–40 kg). A detailed rehabilitation protocol has been developed based on 10 years of clinical experience **(Table 14–1).**

Weight bearing in extension is allowed for patellofemoral lesions. Continuous passive motion (CPM) is used to encourage the appropriate fill of the donor sites and the remodeling of the nonfilled areas of the graft site. Following healing of the bone, progressive weight bearing and functional activity is initiated. Healing and remodeling probably continue for at least 1 year postoperatively, particularly if incomplete fill of the defect is achieved.

Biomechanics of Osteochondral Transfers

Koh et al[15,18–20] have investigated the initial biomechanical parameters of osteochondral grafting under different conditions, such as a single matched plug, multiple plugs, and the result of incongruous grafting (graft–host surface mismatch). Using a porcine knee model, full-thickness articular cartilage defects were created and Fuji pressure-sensitive film was used to measure pressures and contact area profiles of the femoral condyle. Knees were tested with (1) intact cartilage, (2) articular cartilage defect, and (3) defect grafted with either a single or three plugs. Indentation testing of the plugs before and after transplantation demonstrated no change in stiffness. Significant increases (22%) in maximum force were seen in specimens with a full-thickness articular cartilage defect over intact specimens. The maximum pressure significantly decreased to normal levels when the defect was treated with either single or multiple grafts **(Table 14–2).**

Contact pressure distribution changed from an ellipse in intact to a donut in defect specimens, and returned to an ellipse after grafting. Typical false-color digitized pressure scans for single and multiple plug grafts are demonstrated in **Fig. 14–8.**

Smaller size plugs theoretically may be able to fill irregular defects with possibly less donor site morbidity. However, they are more fragile, have lower pullout strength, are more technically difficult to harvest and insert, and in one animal model failed in >10% of grafts.[21] Larger diameter grafts have increased graft stability. If improperly harvested, there may be a minimal increased articular cartilage step-off (<0.145 mm with 8-mm versus 4-mm diameter plug, Bartz et al[22]); but the overall congruity and contact pressure is better with fewer plugs for a circular defect.

TABLE 14–1 Mosaicplasty Rehabilitation Protocol[a]

Activity	Time from surgery
Ambulation[b]	
Two-crutch ambulation, non–weight bearing	Immediate
Two-crutch ambulation, partial loading (30–40 Kg)	2–4 weeks
Discontinue crutches, full weight-bearing	4–5 weeks
Functional exercises	
Form walking, gait evaluation	4–5 weeks
Step-up	4–5 weeks
Step-down	5–6 weeks
Range of motion	
Early range of motion encouraged	
Continuous passive motion (CPM) in case of extended lesions 2–4 cm^2 (in painless range)	Immediate (first week)
Full extension, flexion as tolerated	Immediate
Stationary bicycle	3 weeks
Strength return	
Quadriceps	
Open chain exercises, leg raises	Immediate
Concentric contraction to full extension	1 week (or earlier if tolerated)
Concentric contraction against resistance	2 weeks
Isometric exercises in different angles	Immediate
Excentric exercises against resistance	3–4 weeks
Hamstrings	
Isometric exercises in different angles	Immediate
Concentric and excentric strengthening	1–2 weeks
Against resistance	3–4 weeks
Closed-chain exercises[c]	
Pushing a soft rubber ball with foot	Immediate
Closed-chain exercises with half weight bearing	2–3 weeks
With full weight bearing	5–6 weeks
Stationary bicycle with resistance	2–4 weeks (if 90-degree knee flexion achieved)
Stairmaster	6–8 weeks
Proprioception return	
Balance exercises standing on both feet	5–6 weeks
Standing on one foot (hard ground)	6–8 weeks
Standing on one foot (trampoline or aerostep)	8–10 weeks
Return to activity	
Jogging	10 weeks
Straight line running	3 months
Directional changes	4–5 months
Shear forces	5 months[d]
Sport-specific adaptations	5 months
Sports activity	5–6 months[e]
Special viewpoints:	
Weight bearing at different defects of knee:	

(Continued)

TABLE 14–1 (*Continued*)

Femur or tibia condyle, chondral defect <15 mm	
Non–weight bearing	1 week
Partial weight bearing	1–3 weeks
Femur or tibia condyle, chondral defect, d ≥15 mm	
Non–weight bearing	2 weeks
Partial weight bearing	2–4 weeks
Femur or tibia condyle, osteochondral defect	
Non–weight bearing	3 weeks
Partial weight bearing	3–5 weeks
Patellar defect, d <15 mm	
Partial weight bearing	2 weeks
Patellar defect, d ≥15 mm	
Partial weight bearing	3 weeks
Quadriceps strengthening and patellar mobilization—differences at patellar defects:	
Vastus medialis strengthening	
Isometric exercises in extension	Immediate
Patellar mobilization	Immediate
Isometric exercises in different angles	1 week
Open-chain exercises	2 weeks
Against resistance	3–4 weeks
Excentric exercises against resistance	4–5 weeks
Closed-chain exercises	2–3 weeks
Weight bearing at different defects of ankle:	
Talus, lateral defect, without osteotomy	
Non–weight bearing	2 weeks
Partial weight bearing	2–4 weeks
Talus, med. (or lateral) defect, with osteotomy	
Non–weight bearing	4 weeks
Partial weight bearing	4–6 weeks
Range of motion and muscle strengthening:	
In open chain	While non–weight bearing (see above)
Mainly in closed chain	From the beginning of half-weight
Proprioception return:	
Good proprioception is essential for the good functional result of the ankle.	
Seesaw plateau with partial loading	3–5 weeks
Seesaw plateau with full weight bearing	5–7 weeks
Trampoline and aerostep 5–7	Weeks
Weight bearing at defects of hip:	
Femoral head, osteochondral defect	
Non–weight bearing	3 weeks
Partial weight bearing	3–5 weeks
Range of motion (ROM):	
Early ROM exercises	Immediate
(Gain the full ROM as soon as possible!)	

Strength return:	
Emphasize gluteus medial strengthening	
Open-chain muscle strengthening	1 week
Stationary bicycle and closed-chain exercises	3 weeks
Viewpoints at the defects of upper extremity	
Humeral head and capitulum radii	
Range of motion	
Early range of motion encouraged	
CPM (in painless range)	Immediate, for 2–7 days
ROM exercises, as tolerated	Immediate
Soft tissue mobilization (if needed)	2 weeks
Passive stretching—humeral head	3 weeks
Radius	4 weeks
Strength return	
Muscle strengthening always in the painless range	
Isometric exercises	Immediate
Concentric exercises against resistance	2 weeks
Muscle strengthening using weights, Theraband	3 weeks
The treatment of underlying causes can also modify the rehabilitation program. The most frequent combinations at knee applications are the following:	
ACL reconstruction combined with mosaicplasty:	
Non–weight bearing (up to the mosaicplasty)	2–4 weeks
Partial weight bearing	2 more weeks
5- to 90-degree ROM	4 weeks
Mainly closed chain exercises for quadriceps strengthening	
Hamstring strengthening in open and closed chain	
Proprioceptive training	
Meniscus reinsertion combined with mosaicplasty:	
Non–weight bearing	4 weeks
Partial weight bearing	2 more weeks
5- to 45-degree ROM	4 weeks
Retinaculum patellae reconstruction combined with mosaicplasty:	
Non–weight bearing (up to the mosaicplasty)	2–4 weeks
Partial weight bearing	2 more weeks
0- to 45-degree ROM	4 weeks
HTO combined with mosaicplasty:	
Weight bearing (for 4 weeks only with crutches and only in extension) is up to the mosaicplasty, pain, and degree of the correction of the varus (lower correction—non–weight bearing, overcorrection—early weight bearing)	

[a]Uzsoki Hospital and Sanitas Private Clinic, Budapest, Hungary.
[b]Extent, type (chondral or osteochondral), and location of the defect may modify weight bearing (see text).

[c]Partial loading promotes the transformation of connecting tissue (between transplanted plugs) into fibrocartilage, so these exercises are important, and extremely important in the half-weight bearing period. On the other hand, with some closed chain exercises (e.g., cycling) it is possible to ensure cyclic loading, that makes the fluid- and nutrition-transport much more efficient between synovial-fluid and hyaline cartilage.

[d]Approximately 4–5 months are needed to form a composite hyaline-like surface on transplanted area, which tolerates shear forces.

[e]Depending on depth and extent of the defect. If strength, power, endurance, balance, and flexibility are not satisfactory, sports activity should be delayed.

ACL, Anterior cruciate ligament; HTO, high tibial osteotomy

TABLE 14–2 Initial Contact Pressure after Osteochondral Autografting[27,43]

	Peak pressure: 6.5-mm single plug (kg/cm^2)(*p < .05)	Peak pressure: three 10-mm plugs (kg/cm^2) (*p < .05)
Intact	9.77*	9.43
Defect	11.98*	11.56*
Grafted	8.78*	10.33*

Several authors have investigated the "fingerprint" of articular cartilage collagen and the curvature and thickness of articular cartilage of the knee.[21,22] It remains unclear what role these particular issues may play in choosing the number, type, and alignment of grafts. Indentation testing and contact pressure studies suggest that surface congruity plays a more important role than these parameters.

The effect of incongruity of graft height on contact pressure has also been evaluated using a porcine knee model. As seen in **Fig. 14–9**, osteochondral transplantation with an elevated plug resulted in significantly higher contact pressures, whereas a countersunk plug reduced contact pressures compared with an empty defect.

This suggests that plugs should be placed flush to the surrounding articular cartilage at the time of initial implantation. Pearce et al[17] further confirmed that deliberately proud grafts in a sheep model became flush with surrounding cartilage. However, they also demonstrated persistent clefts at the margins, poor bony incorporation, subchondral cavitation, and fibroplasias.

Animal Studies

Animal studies at Northwestern University compared untreated defects with those treated with an osteochondral plug in a rabbit model. Animals were evaluated at 0, 6, and 12 weeks. Modified O'Driscoll histologic scores[23] were significantly better on the transplanted side (**Fig. 14–10**).

Biomechanical data demonstrated that the plugs had better stiffness and more normal contact pressures than untreated defects. Plugs had excellent bone-to-bone healing, but the articular cartilage graft–host margin remained distinct. The transplanted tissue appeared to be normal viable hyaline cartilage at all time points.

Several animal studies have examined the results of osteochondral grafting, with variable results. Lane et al[24]

conducted an early rabbit study on osteochondral grafting, reporting that over a 12-month period autologous osteochondral grafts remained viable and functionally and structurally intact. The subchondral bone remodeled rapidly but continued to provide structural support.

Hangody[12] has published the results of a canine study in which 18 German shepherd dogs were treated with up to ten 4.5-mm grafts into defects of apparently variable size. Thirty-six operations were performed, with transplantation into the medial femoral condyle in 18 cases and the non–weight-bearing trochlea or patella in 18 cases. Dogs were allowed full activity and walked without a limp 3 to 4 days postoperatively. Significant differences were noted in between the weight-bearing and non–weight-bearing lesions. Non–weight-bearing lesions had 100% surface congruity, with good bony incorporation. Weight-bearing lesions demonstrated subsidence and overgrowth with fibrous or fibrocartilaginous tissue in over one third of the cases. Donor sites were filled with fibrocartilage. Based on these results, Hangody has recommended non–weight-bearing for 6 to 8 weeks following surgery.

Paletta et al[25] in 1998 presented the results of a canine study of nine animals with lesions treated either with three-plug grafting or subchondral drilling, and allowed immediate unrestricted activity. At 6 weeks, bone-to-bone healing had occurred, but there was no articular cartilage healing, and biomechanical properties of the plug were nearly normal. At 12 weeks, there was a persistent cleft between the plug and the surrounding cartilage, and increased stiffness of plugs and some surface irregularity and fibrillation. At 24 weeks the cleft remained, and the plug had decreased cellularity and vacuolization, and the biomechanical properties demonstrated increased stiffness.

Dew and Martin[26] published work on the transplantation of a 5.5-mm osteochondral graft from digit into the canine talus. Grafted animals had significantly better function at postoperative week 6, but no difference was noted by week 20. All grafts restored joint surface congruity, whereas half of the nongrafted lesions had poor congruity.

Desjardins et al[27] examined the results of fresh and frozen autografts in an equine model. Both appeared to maintain a durable weight-bearing surface for 3 months; however, the fresh grafts had better histologic and gross characteristics. They felt that graft stability and articular surface congruity were the determining factors in graft outcome.

The University of Guelph and Toronto Hospital group has evaluated osteochondral transplantation in a sheep model.[17,28,29] Pearce et al[17] studied 13 sheep with proud and flush placement of osteochondral

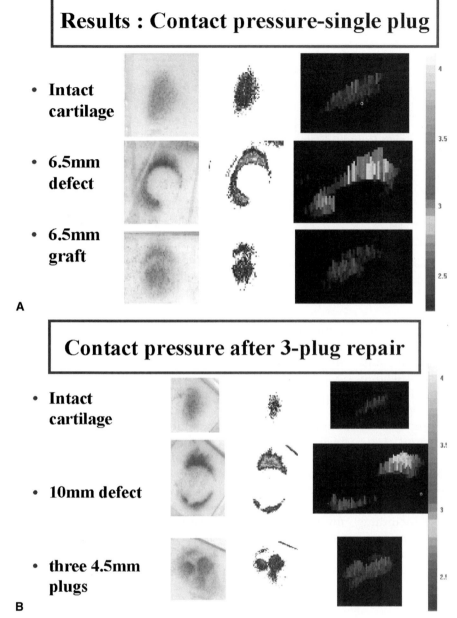

FIGURE 14–8 Single **(A)** and multiple **(B)** osteochondral plug grafting significantly decreased the peak pressure to near-normal loads and re-created near-normal contact pressure patterns. This may contribute to the clinical effectiveness of such treatment in the knee. Single plug grafts were able to more closely duplicate normal biomechanical parameters, despite larger size.

plugs. As previously noted, plugs placed proud developed articular cartilage clefts at the margins and had poor incorporation. Hurtig et al[28] presented results of the treatment of a 15 mm defect with various combinations of grafts, ranging from 2.7 mm × 7 mm, to 4.5 mm × 3 mm, to 6.5 mm × 2 mm. The smaller grafts demonstrated significant failures and cartilage loss, probably due to their intrinsic fragility. The 4.5- and 6.5-mm grafts had intact cartilage at sacrifice at 90 days, with well adherent mature connective tissue in interstices.

Donor-Site Concerns

There are several theoretical disadvantages and limitations of osteochondral autografting. Primary among these is that this technique involves "robbing Peter to pay Paul," because the graft is harvested articular cartilage from the knee. Simonian[30] reported that all donor sites experienced load when cadaver knees were cycled through a range of motion, and Staubli[31] reported contact between the lateral patellar facet and the superolateral trochlea in a combined anatomic, MRI, and

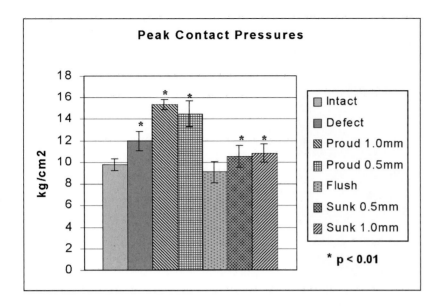

FIGURE 14–9 Osteochondral transplantation with an elevated plug resulted in significantly higher contact pressures, whereas a countersunk plug reduced contact pressures compared with an empty defect.

arthroscopic study. It is unclear what the significance of this load if the pressure is from soft tissue, and multiple authors have reported (Hangody, Bobic, and Koh[6,7,9,11]) minimal or no complications associated with the donor sites at 2- to 5-year follow-up. Hangody at 7 to 10 years has noted a few patients with a small decrease in Bandi scores as a measurement of patellofemoral symptoms, but the etiology of these symptoms is unknown[11.]

The contraindications of the mosaicplasty are existing degenerative changes, the advanced age of the patient, and the presence of a defect of significant size. A small number of complications were observed, including postoperative hemarthrosis and less than 3% long-term donor-site morbidity. Because we found that athletes reported doubled incidence of mild or moderate

donor-site pain (6%) compared with less active patients, it is likely that vigorous exercise increases donor-site pain.

Clinical Results

Clinical results of osteochondral plug autografting have been presented in a few peer-reviewed journals, and several groups have reported good results. Few complications have been noted. However, most of these studies are retrospective and do not have good control populations. In addition, almost all groups analyzed have multiple confounding variables, such as concomitant ligament or realignment surgery. As in most cartilage research, it has been difficult to evaluate results between institutions due to a lack of a standardized scoring sys-

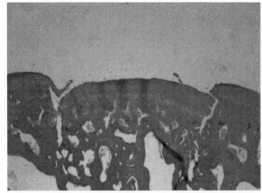
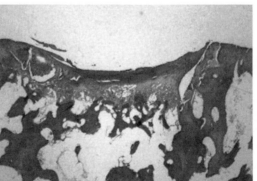

FIGURE 14–10 (A) Histology of articular cartilage defect treated with OAT at 6 weeks. Note excellent bone–bone healing and maintenance of hyaline cartilage. **(B)** Control un-treated articular cartilage defect at 6 weeks. Fibrocartilage partially fills the defect, and there is adjacent articular cartilage damage. (See Color Plate 14–10)

tem for cartilage defects and for outcomes, in addition to the multiple other variables such as age, activity level, chronicity of defects, other injuries, and differences in surgical and rehabilitation techniques.

Fabbriciani et al[32] in 1991 presented work on the transplantation of an osteochondral graft harvested with a Cloward coring instrument from the lateral condyle in 12 patients treated from 1982 to 1988. Lesion size averaged 2.9 cm², and the grafts were fixed with fibrin glue. Follow-up was from 2 to 7 years (average 4.2) and Lysholm II scores improved from 67.8 to 97.1. No patellofemoral degeneration was noted by radiographs, and no patient had complaints of pain.

The most commonly cited reports are from Bobic and Hangody, describing good to excellent results in small series of patients. Bobic's original paper[7] described transplantation of cylindrical autogenous grafts into defects larger than 10 mm diameter in ACL-deficient knees undergoing ligament reconstruction. Four of these patients had failed synthetic grafts. Evaluation criteria included radiographs and MRI demonstrating graft integration and a level surface in 10 patients. The initial two cases had multiple grafts either "too prominent or sunk in, due to inadequate surgical technique." Follow-up arthroscopy was available for nine patients after 1 year, and demonstrated normal cartilage appearance and color. Donor sites were difficult to identify. Clinical evaluation was limited to describing "promising uniform results in ten of 12 cases with 2 years' follow-up." No complications were noted.

Bobic has presented more extensive follow-up information at several meetings.[33] In 1996 he presented a series of 29 patients who underwent osteochondral autografting in conjunction with ACL reconstruction. Nineteen patients underwent second-look arthroscopy at 2 to 3 years with excellent visual and probing results. MRI scans demonstrate fluid content similar to that of surrounding normal articular cartilage. In three patients, grafts were not level with surrounding tissue. Two cases were biopsied at 2 years follow-up and demonstrated hyaline cartilage. No clinical evaluation criteria were provided.

Hangody's initial paper[6] in the English-language literature describes a series of 44 patients treated with mosaicplasty. The majority[25] of these patients had previous surgery, including three ACL reconstructions and seven high tibial osteotomies. Five ACL reconstructions and 19 meniscal ruptures were treated concomitantly with the mosaicplasty procedure. Preoperative Hospital for Special Surgery (HSS) scores averaged 62.18, with postoperative mean 94.23 (range 67–100). This group was compared with 21 patients with "similar conditions" treated with abrasion arthroplasty. The abrasion group pre- and postoperative HSS scores were 59.64 and 78.24, respectively. A prospective study comparing 21

mosaicplasties and 22 abrasion arthroplasties was ended when it was noted that there were significantly improved HSS scores in the mosaicplasty group. Ten patients had arthroscopies demonstrating hyaline-like tissue in the recipient sites with fibrocartilage in the interstices. Biopsies from six patients demonstrated survival of hyaline cartilage and fibrocartilage at donor sites. Three patients developed postoperative hematomas treated with aspiration, and had no subsequent sequelae. No other complications were noted. It was noted that perpendicular graft placement is of great importance.

Hangody has reported follow-up on larger groups of patients at several meetings. In 1998[12] he presented a multicenter study comparing abrasion, microfracture, Pridie drilling, and mosaicplasty, evaluated using Cincinnati scores, in patients of ages 31 to 39. A greater percentage and longevity of good to excellent results was seen with mosaicplasty. Little information is available on this particular series in the English-language literature.

Hangody published a review[16] of a group of 57 patients with >3 year follow-up (mean 48.7, range 36–56 months) in 1998. Average age was 31.4 (range 17 to 45 years). Thirty-nine concomitant procedures were done, including 28.2% ACL, 23.1% meniscectomy, 17.9% patellofemoral realignment, 12.8% femorotibial realignment, 10.3% meniscal reconstruction, and 7.7% debridement. Thirty-five had condylar cartilage defects, seven had chondromalacia patellae, and 15 had osteochondral lesions (condyles in 14, patella in one); 91% of the patients had a good or excellent result on a modified HSS scoring system. The average score was 90.7 (range 64–100). Scores were higher for those with chondral defects compared with osteochondritis dissecans (OCD) lesions, and with condylar lesions compared with patella. No disturbances of the patellofemoral joint were noted using the Bandi scoring system compared with a control group (shaving only).

Second-look arthroscopy was done in 19, with grade II chondromalacia found in three graft sites and the rest normal. Biopsies were obtained in 12, with hyaline cartilage found at graft sites and bordering fibrocartilage. Two patients developed hematomas, and no other complications were noted; 54 of 57 patients returned to their normal activity level.

Later in 1998, Hangody[34] presented a series of 113 patients with greater than 3 years of follow-up. The defect size ranged from 1 to 8.5 cm². An average of eight grafts (range, 2 to 17 grafts) were used; 78% of patients had a concomitant procedure to address "underlying biomechanical disturbance." The majority of defects (n = 83) were on the femoral condyles, with 26 on the patella and four on the talus. The average modified HSS score was 91.1 (52–100). Lower Bandi scores for evaluation of patellofemoral problems were seen in <3% of patients. The number of patients with patellofemoral problems was noted to be higher than the rate at 1-year follow-up, raising concerns about potential long-term morbidity at the donor sites.

Further information was provided in 1999[11] on 52 competitive athletes with follow-up of at least 1 year (mean 26.5 months). The age range was 17 to 50, and good to excellent HSS scores were found in all. Thirteen had ACL repairs, and 10 had meniscal repairs. Overall, 63% returned to full participation and 31% to a lower level of participation. The authors noted that patients ≤30 years of age had a significantly higher (90%) return to full competition, 7% reduced, compared with those >30 years of age, where only 23% returned to full competition and 70% to a reduced level. Several complications were noted, including tourniquet paresthesias (three patients, resolved within 72 hours); clicking and pain with weight bearing due to a nonfilling donor site in a small patient; continued arthritic pain; continued knee degeneration; inadequate filling <75%; and subsidence of grafts with early weight bearing and cycling at 1 week in a noncompliant patient. Kish and Hangody warn that patients with thin or chondromalacic cartilage around a defect may not support the grafts, and that the grafts may fall apart at transfer. Other relative contraindications include those with large (>2 cm) defects associated with synovitis or osteophytes, because these are part of a progressive arthritic process.

Hangody has reported his personal experience with 87 high-level athletes with full-thickness chondral defects who were treated with mosaicplasty. Most of these defects (72 cases) were located in the knee, 13 in the talus, and two in the elbow capitellum. Osteoarthritic degenerative changes of Fairbanks grade I or II were observed in 43% of the affected joints. The average size of the chondral defects in knees treated was an average 2 cm^2 (1–5.5 cm^2) but in three cases it exceeded 4 cm^2. In the talus the mean defect size was 1.5 cm^2 (0.5–2.5 cm^2), whereas in the elbow capitellum the size of the two defects was 1 cm^2 and 1.5 cm^2. The mean follow-up time was 4.1 ± 3.2 years (range 1–9 years). The mean patients' age was 26 ± 6.4 years (range 14–39 years). There were 51 male and 36 female patients. In the knee defect group the mean modified HSS score preoperatively was 61 ± 19.3 (47–82) and at the last postoperative follow-up was 86 ± 18.8 (64–100) points. The mean preoperative Lysholm score was 67 ± 14.5 (49–84) and the last postoperative score was 90 ± 13.1 (68–100). In the talus defect group the mean preoperative Hannover score was 74 ± 12.2 (56–81) and the mean postoperative score was 91 ± 8.4 (84–102). The time to return to the desired level of sports activities averaged 4.3 ± 2.4 months (3–10 months). Sixty-four of 87 patients resumed the same level of athletic activity, 19% a lower

level, and 17% failed to return to sports activities. Only 8% of the athletes rated the postoperative knee function and symptom scores as being worse than that recorded prior to procedure. The author concluded that autologous osteochondral transplantation (mosaicplasty) provides favorable midterm functional results in high-level athletes, even in those with radiographic evidence of osteoarthritic changes or those with large defects as a salvage procedure. The extension of indication is promising, but further follow-up is needed to assess the long-term effects on osteoarthrosis.

Hangody[35] has also published the results of 541 mosaicplasties performed between February 1992 and February 1999; 401 have been of the condyles, 79 of the patella, 22 tibia, and 39 talus. Two thirds were due to chondral lesions; the rest were osteochondral defects. In 84% concomitant procedures were performed. Results were evaluated with HSS, International Cartilage Repair Society (ICRS), Cincinnati, and Lysholm scoring, and good-to-excellent results were found in 92% of femoral condylar lesions, 89% of the tibial, 83% of the patellar, and 95% of the talar lesions. The Bandi score demonstrated abnormalities at the donor site in 3%; 51 of 59 second-look arthroscopies demonstrated good gliding surfaces and survival of hyaline cartilage. Eight patients have had slight degenerative changes. Nineteen have been tested in vivo for stiffness, which showed elasticity to be similar to that of the surrounding cartilage. There were four infections and 29 hemarthroses. Patients older than 35 had less successful outcomes.

Morgan[10] has reported at several meetings on 52 patients with 2- to 4-year follow-up. The average age was 34 (range 18–64). Fourteen were associated with chronic ACL insufficiency; 37 lesions were 1 cm, 15 were 2 cm × 1 cm, four lesions were caused by focal avascular necrosis (AVN), and the rest were chondral defects. Clinical evaluation was performed using International Knee Documentation Committee (IKDC) pain and activity scores. In the pain evaluation, 65% improved two grades, 31% improved one IKDC pain grade, and 4% did not change. In activity evaluation, 27% improved two grades, 50% one grade, and 23% had no change. Mean pre- and postoperative scores were not provided. Morgan indicated that many of the patients preoperatively had only pain complaints, and were already maximally active. No complaints of lateral peripatellar pain were noted.

Gambardella and Glousman[8] have also presented the results of a prospective multicenter study from 10 institutions with >150 patients. Mean follow-up was relatively short (16 months, range 1–36). No specific outcome data have been published. The authors indicated that good-to-excellent results were found with isolated condylar and trochlear lesions, with improvement of multiple clinical indices over time. Outcomes were adversely affected by poor alignment and patellofemoral chondromalacia.

Koh and coauthors[27] have presented the results of a retrospective study performed at the Cleveland Clinic on the first 26 patients undergoing osteochondral autografting. Most of these patients had isolated chondral defects and had failed prior cartilage treatment procedures; 81% had prior surgery. Four patients underwent concomitant procedures: tibial osteotomy in two, open reduction and internal fixation (ORIF) of the patella in one, and patella realignment in one. At an average of 25 months follow-up (range, 13–40 months), statistically significant improvements in patient self-assessment for pain at rest, during activities of daily living, and pain with maximal exertion were found. Patient satisfaction was high, and statistically significant improvements in IKDC pain and activity scores were also found. All patients in this largely salvage population improved, with 36% returning to normal or nearly normal by the rigorous IKDC criteria. No patient had pain or tenderness at the donor sites. Repeat arthroscopy in three patients demonstrated intact grafts with fibrocartilage filling adjacent defects, and fibrocartilage at the donor sites. A nonstudy patient fractured the cartilage cap off a patella graft while road biking at 4 weeks postoperation. The MRI evaluation demonstrated good bony incorporation of the plug with some abnormality of the transplanted cartilage.

■ Conclusion

Osteochondral autografting is a promising technique for the treatment of limited chondral and osteochondral defects. Several groups have reported good clinical results in small series of patients with few complications.[6–11] In vitro data suggest that at least initially, osteochondral grafting may restore normal biomechanical parameters.[26] However, almost all clinical studies lack prospective, randomized assignment to differing treatments. The studies that do exist have extremely limited follow-up, in most cases less than 3 years. Concomitant other surgical procedures such as ACL reconstruction and realignment procedures also make it difficult to isolate the effect of the cartilage transplantation. Evaluation of this technique's efficacy is also confounded by the relatively benign course of many patients who undergo simple debridement of these lesions. Comparison of these results to other techniques is difficult, due in part to a lack of standardized preoperative evaluation and outcome scales.

The long-term outcome of such transfers remains unclear. Case reports on the viability of osteochondral autografts indicate survival of up to 10 years,[35] but long-term data are extremely limited. Similarly, the long-term morbidity at the donor sites is unknown, with one

author[11,35] suggesting that there may be some slight increase (3%) in patellofemoral problems with >3 year follow-up. Alternative donor sites[26] or the use of fresh or cryopreserved allografts[7,27] or engineered tissue may eventually prove to be a more attractive option.

At this time, it appears that osteochondral autografting has good short-term results, and may be a viable technique for the salvage treatment of failed debridement of isolated articular cartilage lesions of up to 2 to 2.5 cm in diameter. In these patients, statistically significant improvements in pain and activity level have been seen. Currently, several long-term studies are underway to further evaluate the results of this technique.[12,19,23,27]

REFERENCES

1. Wilson WJ, Jacobs JE. Patellar graft for severely depressed comminuted fractures of the lateral tibial condyle. J Bone Joint Surg 1952;34-A:436–442

2. Yamashita F, Sakakida K, Suzu F, Takai S. The transplantation of an autogeneic osteochondral fragment for osteochondritis dissecans of the knee. Clin Orthop 1985;201:43–50

3. Outerbridge HK, Outerbridge AR, Outerbridge RE. The use of a lateral patellar autologous graft for the repair of a large osteochondral defect in the knee. J Bone Joint Surg Am 1995;77:65–72

4. Roffman M. Autogenous grafting for an osteochondral fracture of the femoral condyle. A case report. Acta Orthop Scand 1995;66: 571–572

5. Matsusue Y, Yamamuro T, Hama H. Arthroscopic multiple osteochondral transplantation to the chondral defect in the knee associated with anterior cruciate ligament disruption. Arthroscopy 1993;9:318–321

6. Hangody L, Kish G, Karpati Z, Szerb I, Udvarhelyi I. Arthroscopic autogenous osteochondral mosaicplasty for the treatment of femoral condylar articular defects. A preliminary report. Knee Surg Sports Traumatol Arthrosc 1997;5:262–267

7. Bobic V. Arthroscopic osteochondral autograft transplantation in anterior cruciate ligament reconstruction. A preliminary clinical study. Knee Surg Sports Traumatol Arthrosc 1996;3:262–264

8. Gambardella RA, Glousman RE. Autogenous osteochondral grafting: a multicenter review of clinical results. Presented at the 2nd Symposium of the International Cartilage Repair Society, November 16–18, 1998, Boston, and the 18th annual meeting of the Arthroscopy Association of North America, 1999, Vancouver, BC

9. Koh JL, Petty DH, Recht M, Williams J, Bergfeld JA. Osteochondral autografting of articular cartilage defects. Presented at the 20th Annual Meeting, Arthroscopy Association of North America, 2001, Seattle, WA

10. Morgan CD, Carter TR. Osteochondral autograft transfer (OAT) chondral resurfacing. Presented at the 17th annual meeting of the Arthroscopy Association of North America, 1999, Orlando, FL, and at the 25th annual meeting of the American Orthopaedic Society for Sports Medicine, 1999, Traverse City, MI, p. 382

11. Kish G, Modis L, Hangody L. Osteochondral mosaicplasty for the treatment of focal chondral and osteochondral lesions of the knee and talus in the athlete: rationale, indications, techniques, and results. Clin Sports Med 1999;18:45–66

12. Hangody L, Kish G, Karpati Z, et al. Autogenous osteochondral graft technique for replacing knee cartilage defects in dogs. Orthopedics Int Ed 1997;20:525–538

13. Arthrex. Osteochondral Autograft Transfer: Surgical Technique Manual. Naples, FL: Arthrex, 1997

14. Hangody L, Miniaci A, Kish G. Mosaicplasty Osteochondral Grafting: Technique Guide. Andover, MA: Smith and Nephew, 1999

15. Koh JL, Kowalski A, Lautenschlager E. Angled osteochondral grafts-effects on articular contact pressure. Presented at the American Academy of Orthopaedic Surgery, 2004, San Francisco

16. Hangody L, Kish G, Karpati Z, Szerb I, Udvarhelyi I. Mosaicplasty for the treatment of articular cartilage defects: application in clinical practice. Orthopedics 1998;21:751–756

17. Pearce SG, Hurtig MB, Clarnette R, et al. An investigation of 2 techniques for optimizing joint surface congruency using multiple cylindrical osteochondral autografts. Arthroscopy 2001;17: 50–55

18. Koh JL, Wirsing K, Lautenschlager E, Zhang L-Q. The effect of graft height mismatch on contact pressure following osteochondral grafting: a biomechanical study. Am J Sports Med 2004;32: 317–320

19. Koh JL, Kambic H, Valdevit A, Petty D, Bergfeld JA. Osteochondral autografting of an idealized cartilage defect: in vitro evaluation. Presented at the 47th annual meeting of the Orthopaedic Research Society, 2001, San Francisco

20. Koh JL, Petty D, Bergfeld JA. Multiple plug osteochondral grafting for osteochondral defects: biomechanical evaluation. Presented at the International Cartilage Research Society, 2002, Toronto, Canada

21. Below SK, Arnoczky SP, Dodds J, Kooima C, Wessinger S. Fingerprint of the knee joint: a consideration in the orientation of autologous cartilage. Presented at the 18th annual meeting of the Arthroscopy Association of North America, 1999, Vancouver, BC, p. 8

22. Bartz RL, Kamaric E, Noble PC, Lintner D, Bocell J. Geometric incongruity of osteochondral grafts: effects of graft size and donor site selection Presented at the 25th annual meeting of the American Orthopaedic Society for Sports Medicine, 1999, Traverse City, MI, p. 382

23. Nam E, Maksous M, Koh JL, Zhang LQ. Osteochondral transplantation vs. untreated full-thickness defects in a rabbit model. Am J Sports Med 2004;32:308–316

24. Lane JM, Brighton CT, Ottens HR, Lipton M. Joint resurfacing in the rabbit using an autologous osteochondral graft. A biochemical and metabolic study of cartilage viability. J Bone Joint Surg 1977;59-A:218–222

25. Paletta GA, Ibarra C, Wannafin J, Potter HG, Torzilli P. Histologic, biomechanical, and MR image evaluation of autogenous osteochondral plug transplantation using a dog model. Cartilage Study Group Meeting, March 21, 1998, New Orleans, p. 22

26. Dew TL, Martin RA. Functional, radiographic, and histologic assessment of healing of autogenous osteochondral grafts and full-thickness cartilage defects in the talus of dogs. Am J Vet Res 1992;53:2141–2152

27. Desjardins MR, Hurtig MB, Palmer NC. Heterotopic transfer of fresh and cryopreserved autogenous articular cartilage in the horse. Vet Surg 1991;20:434–445

28. Hurtig M, Evans P, Pearce S, Clarnette R, Miniaci A. The effect of graft size and number on the outcome of mosaic arthroplasty resurfacing: an experimental model in sheep. Presented at the 18th annual meeting of the Arthroscopy Association of North America, 1999, Vancouver, BC, p. 16

29. Hurtig MB, Novak K, McPherson R, et al. Osteochondral dowel transplantation for repair of focal defects in the knee: an outcome study using an ovine model. Vet Surg 1998;27:5–16

30. Simonian PT, Sussman PS, Wickiewicz TL, Paletta GA, Warren RF. Contact pressures at osteochondral donor sites in the knee. Am J Sports Med 1998;26:491–494

31. Staubli HU, Durrenmatt U, Porcellini B, Rauschning W. Patellofemoral articular cartilage contact zones and potential trochlear cartilage harvesting sites. Presented at the 2nd Symposium of the International Cartilage Repair Society, November 16–18, 1998, Boston

32. Fabbriciani C, Schiavone Panni A, Delcogliano A, Sagarriga Visconti C. Osteochondral autograft in the treatment of osteochondritis dissecans of the knee. Presented at the 17th annual meeting of the American Orthopaedic Society for Sports Medicine, 1991, pp. 67–68

33. Bobic V. Current methods of treating articular cartilage defects in the knee: an update on arthroscopic osteochondral autograft transplantation in ACL reconstruction. Presented at the 2nd World Congress on Sports Trauma, American Orthopaedic Society for Sports Medicine 22nd annual meeting, 1996, Orlando, FL, and the Meniscus and Articular Cartilage Transplantation Study Group, 1997, San Francisco

34. Hangody L. Medium term results of the clinical practice of the autologous osteochondral mosaicplasty. Presented at the 2nd Symposium of the International Cartilage Repair Society, November 16–18, 1998, Boston

35. Hangody L. Autologous osteochondral mosaicplasty in the treatment of focal chondral and osteochondral defects of the weight-bearing articular surfaces. Osteologie 2000;9:63–69

15

Autologous Chondrocyte Implantation

JEFFREY W. WILEY, TIM BRYANT, AND TOM MINAS

Full-thickness chondral lesions in the knee have been known to be problematic for over two centuries.[1] The incidence and natural history of articular cartilage lesions have not been well defined; however, a lesion in the weight-bearing surface of the knee may progress to osteoarthritis. This is especially thought to be true for larger lesions that are unshouldered. Frequently, chondral injuries are identified incidentally at the time of arthroscopy for the treatment of meniscal or ligamentous injuries.[2,3] Articular cartilage is a unique tissue with limited potential for repair because it lacks vascular, lymphatic, and nerve supply. Subsequently, symptomatic articular cartilage lesions have been difficult management problems for the orthopaedist.

Total knee arthroplasty has proven to be a reliable and durable procedure. However, prostheses begin to fail at an increased rate over the second decade of their use. Thus, young patients who undergo total knee arthroplasty may be subjected to multiple revision surgeries with less predictable results.[4]

There are a variety of treatment options for the orthopaedist treating chondral injuries of the knee. Arthroscopic debridement, or marrow-stimulating techniques including abrasion chondroplasty, microfracture, and drilling may be useful for the patient with symptomatic chondral injuries. Additionally, osteochondral allografting, osteochondral autografting by open or arthroscopic techniques, and autologous chondrocyte implantation have been used to manage the symptomatic patient with chondral injuries.

Patient factors as well as the characteristics of the chondral injury including its size, location, and depth help determine which method is most suitable for a particular patient. Each of these treatments may provide some benefit to properly selected patients. Marrow-stimulating techniques produce a fibrocartilage repair tissue, which has been found to have inferior mechanical properties compared with hyaline cartilage.[5] Only osteochondral autograft/allograft techniques and autologous chondrocyte implantation produce a hyaline cartilage repair tissue. Autologous chondrocyte implantation may lessen the intraarticular donor-site morbidity associated with osteochondral graft transfers and eliminates the concerns of using an allograft if one chose to use an allograft technique. Additionally, the technique may allow for a more homogeneous repair surface compared with the potential "cobblestone" repair surface obtained with osteochondral autograft as per the mosaicplasty technique.

Autologous chondrocyte implantation has produced hyaline repair tissue in experimental models as well as in biopsies taken from second-look arthroscopies,[6] and this technique has produced durable results in a midterm, 2- to 9-year, follow-up report of patients in Sweden. Encouraging results also have been shown at short-term follow-up in a series of patients in the United States.[7] Interestingly, in this series, many of the patients who were significantly improved had multiple or complex cartilage lesions. In select patients, autologous chondrocyte implantation has the benefit of providing end-differentiated chondrocytes to large areas of the injured articular surface. By resurfacing these areas of chondral injury with hyaline cartilage, it is hoped this technique will resolve symptoms and facilitate a return to an active lifestyle for these young patients. Furthermore, the progression of osteoarthritis may be halted or delayed.

■ Healing Process of Autologous Chondrocyte Implantation

Many studies have been performed that explore the healing process of autologous chondrocyte implantation. Rabbit studies have been performed that demonstrate the in vitro cultured chondrocytes to be responsible for the majority of the in vivo repair tissue, and this repair tissue surpassed periosteum alone in quality and quantity.[8,9] Canine studies have revealed that the healing process has distinct phases of healing.[10,11] These stages have been divided into the proliferative stage (0 to 6 weeks), the transition stage (7 to 12 weeks), and a remodeling and maturation stage, which occurs over an extended time frame (13 weeks to 3 years)[12] (Table 15–1).

During the proliferative stage, a primitive cell response occurs with tissue fill of the defect. At this time, the tissue has poor integration to the underlying host bone or adjacent cartilage. This tissue is soft and jelly-like, mostly composed of type I collagen and easily damaged at this stage.[12]

The transition phase is marked by the production of a type II collagen framework. Proteoglycans are produced and imbibe water, giving the articular cartilage its viscoelastic properties. At this stage, the tissue has the consistency of firm gelatin and is milkable when probed arthroscopically, demonstrating that it is not yet well integrated into its surrounding tissues.[12]

During the stage of remodeling and maturation, the collagen matrix is stabilized, by cross-linking, to the underlying bone and adjacent cartilage. At 4 to 6 months, the tissue is integrated to the underlying bone and has a putty-like consistency. It is at this point that patients begin to experience good symptom relief, and they discard their assistive devices. However, the mechanical properties at 4 to 6 months are not yet optimized. It is at this point when symptoms are resolving that excessive activity may cause repair tissue degeneration. Ultimate maturation and stabilization of the repair tissue occurs between 1 and 3 years, depending on patient factors such as patient age and defect size and location.[12]

TABLE 15–1 Time Line for Healing of Autologous Chondrocyte Implantation

Time Stage	0–6 weeks Proliferation	7–12 weeks Transition	>13 weeks–3 years Remodeling and Maturation
Histology	Rapid proliferation of spindle shaped cells with defect fill; mostly type I collagen with early formation of colonies of chondrocytes forming type II collagen	Matrix formation, mostly chondrocytes producing type II collagen and proteoglycans; poor integration to underlying bone and cartilage	Ongoing remodeling of matrix with reorganization and quantity of collagen type II, with integration to bone (arcades of Benninghoff), and adjacent host cartilage; largechain aggregates of proteoglycans, with increased water content of cartilage
Viscoelastic arthroscopic appearance	Filled, soft, white tissue	Jelly-like firmness, with "wave-like" motion when probed, not yet firm and integrated to underlying bone	Firm "indentable," but not "wave-like" when probed by 4–6 months after ACT; graft whiter than host cartilage, may demonstrate periosteal hypertrophy (20%); equal firmness to host cartilage 9–18 months after ACT
Activity level	CPM starts 6 hours after surgery for 6–8 hours/day × 6 weeks Touch WB Isometric muscle exercises and ROM	Discontinue CPM Active ROM Partial graduated WB to full WB by 12 weeks Functional muscle usage, stationary bicycle, treadmill	Discontinue assistive devices 4–5 mos postop if free of pain, catching, swelling Distance walking, resistance walking Nonpivoting running 9–12 mos 14–18 mos pivoting allowed

ACT, autologous chondrocyte transplantation; CPM, continuous passive motion; ROM, range of motion; WB, weight bearing.
Adapted from Minas TM, Peterson L. Autologous chondrocyte transplantation. Oper Tech Sports Med 2000;8:144–157.

■ Patient Presentation and Assessment

Clinical Evaluation

Patients with articular cartilage injuries may present with a variety of symptoms, including prior traumatic injuries, pain, effusion, locking, catching, malalignment of the extremity, and patellar maltracking. To accurately assess if a patient may be a candidate for autologous chondrocyte implantation, a thorough history and physical examination are essential. Prior traumatic injuries are common, and in the senior author's experience, patients who have had anterior cruciate ligament (ACL) injuries are particularly predisposed to chondral injuries. Johnson[13] has noted that 20% of ACL injured knees chronically develop full-thickness cartilage loss. Furthermore, full-thickness chondral injuries have an incidence of between 5% and 10% in patients who have experienced acute work-related or sporting injuries and present with an acute hemarthrosis.[2]

Pain is a frequent complaint, and the location of the pain can help localize the site of chondral injury. Medial or lateral joint line pain focuses attention on the medial or lateral compartments. Locking or catching of the knee may represent the presence of a loose body from an osteochondral injury. These symptoms also may represent a meniscal injury, and this possibility needs to be assessed prior to embarking upon treatment of the chondral injury. Meniscal pathology can then be treated by meniscal debridement, meniscal repair, or meniscal transplantation if it exists at the time of surgery.

Recurrent effusions are also associated with full-thickness chondral injuries. This is particularly true in the case of trochlear lesions. Additional complaints focusing attention on the patellofemoral articulation include anterior knee pain when ascending or descending stairs or inclines, as well as anterior knee pain with prolonged sitting. Pain that is noted in the posterior aspect of the knee also may be related to patellofemoral pathology. Causes of the patellofemoral pathology may be due to prior dislocations or patellar maltracking, resulting in full-thickness chondral injuries. Clinically, evaluation should include evaluation of the Q-angle, hypermobility of the patella, and pain with a patellar grind test. Maltracking must be addressed if one is considering autologous chondrocyte implantation (ACI) to this articulation. Early failures of ACI may have been related to the immature cells continuing to be exposed to increased shear forces due to the maltracking.[6]

Similarly, axial malalignment may also accompany full-thickness chondral weight-bearing injuries. Clinical evaluation may include the observance of genu varum or valgum and the presence of a lateral thrust during gait.

However, long axial alignment x-rays should always be performed to confirm or exclude the clinical impression of alignment. As with the patellofemoral joint, any consideration of ACI must first include correction of any axial malalignment to avoid exposing the immature chondrocytes to increased forces from a malaligned extremity. The decision to perform the realignment procedure concurrently with ACI, or in a staged sequence with the realignment procedure followed at a later date by ACI, is made on a case–by-case basis taking into account individual patient factors.

Ligamentous stability may be just as important to the knee as correct axial alignment when considering ACI as a treatment for a patient with a full-thickness chondral injury. Performing ACI without restoring joint stability may result in the graft site experiencing increased shear forces from recurrent episodes of instability, predisposing the graft to failure. As with realignment procedures, the decision to perform ligament reconstruction concurrently with ACI or in a staged fashion is determined on a case-by-case basis.

Radiographic Evaluation

After obtaining an appropriate history and physical exam, the clinician must then request a radiographic evaluation, which is necessary to diagnose an articular cartilage injury and determine if a patient is a candidate for ACI. A standard radiographic protocol should include weight-bearing anteroposterior and lateral radiographs to assess joint space narrowing and osteophyte formation. Rosenberg et al[14] suggest that standing 45-degree posteroanterior views are also helpful in diagnosing tibiofemoral cartilage loss or osteochondral defect lesions. Additionally, standing 54-inch axial alignment views that include the center of the femoral head and talus are essential to assess the overall axial alignment of the extremity and determine if realignment will be required. Merchant, or sunrise, views assess the patellofemoral articulation for evidence of joint space narrowing or maltracking. Select cases may require a computed tomography (CT) scan of the knee with the leg in extension and the quadriceps contracted, and relaxed, to better assess patellofemoral tracking. Merchant or sunrise views may not reveal some cases of maltracking because the patella engages the trochlea with knee flexion. CT also reveals the rare case of a hypoplastic trochlea that may contribute to patellar maltracking or obvious subluxation. Failed proximal patellar realignment procedures often occur because of unrecognized trochlea dysplasia.

Magnetic resonance imaging (MRI) allows visualization of the articular cartilage as well as the menisci, ligaments, and bone, making it a valuable tool in evaluating patients with suspected articular cartilage injuries. However, technical issues mainly related to spatial resolution and volume averaging can make it difficult to strictly determine exact dimensions of cartilage defects or repair tissues.[15] Newer imaging techniques and protocols have improved the accuracy of evaluating cartilage lesions and repair tissues, and MRI now is a valuable tool in the evaluation of patients with articular cartilage lesions. Winalski and Minas[15] note that the techniques representing state-of-the-art clinical evaluation of articular cartilage include fat-suppressed three-dimensional (3D) T1-weighted gradient echo images, fast spin echo sequences, and magnetic resonance arthrography (MRA). These techniques have improved the sensitivity of detecting cartilage injury to over 85% for moderate to severe cartilage lesions (Outerbridge grade 2–4)[16] while maintaining a specificity of over 90%.[15] However, the availability of these techniques may be limited to specialized centers.

Fat-suppressed 3D T1-weighted gradient echo images cause the articular cartilage to appear bright compared with the surrounding joint fluid and subchondral bone and bone marrow.[15] This produces a very accurate representation of the cartilage-fluid and cartilage bone interfaces,[17] and is therefore a very good method for determining articular cartilage defects. Unfortunately, this technique does not adequately assess the menisci or ligaments.[15]

Fast spin echo techniques facilitate both improved image contrast between cartilage and fluid and assessment of the subchondral bone.[15] Additionally, this technique facilitates evaluation of the menisci and ligaments and minimizes metallic artifact. However, the images are prone to blurring and partial volume averaging inaccuracies.[15]

Magnetic resonance arthrography (MRA) may be performed either directly with intraarticular injection of contrast or indirectly through intravenous administration of contrast.[15] It has been shown to be an excellent method for articular cartilage evaluation.[18] When using indirect arthrography, it is imperative to exercise the joint for a period of time prior to imaging to ensure optimal joint fluid enhancement.[15]

Arthroscopic Evaluation

Traditionally, arthroscopy has been the gold standard when evaluating a patient with a suspected articular cartilage injury, and it continues to play a critical role in evaluating and planning treatment. Arthroscopic evaluation and cartilage biopsy requires a careful and systematic approach. Furthermore, arthroscopy has the benefit of facilitating a staged procedure by harvesting a cartilage biopsy; it also facilitates potential treatment of the

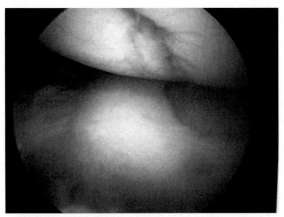

FIGURE 15–1 Arthroscopic photograph of a symptomatic full-thickness chondral injury of the medial femoral condyle.

cartilage injury, depending on the lesion characteristics. The treatment should be discussed with the patient preoperatively.

The arthroscopic examination should begin with an examination of the knee under anesthesia, noting the range of motion and any ligamentous insufficiencies. An arthroscopic probe should be used to determine the extent of grade 3 and 4 chondromalacia[16] **(Fig. 15–1).** The opposing articular surface should also be examined to evaluate if there is cartilage damage on this surface, as ACI has traditionally been reserved for unipolar lesions with no more than grade 2 chondromalacia[16] on the opposing articular surface. The dimensions of the lesion(s) should be recorded to facilitate future planning by obtaining an appropriate volume of cultured chondrocytes. One vial of cultured autologous chondrocytes has a volume of 0.4 mL corresponding to 12 million cells, and this may cover a defect size of about 4 to 6 cm^2.[12] Additionally, a spinal needle can be used to assess the depth and quality of the surrounding cartilage as the bevel of the needle is about 3 mm. This is important for planning the ACI procedure itself, for periosteum will need to be sutured to synovium or through drill holes in the bone if uncontained defects are present.[12] Intraoperative examination of the menisci and ligaments is also important to anticipate the future need for ligamentous repair or possible meniscal allograft transplantation.

If a chondral lesion is found to be appropriate for ACI, surgeons should be prepared to perform a cartilage biopsy, which should be discussed with the patient preoperatively. Loose bodies that may be retrieved during arthroscopy typically are not satisfactory for cell culturing, unless they are large osteochondritis dissecans (OCD) fragments. Biopsies may be performed from the superior medial edge of the trochlea, the superior transverse trochlear margin adjacent to the suprapatellar synovium, or the lateral intercondylar

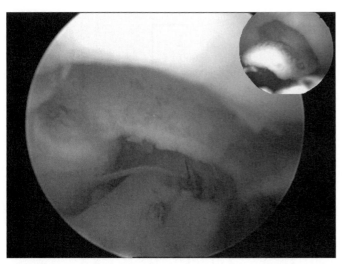

FIGURE 15–2 Biopsy performed at the superolateral aspect of the intercondylar notch.

notch.[12] We choose to perform the biopsy in the superior and lateral intercondylar notch staying anterior to the sulcus terminalis on the lateral condyle **(Fig. 15–2).** This enables the surgeon to perform the biopsy without compromising a weight-bearing surface. The patellofemoral joint also is protected from being involved in the harvest, as the patella typically does not engage the intercondylar notch before 120 degrees of knee flexion. When performing the biopsy, the patient's knee is brought through a range of motion, ensuring that the proposed biopsy site is not involved in tracking of the patellofemoral articulation. We then score the proposed biopsy site with an arthroscopic gouge and elevate the biopsy specimen with a twisting motion, bracing the operative hand against the patient to avoid skiving. The biopsy specimen is then removed. The biopsy should consist of 200 to 300 mg of articular cartilage (about 5 mm wide by 10 mm long), as this is the amount required for enzymatic digestion and cell culturing.[12] This specimen contains about 200,000 to 300,000 cells, which is enzymatically digested and grown to about 12 million cells per 0.4 mL of culture media per implantation vial.[12] In vitro expansion of cells occurs over 3 to 5 weeks and is then suitable to accommodate a defect size of 4 to 6 cm² per implantation vial.[12]

■ Indications

Autologous chondrocyte implantation has been in use in Sweden since 1987.[19] Since the initial report on this technique in the *New England Journal of Medicine* in 1994,[20] ACI has become a recognized technique for the treatment of chondral injuries of the knee. Based on this initial study, the classic indications for ACI have been reserved for symptomatic patients with isolated Outerbridge grade 3 to 4 lesions of the femoral condyle or trochlea in patients between the ages of 15 and 55 with no more than grade 1 to 2 chondromalacia on the opposing articular surface.[19] Osteochondritis dissecans of the medial or lateral femoral condyles has also been an accepted indication. ACI has not been traditionally indicated for kissing lesions or for patients with radiographic evidence of joint space narrowing.

Two reports noted that these isolated lesions are uncommon.[3,7] However, the senior author's experience has extended the indications to include patients with multiple lesions and "salvage" cases with early arthritic change. The results have been encouraging at 2- to 7-year follow-up.[7]

■ Patient Selection

Currently, our approach to treatment includes the findings of the clinical exam, plain radiographs, MRI, and an understanding of the patient's goals and desires **(Fig. 15–3).** This enables us to match an appropriate treatment plan with the patient's expectations to ensure the optimal outcome. Arthroscopy is then used to further evaluate the suspected chondral defect. In general, small grade 3 or 4 lesions (<1.5 cm²) are treated with a chondroplasty technique in relatively sedentary patients. Lesions of similar size in very active athletic patients are more likely to be treated with a microfracture or an osteochondral autograft transplantation system (OATS)™ (Arthrex, Naples, FL) technique using a single plug taken from the periphery of the lateral condyle anterior to the sulcus terminalis to limit donor-site morbidity.

Autologous chondrocyte implantation is used for grade 3 to 4 symptomatic lesions of the femoral condyles, trochlea, and patella when the lesions are 2 cm² or larger or when previous treatment methods have failed. As previously discussed, we carefully examine patients for malalignment, ligamentous insufficiency, and meniscal pathology. We treat patients with these coexisting conditions with staged or combined procedures, depending on patient preferences.

In addition to coexisting orthopaedic issues, general medical comorbidities such as cigarette use and the use of medications that may impair cell proliferation such as nonsteroidals or immunosuppressives are investigated. We do not proceed with ACI until the patient is free from nicotine, as it has been found to impair healing in certain conditions.[21,22] Furthermore, patients frequently are taking narcotic pain medications upon presentation due to numerous prior surgeries. We require patients to eliminate narcotic medications prior to surgery to

Table 1
Algorithm for primary
treatment of chondral injury·

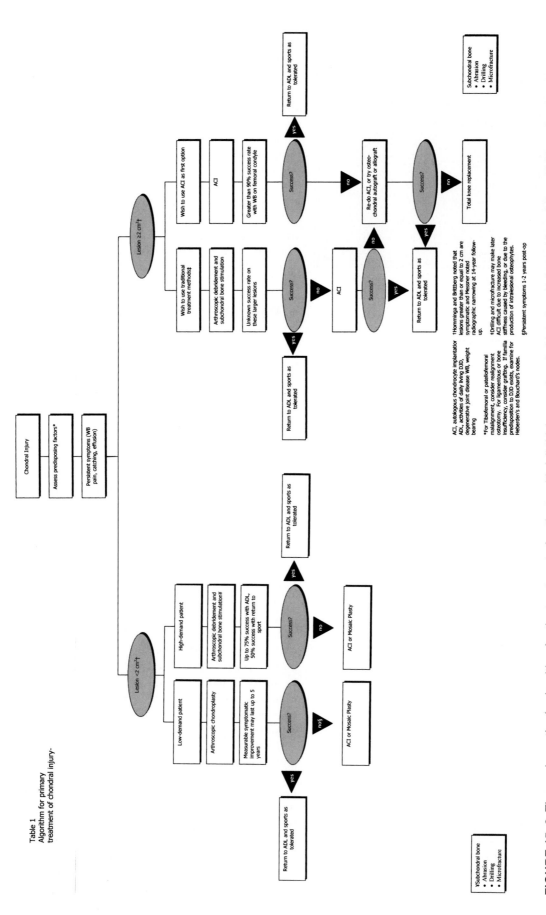

FIGURE 15–3 The senior author's algorithm for the treatment of patients with full-thickness chondral injuries. (Adapted from Minas T. The role of cartilage repair techniques, including chondrocyte transplantation, in focal chondral knee damage. In: American Academy of Orthopedic Surgeons, Zuckerman JD, ed. Instructional Course Lectures, vol. 48. Rosemont, IL: 1999:629–643)

enhance postoperative pain management. If the patient is unable to eliminate nicotine or requires these other medications, other treatment alternatives are considered.

Malalignment is treated with corrective osteotomy. When addressing tibiofemoral malalignment, we aim to restore the mechanical axis to neutral, if there is no evidence of joint space narrowing. We plan for the weight-bearing axis to pass through the lateral tibial spine for patients with a varus deformity if joint space narrowing exists or peripheral osteophytes are present. Similarly, the weight-bearing axis is planned to pass through the medial tibial spine for a valgus deformity in the presence of joint space narrowing or peripheral osteophyte formation. Having the weight-bearing axis pass through the tibial spine results in roughly a 2- to 4-degree overcorrection, thus unloading the affected compartment. We will also overcorrect malalignment in patients with an absent meniscus or when a large (>10 cm^2) weight-bearing lesion is transplanted. The degree of correction is based on our preoperative assessment of angular deformity from the 54-inch films.

Patients with patellar or trochlear lesions typically have associated patellar maltracking and are treated most commonly with a lateral release, medial advancement of the vastus medialis, and possibly a tibial tubercle osteotomy. We have found the Fulkerson[23] tibial tubercle osteotomy to be a very effective osteotomy, as it can correct the maltracking and unload the joint by elevating the tibial tubercle.

Anterior cruciate ligament deficiencies are corrected prior to ACI, as knee instability is detrimental to graft survival. Similarly, patients who have undergone previous subtotal meniscectomy may be considered for allograft meniscal transplantation. Attending to these comorbidities should improve the success of ACI by protecting the graft during the healing stages, and help prevent the progression of degenerative changes.

In the senior author's practice, it is uncommon to have patients with isolated defects. Many patients are found to have multiple defects, and it is not uncommon to place ACI grafts at more than one site at the same surgery **(Fig. 15–4)**. Some young patients have opposing chondral defects. These "kissing" lesions frequently involve the patella and trochlea, and less frequently involve the femur and tibia. These young patients are treated very aggressively with osteotomy as well as ACI to these multiple sites. Additionally, they may have evidence of early arthritic change including joint space narrowing.

Patient education is critical to a successful outcome. There may not be a good treatment option for this type of patient, but in our practice an ACI is considered, provided the patient has a thorough understanding of the rehabilitation process and the potential complications, and desires a biologic approach to the problem. Extensive preoperative counseling is required with these patients to involve them in the decision-making process, for failure rates and complications such as graft hypertrophy and arthrofibrosis may be higher in these salvage cases. If ACI does not appeal to a patient or if it fails, unicondylar knee replacement or patellofemoral arthroplasty is an alternative, as is salvage treatment. Total knee arthroplasty is reserved for tricompartmental disease.

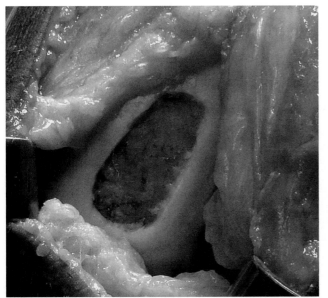
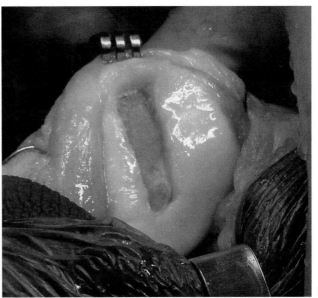

A   B

FIGURE 15–4 Multiple chondral lesions may be present. Medial femoral condyle **(A)** and patellar lesions **(B)** after debridement to stable edges.

■ Surgical Technique

Autologous chondrocyte implantation is performed as a separate procedure after cartilage biopsy and cell expansion have occurred. Preoperative antibiotics are administered, and a tourniquet is usually used during preparation of the graft site and harvesting of the periosteum. A bump is used to allow knee flexion of 90 to 100 degrees, and a post is placed on the lateral aspect of the thigh to allow for a stable extremity when suturing the periosteal graft.

A midline incision is utilized to avoid wound-healing issues if and when future surgeries are indicated. Alternatively, two incisions may also be used—the proximal for the arthrotomy and the distal for the periosteal harvest **(Fig. 15–5)**. Full-thickness medial and lateral skin flaps are raised, thus facilitating adequate exposure when concurrent osteotomy is required. A standard medial parapatellar arthrotomy is performed to access the joint, unless an isolated lateral femoral condylar defect is present warranting a lateral arthrotomy. When previous arthroscopy reveals a lesion that extends to the posterior aspect of the condyle, a meniscal takedown is required to facilitate adequate visualization and debridement of the lesion. The coronary ligament is sharply incised along with the anterior-medial attachment site of

the meniscus. A full-thickness soft tissue sleeve is then elevated in an anterior to posterior direction, providing excellent exposure of the posterior aspect of the femoral condyle.

Radical debridement of the chondral lesion is crucial to the success of ACI **(Fig. 15–6)**. Debridement is performed back to a stable edge of intact articular cartilage with vertical edges **(Fig. 15–7)**. Occasionally, lesions are uncontained, with no peripheral margin of intact articular cartilage. In these instances, the periosteum needs to be sutured to synovium or through small drill holes through bone to contain the cell suspension. In cases where previous marrow stimulating techniques have been performed, there are frequently intralesional osteophytes that must be debrided. Similarly, lesions associated with osteonecrosis have sclerotic bases that must be debrided to viable bone without violating the subchondral bone plate. These debridements are best performed with the use of a high-speed burr. Bone grafting is required if the depth of the lesion is >10 mm; this may be performed either as a staged procedure or during the same setting as the ACI.

After the lesion has been debrided, it is templated most easily with a marking pen to outline the size of the lesion **(Fig. 15–7)**. The wrapping from the surgical

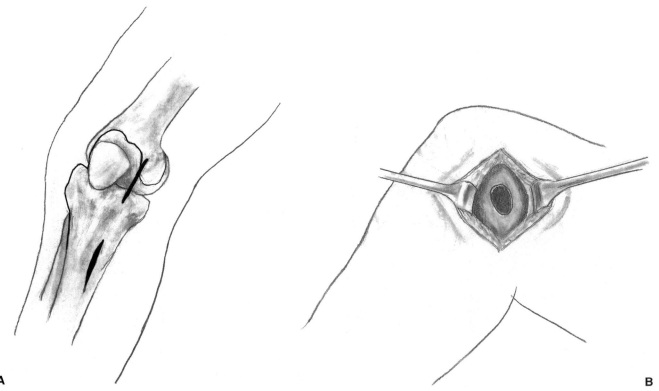

A

B

FIGURE 15–5 A midline incision or two medially based incisions **(A)** may be used, and a medial arthrotomy **(B)** is carried to gain access to the joint.

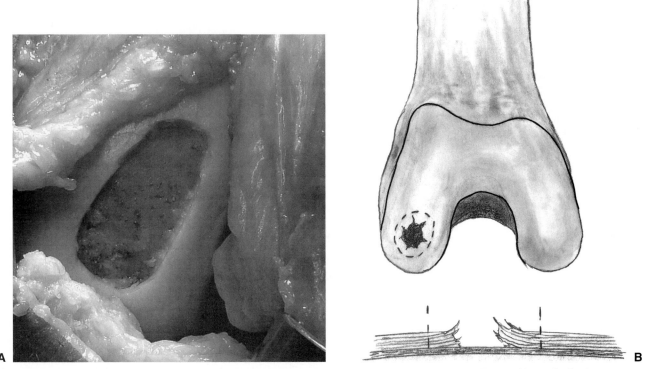

FIGURE 15–6 (A,B) Debridement is performed back to a stable edge of intact articular cartilage with vertical edges.

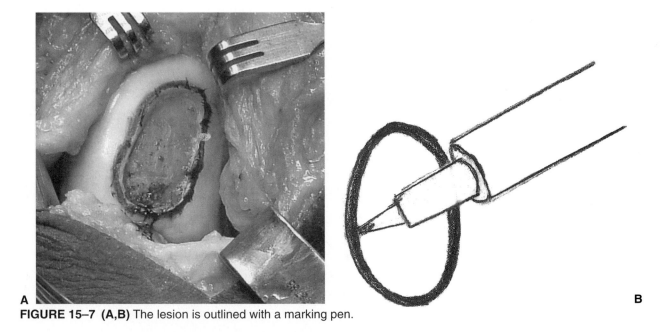

FIGURE 15–7 (A,B) The lesion is outlined with a marking pen.

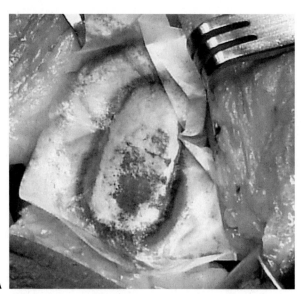

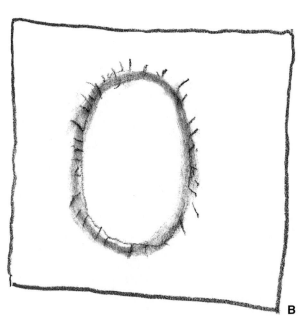

FIGURE 15–8 (A,B) The wrapping from the surgical gloves is then placed over the lesion and the ink is transferred onto the paper.

gloves is then placed over the lesion and the ink is transferred onto the paper **(Fig. 15–8).** The proper orientation of the lesion (12 o'clock position) is marked on the paper. The template is then cut from the glove wrapping about 2 mm larger than the markings **(Fig. 15–9).** A thrombin- and epinephrine-soaked sponge is then placed over the prepared defect to limit bleeding when the tourniquet is deflated **(Fig. 15–10).**

The periosteum is then harvested using a second incision over the medial tibia, distal to the pes anserine insertion. Fat is cleared from the periosteum, and small retractors facilitate exposure of the tibia. The periosteum is sharply incised 1 to 2 mm larger than the prepared template **(Fig. 15–11A).** One must remember to mark the periosteum with a marking pen, similar to the

template, to ensure optimal orientation of the periosteum and superficial surface prior to suturing. With large lesions, multiple lesions, or revision surgeries, it may be difficult to obtain an adequate amount of periosteum from the medial aspect of the tibia. In these cases, additional periosteum can be harvested from the distal medial or lateral aspect of the femur, though this may

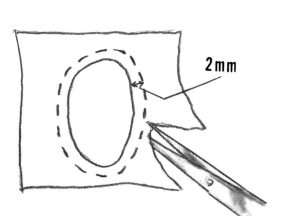

FIGURE 15–9 The template is then cut from the glove wrapping about 2 mm larger than the markings.

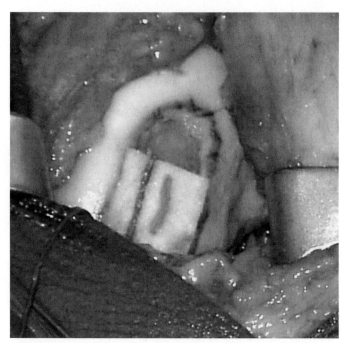

FIGURE 15–10 A thrombin and epinephrine soaked sponge is then placed over the prepared defect to limit bleeding.

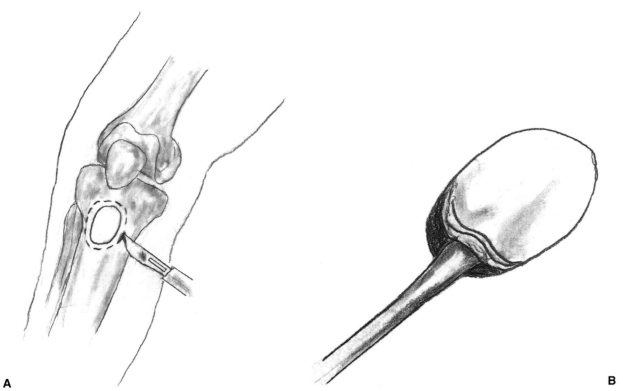

FIGURE 15–11 (A) The periosteum is sharply incised 1 to 2 mm larger than the prepared template. **(B)** A sharp periosteal elevator is then used to elevate the periosteum.

increase the risk of arthrofibrosis. Smooth forceps and a sharp periosteal elevator are then used to elevate the periosteum **(Fig. 15–11B).** If the graft is perforated, the defect is closed with suture when it is placed over the cartilage lesion.

After harvesting the graft, the tourniquet is deflated and hemostasis achieved in the soft tissues and in the prepared defect. The graft is then placed in its correct orientation with the cambium layer facing the defect. Suturing is then performed, at 3- to 5-mm intervals, with 6-0 Vicryl sutures that have been soaking in sterile mineral oil **(Fig. 15–12).** An opening is left to allow insertion of a catheter to test graft integrity and allow injection of the cell suspension **(Fig. 15–13).** Fibrin glue is then placed over the edges of the graft to obtain a watertight seal **(Fig. 15–14).** Sterile saline is injected into the defect to ensure the watertight seal. The saline is then aspirated out of the defect, and the cell suspension is then injected into the defect **(Fig. 15–15).** Finally, the opening at the catheter insertion site is sealed with suture and fibrin glue.

If meniscal takedown was required, the knee is extended and the meniscus reduced. Number 2 braided, nonabsorbable suture is placed through the anterior-medial attachment of the meniscus and is anchored through bone. Suction drains are not placed intraarticularly to avoid injury to the graft. The wound is then closed in layers with a drain in the subcutaneous tissues if a lateral release was performed.

■ Postoperative Care

A knee immobilizer is used to keep the leg in extension for the first postoperative day to allow the chondrocytes to adhere to the underlying subchondral bone and surrounding articular cartilage. Following this, the postoperative rehabilitation is guided by the three healing phases of ACI as identified in canine studies **(Table 15–1** and **Fig. 15–16).**[10–12] The principles of rehabilitation are to protect the graft, retain knee motion, and gradually progress activity and weight bearing. The rehabilitation process is somewhat different for lesions of the patellofemoral joint and lesions of the tibiofemoral joint.

For lesions involving weight-bearing areas of the femoral condyles, rehabilitation involves continuous passive motion (CPM) 6 hours a day,[24] with a goal of 0 to 90 degrees. Touchdown weight bearing is allowed and isometric exercises encouraged during the first 6 postoperative weeks.

Continuous passive motion is discontinued and graduated weight bearing is initiated during postoperative weeks 7 to 12. By 12 weeks, full weight bearing status

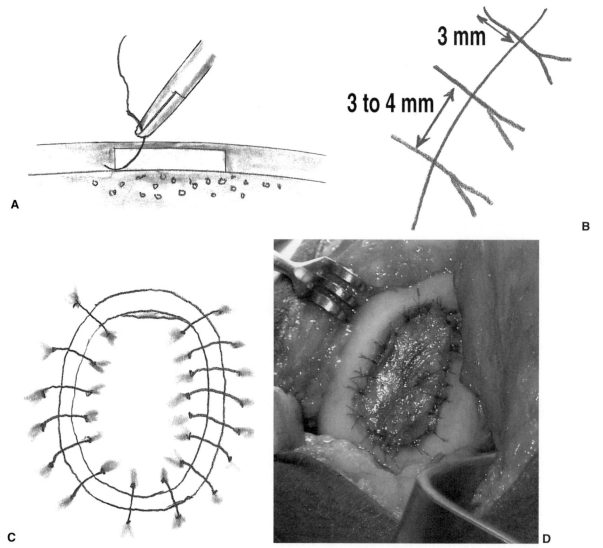

FIGURE 15–12 Suturing is then performed **(A)**, at 3- to 5-mm intervals **(B)**, all around the lesion **(C)**. Full appearance of Sutured periosteal cover prior to cell injection under the periosteum, and sealing margins with fibrin glue **(D)**.

superior opening

FIGURE 15–13 An opening is left at the top for insertion of a catheter for injection of the cell suspension.

is attained, provided that the patient is free of pain and functional muscle usage is encouraged. Stationary bicycling, without resistance, is also helpful during this time.

The maturation phase of healing begins after 12 weeks and can extend to 2 years postoperatively. During this time, assistive devices are discarded and activity levels are increased. Bicycling continues to be encouraged as well as the use of elliptical training machines and treadmill walking. Patients should be encouraged to take an active role in their rehabilitation, and they can begin to use resistive training with the stationary bike and treadmill. Running is not permitted until graft hardness is similar to that of the surrounding cartilage, which may take 12 to 24 months.[12] Activity should be encouraged that fatigues the thigh musculature, but patients should be counseled to lessen their level of activity if they feel knee discomfort.

When ACI is performed on the patellofemoral joint, the rehabilitation differs. These lesions typically

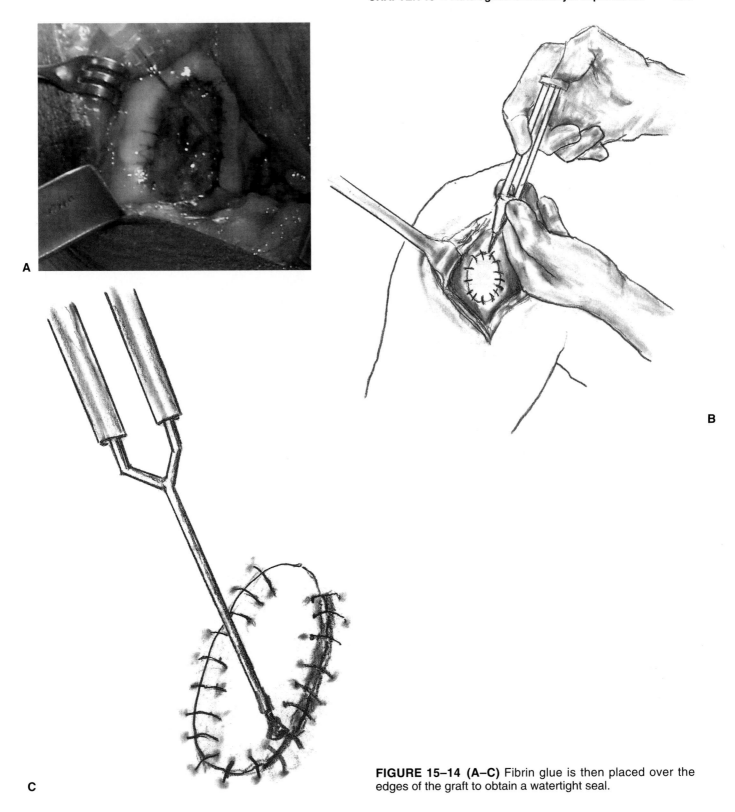

A

B

C

FIGURE 15–14 (A–C) Fibrin glue is then placed over the edges of the graft to obtain a watertight seal.

rehabilitate at a slower pace than lesions of the femoral condyles. Continuous passive motion is used for a range of 0 to 40 degrees during the initial 6 postoperative weeks and full weight bearing is allowed with the knee in full extension. This avoids the maximal contact stresses of the patellofemoral joint that occur between 40 and 70 degrees of flexion. The rest of the motion is gained by dangling the leg over the edge of a bed. Isometric straight leg lifts are instituted postoperatively. Active flexion and passive knee extension is encouraged for the first 6 weeks. Backward treadmill walking, elliptical training machines, and stationary bicycling with

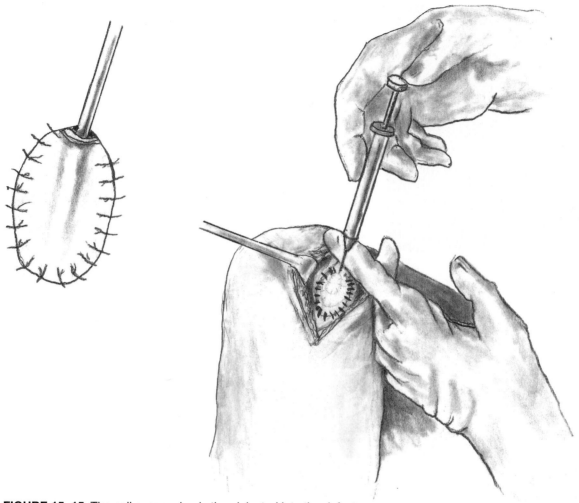

FIGURE 15–15 The cell suspension is then injected into the defect.

minimal resistance are allowed between 6 and 12 weeks. Persistent effusions are common for up to 6 months with trochlear lesions. Kneeling and squatting activities may be allowed 12 to 18 months after surgery.[12]

In the complex, or salvage cases, when multiple grafts are performed at both articulations, rehabilitation is focused on the region that is deemed to be most involved. Similarly, when concomitant procedures such as ligament reconstruction, osteotomy or meniscal transplant are performed, rehabilitation follows the ACI protocol.

■ Complications

Periosteal graft hypertrophy, graft failure or delamination, and arthrofibrosis are the most common complications following ACI.[7] If a patient develops painful catching, new-onset pain, or recurrent effusions in the postoperative period, activity is decreased and an MRI with gadolinium is obtained. Arthroscopy is then performed in select cases. In instances where advanced MRI techniques are not available, diagnostic arthroscopy may be required on a more frequent basis.

In the senior author's experience, second-look arthroscopy for persistent symptoms was required in 25% of patients.[7] Twenty percent were performed due to hypertrophy of the periosteum and 5% performed due to arthrofibrosis following the arthrotomy.

Arthrofibrosis typically develops early (within 3 months) and is treated aggressively with arthroscopic lysis of adhesions, graft assessment, and manipulation under anesthesia. Patients at risk for stiffness were those with a history of keloid formation after prior surgeries, those requiring femoral periosteum for grafts, or those undergoing simultaneous tibial tubercle osteotomy.[7] To limit this complication, we currently do not close the knee arthrotomy below the level of the distal pole of the patella. In addition, though it is an off-label use, we use Seprafilm™ (Genzyme Corp., Cambridge, MA) antiadhesive membrane to possibly reduce the incidence of adhesions, as this has been found to reduce adhesions in abdominal surgeries.[25]

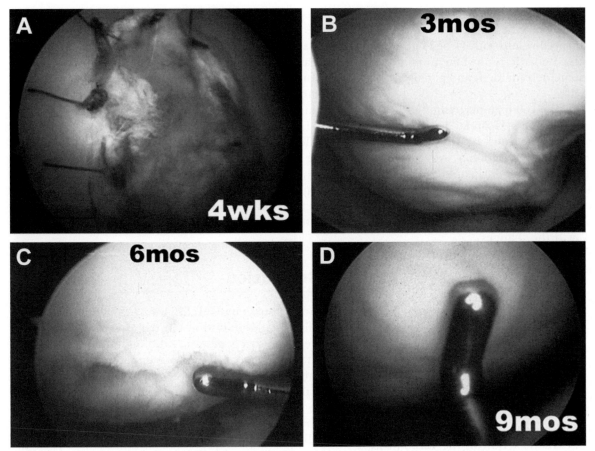

FIGURE 15–16 Arthroscopic photographs of grafts at different stages of healing. **(A)** At 4 weeks, sutures remain present with complete fill of chondral defect with soft, white tissue. **(B)** At 3 months the chondral defect is filled with white, soft, jelly-like tissue, which is not firmly attached to the underlying subchondral bone and has a wave-like consistency. **(C)** At 6 months the graft is putty-like, indentable, and recoils within minutes of being indented. **(D)** At 9 months the graft is firm and has equal viscoelasticity to the adjacent host cartilage. (Adapted from Minas TM, Peterson L. Autologous chondrocyte transplantation. Oper Tech Sports Med 2000;8:144–157)

Periosteal graft hypertrophy usually presents within the first 3 to 9 postoperative months and presents as a new-onset effusion or painful catching. Gentle arthroscopic debridement of the periosteal overgrowth usually relieves symptoms,[6,7] and rarely may be required more than once.

Graft failure has an incidence of 7 to 13% in studies with medium- and short-term results.[6,7] Magnetic resonance imaging frequently reveals progressive or persistent subchondral edema under failing graft sites. Graft failure, or delamination, is heralded by a loose flap at the edge of the graft at second-look arthroscopy. Patients are counseled about the possibility of performing marrow stimulating techniques or autologous osteochondral plug transplant to address areas of possible failure prior to arthroscopy. Either of these techniques is utilized when there is a small area of graft delamination (<1.5 cm^2). If the area of graft failure is larger, consideration is given to revision ACI, fresh osteochondral allograft, or unicompartmental arthroplasty.

■ Results

The first results of ACI were published in 1994 in an initial pilot study from Sweden[20]; 14 of 16 patients treated with ACI for isolated lesions of the femoral condyle obtained good or excellent results. However, patients treated with lesions of the patella did not fare as well, as only two of seven patients obtained good or excellent results. These results prompted further interest in this technique for full-thickness chondral injuries.

The durability of ACI has been confirmed in a 2- to 9-year follow-up study from Sweden that included the patients treated in the initial pilot study.[6] This medium-term retrospective assessment of 101 patients treated with ACI revealed 92% good to excellent results with isolated lesions involving the femoral condyle. The results were further broken down according to diagnosis. Good to excellent results were obtained in 89% of patients treated for osteochondritis dissecans, 75% of patients with concomitant ACL reconstruction, 67% of patients with multiple lesions, and 65% of patients with patellar lesions. The fate of patellar lesions may be improved, however. The authors noted improved results with 11 of 14 good to excellent results with patellar lesions when more attention was given to adequate debridement and patellar realignment when needed.[6]

The results of the first 169 patients treated with ACI at the Brigham and Women's Hospital in Boston were released and were encouraging.[7] In this short-term follow-up study, 87% of the patients were improved, despite the fact that, "simple," isolated lesions of the femoral condyle were unusual in this series. Patients were divided into simple, complex, and salvage groups based on the size and number of lesions as well as the presence of early arthritic changes.

Patients were prospectively evaluated and numerous outcome measures used to assess the results. Short Form (SF-36) scores showed clinical improvement in pain relief and were statistically significant in the complex and salvage groups. The simple category did not achieve statistical significance, although 10 of 12 patients were pain free and returned to participation in sports. The Knee Society scores improved in all groups and were statistically significant at 24 months and were maintained at 4 years. Western Ontario McMaster University Osteoarthritis Index scores showed statistical significance at 24 months. Interestingly, the salvage group reported the highest satisfaction of the three groups, with 93% ($n = 15$ patients at 24 months) reporting they would choose the surgery again.

In general, there was a time-dependent improvement, with maximal improvement occurring by 24 months with femorotibial resurfacing. Patellofemoral resurfacing took longer, 36 months, to reach maximal improvement. Improvements were not as significant when the patellofemoral joint was involved compared with improvements when the tibiofemoral joint was involved. Additionally, when chondral defects were treated with ACI alone, in patients with normal axial alignment, the results seemed superior to those in patients who required osteotomy.

■ Future Developments

Improvements for ACI include substitution for periosteum with an off-the-shelf biologic or synthetic membrane, and substances to prevent adhesions such as hyaluronic acid gels or membranes to eliminate periosteal-related problems and arthrofibrosis. Minimally invasive delivery of ACI will only be available after the next generation development of tissue-engineered cartilage, eliminating the need for microstructuring.

Tissue engineering products that are implanted at a more mature stage of cartilage development along with self-adhering properties to the subchondral bone and adjacent cartilage will dramatically improve clinical outcomes. These will allow arthroscopically performed treatments for small lesions, smaller incisions for large lesions, and a more reproducible histologic repair with a lessened rehabilitation, which translates into less pain, a shorter period of rehabilitation, and a more reproducibly excellent clinical outcome. Tissue engineering will also facilitate a more user-friendly technique that is more widely applicable by the orthopaedist and not as technique sensitive as the present technique of ACI.

■ Conclusion

In the past, patients with full-thickness chondral injuries had few treatment options. Today, these injuries may be treated in a variety of ways. Autologous chondrocyte implantation is a technique with encouraging short-term and midterm results that allows predictable results with hyaline-like repair tissue in young, active patients with large (>2 cm^2) lesions. Care must be taken to assess comorbid conditions such as axial alignment, ligamentous stability, and meniscal pathology to ensure optimal outcomes. Traditional indications for ACI have been reserved for isolated grade 3 to 4 lesions of the femoral condyle or trochlea with no more than grade 2 chondromalacia of the opposing articular surface.[20] However, young, active patients frequently are found to have multiple lesions or early arthritic changes. These injuries can also be treated successfully. Prospective evaluation of patients with validated outcomes analysis suggests that the indications for ACI may be expanded to include complex or salvage patients.[7,12] Preoperative counseling is imperative to ensure that patients understand the extensive rehabilitation process that is required as well as the potential complications that may occur. It is hoped that future technologic developments will make ACI a less invasive procedure with more universal application.

REFERENCES

1. Hunter W. Of the structure and diseases of articulating cartilages. Philosophical Trans 1743;470:514
2. Noyes FR, Bassett RW, Noyes FR, et al. Arthroscopy in acute traumatic hemarthrosis of the knee: incidence of anterior cruciate tears and other injuries. J Bone Joint Surg Am 1980;62A:687–695
3. Curl W, Krome J, Gordon S. Cartilage injuries: a review of 31,516 knee arthroscopies. Arthroscopy 1997;13:456–460
4. Goldberg V. Principles of revision total knee arthroplasty: overview. In: Sim FH, ed. Instructional Course Lectures, vol 50. Rosemont, IL: American Academy of Orthopaedic Surgeons, 2001:357–358

5. Buckwalter JA, Mankin HJ. Articular cartilage: degeneration and osteoarthrosis, repair, regeneration and transplantation. J Bone Joint Surg Am 1997;79A:612–632

6. Peterson L, Minas T, Brittberg M, Nilsson A, Sjogren-Jansson E, Lindahl A. Two to nine year outcome after autologous chondrocyte transplantation of the knee. Clin Orthop Relat Res 2000;374:212–234

7. Minas T. Autologous chondrocyte implantation for focal chondral defects of the knee. Clin Orthop Relat Res 2001;391S:S349–S361

8. Grande DA, Pitman MI, Peterson L. The repair of experimentally produced defects in rabbit cartilage by autologous chondrocyte transplantation. J Orthop Res 1989;7:208–218

9. Brittberg M, Nilsson A, Lindahl A, et al. Rabbit articular cartilage defects treated with autologous cultured chondrocytes. Clin Orthop Relat Res 1996;326:270–283

10. Breinan HA, Minas T, Barone L, et al. Histological evaluation of the course of healing of canine articular cartilage defects treated with cultured autologous chondrocytes. Tissue Eng 1998;4: 101–114

11. Shortkroff S, Barone L, Hsu HP. Healing of chondral and osteo-chondral defects in a canine model: the role of cultured chondrocytes in regeneration of articular cartilage. Biomaterials 1996;17:147–154

12. Minas T, Peterson L. Autologous chondrocyte transplantation. Op Tech Sports Med 2000;8:144–157

13. Personel communication.

14. Rosenberg T, Paulos L, Parker R, et al. The forty-five degree posterior-anterior flexion weight bearing radiograph of the knee. J Bone Joint Surg Am 1988;70A:1479–1483

15. Winalski C, Minas T. Evaluation of chondral injuries by magnetic resonance imaging: repair assessments. Op Tech Sports Med 2000;8:108–119

16. Outerbridge RE. The etiology of chondromalacia patella. J Bone Joint Surg Br 1961;43B:752–757

17. Recht MP, Kramer J, Marcelis S, et al. Abnormalities of articular cartilage in the knee: analysis of available MR techniques. Radiology 1993;187:473–478

18. Vahlensieck M, Peterfy CG, Wischer T, et al. Indirect MR Arthrography: Optimization and clinical applications. Radiology 1996;200:249–254

19. Peterson L. International experience with autologous chondrocyte transplantation. In: Insall JN, Scott WN, ed. Surgery of the Knee, 3rd ed. Philadelphia: Churchill Livingstone, 2001:341–356

20. Brittberg M, Lindahl A, Nilsson A, et al. Treatment of deep cartilage defects in the knee with autologous chondrocyte implantation. N Engl J Med 1994;331:889–895

21. Riebel GD, Boden SD, Whiteside TE, Hutton WC. The effect of nicotine on incorporation of cancellous bone graft in an animal model. Spine 1995;20:2198–2202

22. Raikin SM, Landsman JC, Alexander VA, Froimson MJ, Plaxton NA. Effect of nicotine on the rate and strength of long bone fracture healing. Clin Orthop Relat Res 1998;353:231–237

23. Buuck DA, Fulkerson JP. Anteromedialization of the tibial tubercle: a 4 to 12 year follow-up. Op Tech Sports Med 2000;8:131–137

24. O'Driscoll SW, Salter R. The induction of neochondrogenesis in free intra-articular periosteal autografts under the influence of continuous passive motion. J Bone Joint Surg Am 1984;66A: 1248–1257

25. Vrijland WW, Tseng LN, Eijkman HJ, et al. Fewer intraperitoneal adhesions with use of hyaluronic acid-carboxymethylcellulose membrane: a randomized clinical trial. Ann Surg 2002;235: 193–199

16

Osteochondral Allograft Transplantation

WILLIAM D. BUGBEE AND MICHAEL J. OSTEMPOWSKI

Experience with fresh osteochondral allografting in the management of chondral and osteochondral injuries extends over many decades. In fact, the first documented use of fresh allografts was by Erich Lexer[1] in 1908. In more modern times, the pioneering work by Dr. Alan Gross and Marvin Meyers in the 1970s has led to greater understanding of the indications, outcomes, and basic science of fresh osteochondral allograft transplantation in the treatment of chondral and osteochondral injuries.[2,3] Traditionally, the complexities of allograft surgery, including the recovery, procurement, testing, and storage of fresh tissue, as well as the surgical technique, have limited the use of allografts to specialized centers that have devoted time and effort to overcoming many of the obstacles and difficulties in working with fresh allografts. More recently, however, allografts have become increasingly popular in the orthopaedic community, and as a result the number of allograft procedures is increasing, limited mainly by the availability of fresh allograft tissue. Historically, allografts have been used in the treatment of large chondral or osteochondral defects, particularly in the knee,[2–9] but also in the ankle[10,11] and hip.[12] In the algorithm of cartilage restoration, allografts often are indicated as a salvage treatment in posttraumatic situations after periarticular fracture or in lesions where there is a significant os- seous component, such as osteochondritis dissecans (OCD) or avascular necrosis. Fresh allografts may also be employed after failure of other biologic resurfacing techniques such as microfracture, osteochondral autograft transplantation system (OATS), or autologous chondrocyte implantation. Very occasionally, allografting is considered as an alternative to arthroplasty in the young, active individual. In the athlete, allografts are most useful in those individuals with major trauma, or with large focal or multiple defects, who have failed to respond to more conservative measures.

Current techniques of cartilage repair and restoration generally involve two fundamental strategies. The first is to induce cells to form tissue that can function as an articular surface. Examples of this include abrasion, microfracture, periosteal grafts, autologous chondrocyte implantation, and many tissue-engineering techniques that are not yet clinically available. The second strategy of biologic resurfacing involves the replacement of diseased or absent tissue with architecturally mature articular cartilage. Surgical techniques that fall into this realm include osteochondral autografting, osteochondral allografting, and perhaps in the future, tissue-engineered articular cartilage constructs.

The rationale for fresh allografting thus relies on the consideration that it is a tissue or organ transplantation procedure, utilizing mature hyaline cartilage with underlying bone that functions as a vehicle for attachment, and in some cases to fill an associated osseous defect. The fresh osteochondral graft, therefore, is a composite of living chondrocytes supporting the hyaline matrix and nonliving bone. The chondrocytes survive transplantation and support the hyaline matrix over time, whereas the allograft bone is replaced by host bone, over time, by the process of creeping substitution.[13,14]

Cartilage is an ideal tissue for transplantation. It is avascular, aneural, and by virtue of chondrocytes being embedded within the hyaline matrix, relatively immunoprivileged.[15] Further, cartilage is amenable to storage for a period of time,[16,17] and the cartilage can be fashioned to fit the recipient's anatomy.

Experience with fresh allografts at our institution began in 1983 with an institutional review board–approved protocol. The success of this program was directly related to a close association with a tissue bank and the development of clinical protocols and research programs. Nearly 500 procedures have been performed during this period, and currently about 50 per year are performed, depending on tissue availability. The vast majority of these procedures involve the knee; however, the ankle is another joint that has been successfully treated with allografting.[10,11] Allografting of the hip has been performed, but on a limited basis.[12] Finally, it should be noted that there is no theoretical contraindication to performing allografts on any joint; however, the indications and thus the clinical experience is relatively limited in these situations.

■ Indications

Clinical experience with fresh osteochondral allografting has demonstrated its utility in a wide spectrum of pathology, including osteochondritis dissecans, large or traumatic or degenerative chondral lesions, osteonecrosis, posttraumatic reconstruction after intraarticular fracture, and increasingly, in the salvage of failed cartilage restorative procedures, such as microfracture, osteochondral autografting, or autologous chondrocyte implantation. Additionally, allografts can be utilized in carefully selected cases of patellofemoral disease, such as chondrosis or secondary arthrosis, and in unicompartmental arthrosis of the knee joint. In the ankle, allografts are indicated for the treatment of large OCD lesions and osteonecrosis of the talus, and in the treatment of traumatic arthritis, as an alternative to arthrodesis or arthroplasty.

In our experience, fresh allografts can be utilized in treating defects of any size. In most cartilage restoration algorithms, however, fresh allografts are reserved for lesions larger than 2 cm^2 that have associated osseous defect or abnormality. In practical terms, the most common indication in the athlete is in the treatment of OCD, or as a salvage after failure of another cartilage repair technique **(Table 16–1)**.

■ Patient Selection

Patient selection is critical to the success of the fresh allografting procedure. Careful evaluation of the patient's goals and activity level are vital. Patients should have realistic expectations about the outcome and their ability to return to high-level activity. Patient age is important, because allografting, just like other biologic resurfacing techniques, is less successful in patients over 40 than in those in their 20s. This relates to the important issue of

TABLE 16–1 Indications for Fresh Osteochondral Allografting

Knee
1. Chondral lesions
Traumatic
Degenerative
2. Osteochondritis dissecans
3. Salvage of previous cartilage procedure
4. Posttraumatic reconstruction
Tibial plateau fracture
Femoral condyle fracture
5. Osteonecrosis
6. Patellofemoral chondrosis or arthrosis
7. Unicompartmental arthrosis (selected cases)
Ankle
1. Osteochondritis dissecans
2. Osteonecrosis
3. Posttraumatic arthrosis
Hip
1. Osteonecrosis
2. Osteochondral fracture

the biologic status of the joint, and the concept of the continuum of cartilage disease. One can easily recognize that a focal lesion in a 21-year-old with an otherwise healthy knee is a far different situation from a similar-sized lesion in a 45-year-old with secondary degenerative changes and multiple previous surgeries. As such, it is crucial in the preoperative assessment to perform a careful evaluation of the biologic and mechanical status of the involved limb. This includes attention to the status of ligaments, meniscus, and other compartments of the knee joint, as well as a careful assessment of the mechanical alignment. Instability and mechanical malalignment should always be corrected prior to, or simultaneously with, the allografting procedure. Finally, the lesion size, depth, and location should be evaluated, usually arthroscopically. Most often, patients have had previous surgical intervention, and the status of the knee is fairly well defined.

Imaging studies include the following radiographs: standing anteroposterior (AP), lateral, 45-degree posterior-anterior views, and standing alignment films, as well as patellofemoral views, when indicated. These provide a comprehensive evaluation of the osseous structures, and can characterize the pattern of joint disease. Additionally, advanced imaging studies such as magnetic resonance imaging (MRI) are useful, particularly where there are questions about ligament and meniscus status, or when the disease involves subchondral bone, such as is seen in OCD or osteonecrosis. Finally, and perhaps more importantly with allografting than with any other cartilage-restorative procedure, a careful discussion and informed consent process should be undertaken by the surgeon. This is due to the fact that allograft donor material will be used, and both the surgeon and the patient should understand the unique risks inherent in this procedure, including, but not limited to, viral and bacterial disease transmission.

■ Surgical Technique

Femoral Condyle

Preoperative planning includes careful informed consent, and matching of donor and recipient. Currently, no attempt is made at matching tissue type or blood group. Thus, size is the important parameter in matching donor with recipient. Preoperatively, a standing AP knee x-ray is obtained with a radiographic marker. A corrected size measurement, typically of the tibial plateau width or the femoral condyle width, is made, and this measurement is provided to the tissue bank to obtain a matching donor.[18] Measurements obtained with computed tomography (CT) scans or MRIs may be acceptable, but we have no experience with their accuracy in matching osteochondral grafts, although this technique is used for meniscal allografts.

Once a match is obtained and the tissue becomes available, the surgical technique depends on the site to be grafted. Most commonly, grafting involves the femoral condyle. Arthroscopic evaluation is performed only when indicated, if there is a question about other pathology, or if meniscal or ligament treatment is necessary.

The knee is prepped and draped in standard fashion. Care is taken to place a bolster on the table, to allow the knee to stand free in about 70 to 100 degrees of flexion, to access the femoral condyle easily. A midline incision measuring 6 to 7 cm is made, and a miniarthrotomy is performed, either medially or laterally, depending on the site of the lesion. This incision is extended carefully to the mid- or superior patellar retinaculum, and distally into the fat pad, taking care not to injure the meniscus. In some cases where the lesions are very posterior, typically in the lateral femoral condyle, the meniscus must be taken down to gain access. This can be done by incising the meniscus within a few millimeters of the anterior attachment, leaving enough tissue to perform suture repair at the conclusion of surgery.

Retractors are placed to expose the femoral condyle **(Fig. 16–1).** Careful placement of a retractor in the notch allows mobilization of the patella, but it should be noted that high degrees of flexion decrease the ability

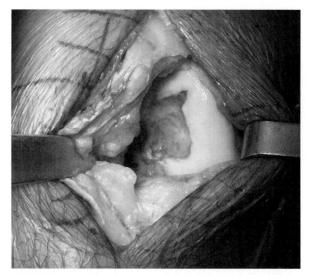

FIGURE 16–1 Miniarthrotomy with exposure of femoral condyle lesion.

to mobilize the patella. This is particularly true in the setting of OCD of the medial femoral condyle, where the lesion extends into the notch, making mobilization of the patella crucial to accessing the lesion. Fortunately, in this setting, the lesions are very anterior, and lower degrees of knee flexion allow easy access with mobility of the patella. Trochlear lesions can be accessed by extending the knee and retracting the patella. Rarely is it necessary to perform a full arthrotomy with patellar eversion unless grafting is to be done on both condyles.

Once the site of the lesion is inspected, a size measurement is obtained. This can be done either with a ruler or by utilizing commercially available instruments **(Fig. 16–2)** (Arthrex, Naples, FL). The availability of instruments to allow preparation of dowel-type allografts from 15 to 35 mm has improved the precision and facilitated the performance of femoral condyle allografts; however, the surgeon should be ready to prepare the

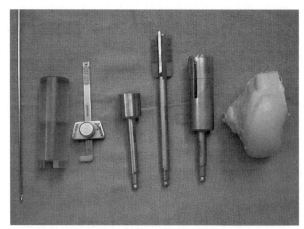

FIGURE 16–2 Typical instruments used for preparation of dowel-type allografts up to 35 mm in diameter.

allograft freehand, utilizing curettes, osteotomes, and high-speed burrs, in situations where dowel grafts are not appropriate.

Once the site is exposed, a guide pin is placed through the center of the lesion, and the size measurement is obtained. The cartilage is then scored, utilizing a special cannulated cartilage cutter, and a router is used to prepare a circular defect. Great care must be taken not to extend this too deep into the subchondral bone. Typically, the depth within the subchondral bone is 3 to 5 mm, making the entire composite depth 5 to 8 mm, including the healthy surrounding cartilage **(Fig. 16–3)**. Occasionally, the preparation needs to be performed deeper, to remove diseased bone. Rarely does this require a depth of greater than 10 to 12 mm.

The next step is to measure the depth of the prepared recipient site, utilizing a depth gauge. These measurements are performed in four quadrants, and transferred to a map, which will be used in preparing the donor material.

On the back table, the fresh graft is removed from its packaging and inspected. (Ideally, this should be done prior to surgery, to ensure the appropriate size and quality of the donor material, prior to incision.) The graft is then placed into a graft holder, and the corresponding position of the lesion on the recipient is marked. Landmarks such as the notch, sulcus terminalis, or other sites can be used to confirm the appropriate position. This becomes critical as graft size increases, to create a graft that has a similar contour to the recipient knee. Once this is performed, a mark is made on a defined position on the graft, to determine rotation after the graft is removed. A cutting guide is placed over the site of the graft, taking care to align this perpendicular to the graft surface and at the same angle that was used to prepare the recipient socket, and a tube saw is utilized to core out the appropriate sized graft. The core is then removed and inspected. The depth measurements made in the recipient are then transferred to the graft core

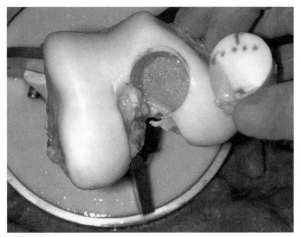

FIGURE 16–4 The allograft is harvested and trimmed to appropriate thickness.

and marked. The allograft is placed in a holder, and an oscillating saw is used to resect portions of the osseous component of the graft until the appropriate thickness in all four quadrants is obtained **(Fig. 16–4)**. A rasp can be used for final contouring. At this point, it is critical to wash the graft thoroughly, utilizing high-pressure lavage, to remove as much marrow element as possible. A final check of measurements should be done to confirm the appropriate thickness of the graft in relationship to the recipient socket. Next, the graft is placed into the site and gently tamped in place **(Fig. 16–5)**. In situations where there is difficulty fitting the graft, dilators are available to dilate the graft; also, a rasp may be used to gently round the corners of the graft, to aid in its fitting.

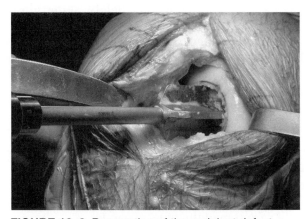

FIGURE 16–3 Preparation of the recipient defect.

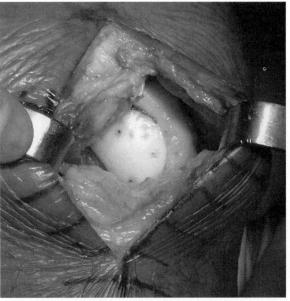

FIGURE 16–5 Final implantation of the allograft prior to placement of polydiaxanone (PDS) pins.

Once the graft is seated, a decision is made regarding whether adjunctive fixation is necessary. We routinely use absorbable pins (Orthosorb, Johnson & Johnson, Raynham, MA), because of concern about micromotion of the graft in the postoperative period. We have seen no deleterious effect from placing 1.3-mm pins through the graft surface; in fact, MRI studies have shown the dissolution of these pins and healing within 3 to 6 months.[19] After the graft is seated, the range of motion should be carefully checked, to ensure that the graft is not catching or unstable. Once this is performed, the knee is irrigated, to remove any debris, followed by routine closure.

Patellofemoral Joint Surgical Technique

The allografting procedure can be performed in the femoral trochlea with a technique quite similar to that for the femoral condyle. In this setting, a slightly larger arthrotomy is necessary, and most lesions are amenable to dowel-type grafting. Great care should be taken in this region, because the complex anatomy can lead to technical errors in preparation and creation of the grafts. On the patellar surface, hemipatellar grafts can be utilized for small lesions. Often we find it necessary to resurface the entire patella, and this is performed in a fashion similar to placing a prosthetic patellar component **(Fig. 16–6).** The entire patellar articular surface is removed, leaving a residual osseous component of 12 to 16 mm. The patellar graft is resected freehand, taking care to include at least 2 mm of subchondral bone with the lateral facet, and placed in the appropriate position on the resected surface, creating a type of sandwich. Tracking then is checked, and fixation of the graft is performed with small-fragment screws from the anterior surface of the patella, in a lag fashion.

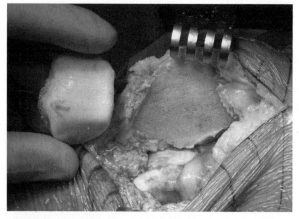

FIGURE 16–6 Patellar allograft.

Tibial Allografts

The majority of tibial allografts involve resurfacing the entire medial or lateral tibial plateau. These are performed in cases of posttraumatic injuries, such as those seen in tibial plateau fractures. Occasionally, focal lesions of the tibia are resurfaced, which present a challenge in accessing the lesions. Anterior detachment of the meniscus is necessary in these cases, and in our experience it has been unusual to require take-down of the collateral ligaments. Flexion and rotation often allows access to the anterior half of the tibial plateau surface where the dowel instrumentation can be utilized. Central lesions can be grafted utilizing a freehand technique, which is technically very challenging. When 50% or more of the tibial surface is involved (the most common scenario), resurfacing the entire plateau is recommended. In cases where the entire tibial plateau is resurfaced, the use of fluoroscopy is necessary. Reciprocating and oscillating saws are used to resect the tibial surface. This can be done either freehand or utilizing Kirschner wires (K-wires) to guide appropriate slope and alignment. Alternatively, a unicompartmental arthroplasty jig can be employed. A minimal resection (2–6 mm) is desired, understanding that typically there is already loss of plateau height from previous trauma. If the recipient meniscus is to be preserved, it is detached anteriorly and protected, and the vertical resection on the plateau is carefully made on the up-slope of the tibial spine, protecting both the posterior attachment of the meniscus and the anterior cruciate ligament. Once the tibial surface is resected, the leg is brought into extension and the measurement of the extension space is performed with a caliper. This gap is typically 10 to 15 mm. Measurements of the anteroposterior and mediolateral dimensions of the prepared defects are also made, and the tibial allograft is carefully marked. Reciprocating and oscillating saws are used to carefully remove the allograft hemiplateau from the tibial graft. Remeasuring and recutting is routine; and trial fittings are performed as the surgeon checks visually and fluoroscopically for restoration of plateau height, slope, graft position, coverage, and stability. When satisfactory fit and stability are obtained, the graft is lavaged. Fixation is obtained with small interfragmentary screws placed in the midcoronal region and anteriorly **(Fig. 16–7).** The meniscus is repaired with nonabsorbable suture. In situations where meniscus allografting is performed in conjunction with the osteochondral allograft, it is important to complete the recipient meniscectomy. Plateau resection is performed closer to the cruciate insertion, and the plateau graft is prepared to include the insertions of the meniscus. All residual soft tissue is removed from the composite allograft, and meniscal suturing is performed after fixation of the tibial allograft.

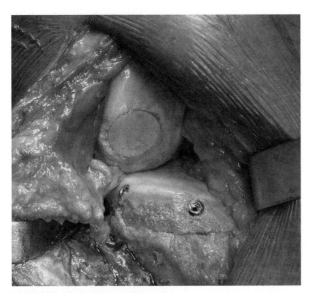

FIGURE 16–7 Tibial allograft.

■ Postoperative Care

For femoral condyle grafts, the postoperative management is straightforward. Patients typically are allowed full range of motion, except in cases where meniscus has been repaired. A continuous passive motion (CPM) machine is used during the brief hospitalization; physical therapy, including quadriceps-setting exercises and crutch training, is performed. Patients undergo a period of 6 to 12 weeks of protected weight bearing, and begin closed-chain exercises at 4 weeks. Unlimited weight bearing is generally allowed at between 2 and 4 months, depending on the size of the graft and the rehabilitation of the knee. Radiographs are obtained at 4 to 6 weeks, 3 months, and 6 months to assess healing of the allograft. Full activity is allowed at 6 months, if functional rehabilitation is complete.

Postoperative management of patellofemoral allografts includes restricted knee flexion (typically 0–45 degrees for the first 4–6 weeks) utilizing a range-of-motion brace. Unrestricted weight bearing is generally allowed in full extension.

Postoperative management of tibial allografts is similar to that for femoral allografts, with attention to meniscal protection and often a longer period (3–4 months) of restricted weight bearing. In addition, range-of-motion braces routinely are utilized, followed by prescription of an unloader brace to be used for at least 1 year. Patients are generally cautioned about excessive impact loading of the allograft, particularly in the first year.

No immunosuppression is utilized with fresh osteochondral allografts, and the use of antiinflammatories is carefully considered, due to concerns with inhibition of osseous healing, which is critical to the success of the allograft.

■ Complications

Early complications unique to the allografting procedure are few. There does not appear to be any increased risk of surgical site infection with the use of allografts as compared with other procedures. The use of a miniarthrotomy in the knee likely decreases the risk of postoperative stiffness. Occasionally, one sees a persistent effusion, which is typically a sign of overuse, but which may also indicate a possible graft-mediated synovitis.

Delayed union or nonunion of the fresh allograft is the most common early finding. This is evidenced by persistent discomfort or visible graft–host interface on serial radiographic evaluation. Delayed union or nonunion is more common in larger grafts, such as those used in the tibial plateau, or in the setting of compromised bone, such as in the treatment of osteonecrosis. In this setting, patience is essential, and complete healing or recovery may take an extended period. Decreasing activities, instituting weight-bearing precautions or the use of braces, and possibly using external bone stimulators may be helpful in the early management of a delayed healing. In such cases, careful evaluation of serial radiographs can provide insight into the healing process; MRI scans are rarely helpful, particularly prior to 6 months postoperatively, as they typically show extensive signal abnormality that is difficult to interpret. It should be noted that with adequate attention to postoperative weight-bearing restrictions and adequate graft fixation, delayed union or nonunion requiring repeat surgical intervention within the first year is extremely uncommon.

The natural history of the graft that fails to osseointegrate is unpredictable. Clinical symptoms may be minimal, or there may be progressive clinical deterioration and radiographic evidence of fragmentation, fracture, or collapse. Typical symptoms of this type of graft failure include increase of pain or sudden onset, often associated with minor trauma. Effusion, crepitus, or focal, localized pain is commonly seen. Careful evaluation of serial radiographs typically will demonstrate collapse, subsidence, fracture, or fragmentation. CT or MRI also can be utilized to confirm graft failure.

Late complications associated with the allografting procedure also usually involve the osseous portion of the graft. The requisite event for a successful fresh allograft procedure is healing of the host–graft bony interface and integration of the host bone into the osseous portion of the allograft. This process of so-called creeping substitution is well described in the paradigm of bone–graft healing. Revascularization of the allograft bone by the host may take many years, and may not be complete.[20] The amount of bone within the allograft may be important in this process, and it is likely that thinner grafts will have more complete revascularization than thicker grafts. Retrieval studies[13,14,20] of failed fresh osteochondral allografts have provided tremendous insight into the allograft healing process, and have led to the understanding that fresh osteochondral allografts rarely fail due to the cartilage portion of the graft; rather, most failures originate within the osseous portion of the graft, or from progression of the host joint disease process, that is, osteoarthrosis. It is likely that late allograft failure, which has been seen at between 2 and 17 years, is the result of graft subsidence collapse or fragmentation due to fatigue failure, very much like that seen with bulk allografts placed under repetitive loading situations. This clinical finding underscores the need to pay close attention to joint alignment and stability in the initial treatment of the patient. Clinically, the patient presents with new pain or mechanical symptoms, of either insidious or acute onset. Radiographs show cysts or sclerosis, or perhaps subchondral collapse, typically in the center of the graft, which may be most distant from the revascularization process, or in an area that has been under higher load due to activity of the patient or malalignment. Again, careful review of serial radiographs is important. MRI also may be useful at this point, and generally is obtained to confirm suspected allograft pathology and to rule out other sources of pain or sites of pathology in the knee joint **(Fig. 16–8).** It is important to note that the allografted joint may suffer from the same pathology that is present in any other joint, such as meniscus or ligamentous injury. It should also be noted that radiographic and magnetic resonance abnormalities are commonly noted, even in well-functioning allografts,[19] and great care must be taken in interpreting and correlating the imaging studies with clinical findings. Finally, it is not yet clear whether allografting alters the natural history of an injured joint. Therefore, over time, progression of cartilage disease and frank osteoarthrosis is possible and likely, particularly in the older population. Further intervention for a previously allografted knee may not be related to the allograft.

Treatment options for failed allografts include observation, if the patient is minimally symptomatic and the joint is thought to be at low risk for further progression of disease. Arthroscopic evaluation and debridement also may be utilized. In many cases, revision allografting is performed, and generally has led to a success rate equivalent to primary allografting. This appears to be one of the particular advantages to fresh osteochondral allografting, in that fresh allografting does not preclude a revision allograft as a salvage procedure for failure of the initial allograft. In cases of more extensive joint disease, particularly in older individuals, conversion to prosthetic arthroplasty is necessary.

■ Case Example

A 17-year-old high school baseball player sustained a noncontact injury to his left knee while running the bases. He presented with mild medial knee pain and mechanical symptoms. Clinical evaluation, including plain radiographs and MRI, revealed a large osteochondritis lesion of the medial femoral condyle, with fragment displacement and loose bodies **(Fig. 16–9A).** He was unable to fully extend the affected knee. Ligament and meniscus exam were unremarkable, and there was no axial malalignment of the limb. His past history was remarkable for occasional knee discomfort for many years that did not interfere with activity and was diagnosed as "growing pains."

The patient underwent arthroscopic debridement and removal of loose bodies. The lesion measured 2.8 by 2.2 cm and 8 mm deep **(Fig. 16–9B).** Because of persistent symptoms, size and depth of the lesion, and his desire to return to sports, he underwent fresh osteochondral allografting. A 3.0 cm by 9 mm dowel graft was harvested, fit into the prepared defect, and fixed with three absorbable pins **(Fig. 16–9C).**

The patient had an uneventful recovery. After 3 months of protected weight bearing, radiographs demonstrated osseous healing. He gradually returned to sports and recreational activities, resuming competitive baseball by 8 months after surgery.

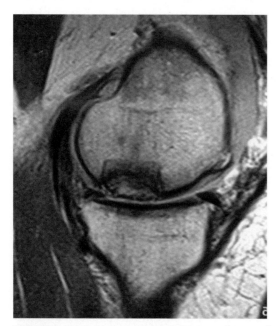

FIGURE 16–8 Failed allograft. Note collapse of subchondral bone and irregularity of articular surface.

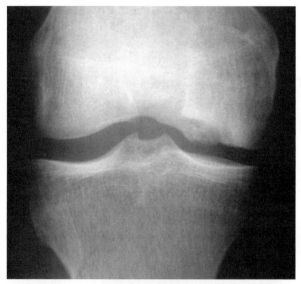

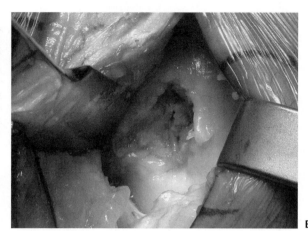

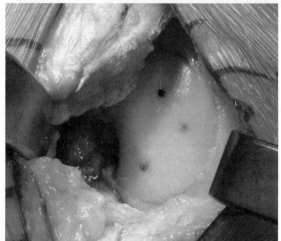

FIGURE 16–9 (A) Anteroposterior (AP) radiograph of osteochondritis dissecans of the medial femoral condyle in a 17-year-old baseball player. **(B)** Osteochondral defect prior to allografting. **(C)** Medial femoral condyle with implanted allograft. Three PDS pins have been placed.

■ Results

The clinical outcome of fresh osteochondral allografting depends on the age and diagnosis of the patient, the size of the lesion, and the number of lesions grafted (**Table 16–2**).

We have reported a series of 69 knees in 66 individuals with OCD of the femoral condyle treated with fresh osteochondral allografts.[21] All allografts were implanted within 5 days of procurement. Patients were prospectively evaluated using an 18-point modified D'Aubigne and Postel scale, and subjective assessment

TABLE 16–2 Results of Fresh Osteochondral Allografting

Author	Site	Diagnosis	Number	Mean Follow-Up (Years)	Successful Outcome
Ghazavi[8]	Knee	Trauma	126	7.5	85% survivorship
Meyers[2]	Knee	Multiple	31	3.5	77%
Chu[4]	Knee	Multiple	55	6.2	84% G/E
Aubin[9]	Femur	Trauma	60	10.0	85% survivorship
Garrett[6]	f. c.	OCD	17	2–9	16/17
Bugbee[21]	f. c.	OCD	69	5.2	80% G/E
Bugbee[7]	Knee	Arthrosis	41	4.5	54% G/E
f.c.,femoral condyle, G/E, good and excellent.					

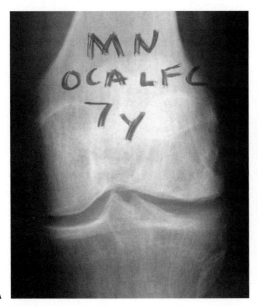
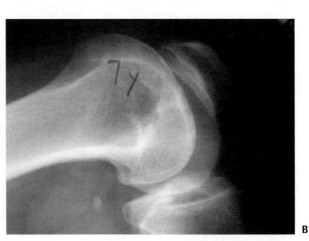

A **B**

FIGURE 16–10 (A,B) Anteroposterior and lateral radiograph 7 years after fresh allograft of lateral femoral condyle in 47-year-old man. Note integration of allograft and evidence of osteoarthrosis. Patient is a recreational triathlete.

was performed with a patient questionnaire. In this group, there were 49 males and 17 females, with a mean age of 28 years (range 15–54). Forty lesions involved the medial femoral condyle, and 29 the lateral femoral condyle. An average of 1.6 surgeries had been performed on the knee prior to the allograft procedure. Allograft size was highly variable, with a range from 1 to 13 cm². The average allograft size was 7.4 cm². Two knees were lost to follow-up. Mean follow-up in the remaining 67 knees was 5.2 years (range 1–14). Overall, 50/69 (72%) knees were rated good or excellent, scoring 15 or above on the 18-point scale; 11/69 (16%) were rated fair; and 2/69 (3%) were rated poor. The average clinical score improved from 13.0 preoperatively to 15.8 postoperatively ($p <. 01$). Six patients had reoperations on the allograft: one was converted to total knee arthroplasty, and five underwent revision allografting at 1, 2, 5, 7, and 8 years after the initial allograft. Thirty-six of 66 patients completed questionnaires: 95% reported satisfaction with their treatment; 86% felt they were significantly improved. Subjective knee function improved from a mean of 3.2 to 7.8 on a 10-point scale. Garrett[6] also reported on treating OCD with fresh allografts. At 2- to 9-year follow-up, 16/17 were reported successful.

Chu et al[4] reported on 55 consecutive knees undergoing osteochondral allografting. This group included patients with diagnoses such as traumatic chondral injury, avascular necrosis, OCD, and patellofemoral disease. The mean age of this group was 35.6 years, with follow-up averaging 75 months (range 11–147 months). Of the 55 knees, 43 were unipolar replacements and 12 were bipolar resurfacing replacements. On an 18-point scale,

42/55 (76%) of these knees were rated good to excellent, and 3/55 were rated fair, for an overall success rate of 82%. It is important to note that 84% of the knees that underwent unipolar femoral grafts were rated good to excellent, and only 50% of the knees with bipolar grafts achieved good or excellent status. No realignment osteotomies were reported in this series. Many of the patients who underwent unipolar replacement were allowed to return to recreational and competitive sports **(Fig. 16–10).**

Ghazavi et al[8] reported on 126 knees in 123 patients with posttraumatic osteochondral lesions of the tibia and femur at an average follow-up of 7.5 years. Eighty-five percent of patients were rated as successful; the remaining 18 patients had failed. Factors related to failure included age over 50 years, bipolar defects, malalignment, and workers' compensation cases. Aubin et al[9] later reported on the long-term results of 60 fresh femoral grafts implanted for posttraumatic lesions. These patients were a subgroup of the cohort reported by Ghazavi et al. Kaplan-Meier survivorship analysis showed 85% graft survival at 10 years and 74% survival at 15 years. Sixty-eight percent of patients underwent simultaneous realignment osteotomy, and 17% had concomitant meniscal transplantation.

■ Fresh Allograft Tissue

The fundamental principle of fresh osteochondral allografting is that fresh allografts, rather than frozen allografts, contain a high percentage of viable chondrocytes, and these chondrocytes will maintain the intact hyaline cartilage matrix. It has been shown in retrieval studies that viable chondrocytes are present for up to 17 years after implantation.[14] In contrast, frozen allografts demonstrate little to no chondrocyte viability,[13,22] and as a result matrix degeneration invariably ensues within a few years after implantation of frozen allografts.[13] This experience supports the fundamental basis of utilizing fresh allografts, in spite of the increased difficulty in tissue recovery and processing. It is thought that the fresh graft provides the maximum chondrocyte viability, leading to the best long-term graft function. Historically, in allograft centers, transplantation has occurred within 7 days of tissue recovery; however, current fresh tissue banking protocols require a period of 14 days for completion of tissue testing. The issue, therefore, becomes one of balance between the safety of fresh tissue and deterioration of tissue during storage.

Storage studies have demonstrated that chondrocyte viability decreases with storage time, and particularly after 14 days of storage in a modified culture medium at 4°C. Between days 14 and 21, chondrocyte viability decreases from percents in the upper 90s to 70%. Additionally, viable cell density decreases dramatically. It has also been shown that sulfate uptake, a measure of metabolic activity of the tissue, declines significantly after only 7 days of storage.[16,17]

The issue of prolonged storage of fresh allografts is evolving. At the present time, there are no clinically relevant studies investigating the outcome of allografting utilizing grafts stored for longer than 7 days. It is therefore unclear whether there are any clinical consequences to prolonged storage. Clearly, further investigation is needed in this area. The storage of osteochondral allografts is an important component of the tissue banking aspects that are so unique to fresh osteochondral allografts. Few tissue banks have developed protocols to screen, recover, test, and process fresh allograft material. These processes are difficult and complex; however, they yield tissue that strikes a balance between safety and graft quality.

Allograft tissue donors are rigorously screened and tested, utilizing American Association of Tissue Banks guidelines.[23] Nonetheless, it is important to recognize that fresh osteochondral allografts cannot be sterilized; more properly, they are harvested aseptically and tested for the presence of bacteria and viral disease. Historically, allografts, including fresh allografts, have been very safe; at our institution we have had no documented cases of disease transmission from allograft to recipient in over 20 years and 500 procedures. Disease transmission and infections from both fresh and frozen allografts have been reported.[24] It is therefore critically important for surgeons to have a careful understanding of the process and the tissue bank with which they work, and communicate the appropriate risk to patients undergoing the procedure.

■ Immunologic Response to Fresh Allografts

The long-term function of fresh allografts depends on the osseous integration of the allograft to the host, the maintenance of the matrix by viable chondrocytes, and the relatively limited immune response and lack of frank rejection of the graft by the recipient. Several basic scientific studies have been performed investigating the immune response to fresh and frozen matched and mismatched osteochondral allografts. Stevenson[25] demonstrated, in a canine study, that fresh canine leukocyte antigen–mismatched grafts generated the most vigorous immune response. Human studies include the histologic evaluation of retrievals of both functioning and failed allografts.[20] These studies typically show osseous integration of the graft to the host with variable replacement and revascularization of the osseous portion of the graft, up to 90% chondrocyte viability, and no evidence of cell-mediated rejection such as lymphocyte infiltration. Conversely, in our series, we have measured anti–human leukocyte antigen (HLA) cytotoxic antibodies in the serum of patients. Approximately 50% of patients undergoing fresh osteochondral allografts generate these antibodies, presumably against the osseous or chondral component of the donor material. Although the clinical consequences of this response are not yet clear, we have demonstrated a correlation with the presence of these antibodies and inferior appearance on postoperative MRI.[19] Additionally, over 90% of failed allografts in our series are antibody-positive. These findings suggest the need for further study on the immunologic response to fresh grafts. It is entirely possible that in the future we will have a better understanding of the immune behavior of fresh allografts, and perhaps perform some type of tissue matching or pharmacologic immune modulation.

■ Conclusion

Fresh osteochondral allografts are extremely useful for a wide spectrum of cartilage pathology, from the focal chondral lesion to extensive articular disease. Most commonly, in the athlete, allografts are utilized in the treatment of focal osteochondral lesions, such as those seen in osteochondritis dissecans, and as a salvage procedure when other cartilage restorative procedures have failed. Additionally, reconstruction of posttraumatic defects, such as those seen in periarticular fractures, is another common indication for fresh allografts in young, active individuals.

The allografting procedure takes advantage of the unique characteristics of both osseous and chondral tissue components. Uniquely, allografts can restore both osseous and chondral defects with a single graft material. Long-term clinical studies have demonstrated success rates of between 75% and 90% in focal femoral condyle lesions. Nonetheless, the allograft procedure presents unique clinical issues that require careful understanding prior to its undertaking. It is anticipated that in the future, advances in tissue banking, basic scientific investigations into the behavior of fresh allografts, and further study of clinical results will improve the outcome and more clearly define the indications for fresh osteochondral allografts.

REFERENCES

1. Lexer E. Joint transplantations and arthroplasty. Surg Gynecol Obstet 1925;40:782–809
2. Meyers MH, Akeson WA, Convery FR. Resurfacing of the knee with fresh osteochondral allograft. J Bone Joint Surg Am 1989;71A:704–713
3. Gross AE, McKee NH, Pritzker KP. Reconstruction of skeletal deficits of the knee: a comprehensive osteochondral transplant program. Clin Orthop 1983;174:96–106
4. Chu CR, Convery FR, Akeson WA, et al. Articular cartilage transplantation: clinical results in the knee. Clin Orthop 1999;36:159–168
5. Bugbee WD, Jamali A, Rabbani R. Fresh osteochondral allografting in the treatment of tibiofemoral arthrosis. Proceedings of the 69th meeting of the American Academy of Orthopaedic Surgeons (AAOS), Dallas, TX, February 2002
6. Garrett JC. Fresh osteochondral allografts for treatment of articular defects in osteochondritis dissecans of the lateral femoral condyle in adults. Clin Orthop 1994;303:33–37
7. Bugbee WD. Fresh osteochondral allografts. Semin Arthroplasty 2000;11:1–7
8. Ghazavi MT, Pritzker RP, Davis AM, et al. Fresh osteochondral allografts for post-traumatic osteochondral defects of the knee. J Bone Joint Surg Br 1997;79B:1008–1013
9. Aubin PP, Cheah HK, Davis AM, Gross AE. Long term follow-up of fresh femoral osteochondral allografts for post-traumatic knee defects. Clin Orthop Relat Res 2001;391(suppl):318–327
10. Gross AE, Agnidis A, Hutchison CR. Osteochondral defects of the talus treated with fresh osteochondral allograft transplantation. Foot Ankle Int 2001;22:385–391
11. Kim CW, Tontz WL, Jamali A, Convery FR, Brage ME, Bugbee WD. Treatment of post-traumatic ankle arthrosis with bipolar tibiotalar osteochondral shell allografts. Foot Ankle Int 2002;23:1091–1102
12. Meyers MH. Resurfacing of the femoral head with fresh osteochondral allografts: long-term results. Clin Orthop 1985;197:111–114
13. Enneking WF, Campanacci DA. Retrieved human allografts: a clinicopathological study. J Bone Joint Surg Am 2001;83:971–986
14. Czitrom AA, Keating S, Gross AE. The viability of articular cartilage in fresh osteochondral allografts after clinical transplantation. J Bone Joint Surg Am 1990;72:574–581
15. Langer F, Gross AE. Immunogenicity of allograft articular cartilage. J Bone Joint Surg Am 1974;56A:297–304
16. Ball S, Amiel D, Williams SK, et al. The effects of storage on fresh human osteochondral allografts. Clin Orthop Relat Res 2004;418:246–252
17. Williams SK, Amiel D, Ball ST, et al. Prolonged storage effects on the articular cartilage of fresh human osteochondral allografts. J Bone Joint Surg Am 2003;85-A:2111–2120
18. Convery FR, Akeson WH, Meyers MH. The operative technique of fresh osteochondral allografting of the knee. Oper Tech Orthop 1997;47:340–344
19. Sirlin CB, Brossman J, Boutin RD, et al. Shell osteochondral allografts of the knee: comparison of MR imaging findings and immunologic responses. Radiology 2001;219:35–43
20. Oakeshott RD, Farine I, Pritzker KP, et al. A clinical and histologic analysis of failed fresh osteochondral allografts. Clin Orthop 1988;233:283–294
21. Bugbee WD, Emmerson BC, Jamali A. Fresh osteochondral allografting in the treatment of osteochondritis dissecans of the femoral condyle. Paper 054. Presented at the 70th annual meeting of the American Academy of Orthopaedic Surgeons (AAOS, New Orleans, LA), February 2003
22. Ohlendorf C, Tomford WM, Mankin HJ. Chondrocyte survival in cryopreserved osteochondral articular cartilage. J Orthop Res 1996;14:413–416
23. American Association of Tissue Banks. Standards for tissue banking. Arlington, VA: American Association of Tissue Banks, 1987
24. Centers for Disease Control. Update. Allograft-associated biochemical infections–United States, 2002. Morb Mortal Wkly Rep 2002;51: 207–210
25. Stevenson S. The immune response to osteochondral allografts in dogs. J Bone Joint Surg Am 1987;69:573–582

Joint-Specific Treatment

17

Osteochondral Lesions of the Talus

MARK E. EASLEY, STEVEN D. SIDES, AND ALISON P. TOTH

Treatment of symptomatic focal talar osteochondral defects has undergone a dramatic evolution over the past decade. Management of symptomatic osteochondral lesions of the talus (OLT) is challenging given the poor healing potential of articular cartilage. The standard of care in surgical management of chronic lesions remains debridement of the OLT in combination with methods of recruiting mesenchymal stems cells to differentiate within the defect (drilling versus microfracture). Intermediate- to long-term results of these techniques have been reported as favorable.[1–3]

Debridement and drilling or microfracture fails to restore the natural articular cartilage surface, instead filling the void with fibrocartilage. Fibrocartilage is less durable than the adjacent physiologic hyaline cartilage and tends to degenerate with mechanical stress. In smaller diameter lesions (10 mm or less), this is probably well tolerated as mechanical symptoms from impingement of the small lesion are relieved by debridement, and sufficient surrounding hyaline cartilage exists to provide mechanical support. In contrast, larger osteochondral defects (greater than 10 mm) filled with fibrocartilage may provide inadequate mechanical support and may distort the natural viscoelastic properties of the talar dome. Small, nondisplaced acute osteochondral injuries to the talar dome may be observed and are typically excised if displaced. Larger acute osteochondral injuries are probably best treated with internal fixation, particularly if displaced. Frequently, acute injuries are not initially detected, and are thus managed as chronic lesions.

Numerous cartilage repair techniques have been described for managing OLTs.[4–7] In general, these techniques are reserved for salvage of failed debridement and drilling or microfracture. As for the knee, two fundamentally different treatment principles have recently been popularized as favored cartilage repair procedures: (1) osteochondral autograft/allograft transplantation,[6,7] and (2) autologous chondrocyte implantation.[4,5]

This chapter addresses current concepts in the management of OLT, reviews the prevalence and pathophysiology of OLTs, discusses the diagnosis and staging systems and the operative and nonoperative treatment, and suggests future directions in the management of these lesions.

■ Prevalence and Pathophysiology

Osteochondral lesions of the talus are rare. Based on the early literature, the reported prevalence of OLTs ranges from 0.09% of all talar fractures[8] to 6.5% of ankle sprains.[9] The prevalence is likely higher; the use of bone scintigraphy[10] and magnetic resonance imaging (MRI)[11] in the evaluation of ankle pain has shown that OLTs are more common than previously indicated. The prevalence of bilateral lesions is ~10%.[12,13] Medial lesions are more common than lateral lesions, and central lesions are relatively uncommon.[14] Arthroscopic evaluation of the talar dome at the time of open reduction and internal fixation of ankle fractures suggests that the prevalence may far exceed what is reported. In a prospective evaluation of 288 ankle fractures assessed arthroscopically, cartilage lesions were identified in 79%.[15] Similarly, ankle arthroscopy in patients with lateral ankle ligament injuries reveals a high prevalence of OLTs.[16]

■ Ankle Joint Characteristics

Ankle articular cartilage is only 1 to 2 mm thick (in comparison, hip and knee cartilage is 3 to 6 mm).[17] Degenerative changes in the ankle are rare in the absence of trauma.[18] Factors that may protect the ankle include favorable cartilage tensile fracture stresses, favorable responses to degradative proteases, joint congruency, and motion.[19]

Although cartilage tensile fracture stress decreases exponentially for the hip over time, it decreases only linearly for the talus, and by middle age, ankle articular cartilage typically can withstand greater tensile loads than hip cartilage.[20] There also are biochemical advantages in the ankle. In contrast to knee articular cartilage, ankle cartilage expresses minimal RNA for cartilage-degrading enzyme matrix metalloproteinase-8 MMP-8[21] and exhibits less proteoglycan degradation in response to the catabolic cytokine interleukin-1β (IL-1β) because of a decreased number of IL-1 receptors.[22]

The advantages described for the intact ankle joint are forfeited following trauma. With a contact area measuring 350 mm^2 in the ankle[23–25] versus 1120 mm^2 in the knee[26] and 1100 mm^2 in the hip,[27] the thinner, stiffer ankle articular cartilage may be less adaptable to articular surface incongruity and increased contact stresses.[19] Localized subchondral plate sclerosis (after trauma) increases contact stresses in the cartilage directly overlying the stiffened bone, and associated joint instability may lead to greater damage.

■ Etiology

Osteochondral lesions of the talus may occur in any location on the talar dome, but typically are observed posteromedially or anterolaterally **(Fig. 17–1).** Lateral OLTs usually are associated with trauma, whereas medial lesions may be traumatic or nontraumatic.[28] Berndt and Harty[12] reported that 88% of patients with OLTs had a history of trauma. Moreover, in a cadaver model, they created lateral OLTs with ankle inversion and dorsiflexion and produced medial OLTs with ankle inversion, plantarflexion, and external rotation. Whereas lateral lesions tend to be shallow and wafer-shaped, medial lesions are generally relatively deep and cup-shaped.

Canale and Belding[29] reported that all lateral lesions and 64% of medial lesions were related to trauma. Likewise, Alexander and Lichtman[30] noted that 100% of lateral lesions and 82% of medial lesions were associated with trauma. In a literature review, Flick and Gould[31] observed a reported history of trauma associated with 98% of lateral OLT and 70% of medial OLT. Other studies that include arthroscopic evaluation document a

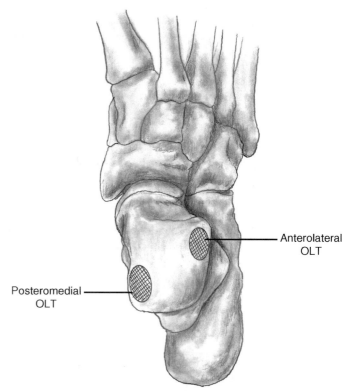

FIGURE 17–1 Schematic of an axial view of the talar dome. Osteochondral defects of the talus occur most typically posteromedially or anterolaterally.

history of antecedent trauma in greater than 75%,[28,32–34] regardless of the location of the OLT. Similarly, an MRI study suggested 50% of lateral ligament injuries have concomitant OLTs.[11] In the absence of trauma, ossification defects, abnormal vasculature, emboli, or endocrine disorders may be responsible for pathologic subchondral fracture of focal areas of the talar dome. Overuse and concentrated pressure increases could produce focal necrosis with formation of a sequestrum or cyst. In the normal ankle joint, considerable stresses are imposed on the medial talar dome; this may explain atraumatic medial dome and bilateral lesions.[14,35]

■ Diagnosis and Staging

The methods of diagnosing OLTs have not changed significantly over the past several years. The patient typically reports an ankle injury such as a sprain that fails to heal in the anticipated time course. Persistent pain with activity and accompanying mechanical symptoms, such as popping, catching, and occasional locking are noted. Acute injuries may demonstrate mechanical symptoms consistent with a loose body. The suspected OLT generally can be detected on plain radiographs, but occasionally

MRI is necessary to reveal the lesion.[36–38] A recent prospective investigation demonstrated that MRI, helical computed tomography (CT), and diagnostic arthroscopy are superior to physical examination and plain radiography in detecting OLTs.[39] However, the authors concluded that diagnostic arthroscopy did not outperform MRI or helical CT for detecting or excluding OLTs.

Recently, more attention has been given to OLTs associated with ankle fractures and ligamentous ankle injuries, and some surgeons are reporting the benefits of ankle arthroscopy at the time of open reduction and internal fixation of ankle fractures and ligament reconstruction, respectively.[15,40,41] Possibly, there is an advantage to the recognition of these lesions in patients with ankle fractures or sprains; fixation or debridement of OLTs may lead to better outcomes following ankle fractures/sprains with associated OLTs.

Staging of OLTs is generally based on the original radiographic classification by Berndt and Hardy[12]: I, small subchondral compression; II, partial fragment detachment; III, complete fragment detachment without displacement; IIIA, complete fragment detachment and rotation without displacement; IV, complete fragment detachment with displacement **(Fig. 17–2).**

An MRI classification has been introduced by Hepple et al[37]: 1, chondral injury only; 2a, cartilage injury with underlying fracture and surrounding bone edema; 2b, the same as stage 2a but without bone edema; 3,

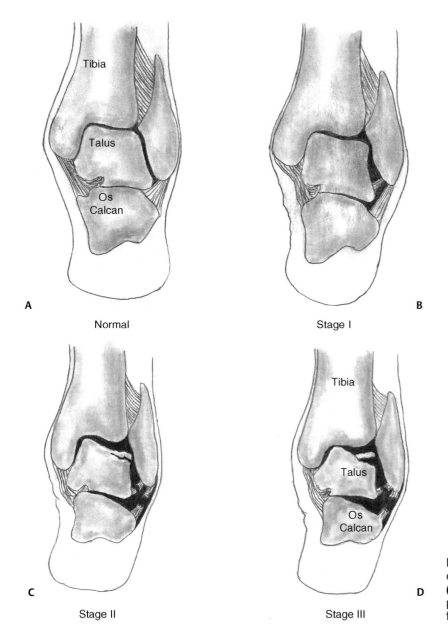

FIGURE 17–2 Berndt and Hardy[12] staging of osteochondral defects of the talus. **(A)** Normal. **(B)** I, small subchondral compression. **(C)** II, partial fragment detachment. **(D)** III, complete fragment detachment without displacement.

(Continued)

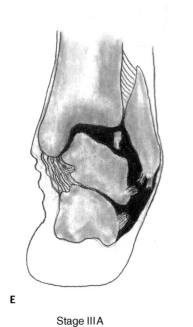

E

Stage IIIA

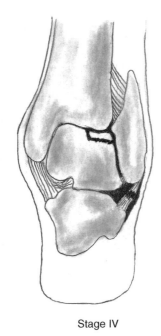

F

Stage IV

FIGURE 17–2 (*Continued*) **(E)** IIIA, complete fragment detachment and rotation without displacement. **(F)** IV, complete fragment detachment with displacement.

detached but undisplaced fragment; 4, detached and displaced fragment; 5, subchondral cyst formation. Ferkel and Sgaglione[42] introduced a CT classification **(Fig. 17–3)**: I, cystic lesion in talar dome with intact roof; IIA, cystic lesion with communication to talar dome surface; IIB, open articular surface lesion with overlying nondisplaced fragment; III, nondisplaced lesion with lucency; IV, displaced fragment. Loomer et al[43] added

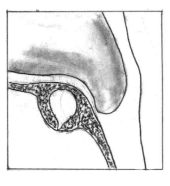

Stage I

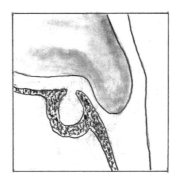

Stage IIA

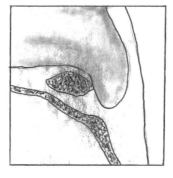

Stage IIB

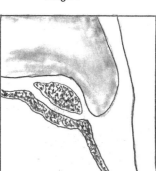

Stage III

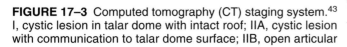

Stage IV

FIGURE 17–3 Computed tomography (CT) staging system.[43] I, cystic lesion in talar dome with intact roof; IIA, cystic lesion with communication to talar dome surface; IIB, open articular surface lesion with overlying nondisplaced fragment; III, nondisplaced lesion with lucency; IV, displaced fragment.

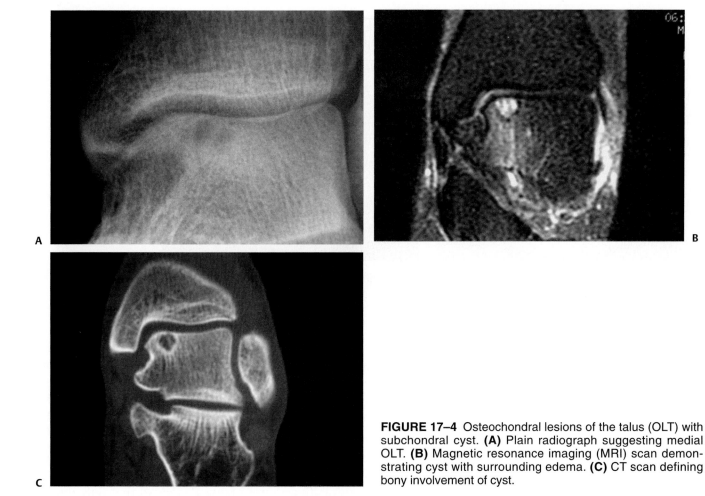

FIGURE 17–4 Osteochondral lesions of the talus (OLT) with subchondral cyst. **(A)** Plain radiograph suggesting medial OLT. **(B)** Magnetic resonance imaging (MRI) scan demonstrating cyst with surrounding edema. **(C)** CT scan defining bony involvement of cyst.

stage V to account for an OLT with a subchondral cyst **(Fig. 17–4)**.

Subchondral cysts are difficult to detect by plain radiographs and are frequently difficult to treat. In fact, Kumai et al[1] reported that regardless of treatment method, results of management in patients with OLTs associated with subchondral cysts are poor. Robinson et al[44] noted a 53% poor outcome in debridement and drilling/curettage of OLTs with subchondral cysts. However, current cartilage resurfacing techniques have shown some promise in management of these deeper lesions.[5,7] Because of the difficulty encountered in detecting subchondral cysts by plain radiographs, MRI and/or CT are often considered essential in directing the appropriate treatment of OLTs.[36,38,45,46] Despite the advantages of advanced imaging techniques, probably the most accurate staging tool remains arthroscopy, although the limited access to some OLTs during arthroscopy may not provide a full appreciation of an associated subchondral cyst[47] **(Fig. 17–5)**.

■ Nonoperative Treatment

Not all OLTs are symptomatic. Smaller lesions that are relatively stable and produce minimal to no symptoms do not warrant any intervention. Skeletally immature patients retain some healing potential, often prompting immobilization and protective weight-bearing status.[48] Most OLTs in skeletally immature patients are caused by trauma. These lesions typically demonstrate favorable healing and outcome. There is a decline with age in the number of pleuripotential mesenchymal cells in the bone marrow, periosteum, and perichondrium. Adult patients rarely demonstrate spontaneous healing. Nevertheless, some OLTs may become asymptomatic despite lack of healing to the surrounding subchondral bone. Surprisingly, a recent report by Shearer et al[49] suggests that 71% of stage V lesions (OLTs associated with subchondral cysts) treated without surgery have good-to-excellent results at an average follow-up of 38 months and an average of 88 months after the onset of symptoms. The investigators concluded that (1) the

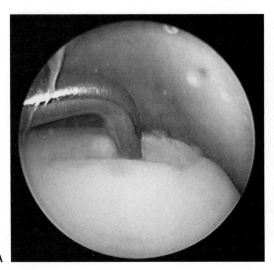
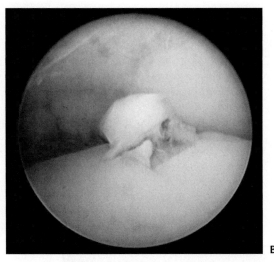

A B

FIGURE 17–5 Arthroscopic view of a medial OLT. The cartilage defect is apparent; however, a subchondral cyst cannot be reliably identified by arthroscopy alone.

general course of stage V OLT is benign in a majority of patients, (2) nonsurgical treatment of stage V lesions does not lead to the development of advanced osteoarthritis of the ankle, (3) the development of mild radiographic changes of osteoarthritis does not correlate with clinical outcome, (4) most lesions remain radiographically stable, and (5) there is a poor correlation between changes in lesion size and clinical outcome. They acknowledge, however, that patients with larger diameter lesions have a less favorable outcome.

Chondroprotective agents typically utilized to treat knee arthrosis, such as orally administered glucosamine and chondroitin sulfate or injectable hyaluronic acid, may have some role in the management of mildly symptomatic OLT, but to the author's knowledge, no objective evidence exists to support their administration for OLT.[50] A single steroid injection may diminish associated symptoms, but its effect is typically transient.

■ Surgical Treatment

Operative treatment of OLTs is reserved for lesions that fail to respond to nonsurgical measures. However, patients with unstable lesions associated with mechanical symptoms should probably not be subjected to a long course of conservative management, as there is little potential for spontaneous improvement.

Debridement and Drilling or Microfracture

Arthroscopic debridement and drilling or microfracture remains the standard in operative care of chronic OLT.[51] The advantage of debridement and drilling is

simplicity. Two to three small arthroscopy portals provide adequate access to the majority of talar dome lesions. Curettage of the unstable cartilage lesions is facilitated by the use of anteromedial, anterolateral, and posterolateral portals. Drilling can be specifically directed to the lesion using a commercially available guide (Microvector, Smith and Nephew, Andover, MA) **(Fig. 17–6).** Should it be necessary to penetrate the malleoli or distal tibia to access the OLT, the ankle can be dorsiflexed and plantarflexed, so that only one or two drill passes through the intact tibial cartilage is necessary **(Fig. 17–7).** Small joint awls are becoming available to perform the microfracture technique through the portals, negating the need for transmalleolar drilling.[3] Retrograde drilling is also possible to avoid damage to both the intact tibial surface and an intact talar dome with underlying osteochondral lesion.[52] A three-dimensional guidance system has been introduced to make drilling these lesions extremely accurate.[45,46] In this technique, the OLT is identified by CT or MRI, and under sterile technique a guidewire is placed retrograde into the OLT. The patient is then transferred to the operating room and the guide pin is overdrilled to decompress the OLT. The investigators concluded that the technique is simple, saves time, and avoids damaging an intact cartilage surface overlying the diseased subchondral bone of an OLT. Additional advantages of debridement and drilling/microfracture are (1) it does not compromise the ability to perform a revision surgery should the primary procedure fail, (2) it is typically cost-effective, and (3) there is no concern for donor-site morbidity, unless bone grafting is performed in conjunction with retrograde drilling (however, even this risk can be avoided by using allograft).

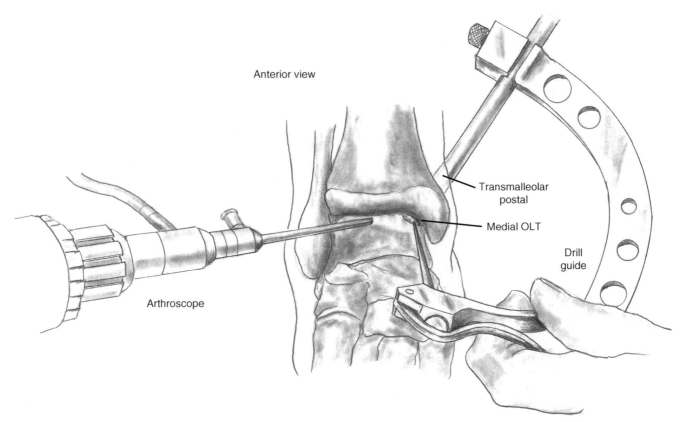

Anterior view

Transmalleolar
postal

Medial OLT

Drill
guide

Arthroscope

FIGURE 17–6 Drilling can be specifically directed to the lesion using a commercially available guide.

Most importantly, the results of debridement and drilling are typically favorable.

Reports reflect the results of previous studies, with good-to-excellent outcomes in 65 to 90% of patients.[1,38] In 1986, Parisien[33] reported 88% good-to-excellent results in 18 patients with OLT debridement and curettage. Based on a meta-analysis, Tol et al[53] suggested that excision and drilling was superior to excision and curettage with good to excellent results of 85% and 78%, respectively. According to a report by Kelberine and Frank,[14] better results can be anticipated with management of acute lesions relative to chronic lesions. Schuman et al[2] reported good-to-excellent results of debridement and drilling in 86% of primary procedures and 75% in revision procedures at an average follow-up of 4.8 years.

Results of retrograde drilling and the microfracture technique have also been reported. Taranow et al[52] reported a mean increase in the American Orthopaedic Foot and Ankle Society (AOFAS) ankle-hindfoot outcome score of 54 to 83 points in 16 patients treated with retrograde drilling of OLTs at a mean follow-up of 2 years. Thermann and Becher[3] managed 32 OLTs (22 acute injuries, 10 chronic lesions) with the microfracture technique; 23 of these patients were examined at a

mean follow-up of 2 years. Using a Hannover scoring system for the ankle, good-to-excellent results were noted in 93% of acute lesions and 78% of chronic lesions. The authors also noted that older age (patients >50 years old) was not a limiting factor.

Despite encouraging results from multiple investigations, shortcomings of the debridement and drilling technique remain. Physiologic restoration of the defect with hyaline cartilage is not achieved; instead fibrocartilage fills the defect. This is probably acceptable for smaller lesions, but less favorable for larger lesions. Furthermore, the surgical management of the type V lesion[43] (subchondral cyst) is less amenable to debridement and drilling as the deeper defect would have only fibrocartilage and lack support of underlying subchondral bone.[1,44] Robinson et al[44] reported a poor outcome in 53% of OLTs treated with arthroscopic debridement and drilling/curettage. In these cases, bone graft could be added such that fibrocartilage could grow on the surface, but packing bone graft into the defect with the limitations of an arthroscopic approach to the ankle may be prohibitive.[54] Nevertheless, bone grafting after excision and curettage has been reported to demonstrate benefit and successful treatment of OLT.[55,56] Larger shoulder

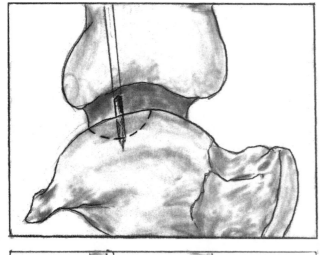

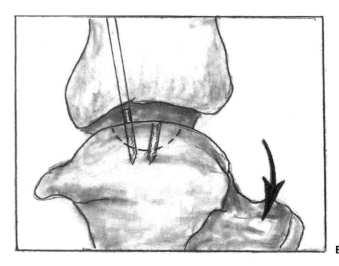

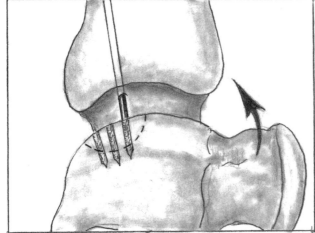

FIGURE 17–7 The neutral ankle **(A)** can be dorsiflexed **(B)** and plantarflexed **(C)**, so that only one or two drill passes through the intact tibial cartilage is necessary.

lesions (transition from superior talar cartilage to medial or lateral cartilage surface) on the talar dome are probably less likely to heal well with debridement and drilling alone. Although fibrocartilage will form, its less favorable mechanical properties may lead to early failure. Finally, Angermann and Jensen[57] suggested that results of debridement and drilling deteriorate over time. After noting 85% satisfactory outcome at short-term follow-up of 20 patients managed with debridement and drilling of OLTs, average follow-up of 9 to 15 years revealed that over half had pain and swelling.

Cartilage Repair Procedures

Cartilage repair procedures that involve tissue transplantation include (1) osteochondral autologous transfer system (OATS)(Arthrex, Naples, FL),[7,49,58] (2) osteochondral allograft transplantation (fresh or fresh frozen, (3) mosaicplasty,[31,59], and (4) autologous chon-

drocyte implantation (ACI).[4,5] Favorable results have been reported in each of the procedures in the knee, and more recently, favorable short-term to intermediate-term results are being reported for the talar dome.[4,5,7,58–62] The challenge in applying these techniques to the ankle is that access to the talar dome is limited, and often osteotomies are required about the ankle to allow for adequate access for the surgeon to perform the procedure and to allow for proper positioning of instrumentation.

Osteochondral Autologous Transfer System/ Mosaicplasty/Allograft

Osteochondral autologous transfer system (OATS) (Arthrex, Naples, FL) and mosaicplasty (Acufex, Mansfield, MA), which have been used successfully in the knee for many years, have been popularized for talar dome lesions for the past several years. In brief, the technique has three steps: (1) recipient site preparation (removal of an osteochondral plug at the OLT), (2) harvest of a donor-site osteochondral plug from the knee (non-weight-bearing cartilage of the lateral femoral trochlea or notch), and (3) transfer of the donor plug into the recipient site. Unless unique shaping of the osteochondral plug becomes necessary, the donor graft never leaves the harvest tube in the OATS procedure; it is directly implanted into the OLT recipient site after harvest. Osteochondral plug sizes range from 5 to 10 mm, with a 1-mm diameter discrepancy from the recipient site, to create an interference fit of the plug (Fig. 17–8).

Results with this technique have been promising in short- to intermediate-term follow-up. Al-Shaikh et al[58] reported good-to-excellent results in 88% of previously nonoperated patients and in 91% of patients with failed surgical procedures. The study group comprised 19 patients with an average follow-up of 16 months. Even in the difficult stage V lesions (subchondral cyst), the technique has been shown to be effective. At preliminary follow-up, Scranton and McDermott[7] demonstrated an average 27-point increase in the AOFAS score in 10 patients treated for stage V lesions.

In the mosaicplasty procedure, the osteochondral graft is routinely removed from the harvesting device and transferred to the device used to implant the graft; osteochondral plug diameters range from 3.5 to 6.5 mm. With smaller diameter grafts, the plugs can be arranged to match the contour of the defect, even if it is located on the shoulder region of the talar dome. Hangody et al[59] have reported 94% good-to-excellent results in 36 patients with 2- to 7-year follow-up, applying the mosaicplasty procedure to OLTs greater than 10 mm in diameter.

The advantages of these techniques are as follows: (1) it is a single-stage procedure; (2) despite the harvest from the knee, no major donor-site morbidity has been reported; (3) despite osteotomies or ligament releases being required, no major complications have been reported in the surgical exposure of the lesions; and (4) talar dome "shoulder" lesions can be effectively managed with harvest from the edge of the lateral femoral trochlea to match the contour of the cartilage adjacent

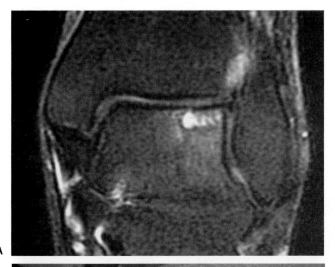

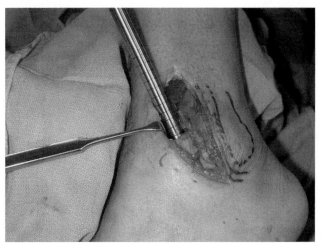

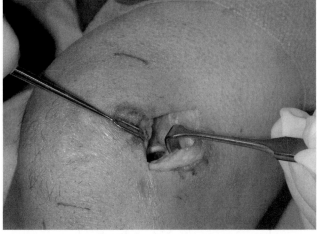

FIGURE 17–8 Patient with lateral ankle instability and lateral OLT. **(A)** MRI scan revealing lateral OLT. **(B)** Lateral approach through the anterior talofibular ligament and osteochondral autograft transplantation system (OATS) instrumentation positioned to insert the osteochondral autograft. **(C)** Superolateral knee donor site for harvesting osteochondral autograft through arthrotomy. After graft transfer, a modified Brostrom procedure is employed to regain lateral ankle stability.

to the OLT or by harvesting multiple smaller diameter plugs to re-create the physiologic anatomy of the talar shoulder **(Fig. 17–9).**

Despite the reported success and low complication rate for the osteochondral autologous transfer procedure in the management of OLTs, some concerns persist: (1) knee and ankle cartilage exhibit different characteristics, (2) donor-site morbidity may occur, and (3) complications may occur from medial and lateral osteotomies. In multiple investigations, Ada Cole and colleagues[21,63–69] have demonstrated considerable differences in ankle and knee cartilage, but the significance of this as it pertains to osteochondral transfer between the two joints remains unclear. Although the donor-site morbidity appears low, regardless of whether the osteochondral graft is harvested arthroscopically or through a small arthrotomy, it does exist. For this reason, some investigators have attempted to transfer local grafts about the ankle, and results using this technique are promising.[70,71] Sammarco and Makwana[71] reported a significant improvement in the AOFAS score at an average follow-up of 25 months in 12 patients treated with this method.

Use of fresh or fresh-frozen osteochondral allograft eliminates the risk of donor-site morbidity as well. Brage[72] reported promising results using fresh talar dome osteochondral allograft at short- to intermediate-term follow-up. Gross et al[73] demonstrated that the majority (six of nine) of these grafts incorporate and function reasonably well at longer-term follow-up. The risk of disease transmission appears to be low, but the use of fresh grafts may require a dedicated team at a well-equipped institution to make such transplantation practical. Furthermore, although donor-site morbidity is nonexistent, osteotomies about the ankle are generally still necessary, no different from the autologous procedures described above.

Autologous Chondrocyte Implantation

Autologous chondrocyte implantation (ACI) has gained recent popularity in treating chondral and osteochondral lesions in the knee. Given the success in the knee, the technique has been applied to the ankle as well. In brief, the procedure is performed in stages. Stage one consists of (1) harvest of a small amount of nonweight-bearing articular cartilage, typically from the knee; and (2) culturing of these chondrocytes. Stage two consists of (1) debridement of the OLT, (2) harvest of a periosteal flap, (3) attachment of the periosteal flap to the intact articular cartilage adjacent to the OLT, and (4) injection of the cultured chondrocyte suspension under the periosteal flap in the cartilage defect.

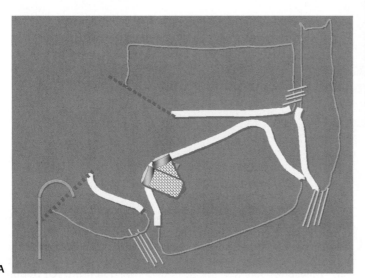
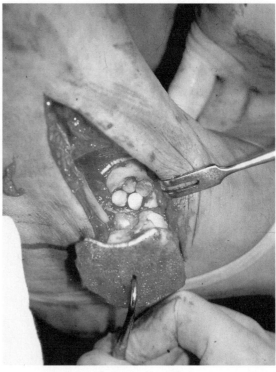

A   **B**

FIGURE 17–9 Medial talar dome shoulder defect managed with the mosaicplasty technique (described by Laslo Hangody, M.D.). **(A)** Schematic diagram shows how to position autologous osteochondral plugs. **(B)** Intraoperative photo through the medial malleolar osteotomy. (Courtesy of Laslo Hangody, M.D.)

The procedure's second stage is rather tedious and typically requires an osteotomy to access the lesion, unless the ankle pathology includes lateral ankle instability. Suturing of the periosteal flap must be performed in a restricted space despite osteotomy. Advantages are as follows: (1) large defects can be easily addressed with this technique, as there really is no limit to the size defect that can be repaired; (2) the periosteal flap is harvested from the adjacent distal tibia; and (3) with careful suture technique, shoulder lesions can also be treated. Disadvantages are as follows: (1) the procedure is Food and Drug Administration (FDA)-approved only for the knee, not for the ankle (as of March 2005); (2) the fee for the chondrocyte culturing process is considerable; and (3) the procedure must be performed in a staged fashion to allow time for the chondrocyte culture. A further concern has been that the technique could not effectively address type V lesions (subchondral cysts) because (1) chondrocytes die if exposed to bleeding; and (2) deeper lesions cannot simply be filled with chondrocytes, but require subchondral support, particularly large diameter lesions. However, advanced techniques of ACI have successfully been applied to stage V lesions as well. A "sand-wich technique" has been employed in which (1) bone graft is packed within the defect after the OLT is debrided and the deeper bone is drilled, (2) the first periosteal flap is sutured on the bone graft with the cambium layer facing the joint, (3) a second periosteal flap is sutured in the traditional fashion at the level of the healthy adjacent articular cartilage with the cambium layer away from the joint, and (4) the chondrocyte suspension is injected between the periosteal flaps[74] (**Fig. 17–10**). Results of ACI are favorable in the ankle. At the time of this publication, Lars Peterson, who developed the procedure, had performed over 30 autologous chondrocyte implantations for OLTs. His group reported results on the first 14 patients, with an average follow-up of 45 months: 12 patients are considered improved, and 11 have good-to-excellent outcomes.[5,75] Giannini et al[4] reported an improvement in the average AOFAS ankle-hindfoot score from 32 to 91 points in eight patients examined at a mean follow-up of 26 months. Histologic examination of biopsies obtained at second-look arthroscopies performed at 12 months suggested physiologic type 2 hyaline cartilage (cartilage thickness, chondrocyte viability, staining) in all eight specimens.[4,59] In Europe, a

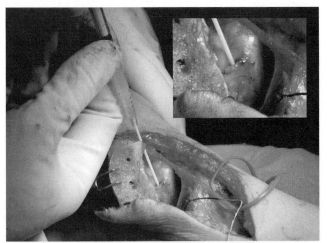

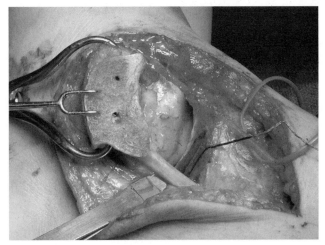

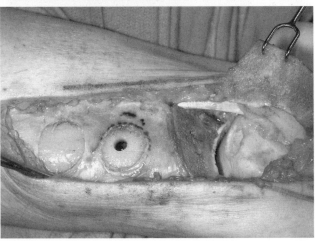

FIGURE 17–10 Autologous chondrocyte implantation for medial talar dome defect performed through a medial malleolar osteotomy. **(A)** Injection of cartilage cells (inset close-up). **(B)** Final view after periosteal flap sealed with fibrin glue. **(C)** Image of "sandwich technique." Two periosteal flaps are harvested from distal medial tibia and a posteromedial defect is visualized through the medial malleolar osteotomy. Note the drill hole in the distal tibia to harvest bone graft to fill the subchondral cyst.

matrix-induced autologous chondrocyte implantation (MACI) system has been developed (Verigen AG, Leverkusen, Germany). The use of the combination of MACI and a purified collagen membrane to treat OLTs has shown favorable preliminary results and may allow for similar results to ACI with less extensive surgical exposure.

Osteotomies

A major concern remains the extensive surgery that the ankle must endure to allow the surgeon adequate exposure to place these osteochondral grafts. Not all lesions require osteotomies; some anterolateral, anteromedial, and posteromedial lesions can be addressed with ankle hyperplantarflexion or hyperdorsiflexion and capsular releases and/or creation of troughs in the distal tibia. Typically, however, medial or lateral malleolar osteotomies are required to permit satisfactory exposure. Risk of nonunion or malunion has prompted development of alternative osteotomies/approaches that may be less morbid. Oznur[76] has described a medial malleolar window; Tochigi et al[77] introduced an anterolateral distal tibial osteotomy, and Sammarco and Makwana[71] have utilized a replaceable anterior tibial plafond bone block. Each of these techniques shows promise, with the medial malleolar window potentially allowing safer access to medial talar dome lesions, the anterolateral distal tibial osteotomy improving access to centrolateral OLTs, and the anterior tibial plafond bone block permitting improved exposure to multiple areas of the talar dome. A fibular window and door have also been described by Hansen[78] and Allen and DiGiovanni.[79] A posteromedial arthrotomy through the posterior tibialis tendon sheath has also been described by Bassett et al.[80] A maximum dorsiflexion lateral radiograph is required in the preoperative workup to ensure the postero- or centromedial lesion can be accessed via this approach. The size of the lesion and the ability to place required instrumentation through this arthrotomy need to be considered. This technique does avoid the possibility of complications from a medial malleolar osteotomy.

Multiple variations of the medial malleolar osteotomy have been described, including chevron, step-cut, and oblique variants. This osteotomy enables access to the central and posterior lesions on the medial talus **(Fig. 17–11).** Technique pearls include the following: (1) Perpendicular instrument access to the lesion is not possible unless the line of the osteotomy is adequately vertical. It must then enter the joint at the junction of the medial malleolus and tibial plafond, so as to not disrupt the weight-bearing surface of the plafond. To avoid damage to the articular cartilage, the osteotomy should be completed with an osteotome. (2) The more oblique the cut, the more eversion and abduction of the talus are needed. The lateral capsule and lateral malleolus are the limiting factors to talar excursion and visualization. (3) The more vertical the cut, the more vertical shear is placed on the fixation during active range of motion through the posterior tibial and Achilles tendons. (4) Fixation of the malleolar fragment should begin with predrilling and tapping of the screw holes prior to osteotomy to avoid loss of orientation and to ensure accurate reduction upon application of final fixation. (5) Necessary and thus available fixation should include 4.0-mm malleolar screws, 2.7- and 3.5-mm cortical screws, and a low-contour plate if apical compression is required.[81]

■ Future Directions

Even though the cartilage repair procedures described above are promising in OLT management, no long-term clinical studies are available to demonstrate the efficacy of these techniques. Arthroscopic evaluation and biopsy of the cartilage repair tissue is most definitive in defining the success of the procedure,[59] but MRI shows promise in follow-up evaluation.[36,38,54] The shoulder lesion in particular remains a difficult problem. Hangody et al[59] and Peterson et al[60] demonstrated techniques for this difficult lesion, but it is hoped that refinement of old and newer techniques will provide better outcomes. As for the knee, ligament stability and joint alignment are essential to avoid excessive contact and shear stresses across the repaired cartilage surfaces. Although distal femoral and high tibial osteotomies are being performed with greater frequency to unload knee compartments with repaired osteochondral defects, the need for periarticular osteotomies about the ankle to unload repaired OLTs has not yet been defined. Clearly there is a role for stabilization of ligamentous instability around the ankle joint to protect the cartilage healing potential just as in the knee.

Pleuripotent cells from other sources may have better potential than mature chondrocytes to repair osteochondral defects and may differentiate and organize into appropriate zones to re-create physiologic subchondral and chondral anatomy. Combined with structural matrices (to support zonal organization of articular cartilage) and growth factors (to promote cell differentiation and bonding of transplanted tissue to adjacent normal cartilage), pleuripotent cells may be the future to promoting a more natural healing response for OLTs.

Mesenchymal progenitor cells may allow for repair of subchondral and cartilage defects. These cells may be cultured similarly to chondrocytes as in autologous chondrocyte transfer. Current research has focused on

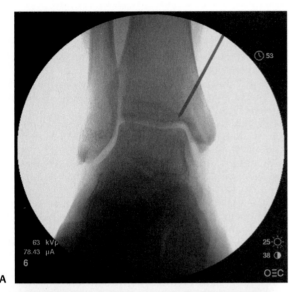

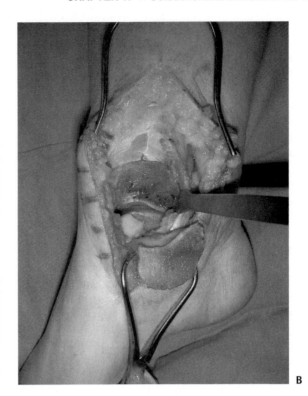

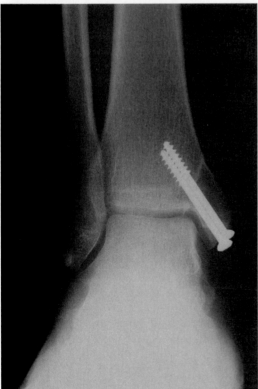

FIGURE 17–11 Medial malleolar osteotomy. **(A)** Intraoperative fluoroscopy to determine the proper plane for the oblique osteotomy. **(B)** Intraoperative photo of exposure of a large OLT obtained with a medial malleolar osteotomy. **(C)** Postoperative radiograph with healed medial malleolar osteotomy.

development of matrices that could serve as effective delivery systems for these progenitor cells. To our knowledge, this technique has yet to be described specifically for OLT. Fibrin clot containing mitogenic growth factors (basic fibroblast growth factor, transforming growth factor-(1, epidermal growth factor, insulin-like growth factor-1, and growth hormone) has been used as a scaffold for the migration of reparative cells.[82]

Artificial structural matrices are designed to act as scaffolding for cartilage growth within an osteochondral defect. The ideal matrix has yet to be developed, but it should meet the following requirements: (1) it should have appropriate porosity to allow for cell migration; (2) it should serve as a carrier for hormonal substances that direct cell maturation and proliferation; (3) it should allow for cell adhesion; (4) it should provide a malleable contour permitting maximum contact with the host tissue; (5) it should enhance the binding of the repair tissue to the host tissue; (6) it should have sufficient biodegradability to allow for remodeling of the repair tissues; (7) it should provide matrix cohesiveness; (8) it should have sufficient resiliency to allow for dynamic and static deformation; and (9) it should bond adequately to prevent displacement. Absorbable polymers that can be locally implanted into defects would likely be most useful. A collagen sponge has been developed that can serve as a scaffold in an osteochondral defect. A polyglycolic acid implant has been utilized in animal studies. Carbon fiber scaffolds have also been evaluated, though they seem to provide only fibrous tissue within osteochondral defects. Teflon, Dacron, Gore-Tex, and several other polymers have been studied, although none has demonstrated the ability to generate healing of cartilage in the animal models employed.

Until gene-modified tissue engineering becomes available to activate an appropriate healing response in humans, osteochondral transfer and autologous chondrocyte implantation represent attractive alternatives.

REFERENCES

1. Kumai T, Takakura Y, Higashiyama I, Tamai S. Arthroscopic drilling for the treatment of osteochondral lesions of the talus. J Bone Joint Surg Am 1999;81:1229–1235

2. Schuman L, Struijs PA, van Dijk CN. Arthroscopic treatment for osteochondral defects of the talus: results at follow-up at 2 to 11 years. J Bone Joint Surg Br 2002;84:364–368

3. Thermann H, Becher C. [Microfracture technique for treatment of osteochondral and degenerative lesions of the talus: 2-year results of a prospective study.] Unfallchirurg 2004;107:27–32

4. Giannini S, Buda R, Grigolo B, et al. Autologous chondrocyte transplantation in osteochondral lesions of the ankle joint. Foot Ankle Int 2001;22:513–517

5. Peterson L, Brittberg M, Lindahl A. Autologous chondrocyte transplantation of the ankle. Foot Ankle Clin 2003;8:291–303

6. Hangody L, Kish G, Modis L, et al: Mosaicplasty for the treatment of osteochondritis dissecans of the talus; two to seven year results in 36 patients. Foot Ankle Int 2001;22:552–558

7. Scranton PE Jr, McDermott JE. Treatment of type V osteochondral lesions of the talus with ipsilateral knee osteochondral autografts. Foot Ankle Int 2001;22:380–384

8. Coltart WD. Aviator's astragalus. J Bone Joint Surg Am 1952;34:545–566

9. Bosien WR, Staples OS, Russell SW. Residual disability following acute ankle sprains J Bone Joint Surg Am 1955;37:1237–1243

10. Urman M, Ammann W, Sisler J, et al. The role of bone scintigraphy in the evaluation of talar dome fractures. J Nucl Med 1991;32:2241–2244

11. Hepple S, Winson IG, Glew D. Lateral ligament injuries and osteochondral lesions in MRI of the ankle. In: Programs and Abstracts of the 13th annual summer meeting of the American Orthopaedic Foot and Ankle Society, Monterey, CA, 1997

12. Berndt A, Hardy M. Transchondral fractures (osteochondritis dissecans) of the talus. J Bone Joint Surg Am 1959;41:988–1020

13. Blom JM, Strijk SP. Lesions of the trochlea tali: osteochondral fractures and osteochondritis dissecans of the trochlea tali. Radiol Clin (Basel) 1989;44:387–399

14. Kelberine F, Frank A. Arthroscopic treatment of osteochondral lesions of the talar dome: a retrospective study of 48 cases. Arthroscopy 1999;15:77–91

15. Hintermann B, Regazzoni P, Lampert C, et al: Arthroscopic findings in acute fractures of the ankle. J Bone Joint Surg Br 2000.;82:345–351

16. Takao M, Ochi M, Uchio Y, Naito K, Kono T, Oae K. Osteochondral lesions of the talar dome associated with traum. Arthroscopy 2003;19:1061–1067

17. Athanasiou KA, Niederauer GG, Schenck RC Jr. Biomechanical topography of human ankle articular cartilage. Ann Biomed Eng 1995;23:697–701

18. Huch K, Kuettner KE, Dieppe P. Osteoarthritis in knee and ankle joints. Semin Arthritis Rheum 1997;26:667–674

19. Buckwalter JA, Saltzman CL. Ankle osteoarthritis: distinctive characterisics. Instr Course Lect 1999;48:233–241 (AAOS)

20. Kempson GE. Age-related changes in the tensile properties of human articular cartilage: a comparative study between the femoral head of the hip joint and the talus of the ankle joint. Biochim Biophys Acta 1991;1075:223–227

21. Chubinskaya S, Huch K, Mikecz K, et al. Chondrocyte matrix metalloproteinase-8: up-regulation of neutrophil collagenase by interleukin-1 beta in human cartilage from knee and ankle joints. Lab Invest 1996;74:232–240

22. Hauselmann HJ, Fletcenmacher J, Gitelis SH, et al. Chondrocytes from human knee and ankle joints show differences in response to IL-1 and IL-1 reception inhibitor. Trans Orthop Res Soc 1993;17:710

23. Alexander AH, Lichtman DM. Surgical treatment of transchondral talar dome fractures: long-term follow-up. J Bone Joint Surg Am 1980;62:646–652

24. Beaudoin AJ, Fiore SM, Krause WR, et al. Effect of isolated talocalcaneal fusion on contact in the ankle and talonavicular joints. Foot Ankle 1991;12:19–25

25. Kimizuka M, Kurosawa H, Fukubayashi T. Loadbearing pattern of the ankle joint: contact area and pressure distribution. Arch Orthop Trauma Surg 1980;96:45–49

26. Ihn JC, Kim SJ, Park IH. In vitro study of contact area and pressure distribution in the human knee after partial and total meniscectomy. Int Orthop 1993;17:214–218

27. Brown TD, Shaw DT. In vitro contact stress distributions in the natural human hip. J Biomech 1983;16:373–384

28. Van Buecken K, Barrack RL, Alexander AH, et al. Arthroscopic treatment of transchondral fractures of the talar dome. Am J Sports Med 1989;17:350–355

29. Canale ST, Belding RH. Osteochondral lesions of the talus. J Bone Joint Surg Am 1980;62:97–102

30. Alexander AH, Lichtman DM. Surgical treatment of transchondral talar dome fractures: long-term follow-up. J Bone Joint Surg Am 1980;62:646–652

31. Flick AB, Gould N. Osteochondritis dissecans of the talus (transchondral fractures of the talus): review of the literature and new surgical approach for medial dome lesions. Foot Ankle Int 1985;5:165–185

32. Baker CL, Andrews JR, Ryan JB. Arthroscopic treatment of transchondral talar dome fractures. Arthroscopy 1986;2:82–87

33. Parisien JS. Arthroscopic treatment of osteochondral lesions of the talus. Am J Sports Med 1986;14:211–217

34. Pritsch M, Hroashovski H, Farine I, et al. Arthroscopic treatment of osteochondral lesions of the talus. J Bone Joint Surg Am 1986;68:862–865

35. Vrahas M, Fu F, Veenis B. Intraarticular contact stress with simulated ankle malunions. J Orthop Trauma 1999;82:159–166

36. Assenmacher JA, Kelikian AS, Gottlob C, Kodros S. Arthroscopically assisted autologous osteochondral transplantation for osteochondral lesions of the talar dome: an MRI and clinical follow-up study. Foot Ankle Int 2001;22:544–551

37. Hepple S, Winson IG, Glew D. Osteochondral lesions of the talus: a revised classification. Foot Ankle Int 1999;20:789–793

38. Higashiyama I, Kumai T, Takakura Y, Tamail S. Follow-up study of MRI for osteochondral lesion of the talus. Foot Ankle Int 2000;21:127–133

39. Verhagen RA, Maas M, Dijkgraaf MG, et al. Prospective study on diagnostic strategies in osteochondral lesions of the talus. Is MRI superior to helical CT? J Bone Joint Surg Br 2005;87:41–46

40. Loren GJ, Ferkel RD. Arthroscopic assessment of occult intra-articular injury in acute ankle fractures. Arthroscopy 2002;18: 412–421

41. Hintermann B, Bos A, Schafer D. Arthroscopic findings in patients with chronic ankle instability. Am J Sports Med 2002;30: 402–409

42. Ferkel RD, Sgaglione N. Arthroscopic treatment of osteochondral lesions of the talus: long-term results. Trans Orthop Res Soc 1990;14:172–178

43. Loomer R, Fisher C, Lloyd-Smith R, Sisler J, Cooney T. Osteochondral lesions of the talus. Am J Sports Med 1993;21:13–19

44. Robinson DE, Winson IG, Harries WJ: Arthroscopic treatment of osteochondral lesions of the talus. J Bone Joint Surg 2003;85-B:989–993

45. Bale RJ, Hoser C, Rosenberger R, Rieger M, Benedetto KP, Fink C. Osteochondral lesions of the talus: computer-assisted retrograde drilling–feasibility and accuracy in initial experiences. Radiology 2001;218:278–282

46. Fink C, Rosenberger RE, Bale RJ, et al. [Computer-assisted retrograde drilling of osteochondral lesions of the talus.] Orthopade 2001;30:59–65

47. Schimmer RC, Dick W, Hintermann B. The role of ankle arthroscopy in the treatment strategies of osteochondritis dissecans lesions of the talus. Foot Ankle Int 2001;22:895–900

48. Higuera J, Laguna R, Peral M, Aranda E, Soleto J. Osteochondritis dissecans of the talus during childhood and adolescence. J Pediatr Orthop 1998;18:328–332

49. Shearer C, Loomer R, Clement D. Nonoperatively managed stage 5 osteochondral talar lesions. Foot Ankle Int 2002;23:651–654

50. Marshall KW. Intra-articular byaluronan therapy. 2003;8:221

51. Struijs PA, Tol JL, Bossuyt PM, Schuman L, van Dijk CN. [Treatment strategies in osteochondral lesions of the talus. Review of the literature.] Orthopade 2001;30:28–36

52. Taranow WS, Bisignani GA, Towers JD, et al. Retrograde drilling of osteochondral lesions of the medial talar dome. Foot Ankle Int 1999;20:474–480

53. Tol JL, Struijs PA, Bossuyt PM. Treatment strategies in osteochondral defects of the talar dome: A systematic review. Foot Ankle Int 2000;21:119–126

54. Lahm A, Erggelet C, Steinwachs M, Reichelt A. Arthroscopic management of osteochondral lesions of the talus: results of drilling and usefulness of magnetic resonance imaging before and after treatment. Arthroscopy 2000;16:299–304

55. Bruns J. Osteochondrosis dissecans. Orthopade 1997;26: 573–584

56. Draper SD, Fallat LM. Autogenous bone grafting for the treatment of talar dome lesions. J Foot Ankle Surg 2000;39:15–23

57. Angermann P, Jensen P. Osteochondritis dissecans of the talus: long-term results of surgical treatment. Foot Ankle 1989;10: 161–163

58. Al-Shaikh RA, Chou LB, Mann JA, Dreeben SM, Prieskorn D. Autologous osteochondral grafting for talar cartilage defects. Foot Ankle Int 2002;23:381–389

59. Hangody L, Kish G, Modis L, et al. Mosaicplasty for the treatment of osteochondritis dissecans of the talus: two to seven year results in 36 patients. Foot Ankle Int 2001;22:552–558

60. Petersen L, Brittberg M, Lindahl A. Autologous chondrocyte transplantation of the ankle. Foot Ankle Clin 2003;8: 291–303

61. Ferkel RD. AAOS Annual Meeting, 2004(publication pending)

62. Hangody L. The mosaicplasty technique for osteochondral lesions of the talus. Foot Ankle Clin 2003;8:259–273

63. Chubinskaya S, Kuettner KE, Cole AA. Expression of matrix metalloproteinases in normal and damaged articular cartilage from human knee and ankle joints. Lab Invest 1999;79: 1669–1677

64. Eger W, Schumacher BL, Mollenhauer J, Kuettner KE, Cole AA. Human knee and ankle cartilage explants: catabolic differences. J Orthop Res 2002;20:526–534

65. Homandberg GA, Kang Y, Zhang J, Cole AA, Williams JM. A single injection of fibronectin fragments into rabbit knee joints enhances catabolism in the articular cartilage followed by reparative responses but also induces systemic effects in the non-injected knee joints. Osteoarthritis Cartilage 2001;9:673–683

66. Kang Y, Koepp H, Cole AA, Kuettner KE, Homandberg GA. Cultured human ankle and knee cartilage differ in susceptibility to damage mediated by fibronectin fragments. J Orthop Res 1998;16:551–556

67. Koepp H, Eger W, Muehleman C, et al. Prevalence of articular cartilage degeneration in the ankle and knee joints of human organ donors. J Orthop Sci 1999;4:407–412

68. Schumacher BL, Su JL, Lindley KM, Kuettner KE, Cole AA. Horizontally oriented clusters of multiple chondrons in the superficial zone of ankle, but not knee articular cartilage. Anat Rec 2002;266:241–248

69. Treppo S, Koepp H, Quan EC, Cole AA, Kuettner KE, Grodzinsky AJ. Comparison of biomechanical and biochemical properties of cartilage from human knee and ankle pairs. J Orthop Res 2000;18:739–748

70. Lee MS. Anterior talar dome as an alternative donor site for osteochondral transplantation for medial talar dome lesions. Clin Podiatr Med Surg 2001;18:545–549

71. Sammarco GJ, Makwana NK. Treatment of talar osteochondral lesions using local osteochondral graft. Foot Ankle Int 2002;23:693–698

72. Brage M. Osteochondral grafting of osteochondral lesions of the talus. In: Proceedings of the International Federation of Foot and Ankle Societies: Triennial Scientific Meeting, 2002;146–147

73. Gross AE, Agnidis Z, Hutchison CR. Osteochondral defects of the talus treated with fresh osteochondral allograft transplantation. Foot Ankle Int 2001;22:385–391

74. Minas T, Peterson L. Advanced techniques in autologous chondrocyte transplantation. Clin Sports Med 1999;18:13–44 v–vi.

75. Peterson L. Treatment of Cartilage Injuries in the Ankle. In: Proceedings of the International Federation of Foot and Ankle Societies: Triennial Scientific Meeting, 2002;147–148

76. Oznur A. Medial malleolar window approach for osteochondral lesions of the talus. Foot Ankle Int 2001;22:841–842

77. Tochigi Y, Amendola A, Muir D, Saltzman C. Surgical approach for centrolateral talar osteochondral lesions with an anterolateral osteotomy. Foot Ankle Int 2002;23:1038–1039

78. Hansen ST Jr. Functional Reconstruction of the Foot and Ankle. Philadelphia: Lippincott Williams & Wilkins, 2000:494–497

79. Allen SD, DiGiovanni CW. Distal fibular window osteotomy for exposure of lateral talar osteochondral lesions. Tech Foot Ankle Surg 2003;2:129–134

80. Bassett FH, Billys JB, Gates HS. A simple surgical approach to the posteromedial ankle. Am J Sports Med 1993;21:144–147

81. Kish G. Mosaicplasty for osteochondral lesions of the talus. In: Masters Techniques in Orthopaedic Surgery: The Foot and Ankle, 2nd ed. Philadelphia: Lippincott Williams & Wilkins, 2002: 643–664

82. Hunziker EB, Kapfinger E. Removal of proteoglycans from the surface of defects in articular cartilage transiently enhances coverage by repair cells. J Bone Joint Surg Br 1998;80:144–149

18

Acute Osteochondral Defects in the Knee

*JOHN G. COSTOUROS, MARC R. SAFRAN,
AND GREGORY B. MALETIS*

Despite surgical and technologic advancements, the treatment of osteochondral defects continues to challenge orthopaedic surgeons. Articular cartilage lesions are common and have been reported in 63% of over 31,000 arthroscopic procedures in one series.[1] Although 20% have been documented to extend to the subchondral bone at the time of surgery, few studies exist delineating the actual incidence of osteochondral lesions of the knee following acute injury. This is complicated by the lack of differentiation in much of the literature between osteochondritis dissecans and other osteochondral lesions or fractures. The injury may go undiagnosed after subtle injury, or if severe enough, may cause significant effusion, hemarthrosis, and dysfunction. Although the natural history of isolated osteochondral defects is unknown, it is hypothesized that untreated lesions may progress and lead to the development of generalized osteoarthritis.[2]

Osteochondral injury sets off a cascade of events within the joint that extend beyond the immediate zone of injury and stimulate chondrocyte death. Chondrocyte death and presumed progression to degenerative joint disease may occur primarily as a result of mechanical trauma and altered biomechanics, or as a consequence of exposure to known mediators of chondrocyte loss including hemarthrosis, reactive oxygen species, inflammatory cytokines, and matrix degradative enzymes.[3–6] Injury due to severe impact or repetitive trauma decreases proteoglycan concentration in the matrix, increases tissue hydration, alters the fibrillar organization of collagen, and alters the ability of chondrocytes to

perform synthetic and degradative homeostatic functions. Chondrocyte preservation is paramount in preventing subsequent disability as native hyaline cartilage possesses superior durability and wear characteristics and has a poor capacity for healing.[7,8] Recent advances in understanding the complex intracellular biochemistry as well as joint and tissue biomechanics may improve the outcomes of existing treatment modalities that have failed to consistently restore osteochondral defects with native hyaline cartilage and promote "edge-healing." Current operative treatment includes debridement and stabilization, stimulation of intrinsic repair mechanisms, and repair or transplantation of chondral and osteochondral tissue.

Acute mechanical injury within the knee may produce osteochondral defects by three distinct mechanisms: impaction, shear, and avulsion. Under normal physiologic conditions, articular cartilage is able to accommodate external loading by viscoelastic deformation, which serves to effectively increase joint contact area and decrease contact stresses.[9] Loading and deformation generate a combination of tensile, compressive, and shear stresses within the tissue, which, if exceeded, lead to failure. Impact loading has been shown to instigate both acute and progressive damage to articular cartilage of the knee joint in animal models.[10–15] Animal studies have also found that repetitive loading of articular cartilage in knees results in subchondral plate fractures and tidemark advancement that is mechanically less compliant.[12] The proteoglycan matrix and water content are the primary constituents of articular cartilage responsible for resisting compressive loads. High compression forces manifest clinically as surface cracks in articular cartilage, which can propagate to the tidemark and result in delamination and production of an osteochondral fragment.[16,17] Such forces can occur acutely, as when the distal femoral condyles strike a dashboard during a motor vehicle accident, or secondary to repetitive microtrauma and progressive loss of the intrinsic viscoelasticity of hyaline cartilage. Generally speaking, high-energy compressive forces produce greater injury to articular and superficial tangential zone (STZ) chondrocytes, whereas low-energy, low-velocity compressive forces produce selective injury to the deeper structures (e.g., deep zone of cartilage and tidemark).[14,16,18]

Shear forces can also generate damage to articular cartilage by creating surface irregularities, but place the greatest strain at the interface between calcified cartilage and subchondral bone. Type II collagen, which comprises 90 to 95% of total collagen in articular cartilage, is the primary constituent responsible for resisting shear stress.[9,19] Normal shear forces are generated under physiologic conditions with femoral rollback or in athletes involved in pivoting sports. Abnormal shearing can occur in athletes involved in sports that require aggressive pivoting, following patellar dislocation, or in the setting of ligamentous laxity or meniscal pathology. The vertical orientation of collagen fibrils at the tidemark are poorly suited to resist shear stresses and result in progressive chondral delamination and potentially osteochondral fragmentation. Experimental models of osteoarthritis that simulate nonphysiologic shear forces following anterior cruciate ligament (ACL) transection or meniscectomy show evidence of acute and chronic forms of cartilage degeneration.[5,20–26]

When cartilage is loaded in tension, collagen and proteoglycan molecules align and stretch along the axis of loading. Surface zone articular cartilage is much stiffer than middle and deep zone cartilage, and this is attributed to the parallel orientation of collagen fibers at the articular surface. Collagen cross-linking is the primary determinant of the tensile properties of cartilage, and any agents such as proteolytic enzymes that disrupt this architecture dramatically reduce the tensile strength of articular cartilage.[27] Avulsion injuries to articular cartilage, such as in the setting of tibial eminence fractures, occur when tensile forces exceed the tensile modulus.

The amount of bone that is part of an acute osteochondral fragment is dependent on the mechanism of injury, with shearing types of forces generally producing a smaller percentage of attached subchondral bone and avulsion types of forces producing a greater percentage of subchondral bone. In addition, the amount of bone that is attached to the cartilage fragment is dependent on the age of the patient. In the immature skeleton, where there is no calcified zone, shearing forces are transmitted directly to subchondral bone producing a higher percentage of bone within the fragment. The quantity of bone in the osteochondral fragment is also dependent on bone density and the quality of overlying hyaline cartilage. In summary, mechanical trauma can manifest as microdamage to otherwise intact cartilage, damage to cartilage with intact subchondral architecture, or fracture of the cartilage and underlying subchondral bone.

■ Classification

Osteochondral fragments have been well recognized and described for over 250 years, whereas isolated chondral fragment have been reported only in the past 20 years.[28–30] Aside from providing an anatomic basis for classification, it is important to distinguish between chondral and osteochondral lesions, as the natural history and potential for healing varies dramatically between the two entities. It is well recognized that isolated chondral defects have a poor intrinsic capacity for healing, whereas osteochondral defects are able to regenerate a fibrocartilaginous cartilage-like substitute.[30–40] The primary impediment toward the healing of chondral lesions is the inherently poor vascularity of articular cartilage and the inability to recruit mesenchymal precursors into the defect, which can create this fibrocartilaginous repair tissue. Articular defects that penetrate through the highly vascularized subchondral bone elicit an aggressive healing response with creation of a hematoma, fibrin clot formation, and influx of inflammatory cytokines and mesenchymal precursors into the lesion. Of course, the repair tissue, which is "hyaline-like" at best and rich in type I collagen, has inferior wear characteristics and durability when compared with native articular hyaline cartilage.[41]

An effective classification system is characterized by simplicity, interobserver reliability, and the ability to delineate prognosis and guide clinical decision making. Although several classification systems exist for isolated chondral lesions and osteochondritis dissecans (OCD), the literature interestingly lacks a classification system devoted to acute osteochondral lesions.

The most commonly used operative classification system for isolated cartilage lesions continues to be the Outerbridge system, first presented in 1961.[42] The Outerbridge, International Cartilage Repair Society (ICRS), and Noyes and Stabler scales describe articular cartilage changes, with the last stage including exposed bone or an osteochondral defect.[43,44] Criticisms of these classification systems include a lack of detailed discussion on lesion depth or diameter, articular surface appearance, and location.

In 1959 Berndt and Harty[45] reviewed 24 cases and presented a classification system for OCD of the talus that continues to be used based on radiographic findings: stage 1, a small compression fracture, with some authors restricting the size of the fracture to between 1 and 3 cm in diameter; stage 2, an incomplete avulsion of an osteochondral fragment; stage 3, complete avulsion of an osteochondral fragment without displacement; and stage 4, an avulsed fragment and loose body within the joint. This classification system has been extrapolated for use for OCD of the knee.

The classification of osteochondral lesions using magnetic resonance imaging (MRI) is gaining popularity as improvements in imaging techniques have greatly enhanced the sensitivity and specificity of this diagnostic modality. Bohndorf[46] reported on a new MRI classification system composed of two distinct stages: stage 1, intact cartilage, contrast enhancement of the lesion, and no cystic defects; stage 2, a cartilage defect with or without incomplete separation of the fragment, fluid around an undetached fragment, and a dislodged fragment.

Osteochondral lesions have traditionally been characterized based on classification schemes applied to OCD lesions, which differ significantly in etiology, epidemiology, clinical presentation, and response to treatment. We propose that acute osteochondral lesions be described based on the following parameters at the time of arthroscopy: (1) location (patella, femur, tibia, weight bearing versus non–weight bearing versus meniscal-bearing regions); (2) size; (3) amount of attached bone (partial chondral, at junction of cartilage to subchondral bone, through subchondral bone into trabecular bone); (4) amount of articular cartilage attached to bone (0–25%, 26–50%, 51–75%, >75%); (5) nondisplaced versus displaced versus free-body; (6) well-fitting versus size or contour mismatch; and (7) integrity of adjacent cartilage in the zone of injury.

■ Diagnosis

Although the presentation of patients with acute osteochondral injury is variable, most complain of pain, joint effusions, and mechanical symptoms. The elicitation of a detailed patient history usually reveals a single traumatic antecedent event associated with the onset of symptoms. This can consist of ligamentous or meniscal injury, blunt contusion, axial loading, or a pivoting event. Pain is by far the most common clinical complaint, and frequently it limits weight bearing. Joint effusions due to hemarthrosis or the influx of inflammatory mediators are quite common and can result in restricted range of motion. Patients with subacute osteochondral fractures may complain of mechanical symptoms such as clicking, popping, and locking, which may be superimposed on an underlying meniscal tear or ligamentous injury.

Physical examination should be done in a systematic manner, with careful observation of gross morphology, the presence of an effusion, and alignment, and it should include palpation of structures, assessment of range of motion, stability testing, and the use of specialized provocative tests. Tenderness at the joint line may be associated with far anterior lesions of the femoral condyles or may occur in the context of underlying meniscal pathology, whereas focal femoral condylar tenderness or a palpable defect more often indicates the presence of an osteochondral defect. Osteochondral lesions secondary to patellar dislocation can result following avulsion of the medial patellofemoral ligament or due to shear and impaction forces with reduction. This subset of patients displays focal tenderness along the medial retinaculum. Following lateral patellar dislocation, up to 50% of patients show evidence of osteochondral lesions of the lateral femoral condyle, medial patellar facet, or both.[47] Concomitant ligamentous laxity must be diligently assessed. For the most part, however, the diagnosis is made based on history, advanced imaging studies, and arthroscopic evaluation, as plain radiographs may not always reveal the underlying fragment.

Plain radiographs can be helpful in the diagnosis of osteochondral lesions. A standard trauma series including anteroposterior (AP), lateral, oblique, and Merchant views should be obtained. These views enable the clinician to assess the presence or absence of fractures as well as joint space congruity and narrowing, malalignment, and OCD. However, the amount of bone associated with an osteochondral injury is often small and not detected through the use of routine plain radiographs.

Continuing improvements in MRI enhance its ability to detect articular cartilage pathology and osteochondral injury.[48] Proton-density imaging of thin (3–4 mm) sections, T1-weighted fat-suppressed three-dimensional (3D) gradient echo, and T2-weighted fast spin-echo sequences optimize resolution of the articular cartilage and underlying subchondral bone.[49,50] The osteochondral fracture may parallel the joint surface or it may present as a periarticular osseous fracture that extends and crosses perpendicular to the articular cartilage. High signal intensity is frequently identified underlying the fracture segment in acute injuries, whereas intermediate intensity signal in cartilage or fibrous tissue is more characteristic of chronic lesions. Absence of hyperintensity of the fragment in the junctional zone is associated with fracture stability.[50] High signal intensity fluid surrounding the fragment indicates instability and loosening. MRI is also especially useful in detecting osteochondral loose bodies and chondral fragments. MRI continues to be a highly effective diagnostic tool for the assessment of ligamentous and meniscal pathology as its role in the diagnosis of osteochondral injury continues to evolve.[51,52]

Compaction injuries or bone bruises represent subchondral microtrabecular fractures and can usually only be diagnosed by MRI scan. These injuries can occur in isolation or more commonly they are seen in association with either an ACL tear or a medial collateral ligament tear. As the knee subluxes due to an ACL tear, impaction occurs between the posterior aspect of the lateral tibial plateau and the sulcus terminalis of the lateral femoral condyle, and increased signal is typically noted on the T2 image at these areas. Johnson et al[53] reported that these injuries occur in 80% of complete ACL tears. They described these lesions as being either reticular (limited to the medullary bone) or geographic (extending to the articular surface).[53]

Computed tomography (CT) can be a useful adjunct to the other imaging methods described earlier, especially in defining the degree of bony involvement. CT is able to demonstrate excellent definition of bony fragments and detailed delineation of size, location, and degree of displacement of the fragment. CT, however, is less sensitive than MRI in defining subtle subchondral microfractures and is limited in the assessment of articular cartilage integrity.

Diagnostic arthroscopy continues to be the gold standard in the assessment, evaluation, and characterization of osteochondral lesions. However, accurate assessment of size may be difficult arthroscopically.

■ Surgical Treatment

The ultimate goal in the treatment of osteochondral defects is the restoration of a smooth surface of normal hyaline cartilage bound to a restored subchondral plate and integrated with the adjacent native articular cartilage. This goal has eluded orthopaedic surgeons to this day, yet the current treatment options aim to reduce pain and swelling and improve function. The options currently available to orthopaedic surgeons for the treatment of osteochondral defects can be divided into three broad categories: (1) resection, (2) repair, and (3) replacement.

Resection

The surgical treatment of osteochondral lesions began historically with simple joint debridement. Magnuson[54] first coined the term *debridement* in 1941 for the treatment of osteoarthritis of the knee, which included removal of osteophytes, loose bodies, pathologic cartilage, and hypertrophic synovial tissue. With the advent of arthroscopy and improved techniques and instruments, arthroscopic debridement has evolved considerably in the diagnosis and treatment of osteochondral injury. Although the goals of arthroscopic debridement have remained constant over time (e.g., to reduce pain, improve function, and delay the progression of osteoarthritis), the surgical indications have been variable and continue to generate considerable controversy.[55] The lack of prospective, randomized, double-blinded studies examining the role of arthroscopic debridement in the treatment of osteochondral injuries make it difficult to establish well-defined criteria for surgery and for assessing efficacy.

Arthroscopic debridement enables the clinician to systematically examine the knee in detail. Irrigation with lactated Ringer's solution or normal saline is believed to effectively dilute the synovial fluid of proteolytic and other degradative enzymes, inflammatory mediators, and loose bodies that may contribute to third body wear. Excision of damaged portions of articular cartilage may decrease mechanical symptoms and reduce the release of free particles that can irritate synovial tissue and stimulate inflammation and pain. The pain associated with osteochondral lesions is also attributed to the free nerve endings found in the subchondral bone, which may be sensitive to mechanical irritation by unstable chondral flaps and loose bodies as well as circulating inflammatory mediators.

The decision to perform simple debridement as opposed to repair or replacement is based on a variety of factors such as lesion size, quality of the osteochondral fragment and defect, and patient-specific factors. In general, resection is suitable for osteochondral lesions that (1) are <1 cm in diameter; (2) have comminuted cartilage with or without subchondral bone; and (3) occur in patients who are noncompliant, unmotivated, or otherwise unable to adhere to stringent postoperative rehabilitation protocols. Relative contraindications include (1) age >50, (2) smokers, (3) instability not amenable to reconstruction or repair, (4) intact cartilage with no subchondral bone, and (5) nonambulatory patient.

Debridement can be performed by mechanical methods using a variety of devices such as rotatory shavers and resectors. Debridement to a "stable rim" is a poorly defined term, yet objective data indicate that vertical edges are mechanically advantageous relative to tapered chondral edges.[56] Of note, investigators have shown that a visible osteochondral defect averages approximately one-third the final size of the lesion following debridement.[29,57] The benefits of arthroscopic debridement include a relatively benign postoperative rehabilitation protocol, with unrestricted weight bearing and range of motion immediately following surgery.

Osteochondral resection can be facilitated by the following technical considerations: Removal of a loose body may be aided by placing the suction on medium-low on the arthroscope or turning the inflow off, and capturing the fragment such that the smallest diameter is longitudinal to the axis of the grasping device. In addition, it is important to make sure that the portal is large enough to enable extraction of the fragment prior to attempting the maneuver. Loose particles are often found in the posteromedial or posterolateral compartments of the knee. They are best visualized by placing the arthroscope through the intercondylar notch between the ACL and lateral femoral condyle when the arthroscope is in the anteromedial portal, and between the posterior cruciate ligament (PCL) and medial femoral condyle when the arthroscope is in the anterolateral portal. An accessory posteromedial or posterolateral portal is often necessary for loose body removal. Finally, when debriding the borders of the osteochondral defect, use a hooded shaver to limit overaggressive debridement.

Repair

Internal fixation is usually indicated for larger osteochondral fragments ($\geq$1 cm diameter) with minimal damage to the articular cartilage. A variety of methods are available, all of which have as a goal anatomic and stable restoration of the articular surface with minimal preparation of the donor and recipient tissue. To optimize articular congruity and wear kinematics, the appropriate height must be reestablished following fixation of the osteochondral fragment. If necessary, iliac crest or proximal tibial autograft or allograft can be placed into the bed of the defect to achieve the appropriate height of the fragment.[58]

The surgeon has in his arsenal a variety of implants to facilitate stable fixation of the osteochondral fragment including Kirschner wires (K-wires), standard and cannulated AO screws, and lower profile headless, variable-pitch compression screws and bone pegs. In addition, bioabsorbable implants consisting of polylactic acid (PLA), polyglycolic acid (PGA), mixed PLA and PGA, and poly-p-dioxanone (PDS) polymers in the form of pins, screws, and tacks are gaining popularity in the fixation of osteochondral defects.

Fixation of osteochondral fragments began historically with the use of 0.062-inch K-wires placed through the fragment and into subchondral bone.[59–61] Rotational stability can be achieved with the use of multiple K-wires placed in tandem; however, wire subsidence can occur. In addition, this technique does not enable compression at the fracture site. To prevent migration and achieve more stable fixation, Hughston et al[62] advocated bending the K-wires 1 mm from the tip and seating the wire into the articular cartilage and subchondral bone.

Standard AO screws (small or minifragment) are commonly used, but must be countersunk into the articular cartilage and require a second surgery for hardware removal (Fig. 18–1). The head of the screw may continue to be prominent and damage the opposing articular cartilage, effectively making a unipolar into a bipolar chondral lesion. The Acutrak (Acumed, Beaverton, OR), Herbert (Zimmer, Warsaw, IN), and Heune (Special Devices, Grass Valley, CA) screws are low-profile, headless screws that achieve compression at the fracture site by variable pitch construction, yet are not easily removed and have as a drawback retention of exposed metal in the joint.

Bioabsorbable implants are gaining increased popularity due to progressive load transfer at the osteochondral fracture site as well as the elimination of a required second surgery for hardware removal. PGA polymers, which are the most durable, are characterized by a high rate of resorption. Unfortunately, reports of adverse reactions including late aseptic inflammatory reactions and persistent pain have been found in 6 to 22% of patients.[63,64] A lower incidence of these side effects has been found in the PLA, composite, and PDS polymers, given their slower resorptability. The OrthoSorb (Depuy Ace, Warsaw, IN) device carries a resorption profile in between PGA and PLA polymers and is available in 1.3- and 2.0-mm-diameter sizes, but does not allow compression at the fracture site. The SmartNail (Bionx, Tampere, Finland) is a bioabsorbable device composed of a proprietary polymer that is able to function as a compression device in appropriate osteochondral defects (Fig. 18–2).

Indications for repair of an osteochondral defect include (1) lesion size $\geq$1 cm diameter, (2) fragment with intact articular cartilage with subchondral bone, and (3) compliant patient able to adhere to strict postoperative rehabilitation protocols and weight-bearing restrictions. Relative contraindications include (1) smokers, (2) age >50, and (3) size mismatch of the defect and fragment. Absolute contraindications include (1) uncorrectable ligamentous instability or malalignment, (2) fragment with damaged or comminuted articular cartilage, and (3) noncompliant patients.

Repair may be facilitated by the use of accessory portals as needed, including transpatellar tendon portals to allow correct alignment for placement of pins, screws, and K-wires. Meticulous anatomic reduction as well as compression of the osteochondral fragment must be achieved. In the subacute setting, the subchondral bed should be prepared in an appropriate manner to stimulate bleeding prior to repair of the osteochondral fragment. Provisional fixation using K-wires may be placed into the fragment to prevent rotation prior to placement of the screw. Finally, the surgeon should have a low threshold to convert from an arthroscopic to open procedure if anatomic reduction cannot be obtained.

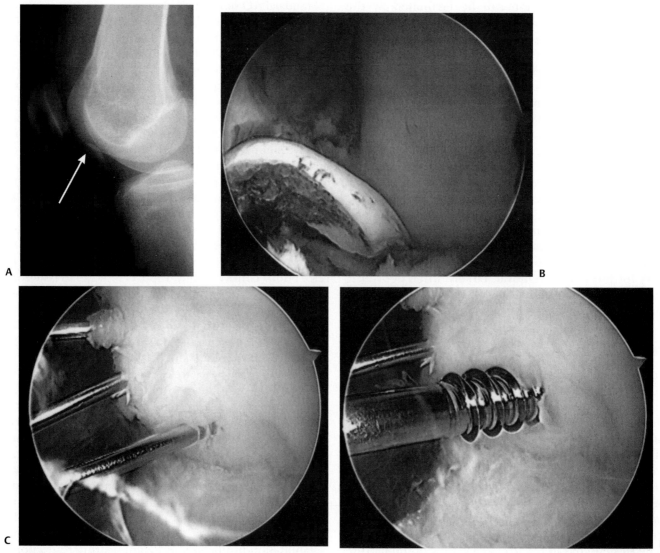

FIGURE 18–1 **(A)** A 16-year-old high-level ballet dancer sustained an injury pivoting during dance. She noted immediate pain and swelling and was brought to the emergency room, where a bony fragment and effusion could be seen within an otherwise normal radiograph. Examination was suggestive of a reduced patellar dislocation with a fracture from the lateral femoral condyle. Lateral radiograph revealed a loose body (arrow pointing to loose body, seen as a double shadow at the notch). **(B)** Arthroscopy revealed the osteochondral fracture involving a significant portion of the meniscal bearing area of the lateral femoral condyle. The osteochondral fragment had cancellous bone on the lower half of the fragment, which was approximately 12 mm wide, and only cartilage on the upper half, which was only 6 mm wide. **(C)** The bony bed was drilled to help stimulate healing. The fragment was then reduced within the defect and held with guidewires for the cannulated 3.5-mm lag screws and for the bioabsorbable pins. **(D)** The wires for the bioabsorbable pins were maintained to help prevent fragment rotation while drilling and inserting the cannulated screws. The screws were placed first to prevent unnecessary forces on the bioabsorbable pins. **(E)** Arthroscopic view of the lower half of the reduced fragment with a cannulated screw countersunk is outlined with arrows. Note the anatomic reduction and articular surface congruity of the superomedial edge of the reduced fragment. Arrows point to the edge of the reduced fragment. Lateral **(F)** and anteroposterior (AP) **(G)** radiographs 6 weeks following arthroscopic assisted internal fixation of the acute osteochondral fracture. However, also note the healing of the entire lesion, including the upper half, where nearly no bone remained on the fragment. At 2-year follow-up the patient is asymptomatic, has returned to high-level ballet dancing, and full activities without restriction. Her knee examination is normal. Radiographs reveal maintenance of joint space.

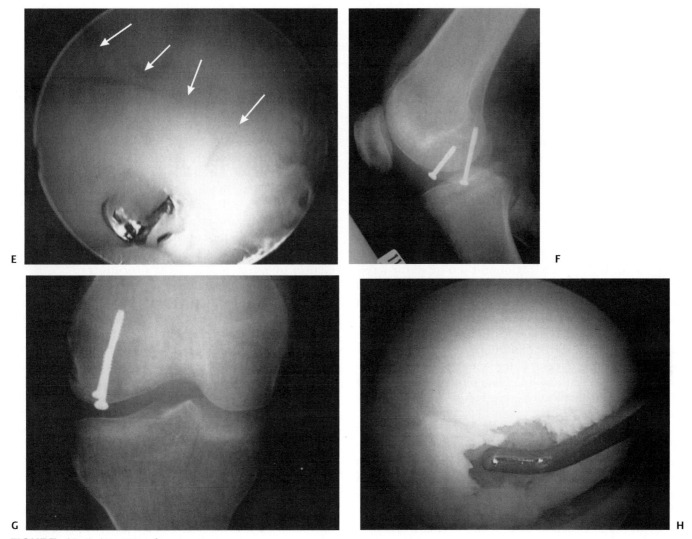

FIGURE 18–1 (*Continued*)

The authors' preferred method of treatment for repairable osteochondral defects is use of a countersunk AO screw with an OrthoSorb pin (Depuy Ace, Warsaw, IN) or SmartNail (Bionx, Tampere, Finland). Patients are placed into immediate continuous passive motion and given non–weight-bearing restrictions for 6 to 8 weeks. Hardware removal and assessment of healing is performed with second-look arthroscopy at 6 to 8 weeks

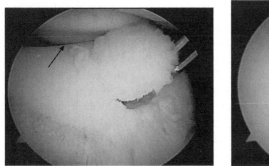
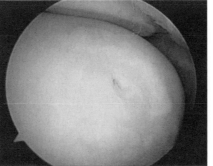

FIGURE 18–2 (A) A 16-year-old boy with an osteochondral injury to the trochlear region of his knee. The lesion is readily identifiable arthroscopically. **(B)** The bed was exposed arthroscopically to allow for debridement and drilling but maintaining the attachment, like a trapdoor. This lesion was then fixed with an absorbable tack that allows for some compression without the need for removal. Care is taken to ensure that the head of this tack is countersunk to avoid injury to the opposing articular surface.

postoperatively. The absorbable devices are used to help provide rotational control of the fragment.

Osteochondral tibial eminence avulsion fractures usually occur in skeletally immature athletes. These fractures can often include a significant portion of the medial or lateral tibial plateau. They can be reduced arthroscopically and fixed with either cannulated screws or sutures. Often the anterior horn of the lateral meniscus or the intermeniscal ligament blocks the reduction and needs to be retracted prior to reducing the fragment. The ACL tibial guide is often useful for holding the reduction. Using an accessory portal just off the medial or lateral border of the patella, a guidewire can be inserted and a screw placed. An image intensifier should be used and care must be taken not to cross the physes with the screws in a skeletally immature patient **(Fig. 18–3).** If the bone fragment is too small for screw fixation, sutures may be arthroscopically placed through the ligament stump and brought out through drill holes through the fragment bed and tied over the anteromedial tibia. Cannulated screw fixation has the advantage of facilitating early range of motion. Arthroscopically assisted reduction and cannulated screw fixation is technically much more difficult in tibial eminence avulsions in adults, and usually mini-open reduction and fixation is preferred for adults.

Osteochondral fractures of the patella are usually a result of a patellar dislocation and often involve the medial facet of the patella. This type of fracture is often not amenable to arthroscopic fixation. If the fragment is reparable, an arthrotomy can be made and the osteochondral fragment fixed using screws or bioabsorbable pins as previously described. Suture fixation has also been described for this type of fracture.[65] Keith needles can be drilled from the articular surface through the reduced fragment and brought out the anterior surface of the patella. The skin and subcutaneous tissue is dissected off the anterior surface of the patella and the needles are identified. Sutures are then passed through the needle eyelets and the needles are brought out the anterior surface of the patella. The sutures can then be tied over the anterior surface of the patella. If four needles are used, then two sutures can be used in a cross pattern, which provides stable fixation for the osteochondral fragment **(Fig. 18–4).**

Replacement

The replacement of damaged osteochondral articular defects is indicated for those lesions greater than 1 cm in diameter that are not amenable to primary repair. As discussed in detail elsewhere in this book, it can be achieved by two specific strategies: (1) intrinsic replacement, and (2) transplantation. Intrinsic replacement is based on stimulating intrinsic repair mechanisms within the articular cartilage and subchondral bone to regener-

ate or reconstitute the osteochondral defect. An alternative approach is the transplantation of autologous or allogeneic chondrocytes, chondrogenic cells, or tissue that have the potential to grow into new cartilage and repair the defect.

Intrinsic replacement can be induced by subchondral drilling, abrasion, or microfracture techniques, which differ mainly in their method of achieving subchondral penetration. The theoretical goal is the recruitment of mesenchymal pluripotential cells into the defect by penetrating the subchondral bone, which can reconstitute a hyaline-like repair tissue.

Subchondral drilling was first reported by Smillie[61] in the open treatment of an osteochondral fragment in 1957. Several investigators have subsequently advocated subchondral drilling in isolation or in conjunction with fixation or other replacement procedures.[56,60–62,66–69] This technique poses the risk of thermal necrosis to articular cartilage and subchondral bone and has been supplanted by newer methods such as abrasion chondroplasty or microfracture.

Abrasion chondroplasty was pioneered by Johnson[70] and is a variation in concept of the subchondral drilling technique. Abrasion chondroplasty involves abrasion of the articular sclerotic defect with an arthroscopic burr to enable bleeding into the articular defect and promote a fibrocartilaginous repair tissue to reconstitute the lesion; however, this was proposed as a treatment for chondral injury with intact subchondral plate. A study has indicated that the integrity of this repair tissue can be maintained for up to 6 years postoperatively.[70] Other studies have reported less favorable outcomes with a rapid deterioration of improvement over time.[71,72] Although this technique has been advocated for chondral lesions with intact subchondral bone, the concept has been extrapolated to the treatment of osteochondral lesions; however, scientific confirmation is lacking.

The microfracture technique, popularized by Steadman, is performed by creating multiple small holes into the subchondral bone using specialized awls that results in "microfracture" of the trabeculae rather than destruction of bone.[73,74] The lesion is debrided and subchondral bone exposed. The arthroscopic awls are used to make microfractures by picking three or four holes per square centimeter to a depth of ~4 mm. Heat necrosis is avoided and the integrity of the subchondral bone shape is maintained, whereas the roughened subchondral surface allows better adherence of the clot. Continuous passive motion and no weight bearing for 6 to 8 weeks is essential for fibrocartilaginous tissue maturation, adherence, and pain relief. Steadman et al[74] reported a 75% improvement at 3- to 5-year follow-up using this technique. Again, while this technique has been extensively investigated in the treatment of isolated chondral lesions, the concept may be applied in the setting of subchondral bone loss.

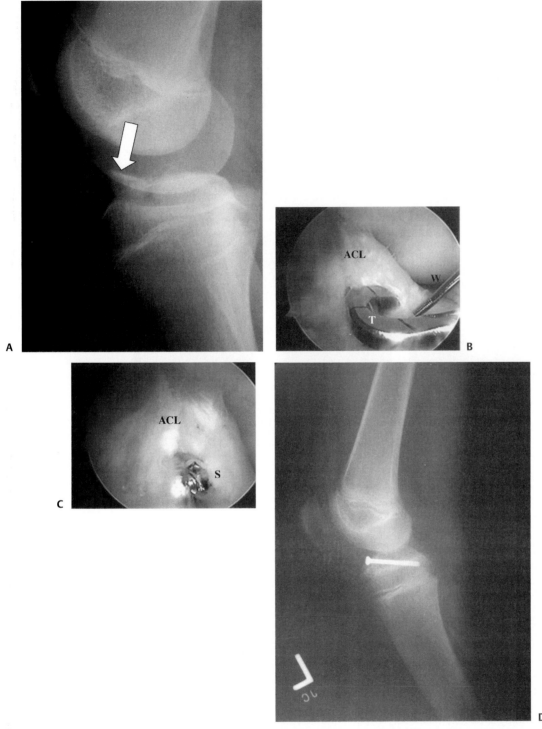

FIGURE 18–3 (A) A 12-year-old boy with a type II tibial eminence avulsion fracture sustained while skateboarding. The fracture fragment (tibial eminence) is outlined by solid straight arrow. **(B,C)** The anterior cruciate ligament (ACL) tibial guide (T) is helpful in holding the reduction while the guidewire (W) is inserted. A 4.0-cannulated screw (S) is the inserted over the guidewire. **(D)** Postoperative lateral radiograph. Care must be taken to keep the screw above the physis in a skeletally immature patient.

Transplantation of osteochondral autograft was first reported by Judet and Henri[75] in 1908 for the treatment of OCD. The osteochondral autograft transplantation system (OATS) (Arthrex, Naples, FL) procedure involves harvest and implantation of a single osteochondral cylinder, whereas mosaicplasty (Acufex, Mansfield, MA), popularized by Hangody in 1994, involves the harvest and implantation of multiple osteochondral

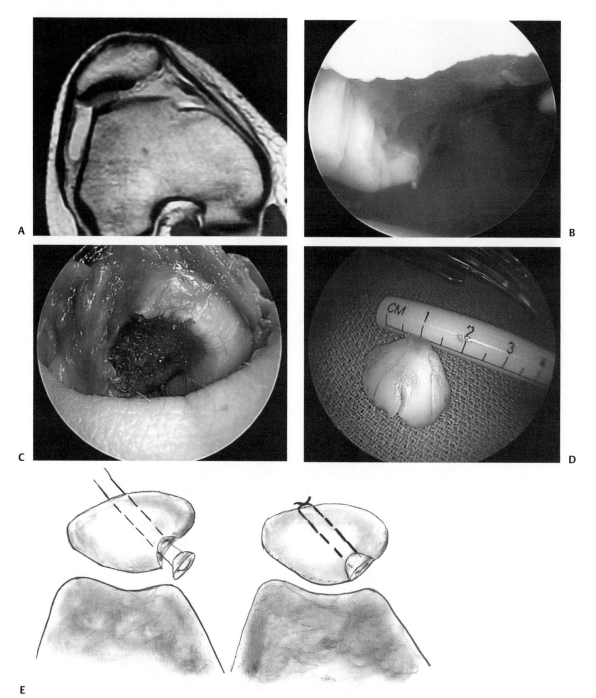

FIGURE 18–4 (A) Medial facet patella (arrow) fracture seen on MRI after patella dislocation. **(B)** Arthroscopic view of patellar defect. **(C)** An arthrotomy is usually necessary when fixing an osteochondral fracture of the patella. **(D)** Fracture fragment is measured on the back table. **(E)** Keith needles can be used to hold the fracture reduced. The needles are then used to pass poly-p-dioxanone (PDS) sutures that can be tied to secure the fragment.

(*Continued*)

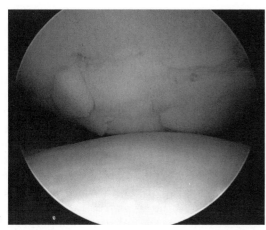

FIGURE 18–4 (*Continued*) **(F)** Medial facet patella osteochondral fracture reduction using suture fixation. (Photo courtesy of Raffy Mirzayan, M.D.)

cylinders that are press-fit into drill holes.[76] Mosaicplasty has been recommended for much larger and deeper osteochondral lesions (1 to 8 cm²). The donor site is usually a relatively non–weight-bearing region of the knee such as the edge of the patellar groove or the area just proximal to the intercondylar notch.

A key component of considering this line of treatment is the necessity for normal knee biomechanics and stability. If abnormal knee alignment or instability is present, it requires simultaneous treatment at the time of osteochondral implantation. Conventional instrumentation systems facilitate arthroscopic osteochondral autografting for limited lesions of the femoral condyles, whereas open arthrotomy is required for lesions of the patella, trochlea, and posterior femoral condyles. Many surgeons find it easier to place the graft perpendicular to the defect using an open or miniarthrotomy approach. Complications of the two procedures include hemarthrosis, effusion, donor-site pain, graft fracture, and osteochondral loose bodies, which can exacerbate the above symptoms.

Osetochondral allografts were first reported in 1925 with the work of Lexer,[77] who reported on osteochondral transplantation of articular cartilage in knees, fingers, and elbows. As increased understanding of the immune system emerged, so did a greater interest in transplantation techniques in the 1960s. Osteochondral allografts may be used for larger osteochondral lesions that are not candidates for autologous replacement or have failed prior restorative efforts. This technique is attractive due to the lack of donor-site morbidity, but it carries the risk of disease transmission, graft settling, poor incorporation, and difficulty with availability. Fresh allografts, obtained within 72 hours, carry the greatest chance of chondrocyte survival and likelihood of integration, yet they also carry the risk of higher disease transmission and immunogenicity. The use of shell allografts, or allografts with less than

1 cm of subchondral bone, reduces the chance of disease transmission by decreasing exposure to leukocytes found in cancellous bone. The preservation of osteochondral allografts is an area of ongoing research, but currently fresh grafts can be preserved to near 100% viability for up to 4 days at 4°C. Fresh grafts are stored for up to 21 days following appropriate harvesting. Frozen grafts are also available, but they show an increased prevalence of fissuring, delamination, fibrosis, and generalized breakdown of the articular surface, making them less attractive for implantation.

The success of osteochondral allografts is dependent on the viability and fixation of the subchondral bone of the graft to native bone. Despite improvements in immunosuppressive techniques, "creeping substitution" is a major impediment to allograft viability as the host immune system can initiate significant tissue remodeling of the allograft. The speed of this process is reduced by "cork" fixation of the allograft, where the graft is shaped like a tapered cone and press-fitted into the defect. Creeping substitution, however, is increased when fixation penetrates the entire graft, with either permanent or bioabsorbable implants.[78]

In autologous chondrocyte implantation (ACI), chondrocytes are harvested arthroscopically, expanded in culture, and transplanted into the defect beneath a periosteal flap 2 to 5 weeks thereafter. This technique was initially described by Brittberg et al[79] for the treatment of symptomatic full-thickness chondral injuries in select patients. The technique has also been advocated in the treatment of osteochondral lesions in OCD, with Peterson et al[80] and Minas and Nehrer[81] recommending bone grafting for lesions greater than 8 mm in depth. Little data exists as to the efficacy of ACI in the treatment of acute osteochondral defects of the knee.

Rib perichondrium has been used as an autologous graft source in the treatment of osteochondral defects in young patients, but it has fallen out of favor due to the high incidence of calcification of the perichondrium.

Technical impediments characteristic of all replacement techniques include difficulty with perpendicular graft placement, graft impaction forces, cartilage thickness and stiffness mismatch, and radius of curvature differences.

The use of periosteum in the treatment of osteochondral lesions is based on the ability of the cambium layer to differentiate into chondrocytes and form hyaline cartilage.[7] Prior investigators have shown that when periosteal tissue is sutured into the base of an osteochondral lesion, a hyaline-like repair tissue (87% type II collagen) is generated with similar biomechanical characteristics of hyaline cartilage. Success of this technique is augmented with the use of continuous passive motion postoperatively, and this has been confirmed in animal studies.[82] This technique has been successful in the treatment of lesions of the patella and femoral condyle as well as diminishing pain in select patients. There continues to be controversy regarding the orientation of the cambium layer into the defect.

A restorative procedure is indicated for those lesions larger than 1 cm in diameter that do not meet the criteria for repair due to the quality of the articular cartilage of the fragment, lack of suitable subchondral bone attached to the fragment, or a lack of suitable implants. Contraindications continue to include smokers and noncompliant patients. In addition, given the absence of any scientific data confirming the benefit of one technique over another, the preferred intervention should be based on surgeon technical experience and comfort. Osteochondral lesions less than 2.5 cm in diameter may be repaired with multiple 1-cm autologous osteochondral grafts obtained from a non–weight-bearing portion of the knee with approximately two-thirds the height of the plug buried within the subchondral bone at the base of the defect. The authors' preference for lesions greater than 2.5 cm in diameter is to use fresh allograft tissue or autologous chondrocyte implantation.

■ Postoperative Care

Continuous Passive Motion

Salter[83,84] introduced the use of continuous passive motion (CPM) of knees for the postoperative treatment of full-thickness articular cartilage lesions as well as intraarticular fractures. In one of Salter's studies, four 1-mm drill holes were created in rabbit knees; hyaline cartilage healing occurred in 60% of rabbits receiving CPM as compared with 10% in those that were immobilized or allowed unrestricted cage activity.[83] Although subsequent studies have shown that CPM is less effective in defects larger than 3 mm in diameter, it is generally regarded to be adjunctive in any procedure directed toward chondral and osteochondral healing.[85–87]

■ Complications

Apoptosis and Osteochondral Injury

Studies have shown that chondrocyte apoptosis, or programmed cell death (PCD), is associated with osteochondral injury and may lead to the development of posttraumatic arthritis.[15,88–93] Experimental cartilage injuries such as compression, drilling, and trephine wounding can stimulate significantly increased levels of chondrocyte apoptosis in vitro.[94] Even the presence of a hemarthrosis is deleterious to chondrocyte viability and stimulates apoptosis.[6] Given the poor intrinsic regenera-

tive capacity of hyaline articular cartilage, there has been increasing interest in the possibility of preserving chondrocytes following injury by inhibiting key enzymes in the apoptotic cascade.[95]

Commonly performed arthroscopic procedures such as chondral shaving, debridement, and laser abrasion lead to death of chondrocytes extending beyond the border of the treatment site and may have a deleterious effect on articular cartilage long-term.[96,97] In a recent study, Hunziker and Driesang[98] reported significant chondrocyte loss at the wound edge of partial-thickness chondral defects in pigs repaired with an autologous fascial flap sutured over a fibrinous matrix. Even seemingly benign procedures such as the suturing of a periosteal flap during ACI may result in chondrocyte death along the path of the suture needle. Thus, the iatrogenic creation of an acellular or hypocellular zone of cartilage may be a major factor affecting edge healing and incorporation of transplanted repair tissue. Future research is needed to determine whether apoptosis inhibition may be a useful adjunct in the treatment of acute osteochondral injury by limiting chondrocyte death following trauma and in improving the results of current cartilage repair and replacement techniques.

■ Conclusion

Not enough studies have been done yet to provide the scientific validation needed to guide the treatment of acute osteochondral defects of the knee. Basic tenets of articular fracture management prevail and guide the current treatment algorithms, emphasizing anatomic and stable reduction of the fragment, establishment of articular surface congruity, and the use of compressive techniques to facilitate fracture healing. Early range of motion, the use of continuous passive motion, and accelerated rehabilitation protocols are beneficial for articular cartilage viability and have been shown to accelerate healing. Future developments in stimulating bone and cartilage healing on the cellular level, in limiting programmed cell death following injury and iatrogenic preparation of the defect, and in implant options will likely enable the orthopaedic surgeon to improve surgical outcomes.

REFERENCES

1. Curl WW, Krome J, Gordon ES, Rushing J, Smith BP, Poehling GG. Cartilage injuries: a review of 31,516 knee arthroscopies. Arthroscopy 1997;13:456–460
2. Messner K, Maletius W. The long-term prognosis for severe damage to weight-bearing cartilage in the knee: a 14-year clinical and radiographic follow-up in 28 young athletes. Acta Orthop Scand 1996;67:165–168

3. Blanco FJ, Ochs RL, Schwarz H, Lotz M. Chondrocyte apoptosis induced by nitric oxide. Am J Pathol 1995;146:75–85

4. Frenkel J, Sherman D, Fein A, et al. Accentuated apoptosis in normally developing p53 knockout mouse embryos following genotoxic stress. Oncogene 1999;18:2901–2907

5. Hashimoto S, Takahashi K, Amiel D, Coutts RD, Lotz M. Chondrocyte apoptosis and nitric oxide production during experimentally induced osteoarthritis. Arthritis Rheum 1998;41:1266–1274

6. Hooiveld M, Roosendaal G, Wenting M, van den Berg M, Bijlsma J, Lafeber F. Short-term exposure of cartilage to blood results in chondrocyte apoptosis. Am J Pathol 2003;162:943–951

7. Buckwalter JA, Mow VC, Ratcliffe A. Restoration of injured or degenerated articular cartilage. J Am Acad Orthop Surg 1994;2:192–201

8. Buckwalter JA, Martin JA, Olmstead M, Athanasiou KA, Rosenwasser MP, Mow VC. Osteochondral repair of primate knee femoral and patellar articular surfaces: implications for preventing post-traumatic osteoarthritis. Iowa Orthop J 2003;23:66–74

9. Zhu W, Mow VC, Koob TJ, Eyre DR. Viscoelastic shear properties of articular cartilage and the effects of glycosidase treatments. J Orthop Res 1993;11:771–781

10. Donohue JM, Buss D, Oegema TR Jr, Thompson RC Jr. The effects of indirect blunt trauma on adult canine articular cartilage. J Bone Joint Surg Am 1983;65:948–957

11. Radin EL, Paul IL. Response of joints to impact loading. I. In vitro wear. Arthritis Rheum 1971;14:356–362

12. Radin EL, Parker HG, Pugh JW, Steinberg RS, Paul IL, Rose RM. Response of joints to impact loading. 3. Relationship between trabecular microfractures and cartilage degeneration. J Biomech 1973;6:51–57

13. Repo RU, Finlay JB. Survival of articular cartilage after controlled impact. J Bone Joint Surg Am 1977;59:1068–1076

14. Vener MJ, Thompson RC Jr, Lewis JL, Oegema TR Jr. Subchondral damage after acute transarticular loading: an in vitro model of joint injury. J Orthop Res 1992;10:759–765

15. D'Lima DD, Hashimoto S, Chen PC, Colwell CW Jr, Lotz MK. Impact of mechanical trauma on matrix and cells. Clin Orthop 2001;391(suppl):S90–99

16. Tomatsu T, Imai N, Takeuchi N, Takahashi K, Kimura N. Experimentally produced fractures of articular cartilage and bone. The effects of shear forces on the pig knee. J Bone Joint Surg Br 1992;74:457–462

17. Li X, Haut RC, Altiero NJ. An analytical model to study blunt impact response of the rabbit P-F joint. J Biomech Eng 1995;117:485–491

18. Borrelli J Jr, Torzilli PA, Grigiene R, Helfet DL. Effect of impact load on articular cartilage: development of an intra-articular fracture model. J Orthop Trauma 1997;11:319–326

19. Simon SR, American Academy of Orthopaedic Surgeons. Orthopaedic Basic Science. Rosemont, IL: American Academy of Orthopaedic Surgeons, 1994

20. Setton LA, Mow VC, Howell DS. Mechanical behavior of articular cartilage in shear is altered by transection of the anterior cruciate ligament. J Orthop Res 1995;13:473–482

21. Moskowitz RW, Davis W, Sammarco J, et al. Experimentally induced degenerative joint lesions following partial meniscectomy in the rabbit. Arthritis Rheum 1973;16:397–405

22. Aizawa T, Kon T, Einhorn TA, Gerstenfeld LC. Induction of apoptosis in chondrocytes by tumor necrosis factor-alpha. J Orthop Res 2001;19:785–796

23. Hashimoto S, Creighton-Achermann L, Takahashi K, Amiel D, Coutts RD, Lotz M. Development and regulation of osteophyte formation during experimental osteoarthritis. Osteoarthritis Cartilage 2002;10:180–187

24. Lucchinetti E, Adams CS, Horton WE Jr, Torzilli PA. Cartilage viability after repetitive loading: a preliminary report. Osteoarthritis Cartilage 2002;10:71–81

25. Kobayashi K, Mishima H, Hashimoto S, et al. Chondrocyte apoptosis and regional differential expression of nitric oxide in the medial meniscus following partial meniscectomy. J Orthop Res 2001;19:802–808

26. Asada S, Fukuda K, Nishisaka F, Matsukawa M, Hamanisi C. Hydrogen peroxide induces apoptosis of chondrocytes; involvement of calcium ion and extracellular signal-regulated protein kinase. Inflamm Res 2001;50:19–23

27. Kempson GE, Muir H, Pollard C, Tuke M. The tensile properties of the cartilage of human femoral condyles related to the content of collagen and glycosaminoglycans. Biochim Biophys Acta 1973;297:456–472

28. Sokolof L. The Biology of Degenerative Joint Disease. Chicago: University of Chicago Press, 1969

29. Terry GC, Flandry F, Van Manen JW, Norwood LA. Isolated chondral fractures of the knee. Clin Orthop 1988;234:170–177

30. Hunter W. Of the structure and disease of articulating cartilages. Clin Orthop 1995;317:3–6

31. Bennett G, Baur W, Maddock SJ. A study of the repair of articular cartilage and the reaction of normal joints of adult dogs to surgically created defects of articular cartilage, "joint mice," and patellar displacement. Am J Pathol 1932;8:499–524

32. Bennett G, Baur W. Further studies concerning the repair of articular cartilage in dog joints. J Bone Joint Surg Am 1935;17:141–150

33. Calandruccio R, Gilmer WS. Proliferation, regeneration, and repair of articular cartilage of immature animals. J Bone Joint Surg Am 1962;44A:431–455

34. Campbell CJ. The healing of cartilage defects. Clin Orthop Relat Res 1969;64:45–63

35. DePalma AF, McKeever CD, Subin DK. Process of repair of articular cartilage demonstrated by histology and autoradiography with tritiated thymidine. Clin Orthop 1966;48:229–242

36. Fuller JA, Ghadially FN. Ultrastructural observations on surgically produced partial-thickness defects in articular cartilage. Clin Orthop 1972;86:193–205

37. Ito L. The nutrition of articular cartilage and its method of repair. Br J Surg 1924;12:31–42

38. Mankin HJ. Localization of tritiated thymidine in articular cartilage of rabbits. II. Repair in immature cartilage. J Bone Joint Surg Am 1962;44A:688–698

39. Mankin HJ. The reaction of articular cartilage to injury and osteoarthritis (second of two parts). N Engl J Med 1974;291:1335–1340

40. Paget J. Healing of cartilage. Clin Orthop 1969;64:7–8

41. Moskowitz RW. Osteoarthritis, Diagnosis and Medical/Surgical Management, 2nd ed. Philadelphia: Saunders, 1992:71–107

42. Outerbridge RE. The etiology of chondromalacia patellae. J Bone Joint Surg Br 1961;43-B:752–757

43. Noyes FR, Stabler CL. A system for grading articular cartilage lesions at arthroscopy. Am J Sports Med 1989;17:505–513

44. Brittberg M, Winalski CS. Evaluation of cartilage injuries and repair. J Bone Joint Surg Am 2003;85-A(suppl 2):58–69

45. Berndt AL, Harty M. Transchondral fractures (osteochondritis dissecans) of the talus. Am J Orthop 1959;41-A:988–1020

46. Bohndorf K. Osteochondritis (osteochondrosis) dissecans: a review and new MRI classification. Eur Radiol 1998;8:103–112

47. Boden BP, Pearsall AW, Garrett WE Jr, Feagin JA Jr. Patellofemoral instability: evaluation and management. J Am Acad Orthop Surg 1997;5:47–57

48. Potter HG. Imaging of posttraumatic and soft tissue dysfunction of the elbow. Clin Orthop 2000;370:9–18

49. Kibler WB, Herring SA, Press JM. Functional Rehabilitation of Sports and Musculoskeletal Injuries. Gaithersburg, MD: Aspen, 1998:20–56

50. Stoller DW. Magnetic Resonance Imaging in Orthopaedics and Sports Medicine, 2nd ed. Philadelphia: Lippincott-Raven, 1997:419

51. Rangger C, Klestil T, Kathrein A, Inderster A, Hamid L. Influence of magnetic resonance imaging on indications for arthroscopy of the knee. Clin Orthop 1996;330:133–142

52. Jackson DW, Jennings LD, Maywood RM, Berger PE. Magnetic resonance imaging of the knee. Am J Sports Med 1988;16:29–38

53. Johnson DL, Urban WP Jr, Caborn DN, Vanarthos WJ, Carlson CS. Articular cartilage changes seen with magnetic resonance imaging-detected bone bruises associated with acute anterior cruciate ligament rupture. Am J Sports Med 1998;26:409–414

54. Magnuson PB. The classic: joint debridement: surgical treatment of degenerative arthritis. Clin Orthop 1974;101:4–12

55. Moseley JB, O'Malley K, Petersen NJ, et al. A controlled trial of arthroscopic surgery for osteoarthritis of the knee. N Engl J Med 2002;347:81–88

56. Dzioba RB. The classification and treatment of acute articular cartilage lesions. Arthroscopy 1988;4:72–80

57. Levy AS, Lohnes J, Sculley S, LeCroy M, Garrett W. Chondral delamination of the knee in soccer players. Am J Sports Med 1996;24:634–639

58. Gillespie HS, Day B. Bone peg fixation in the treatment of osteochondritis dissecans of the knee joint. Clin Orthop 1979;143: 125–130

59. Guhl JF. Arthroscopic treatment of osteochondritis dissecans: preliminary report. Orthop Clin North Am 1979;10:671–683

60. Lipscomb PR Jr, Lipscomb PR Sr, Bryan RS. Osteochondritis dissecans of the knee with loose fragments. Treatment by replacement and fixation with readily removed pins. J Bone Joint Surg Am 1978;60:235–240

61. Smillie IS. Treatment of osteochondritis dissecans. J Bone Joint Surg Br 1957;39-B:248–260

62. Hughston JC, Hergenroeder PT, Courtenay BG. Osteochondritis dissecans of the femoral condyles. J Bone Joint Surg Am 1984;66:1340–1348

63. Song EK, Lee KB, Yoon TR. Aseptic synovitis after meniscal repair using the biodegradable meniscus arrow. Arthroscopy 2001;17: 77–80

64. Menche DS, Phillips GI, Pitman MI, Steiner GC. Inflammatory foreign-body reaction to an arthroscopic bioabsorbable meniscal arrow repair. Arthroscopy 1999;15:770–772

65. Dhawan A, Hospodar PP. Suture fixation as a treatment for acute traumatic osteochondral lesions. Arthroscopy 1999;15:307–311

66. Aglietti P, Buzzi R, Bassi PB, Fioriti M. Arthroscopic drilling in juvenile osteochondritis dissecans of the medial femoral condyle. Arthroscopy 1994;10:286–291

67. Anderson AF, Richards DB, Pagnani MJ, Hovis WD. Antegrade drilling for osteochondritis dissecans of the knee. Arthroscopy 1997;13:319–324

68. Bradley J, Dandy DJ. Results of drilling osteochondritis dissecans before skeletal maturity. J Bone Joint Surg Br 1989;71:642–644

69. Rae PJ, Noble J. Arthroscopic drilling of osteochondral lesions of the knee. J Bone Joint Surg Br 1989;71:534

70. Johnson LL. Arthroscopic abrasion arthroplasty historical and pathologic perspective: present status. Arthroscopy 1986;2:54–69

71. Bert JM. Electrocautery. Arthroscopy 1991;7:414–415

72. Bert JM. Role of abrasion arthroplasty and debridement in the management of osteoarthritis of the knee. Rheum Dis Clin North Am 1993;19:725–739

73. Steadman JR, Rodkey WG, Rodrigo JJ. Microfracture: surgical technique and rehabilitation to treat chondral defects. Clin Orthop 2001;391(suppl):S362–369

74. Steadman JR, Rodkey WG, Briggs KK. Microfracture to treat full-thickness chondral defects: surgical technique, rehabilitation, and outcomes. J Knee Surg 2002;15:170–176

75. Henri JA, Judet. Essai sur la greffe des tissues articulares. Comp Rend Acad D Sci. 1908;146:193–196

76. Hangody L, Kish G, Karpati Z, Udvarhelyi I, Szigeti I, Bely M. Mosaicplasty for the treatment of articular cartilage defects: application in clinical practice. Orthopedics 1998;21:751–756

77. Lexer E. Joint transplantations and arthroplasty. Surg Gynecol Obstet 1925;40:782–809

78. Browne JE, Branch TP. Surgical alternatives for treatment of articular cartilage lesions. J Am Acad Orthop Surg 2000;8:180–189

79. Brittberg M, Lindahl A, Nilsson A, Ohlsson C, Isaksson O, Peterson L. Treatment of deep cartilage defects in the knee with autologous chondrocyte transplantation. N Engl J Med 1994;331: 889–895

80. Peterson L, Minas T, Brittberg M, Lindahl A. Treatment of osteochondritis dissecans of the knee with autologous chondrocyte transplantation: results at two to ten years. J Bone Joint Surg Am 2003;85-A(suppl 2):17–24

81. Minas T, Nehrer S. Current concepts in the treatment of articular cartilage defects. Orthopedics 1997;20:525–538

82. Delaney JP, O'Driscoll SW, Salter RB. Neochondrogenesis in free intraarticular periosteal autografts in an immobilized and paralyzed limb. An experimental investigation in the rabbit. Clin Orthop 1989;248:278–282

83. Salter RB, Simmonds DF, Malcolm BW, Rumble EJ, MacMichael D, Clements ND. The biological effect of continuous passive motion on the healing of full-thickness defects in articular cartilage. An experimental investigation in the rabbit. J Bone Joint Surg Am 1980;62:1232–1251

84. Salter RB. Continuous Passive Motion (CPM): A Biological Concept for the Healing and Regeneration of Articular Cartilage, Ligaments, and Tendons: From Its Origination to Research to Clinical Applications. Baltimore: Williams & Wilkins, 1993

85. O'Driscoll SW, Keeley FW, Salter RB. The chondrogenic potential of free autogenous periosteal grafts for biological resurfacing of major full-thickness defects in joint surfaces under the influence of continuous passive motion. An experimental investigation in the rabbit. J Bone Joint Surg Am 1986;68:1017–1035

86. O'Driscoll SW, Salter RB. The repair of major osteochondral defects in joint surfaces by neochondrogenesis with autogenous osteoperiosteal grafts stimulated by continuous passive motion. An experimental investigation in the rabbit. Clin Orthop 1986;208: 131–140

87. Rodrigo JJ, Steadman JR, Syftestad G, Benton H, Silliman J. Effects of human knee synovial fluid on chondrogenesis in vitro. Am J Knee Surg 1995;8:124–129

88. Blanco FJ, Guitian R, Vazquez-Martul E, de Toro FJ, Galdo F. Osteoarthritis chondrocytes die by apoptosis. A possible pathway for osteoarthritis pathology. Arthritis Rheum 1998;41: 284–289

89. Hashimoto S, Ochs RL, Komiya S, Lotz M. Linkage of chondrocyte apoptosis and cartilage degradation in human osteoarthritis. Arthritis Rheum 1998;41:1632–1638

90. D'Lima DD, Hashimoto S, Chen PC, Lotz MK, Colwell CW Jr. Prevention of chondrocyte apoptosis. J Bone Joint Surg Am 2001;83-A(suppl 2, pt 1):25–26

91. D'Lima DD, Hashimoto S, Chen PC, Colwell CW Jr, Lotz MK. Human chondrocyte apoptosis in response to mechanical injury. Osteoarthritis Cartilage 2001;9:712–719

92. D'Lima DD, Hashimoto S, Chen PC, Lotz MK, Colwell CW Jr. In vitro and in vivo models of cartilage injury. J Bone Joint Surg Am 2001;83-A(suppl 2, pt 1):22–24

93. Kim HT, Lo MY, Pillarisetty R. Chondrocyte apoptosis following intraarticular fracture in humans. Osteoarthritis Cartilage 2002; 10:747–749

94. Tew SR, Kwan AP, Hann A, Thomson BM, Archer CW. The reactions of articular cartilage to experimental wounding: role of apoptosis. Arthritis Rheum 2000;43:215–225

95. Costouros JG, Dang AC, Kim HT. Inhibition of chondrocyte apoptosis in vivo following acute osteochondral injury. Osteoarthritis Cartilage 2003;11:756–759

96. Hunziker EB. Articular cartilage repair: are the intrinsic biological constraints undermining this process insuperable? Osteoarthritis Cartilage 1999;7:15–28

97. Hunziker EB, Quinn TM. Surgical removal of articular cartilage leads to loss of chondrocytes from cartilage bordering the wound edge. J Bone Joint Surg Am 2003;85-A(suppl 2): 85–92

98. Hunziker EB, Driesang IMK. Surgical suturing of adult articular cartilage is associated with a loss of chondrocytes and an absence of wound healing. Transactions of the 49th annual meeting of the Orthopaedic Research Society. 2003.

19

Osteochondral Defects in the Elbow

RUSSELL S. PETRIE AND JAMES P. BRADLEY

Treatment of articular cartilage injuries remains difficult and frustrating in virtually every joint in which these maladies occur. This is particularly true of young athletes who continue to place high demands on their joints. Due to the poor biologic properties of articular cartilage, these lesions have minimal potential for healing, making them susceptible to progression with repetitive trauma. Many of the injuries develop prior to skeletal maturity and are underappreciated or missed. Osteochondritis dissecans is the prototypical chondral lesion of the elbow affecting young athletes. This condition is seen primarily in throwing athletes as well as gymnasts, although it may occur in any number of sports.

When treating osteochondral injuries, consideration must be given to the skeletal maturity of the individual. Treatment differs to some extent between skeletally immature and mature patients. This chapter focuses on the etiology, presentation, imaging, and treatment of osteochondritis dissecans, as this is perhaps the most difficult articular problem to treat in the skeletally immature athlete's elbow.

Treatment has evolved from removal of loose bodies, first described more than 150 years ago,[1] to nonoperative treatment,[2–4] arthroscopic debridement,[5,6] arthroscopic subchondral drilling,[3,4,7] open drilling,[2,8] abrasion chondroplasty,[9] and internal fixation with bone pegs,[7] bioabsorbable or metal screws,[10,11] pull-out wire,[12] compression staples,[13] and most recently tissue engineered cartilage gels.[14] Most authors would agree there is no indication for reduction and fixation of loose bodies. Excision of the fragment only with debridement of the bed is the mainstay of treatment.[2–8] Long-term re-

sults have shown that about half of the affected adolescents will develop symptomatic degenerative joint disease.[4] Magnetic resonance imaging (MRI) with and without contrast has been shown to help with early detection, which may allow for earlier intervention and improved long-term outcome.[15] Although most of the attention in the orthopaedic literature focuses on osteochondritis dissecans of the capitellum, the process has been reported in the trochlea,[16] radial head, and olecranon.[17,18]

Reconstructive options such as interposition arthroplasty and total elbow arthroplasty are not discussed here, as these are primarily salvage procedures not designed for the athletic population, but they remain an important part of the armamentarium of elbow surgeons.

■ Etiology

Osteochondritis dissecans (OCD) occurs predominantly in immature athletes and is rarely found in adults, although the sequelae are often seen in adults. It is a localized injury or condition to the subchondral bone resulting in loss of support for the overlying articular cartilage, which leads to breakdown and fragmentation of the cartilage and underlying bone.[19] Various theories regarding etiology have been proposed, but no single etiology is universally accepted.[20] König[21] is credited with the original description and naming of the lesion. The term is somewhat inaccurate as the name implies inflammation of the bone and cartilage. No inflammatory cells have been shown on histologic sections of excised fragments or surrounding synovium.[22,23] However, dissecans comes from the Latin *dissec-*, meaning to separate, and it accurately describes the separation of osteochondral fragments seen in the late stages of the process.

There are two similar disorders of the humeral capitellum that occur in immature individuals with similar radiographic findings: Panner's disease and OCD. The age at presentation and the prognosis are different, and therefore they should be distinguished as separate but related entities. Panner's disease typically presents in patients between 7 and 12 years of age, with a peak age of 9 years.[24,25] It is not associated with repetitive trauma, and it demonstrates flattening and patchy sclerosis of the entire humeral capitellum on x-ray. The capitellum reconstitutes with time and results in no demonstrable long-term sequelae.[26,27] OCD, in contradistinction, presents between 11 and 15 years of age and is associated with repetitive trauma, especially baseball and gymnastics, but has been seen in ice and roller hockey. Radiographically, the lesion is more focal with capitellar rarefaction **(Fig. 19–1)**. As the lesion progresses, capitellar flattening and subsequent fragmentation occur. Long-term degenerative joint disease affects nearly half of the elbows.[4,27–29]

Most authors agree that a combination of injury from repetitive trauma and a tenuous blood supply to the humeral capitellum leads to OCD.[20] Schenk et al[30] have demonstrated biomechanical differences between the capitellar and the radial head articular cartilage, which may play a role in the genesis of OCD. Significantly stiffer radial head cartilage compared with the

lateral capitellum creates a mechanical mismatch, which may cause injury to the capitellum that explains the creation of an OCD lesion.[20,30] Some individuals may have a genetic predilection to OCD, as evidenced by reports of bilateral and multiple joint involvement.[10,18] Review of the literature reveals that OCD of the capitellum predominantly affects the dominant arm of Little League male pitchers and helps support an etiology with trauma as a major component[2–4,6,15,22,31–33] High stresses are applied to the elbow during early and late cocking of the throwing cycle. A significant distraction force is applied to the medial aspect of the elbow.[32,34] Compression and shear forces occur at the radiocapitellar articulation in late cocking.[33–37] Reports of OCD in young female gymnasts seems to corroborate this assertion.[2] In gymnastics, the elbow becomes a weight-bearing joint as the radiocapitellar joint transmits 60% of the force across the elbow.[2,38]

The ischemic component is based on Haraldsson's[39] description of the vascular anatomy supplying the distal humerus and in particular the capitellum. The capitellar epiphysis receives blood from only one or two isolated vessels that enter posteriorly and traverse the cartilaginous capitellum. No metaphyseal collateral flow exists, resulting in a tenuous blood supply. Thus, the ability of the epiphysis to heal between traumatic events may be limited, rendering it susceptible to osteonecrosis. The histopathology is more consistent with necrosis than an inflammatory event.[23] Hyperemia and edema are the earliest changes. Loss of subchondral bone support results in articular cartilage breakdown and the formation of loose bodies.[26] Takahara et al[3,15] believe that the new healing subchondral bone exposed to stress will fracture, leading to articular cartilage fragmentation. Furthermore, removal of stress early in the process can prevent progression of the disease.

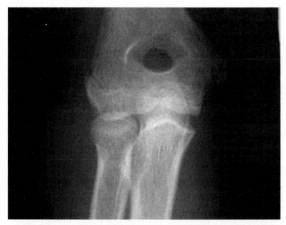

FIGURE 19–1 A 14-year-old female roller hockey player demonstrating capitellar rarefaction of early stable osteochondritis dissecans (OCD) on 45-degree flexion anterior posterior view.

■ History

The typical patient is an adolescent baseball pitcher between 11 and 15 years of age who has been pitching for 3 to 5 years prior to the onset of symptoms.[15] Patients often seek medical attention only after several months of pain.[2,15] Pain is often localized to the lateral aspect of the elbow and relieved by rest. Catching or locking of the elbow are late symptoms and are indicative of articular cartilage fragmentation and loose body formation.[4,15] It is important to note that pain may not be present or may be poorly localized, as the presenting symptoms can be variable and benign in appearance.

■ Examination

Tenderness laterally over the radiocapitellar joint is often present but may be poorly localized. Loss of extension is more common than loss of flexion; however, early in the disease process no motion loss may be present.[15] Provocative maneuvers include the active radiocapitellar compression test,[19] which involves having the patient pronate and supinate the forearm in full extension. Compression across the radiocapitellar joint from muscular forces may reproduce symptoms.[19]

■ Diagnostic Evaluation

Plain radiographs are the initial diagnostic test of choice. Very early in the disease process, radiographs may be negative or show very subtle changes.[15] Anterior-posterior radiographs with the elbow in full extension may not demonstrate the lesion. Takahara et al[3] have shown that obtaining anterior-posterior radiographs in 45 degrees of flexion is more helpful **(Fig. 19–1)**. As the disease progresses, flattening of the capitellar subchondral bone along with subchondral bone rarefaction and isolation of the OCD fragment by the zone of rarefaction are seen and loose body formation occurs.[3,40] The classic lesion occurs on the anterolateral aspect of the capitellum. Widening of the radial head and medial osteophyte formation are seen late in the disease process. The traditional classification on which discussion and treatment have been based is an adaptation of Minami et al's description.[7,41] Lesions are graded on the anterior-posterior view of the elbow and stratified into three grades. Grade I lesions demonstrate a translucent cystic shadow in the lateral or middle capitellum. Grade II lesions demonstrate a clear zone, or a split line is seen between the lesion and the adjacent subchondral bone. Grade III elbows have loose bodies.

Three basic types of lesions have been identified: stable, unstable but attached, unstable and loose (i.e., loose bodies). These types correspond roughly to the radiographic classification. Stable lesions by definition are in situ and have intact articular cartilage. Unstable lesions are those in which the overlying articular cartilage is broken. The lesions may remain attached as in situ unstable lesions or they may detach and become loose bodies.[26,42]

The size of the lesion according to Takahara et al[4] has predictive value and should be evaluated. The defect is sized on the anterior-posterior radiograph as a percent of the entire capitellum **(Fig. 19–2A)**. Additionally, the defect angle can be measured on the lateral x-ray **(Fig. 19–2B)**. A large defect measured >70% with a defect angle of 90 degrees. A small defect measured <55% with a defect angle of <60 degrees. All others were classified as moderate. According to Takahara et al,

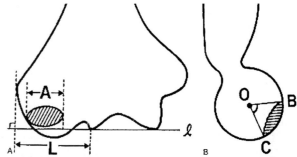

FIGURE 19–2 Diagrams of **(A)** anteroposterior (AP) and **(B)** lateral radiographs showing osteochondral defect in the capitellum. **(A)** Defect size (%) = $A/L \times 100$. A = length (mm) of the osteochondral defect, paralleling the line l; L = length of capitellum (mm). **(B)** Defect angle B = superior aspect, C = inferior aspect of the defect, and O = the center of the capitellum. (From Takahara M, Ogino T, Sasaki I, Kato H, Minami A, Kaneda K. Long term outcome of osteochondritis dissecans of the humeral capitellum. Clin Orthop 1999;363: 108–115, with permission.)

all small lesions do well and all large lesions do poorly. Moderate-size lesions have variable outcome.

In an attempt to elucidate the early pathologic changes in the humeral capitellum, Takahara et al[15] used MRI and ultrasound to evaluate the early changes in OCD, prior to fragmentation. They had minimal radiographic changes best seen on 45 degrees flexion view. Demonstrable changes were seen only on T1-weighted MRI scans and consisted of a low signal intensity at the capitellar surface. In contrast to more advanced lesions no abnormality was seen on T2-weighted images. Ultrasound was used to confirm that capitellar flattening was present. Having the patient refrain from throwing (i.e., the offending force) was necessary to obtain healing. Takahara et al's series was limited to three patients and therefore should be considered presumptive evidence. Early stable lesions can be seen as an increased signal on two-dimensional (2D) fast spin-echo sequences **(Fig. 19–3)**.

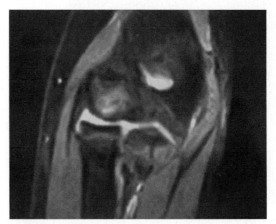

FIGURE 19–3 Magnetic resonance imaging (MRI) (corresponding to x-ray in Fig. 19–1) without contrast of an early stable OCD lesion in an immature elbow.

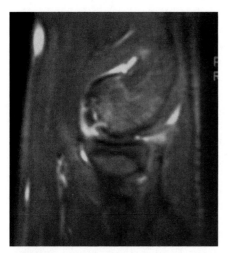

FIGURE 19–4 MRI with intraarticular gadolinium of an unstable OCD lesion in an elbow, sagittal view. Notice dye tracking into subchondral cleft indicating an unstable lesion. (Photo courtesy of Karenze Chan, M.D.)

The normal MRI anatomy of the elbow has been reported as well as the MRI findings in typical OCD of the elbow.[43–47] Loose in situ lesions may be diagnosed by the appearance of a cyst under the lesion.[45] Staging accuracy can be improved with MR arthrography.[48] Intraarticular contrast has been used in an attempt to assess stability of the OCD fragment as it relates to the integrity of the articular surface and loose body formation. Both saline and dilute gadolinium have been used.[47] Dye tracking into the interface between the fragment and proximal bone suggests a break in the articular surface and hence an unstable lesion[44] (**Figs. 19–4** and **19–5**). However, not all loose fragments demonstrate these MRI findings and may be mistaken for a stable fragment.[40]

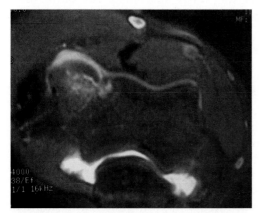

FIGURE 19–5 MRI with intraarticular gadolinium of an unstable OCD lesion in an elbow. Notice the dye tracking between the OCD fragment and the underlying subchondral bone and into the subchondral cleft. Image corresponds to sagittal MRI in Fig. 19–4. (Photo courtesy of Karenze Chan, M.D.)

The use of intravenous gadopentetate-dimeglumine has been described in an attempt to evaluate the stability and viability of attached OCD fragments and may improve the diagnostic and prognostic capabilities of MRI.[40] Fragment enhancement following intravenous contrast (i.e., gadopentetate-dimeglumine) signifies blood supply and hence viability of the fragment. A diffusely enhancing lesion at the fragment subchondral bone interface suggests granulation tissue is present, indicating that the fragment is unstable. This technique, however, has limited potential to assess the integrity of the articular surface in comparison to intraarticular contrast.

A potential MRI pitfall is the pseudodefect of the capitellum that is occasionally mistaken for OCD.[45] The normal articular portion of the capitellum is an anteriorly directed hemisphere. The pseudodefect occurs at the posteroinferior junction of the articular and nonarticular portions for the capitellum.[45,49] True OCD of the capitellum is directed anteriorly.

Computed tomography (CT) arthrography has also been employed with intraarticular gadolinium to evaluate articular cartilage.[28] It is perhaps better than MRI at detecting loose bodies, although relatively less effective at assessing the articular cartilage.

■ Review of the Literature

Interpreting the literature is difficult. Studies often do not distinguish between very early, early, and late presenting OCD. No universally accepted classification exists, and not all studies include MRI findings. In addition, surgical techniques have changed dramatically over the past 15 years. Therefore, comparisons of more recent studies to historical studies are difficult.

Central to the treatment of OCD fragments is their size, stability, viability, and location. To date only one study has addressed the viability of an OCD fragment[40]; these results, however, are preliminary. None of the other larger studies in the literature incorporate this issue into their treatment algorithm. Presumably, a viable fragment would have the best chance of healing.

In 1985, McManama et al[8] reported on 14 adolescents with OCD of the elbow. Thirteen had good or excellent results after loose or attached capitellar segment was removed and shaved to bleeding bone. This was done via a lateral arthrotomy, without an attempt at fixation. The lesions were not sized.

In 1992, Bauer et al[29] reported average 23-year follow-up (range 11 to 35 years) on 31 patients. Eight were less than 16 years of age and 23 were older than 16 years. About half the elbows were symptomatic at follow-up. No stratification was done based on radiographic criteria.

Only six patients had demarcated islands of bone, and 20 had loose bodies. Twenty-three of 31 were treated surgically, 19 for removal of loose bodies. Advanced lesions were seen in over half the cases. A 10-degree flexion and extension loss was noted. Twenty-seven of 31 had increased radial head diameter, and 19 of 31 had signs of degenerative joint disease.

In 1989 Jackson et al reported 10 cases of OCD in female gymnasts. The average age was 12.5 years (range 8–17 years). Nine out of the 10 underwent curettage of loose articular cartilage and drilling of the bed and removal of loose bodies. Follow-up averaged 2.9 years (7 months to 7 years). Only one athlete returned to sports, but participated with discomfort. Average loss of extension was 9 degrees and flexion was 2 degrees. The authors felt that once radiographs are positive and nonoperative treatment fails, surgical intervention can improve symptoms, but return to gymnastics was unlikely.

Peiss et al[40] in 1995 published their initial experience of three patients treated based on an MRI with intravenous gadopentetate-dimeglumine contrast. They felt enhancement of the lesion itself, as opposed to around the lesion, indicated blood supply to the lesion and hence viability. Their article is largely anecdotal, due to the small number of patients involved, but it does raise the question as to whether or not the viability of the fragment should be taken into account when deciding treatment.

Klekamp et al[11] in 1997 published a series of seven cases with an average age of 13 years, in whom OCD of the humeral capitellum led to posterolateral rotatory instability. Treatment involved open reduction and internal fixation with 1.5-mm metal screws. At an average of 3.2 years follow-up, range of motion had improved in extension 17 degrees and the elbows were stable.

Janarv et al[9] reported on 13 consecutive patients who underwent shaving and/or drilling of the OCD bed, and loose body removal was done in 11 of the 13. The patients averaged 13.5 years of age (range 11–16 years), with follow-up of 1.3 years. The lesions measured between 10 and 20 mm, were round, and located on the anterior inferior capitellum and radial head. Procedures were done both open and arthroscopically, and all 13 improved. Twelve returned to their desired level of activity; however, none were gymnasts and five of the 11 treated surgically participated with symptoms. Range of motion improved. The authors noted radial head OCD in combination with capitellar OCD lesions in three of the 13 patients, and one had isolated radial head OCD. MRI detected only two of the four patients with radial head involvement. Preoperative MRIs clearly demonstrated the pathologic cartilage on the capitellum confirmed at the time of surgery. No comment in regard to fragment size, stability, or viability was made. No intravenous contrast was used. In six patients, dorsally based flaps were noted and debrided. Flaps or loose bodies were noted in patients with symptoms of locking and indicated advanced disease.

Ruch et al[6] reported on 12 patients, average age of 14.5 years, who underwent arthroscopic debridement alone. Follow-up was 3.2 years. Flexion contractures improved on average from 23 to 10 degrees. All had remodeling of the capitellum, with five of 12 demonstrating enlargement. Five patients had a triangular avulsion fragment off the lateral condyle that was seen radiographically. Interestingly, this was not demonstrable at arthroscopy but correlated with a poor outcome. Lesions ranged from 0.75 to 4.2 cm^2 with an average square area of 2.5 cm^2. Seven of 12 patients had detached lesions, whereas five had hinged lesions. All lesions were debrided. Total arc of elbow motion improved from 110 to 127 degrees. Flexion contractures improved, on average, from 23 to 11 degrees. All patients demonstrated remodeling of the capitellum.

Baumgarten et al[5] reported an arthroscopic classification (**Fig. 19–6**) based on a review of 17 elbows (16 patients) with an average follow-up of 48 months (range 24–75 months). Average age was not reported. Their classification separated lesions into five categories and gave suggestions regarding treatment based on the grade of the lesion: Type 1 had intact chondral surface, and observation or drilling of lesion was advocated. Type 2 had fissuring of the articular cartilage identified by probing, and treatment involved resection back to stable cartilage. Type 3 had a fragment that was loose on probing, and the fragment was removed with the aid of an osteotome. Type 4 had a grossly loose fragment and was removed. Type 5 had an empty crater that was burred to bleeding bone, and the loose bodies were removed. Lesion size was not mentioned. At follow-up, the average flexion contracture improved from 19 to 5 degrees. Four of the 17 elbows had pain; however, no correlation with the lesion type was made. Two of the nine throwers and one of the five gymnasts did not return to sports. Eight of 17 demonstrated flattening of the capitellum but no degenerative joint disease at 48 months.

Recently, Byrd and Jones[50] reported on 10 patients with 3.9-year follow-up using the above classification. The average age was 13.8 years (range 11–16 years) and were skeletally immature. All patients had pain as a presenting symptom. Loss of extension was more significant (18 degrees) than loss of flexion (11 degrees) when motion loss was a presenting symptom. Four of 10 had locking symptoms at presentation. Objective findings correlated poorly with stage of lesion. The OCD lesion was present on all x-rays. However, the size of the lesion was never reported. All patients were treated arthroscopically and included synovectomy, abrasion chondroplasty, and loose body removal depending on the nature of the

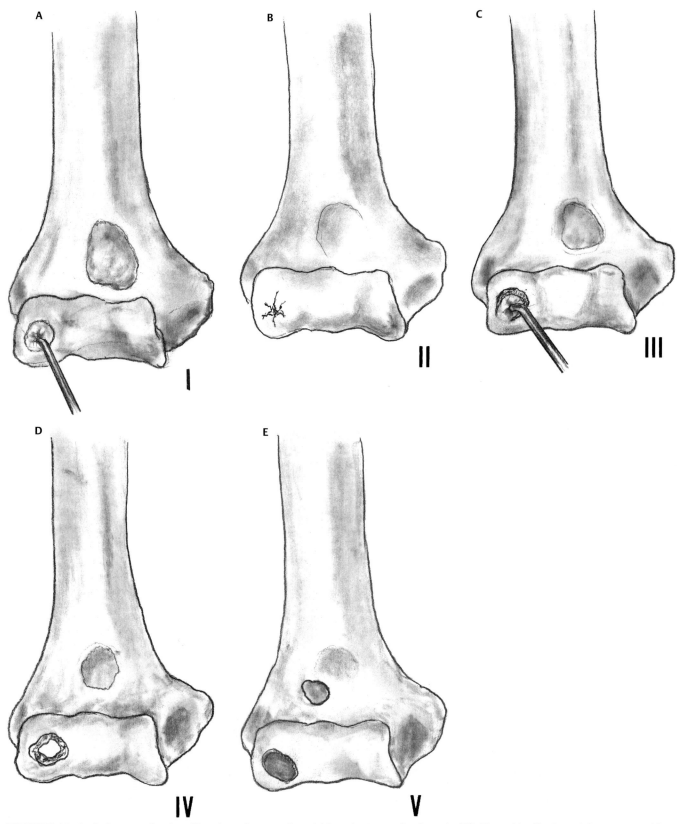

FIGURE 19–6 Arthroscopic classification of osteochondritis dissecans of the capitellum. **(A)** Type I: the cartilage is intact but is soft and ballotable. **(B)** Type II: fissuring of the cartilage. **(C)** Type III: exposed bone with a partially attached osteochondral flap. **(D)** Type IV: completely detached fragment but nondisplaced. **(E)** Type V: displaced fragment with a loose body. (Adapted from Baumgarten T, Andrews J, Satterwhite V. The arthroscopic classification and treatment of osteochondritis dissecans on the capitellum. Am J Sports Med 1998;26:520–523.)

individual lesion. Postoperative results were excellent. However, the follow-up was limited. All patients returned to some competitive sport but only 40% returned to their original sport.

To elucidate the early pathologic changes seen in OCD, Takahara et al[15] in 1998 used MRI and ultrasound to diagnose very early OCD when radiographic changes were subtle. T1-weighted MRI demonstrated a low signal in the superficial aspect of the capitellum, with no demonstrable change on T2-weighted images. The authors felt that this represented the earliest changes seen in OCD of the capitellum. Cessation of pitching in two of the three patients resulted in diminution in symptoms and subsequently normal x-rays and elbow function. The third patient continued to throw and went on to develop classic OCD with a painful elbow. Takahara et al also reported a series of 15 patients, average age of 13.3 years (range 11–16 years) with an average of 5.2 years of follow-up. All patients were advised to stop the inciting trauma for 6 months. At follow-up 17% had no pain, 29% had mild pain with heavy activity, and 54% had pain with activities of daily living. Five of the 11 early lesions, classified by radiographs demonstrating rarefaction and flattening of subchondral bone, improved, demonstrating that there is a propensity to heal early lesions but in only 50% of the cases. All four of the advanced lesions showed no improvement radiographically. More recently, they reported a series of 53 patients, 39 of whom underwent operative and 14 of whom underwent nonoperative treatment.[4] The average age was 16.6 with 12.6-year follow-up. Surgical treatment involved removal of loose bodies and debridement of the fragment. This is the first report to correlate lesion size with outcome. The defect was sized by percent defect size and defect angle **(Fig. 19–7)**. A large

defect measured >70% with a defect angle of 90 degrees. A small defect measured <55% with a defect angle of <60 degrees; all others were classified as moderate. The chronicity of the lesion had no value in predicting outcome as six of 19 early lesions (32%) and 13 of 26 late lesions (50%) had a poor outcome. No very early lesions were reported in this series. Predictors of a poor radiographic outcome included early degenerative joint disease in nine of 14 (64%) as opposed to 10 of 32 (31%) without degenerative joint disease. Defect size correlated with outcome; seven of seven large lesions, six of 19 moderate lesions, and zero of six small lesions had a poor outcome. According to Takahara et al, these results suggest that large lesions should be addressed. They recommended using drilling, reduction and fixation, allograft or autologous chondrocyte implantation.[4,31,51–53]

Oka et al[7] reported on bone peg grafting of an OCD fragment with autologous cortical bone taken from the proximal ulna at the time of open arthrotomy. They classified the lesions using a modification of the Minami classification: Type I lesions showed a translucent window in the lateral or middle capitellum. Type II lesions showed a clear zone or line between the OCD and the capitellar subchondral bone. Type III lesions demonstrated loose bodies. There were 32 patients from 4.8 to 20 years of age. Twenty-one of the 32 patients played baseball. Type I or II lesions occurred in 20 elbows and underwent grafting with two cortical bone pegs, measuring $3 \times 3 \times 30$ mm. A pilot hole was drilled with a 2.5-mm Kirschner wire to a depth of 30 mm. Bone pegs were then tapped into place and sheared flush with the chondral surface. Ten elbows underwent nonoperative treatment initially, four of which later underwent bone peg grafting. Six elbows had a loose body only. Six of the 20 that had bone peg grafting

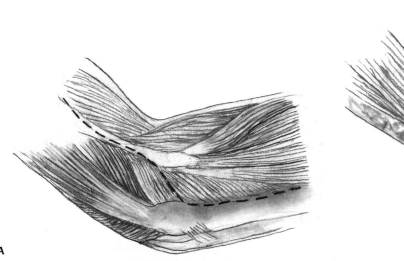
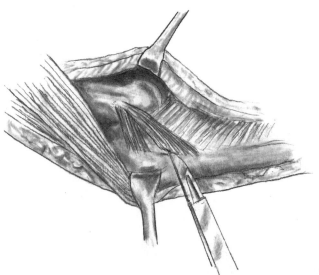

A   B

FIGURE 19–7 Posterior Boyd approach to the capitellum. **(A)** A posterior skin incision is used and deep incision is started from the lateral column and carried distally under the anconeus. **(B)** The lateral collateral ligament complex is then sharply elevated off of the ulna using a sharp blade or needle tip cautery.

(Continued)

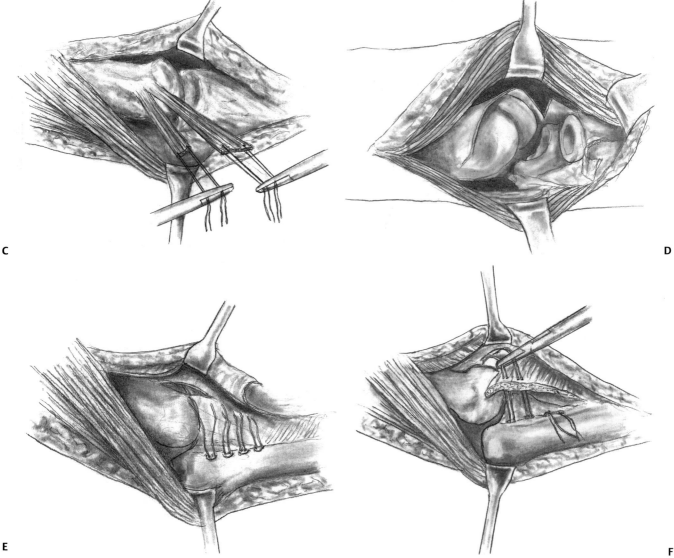

C

D

E

F

FIGURE 19–7 (*Continued*) **(C)** Tagging sutures are placed through the ligament complex. **(D)** By releasing the lateral collateral ligament complex, the radiocapitellar joint can easily be opened allowing easy access to the capitellum.

(E) Once the capitellar lesion is addressed, suture anchors are placed in the ulna along the crista supinatoris. **(F)** The sutures are passed through the ligament complex and repaired back down to the ulna.

also had loose body removal. Range of motion improved 7 degrees in patients who had bone peg grafting only, 15 degrees in patients with combined bone peg grafting and loose body removal, and 8 degrees with loose body removal only. Patients undergoing nonoperative treatment lost 2 degrees. Five of the 10 with nonoperative treatment healed similarly to the patents reported by Takahara et al. Four patients did not improve and subsequently underwent bone peg grafting. Fifteen of the 16 patients with bone pegs healed. Fifteen patients were followed for 5 to 10 years. Radiographs revealed osteoarthritis with spur formation. Bone pegs were used in two type I and six type II lesions. The bone peg group did much better but statistically this was not significant.

Takeda et al[12] reported on a technique using curettage and local bone grafting with removable wire fixation for unstable OCD lesions in 11 skeletally immature baseball players. Average age was 14.7 years and follow-up averaged 57 months. Bony union averaged 17 weeks. Ten of the 11 patients returned to their previous level of activity. The procedure was done through an open lateral approach to the elbow, and required detaching the lateral ulnar collateral ligament complex from the lateral epicondyle. The wire was removed as an outpatient procedure under local anesthesia following bony union.

Harada et al[13] reported on four patients treated with curettage and local bone grafting secured with a compression staple applied from the lateral aspect of the elbow.

Follow-up averaged 7.5 years (range 2–11 years); three of the four were able to return to throwing without pain.

Sato et al[14] recently published a case report on a modification of autologous chondrocyte transplantation described by Brittberg et al.[54] Sato et al implanted a gel impregnated with chondrocytes under a periosteal patch. Follow-up arthroscopy was performed at 3 and 24 months. The patient was pain free and performing activities of daily living without restriction.

■ Treatment Guidelines for Skeletally Immature Athletes

The term *skeletally immature* is variable at a biologic level. It is a continuum, as adolescent athletes mature at different rates. For example, a 14-year-old female athlete who has not started menses is considerably less skeletally mature than another female athlete who has been menstruating for 1½ years despite open growth plates seen on radiographs. There can be big differences in the male population as well. Despite this, some attempt needs to be made to assess skeletal maturity. We have traditionally used radiographs, noting the presence or absence of open physes. But as noted above, the onset of menses as well as the development of secondary sexual characteristics are also helpful but difficult to factor into a treatment regimen. In general, we are less aggressive surgically with skeletally immature patients based on the assumption that there is a greater propensity to heal prior to physeal closure and skeletal maturity.

When treating a young athlete with elbow pain, one must have a high index of suspicion for OCD, particularly if he or she is a baseball pitcher or gymnast. Our approach to this problem is still evolving, as some controversy exists as to the best imaging modality and treatment. The following discussion is intended as a guide, not as the only approach to OCD of the elbow in the immature athlete.

We recommend obtaining anterior-posterior and lateral radiographs of the elbow. Negative radiographs or radiographs with very subtle findings warrant 45-degree flexion anterior-posterior and contralateral views, paying close attention to subtle rarefaction and flattening of the capitellum.[15] In the high-risk athlete, such as a pitcher or gymnast, we obtain an MRI. The use of intravenous and intraarticular contrast depends largely on radiographic findings and symptoms.

Traditional treatment guidelines are based on whether the lesion is intact, partially attached, or completely detached, and is based primarily on radiographic evaluation.[26] We agree with this approach. Information obtained from MRI and in particular intravenous and intraarticular contrast can help guide treatment as these modalities have the potential to pick up unstable lesions that might otherwise be considered stable on conventional radiographs. However, they have not been shown in the literature to have prognostic value, as the reports using these modalities have limited numbers.[15,40] Nevertheless, we feel they are beneficial as they provide information not obtained using conventional radiographs.

We have expanded the traditional classification to include subtyping of type I lesions, and we added a type IV lesion **(Table 19–1)**. Takahara's work suggests that

TABLE 19–1   Classification of Osteochondritis Dissecans of the Capitellum

Type	Radiographs	MRI	Treatment
IA	Normal	Low T1, normal T2	Rest for 6 months
IB flattening ± sclerosis	Capitellar rarefaction	Increased T2	Immobilize × 3 weeks, rest × 6 months, surgery if not improved
II	Clear zone between OCD fragment and subchondral bone	Fluid between OCD and subchondral bone	If stable (hinged): internal fixation
III	Loose body	Loose body	Loose body removal, fixation of fragment if large, removal and curettage of base (±microfracture) if not able to fix
IV	Capitellar and radial head involvement	Capitellar and radial head involvement	Address both sides; see text for details

Based on Oka Y, Ohta K, Fukuda H. Bone peg grafting for osteochondritis dissecans of the elbow. Int Orthop 1999;23:53–57; and Takahara M, Ogino T, Sasaki I, Kato H, Minami A, Kaneda K. Long term outcome of osteochondritis dissecans of the humeral capitellum. Clin Orthop 1999;363:108–115.

with the advent of MRI, there is a subset of early lesions, with essentially normal or nearly normal radiographs, that can be identified by MRI or ultrasound early enough so that nonoperative treatment has a better prognosis.[15] For this reason we divide type I lesions into A and B subtypes. Type IA lesions represent those lesions with essentially normal radiographs and MRI findings of low signal on T1-weighted images and normal T2-weighted images consistent with very early OCD. Type IB lesions have the more classic radiographic findings of early OCD with capitellar rarefaction, flattening, or sclerosis, and MRI findings of classic OCD with increased signal on T2-weighted images. The recognition of associated radial head lesions warrants, in our opinion, expanding the traditional classification to take into account these "bipolar" lesions.[9] Because this adds a dimension of difficulty in treating patients and likely represents a more advanced lesion, we designated it a type IV lesion. This modification of the traditional classification has been presented elsewhere.[55]

Treatment should take into account many variables, including skeletal maturity, size of lesion, the stability or presumed stability, viability of the fragment, the presence or absence of mechanical symptoms, and response to nonoperative treatment. Lastly, the precise surgical intervention will be made on the merits of the capitellum and overlying articular cartilage seen at surgery. No one piece of information or test can be used to make treatment decisions. The following discussion is a guideline for treatment and has been put in table and algorithm form (**Table 19–1** and **Fig. 19–8**). This does not represent the only approach to this problem.

Type IA: Very Early Lesions

These lesions have essentially normal or near normal radiographs. The diagnosis is confirmed by MRI, which demonstrates a low signal in the superficial capitellum on T1-weighted images and normal T2-weighted images.[15] If an OCD is picked up at this point, we feel that it represents a very early lesion and is therefore stable and the capitellum is viable. Contrast is unlikely to be helpful as the capitellar viability is high. This subset is likely to do well with nonoperative treatment alone. A near-normal joint may result. Treatment includes activity modification, that is, complete cessation of the inciting trauma. Strengthening is begun once symptoms have abated. The athlete is not returned to sports for at least 6 months and then only if symptoms have completely resolved. Follow-up radiographs at 3 and 6 months are obtained to assess progression. Follow-up may be required for a period of years. Pitchers are counseled to stop pitching but may return to another fielding position. Gymnastics is more difficult as the elbow becomes a weight-bearing joint, and there is no op-

tion to return to a modified program and remain highly competitive. Return to sports is predicated on symptoms, as radiographic changes may be present for years.[3,15,26] We monitor these patients very carefully. Return of symptoms warrants additional time off from sports. Patients with a normal T1-weighted MRI scan do not return to sports activities until resolution of symptoms, as the diagnosis is likely a soft tissue overuse injury, such as lateral epicondylitis.

Type IB: Early Lesions

Athletes with early lesions demonstrate the more classic early findings of OCD on radiographs, such as capitellar rarefaction, mild flattening, and sclerosis. Once obvious radiographic findings are apparent, we feel it is important to assess the stability and viability of the fragment. Type IB lesions are at risk for articular cartilage breakdown and fragment instability. Mechanical symptoms, however, are notably absent. Therefore, these patients also undergo an MRI. A conventional MRI is adequate for assessing subchondral cysts and fluid, which would indicate an unstable lesion. However, it is in this setting that intravenous contrast and intraarticular contrast have potentially the most benefit. Although neither is mandatory, we have traditionally favored the use of intraarticular contrast. Dye leaking between the fragment and adjacent subchondral bone suggests an unstable lesion and hence a break in the articular cartilage. However, an argument can be made for using intravenous contrast, in which case enhancement as a halo around the fragment suggests perifragment scarring and hence instability of the lesion. Enhancement of the lesion itself suggests viability. In the situation that the MRI demonstrates no instability and viability of the fragment, the arm is immobilized for no more than 3 weeks to allow any acute symptoms to resolve. Following this, we institute the aforementioned physical therapy with the initial goal of obtaining full range of motion. Patients are followed clinically, and radiographs are obtained at 3-month intervals to evaluate progression of healing. Return to play is predicated on resolution of symptoms, but a minimum of 6 months of rest is instituted. Patients are counseled as to the long-term implications of this problem and the unpredictability of nonoperative treatment.

Patients who have failed 6 months of nonoperative treatment, as defined by persistent symptoms of pain, or who have demonstrable instability of the OCD fragment on MRI, undergo surgical intervention. We recommend arthroscopy first, and if necessary, conversion to an open procedure through an anterolateral approach. The actual procedure performed and the method by which it is done, that is, open or arthroscopic, depend on the nature of the lesion and the surgeon's skill. Very small lesions will probably do well, irrespective of the treatment. Lesions measuring less than 55% of the

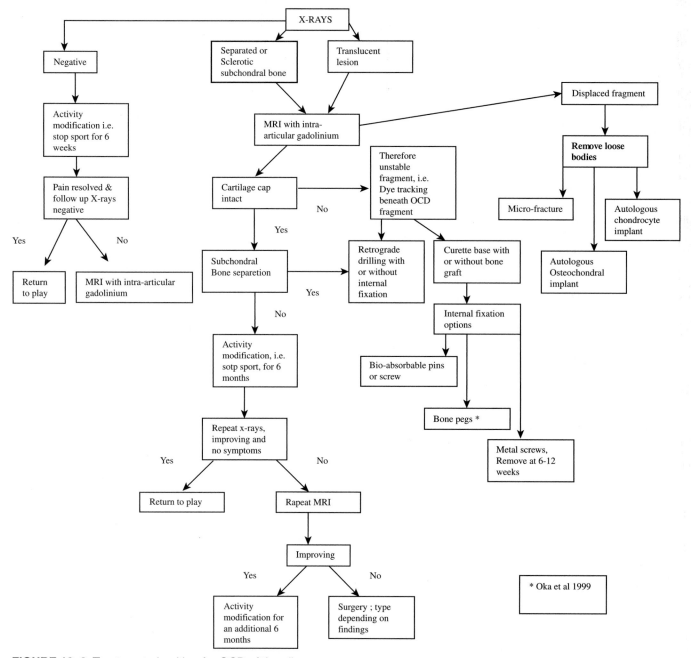

FIGURE 19–8 Treatment algorithm for OCD of the elbow.

capitellum with less than a 60-degree defect angle should undergo subchondral drilling as described by Bradley and Dandy.[31] Damaged articular cartilage should be debrided to bone with stable articular cartilage edges. We do not recommend the use of thermal techniques as recent evidence suggests this may be detrimental to remaining chondrocytes (James P. Bradley, M.D., personal communication).

In medium-sized defects, the status of the overlying articular cartilage and the integrity of the underlying bone determine the treatment. We attempt to internally fix acute lesions if possible. Chronic defects with fragmentation are debrided. Subchondral drilling or microfracture may also be performed. Internal fixation can be considered in some of these lesions with a single fragment. Acceptable choices include metal screws, bioabsorbable screws, cortical bone pegs, and pull-out wires. Machined allograft cortical screws are now available and raise the possibility of compression with biointegration. We have no experience using these devices. We prefer metal or bioabsorbable implants; however, concern over the absorption of bioabsorbable devices across an area with unequal blood flow has limited their use, along with the difficulty in obtaining compression. Osteochondral autograft transplantation is considered. The relative risks and benefits make it difficult to make a definitive recommendation in this population. It is reasonable to consider a two-staged treatment program based on clinical follow-up. If patients continue to have symptoms at 6 to 9 months following debridement and subchondral drilling or microfracture, then consideration is given to additional intervention in the form of osteochondral autograft or autologous chondrocyte implantation.

Large defects measuring greater than 70% of the anterior-posterior capitellar dimension and greater than 90 degrees on the lateral have a poorer long-term outcome.[4,15] With these large defects particularly with subchondral bone loss, we attempt to reconstitute the capitellum. In some cases, a large fragment remains hinged and attached. The sclerotic bone bed is debrided with a curette. This is done in an open fashion. Autograft cancellous bone is obtained from the ulna and packed into the defect. Metal compression screws are used to secure the fragment. The patient is followed with serial radiographs to ensure reformation of subchondral bone. Removable wires can also be used.[12] Screws are removed 3 to 5 months later. Alternatively, bioabsorbable screws can be used, in which case removal is typically not necessary. However, obtaining compression can be difficult. Headless variable pitch metal screws are available and allow for compression, and they represent another option, although we have not used them. Comminuted fragmented OCD lesions are debrided. Immediate consideration is given to autograft osteochondral transplantation, particularly if significant subchondral bone loss is present. Recently, synthetic grafts (Osteobiologics Inc., San Antonio, TX) have been developed for bone and articular cartilage, raising the possibility of addressing these lesions without donor-site morbidity. We have no experience using these grafts and no clinical studies have been published, but the animal studies are encouraging. This procedure is done in an open fashion. It is difficult to obtain congruency of the joint. However, it must be kept in mind that this is a salvage situation. We have not used allograft, autologous chondrocyte implantation,[54] or tissue engineered cartilage,[14] although these remain viable alternatives.

Surgical Technique

Open Technique

The patient is placed in a supine position. A lateral incision is made and the Kocher interval is entered. [*Editor's note*: The book editor uses the posterior Boyd[56] approach to gain access to the capitellum **(Fig. 19–7).**] Either a lateral or a posterior incision is made. The deeper incision is started from the lateral column proximally and taken distally posterior to (under) the anconeus. This is different from the Kocher approach, which enters the interval between the anconeus and extensor carpi ulnaris. Next, the insertion of the lateral collateral ligament complex onto the ulna, including the annular ligament, is subperiosteally elevated off of bone (crista supinatoris). Tagging sutures are placed in the ligament for future repair back down to bone. By the surgeon's supinating the patient's forearm and flexing the elbow, the radial head can be subluxated laterally, facilitating access to the capitellum. At this point, either an osteochondral transfer or an autologous chondrocyte implantation procedure can be performed. Once the procedure is completed, three to four suture anchors are placed into the ulna, and the lateral collateral ligament is repaired back down to the ulna. [The book editor prefers 3.5-mm metal corkscrew anchors loaded with No. 2 Fiberwire suture (Arthrex, Naples, FL).]

Type II

These lesions are distinguished from type IB lesions by more advanced changes on x-ray and in particular a sclerotic margin around a well-defined fragment. In reality this distinction is extremely difficult, and the two lesions are approached in essentially the same manner. Mechanical symptoms may be present from a loose attached lesion. They are distinguished from type III lesions by the lack of loose bodies. Similar to the management of type IB lesions, an MRI is obtained. In our opinion type II lesions are more likely to be unstable and lack viability. We favor intravenous contrast or intraarticular contrast over conventional MRI. Patients with mechanical symptoms or lesions demonstrating instability on MRI are in our opinion unlikely to heal. We are surgically more aggressive with this population of patients. Surgical intervention is essentially the same as that employed for type IB lesions. Hinged fragments are left attached if large enough to accept internal fixation. The subchondral bed is curetted and bone grafted usually from the proximal ulna. Internal fixation is then used. We recommend routinely removing headed metal screws. Enhancing lesions with evidence of instability have not been encountered in our experience, neither has it been reported in the literature.

Type III Chronic Lesions with Loose Bodies

The presence of loose bodies usually indicates a long-standing lesion, although acute dislodging of an in situ lesion can occur. Diagnostic workup proceeds in the same manner as for types IB and II lesions. Intraarticular contrast is helpful in detecting loose bodies and as such may have benefit over intravenous contrast. Most authors agree that removal of loose bodies is indicated, and there is no role for reduction and internal fixation. There is no consensus regarding reduction and internal fixation of an acutely dislodged fragment. However, we would favor fixation depending on the size, location, and integrity of the fragment and if the acuteness of the injury could be well established. Chronic loose bodies are removed. Treatment of the capitellar lesion is based on the principles of treating unstable types IB and II lesions. Patients and family should be counseled appropriately as to the expected outcome. We do not recommend returning patients to sports.

Type IV Associated Radial Head Osteochondral Defects

Radial head lesions occasionally accompany the more common capitellar lesions.[9] We have not had the occasion to treat this combination of injury. As in the knee, this represents a bipolar lesion, and it makes treatment more difficult. Obtaining access to the face of the radial heads is difficult without dislocating the elbow. The value of reconstituting the articular surface of the capitellum in this setting is unknown. If the radial head lesion is small, we would favor treating the capitellar lesion. There is no consensus as to what "small" constitutes, but less than 30% of the articular surface is probably reasonable. With large degenerative bipolar lesions, simple debridement, curettage, and subchondral drilling or microfracture is likely to be more prudent, although we have no experience in this setting. In those patients with severe advanced degenerative changes at the radiocapitellar joint, particularly in adulthood, consideration is given to radial head excision.

■ Treatment Guidelines for Skeletally Mature Athletes

Our approach is essentially the same in the skeletally mature athlete. However, once early degenerative changes occur, we advise our patients that early arthritis is likely to occur. Nonoperative treatment is less likely to be effective, and surgical intervention is consider early in the treatment regimen.

Our approach to the focal lesion attempts to take into account the size and depth location and acuteness of the lesion. Most of these lesions are chronic, and thus

open reduction and internal fixation of the acute dislodged OCD is not done. We try to stair-step the approach beginning with subchondral drilling or microfracture for small lesions. We avoid abrasion chondroplasty in an attempt to maintain some of the subchondral plate if possible. With medium-size and large lesions, consideration is given to osteochondral transplantation using fresh-frozen allograft or autograft from the lateral aspect of the ipsilateral knee. Autologous chondrocyte implantation (ACI) can certainly be considered, but we have no experience with this procedure in the elbow.

■ Future Directions

There are several current controversies in the diagnosis and treatment of OCD of the humeral capitellum. The use of intravenous or intraarticular gadolinium to assess fragment viability and stability remains a subject of debate. We have no experience with intravenous gadolinium. Currently, intraarticular contrast is favored in the United States. Traditional treatment consists primarily of removal of loose bodies and debridement of the lesion.[26] This approach is supported by the literature. However, most of the studies this approach is based on have not used newer diagnostic or treatment modalities. More research needs to be done to determine whether accurate prognostic data can be obtained from intravenous contrast as it relates to fragment viability. Just because a fragment enhances does this mean it is viable? Can it be treated nonoperatively? Or is there another variable such as size in conjunction with gadolinium enhancement that should dictate treatment?

Moreover, once operative treatment has been selected what factors should dictate the procedure used? If fixation is selected should metal, bone, or a bioabsorbable device be used? Each has a particular advantage and disadvantage. We have concerns regarding the use of bioabsorbable devices for articular cartilage injuries. In theory degradation could occur from proximal to distal. When the humeral aspect of the screw has resorbed, the OCD part of the screw may still be present. As such there is the potential for developing an intraarticular loose body or simply loosening of the fragment. To our knowledge, this issue has not been addressed by the manufacturers producing these devices, nor has it been addressed in the orthopaedic literature. This concern may be overstated, as most of the bioabsorbable devices are degraded by hydrolysis and should degrade in synovial fluid. Recently, however, MRI evidence has surfaced corroborating this potential pitfall in the knee, although it remains anecdotal (Dr. Christopher Harner, personal communication). Cortical bone pegs provide an alternative that would allow all biologic fixation presumably without the need for removal.[7] No compression can be obtained with this method, and additional dissection is needed to harvest the grafts. However, with the anatomy of the elbow, compression may not be a major issue as muscle forces acting through the radial head may provide enough compression. Cortical screws machined from cadaveric cortical bone can potentially provide compression and allow for biointegration as they incorporate as bone. Such screws would have to be advanced to at least the level of the OCD fragment calcified cartilage layer. They are, however, expensive, and some surgeons believe the use of allograft tissue in adolescents is undesirable. Furthermore, the screws do not have a variable pitch, so the amount of compression is likely to be minimal, and they are headed screws similar to traditional screw designs and have the potential to be prominent. The distinction between bioabsorption and biointegration is a subtle but potentially important point that may direct future research. The ideal fixation device is one that incorporates into bone, allows for compression, and is inexpensive.

The location and presence of bipolar lesions are largely ignored in most series. Does having an associated radial head OCD affect outcome? And if so, what is the ideal treatment in this setting?

The future of treating established lesions with some osteochondral replacement remains the objective of operative intervention. Sellers et al[57] improved treatment of articular cartilage defects with a recombinant human bone morphogenic protein-2 (rh-BMP-2)-impregnated collagen sponge in New Zealand white rabbits. One year follow-up demonstrated that the repair process held up with time and had improved the graft–host cartilage interface, one of the most difficult areas to address. Potential future options include chondrocyte-impregnated collagen gels. Recently synthetic grafts have been developed to address both bone and articular cartilage defects. These grafts are composed of various polymers (Osteobiologics Inc., San Antonio, TX) may prove beneficial in the treatment of OCD by avoiding the morbidity associated with osteochondral transplant procedures.

■ Conclusion

Osteochondritis dissecans of the humeral capitellum remains a difficult problem to treat. Controversy still exists with respect to the optimal treatment of loose in situ lesions (i.e., loose but attached). Rest is the treatment of choice for very early lesions, and studies suggest that if diagnosed early enough, a near-normal elbow can result.[15] However, early detection and intervention remain difficult as early OCD may or may not present with pain and discomfort significant enough for the athlete to seek medical attention early enough in the process where intervention has a pre-

dictably positive outcome. Nevertheless, elbow pain in the at-risk athlete, such as a baseball pitcher or gymnast, should raise the suspicion of an OCD. Radiographs may be unrevealing or show very subtle changes. Contralateral elbow views are very helpful. The advent of MRI now allows the practicing orthopaedic surgeon to effectively assess very early lesions that might otherwise be missed on x-ray.

With more advanced lesions, x-ray findings are more obvious and demonstrate the more classical capitellar fragment with a surrounding zone of lucency. MRI in this setting is helpful in assessing the overlying articular cartilage and hence the stability of the fragment. In this setting, prior to obvious loose bodies or mechanical symptoms, rest is the first step in the treatment algorithm. If symptoms persist, then operative intervention is indicated. About half of these patients heal with nonoperative treatment. Pretreatment assessment of fragment viability has not traditionally been incorporated into the treatment algorithm. Recent anecdotal evidence suggests that not only stability but viability of a fragment can be assessed using intravenous contrast. Knowledge of the fragment viability may allow distinction between those lesions likely to heal without surgical intervention versus those requiring surgical intervention.

Most authors would agree that there is no role currently for reduction and fixation of long-standing free loose bodies. There is no consensus regarding acute dislodging of an in situ loose fragment.

Long-term results, after radiographic changes are present, suggest a degenerative course in about half the patients. Whether or not newer techniques to address osteochondral defects will have an effect on the natural history remains to be seen.

REFERENCES

1. Paré A. *Oeuvres Completes,* vol. 3. Paris J.B. Ballière, 1840–1841:32
2. Jackson D, Silvino N, Reimen P. Osteochondritis in the female gymnast's elbow. Arthroscopy 1989;5:129–136
3. Takahara M, Ogino T, Fukushima S, Tsuchida H, Kaneda K. Nonoperative treatment of osteochondritis dissecans of the humeral capitellum. Am J Sports Med 1999;27:728–732
4. Takahara M, Ogino T, Sasaki I, Kato H, Minami A, Kaneda K. Long term outcome of osteochondritis dissecans of the humeral capitellum. Clin Orthop 1999;363:108–115
5. Baumgarten T, Andrews J, Satterwhite V. The arthroscopic classification and treatment of osteochondritis dissecans on the capitellum. Am J Sports Med 1998;26:520–523
6. Ruch D, Cory J, Poehling G. The arthroscopic management of osteochondritis dissecans of the adolescent elbow. Arthroscopy 1998;14:797–803
7. Oka Y, Ohta K, Fukuda H. Bone peg grafting for osteochondritis dissecans of the elbow. Int Orthop 1999;23:53–57
8. McManama GB Jr, Micheli LJ, Berry MV, Sohn RS. The surgical treatment of osteochondritis of the capitellum. Am J Sports Med 1985;13:11–21

9. Janarv P-M, Hesser U, Hirsch G. Osteochondral lesions in the radiocapitellar joint in the skeletally immature: radiographic, MRI, and arthroscopic findings in 13 consecutive cases. J Pediatr Orthop 1997;17:311–314

10. Inoue G. Bilateral osteochondritis dissecans of the elbow treated by Herbert screw fixation. Br J Sports Med 1991;25:142–144

11. Klekamp J, Green N, Mencio G. Osteochondritis dissecans as a cause of developmental dislocation of the radial head. Clin Orthop Relat Res 1997;338:36–41

12. Takeda H, Watari K, Matsushita T, Saito T, Terashima Y. A surgical treatment for unstable osteochondritis dissecans lesions of the humeral capitellum in adolescent players. Am J Sports Med 2002;30:713–717

13. Harada M, Ogino T, Takahara M, Ishigaki D, Kashiwa H, Kanauchi Y. Fragment fixation with a bone graft and dynamic staples for osteochondritis dissecans of the humeral capitellum. J Shoulder Elbow Surg 2002;11:368–372

14. Sato M, Ochi M, Uchio Y, Agung M, Baba H. Transplantation of tissue-engineered cartilage for excessive osteochondritis dissecans of the elbow. J Shoulder Elbow Surg 2004;13:221–225

15. Takahara M, Shundo M, Kondo M, Suzuki K, Nambu T, Ogino T. Early detection of osteochondritis dissecans of the capitellum in young baseball players. Report of three cases. J Bone Joint Surg 1998;80-A:892–897

16. Vanthournout I, Rudelli A, Valenti P, Montagne JP. Osteochondritis of the trochlea of the humerus. Pediatr Radiol 1991;21: 600–601

17. Chess T. Osteochondritis. In: Savoie F, ed. Arthroscopy of the Elbow. New York: Churchill-Livingstone, 1996:77–86

18. Bednarz P, Paletta GJ, Stanitski C. Bilateral osteochondritis dissecans of the knee and elbow. Orthopedics 1998;21:716–717

19. Peterson R, Savoie F, Field L. Osteochondritis dissecans of the elbow. Instr Couse Lecture 1999;48:393–398

20. Schenck R. Current concepts review: osteochondritis dissecans. J Bone Joint Surg 1996;78-A:439–455

21. König F. Ueber freie köper in den gelenken. Deutsche Zeitchr Chir 1887;27:90–109

22. Schenck RJ, Goodnight J. Osteochondritis dissecans. J Bone Joint Surg 1996;78-A:439–456

23. Nagura S. The so-called osteochondritis dissecans of König. Clin Orthop 1960;18:100–122

24. Panner HJ. A peculiar affection of the capitellum humeri, resembling Calve-Perthes disease of the hip. Acta Radiol 1927;8:617–618

25. Omer GE Jr. Primary articular osteochondroses. Clin Orthop Relat Res 1981;158:33–40

26. Shaughnessy W. Osteochondritis dissecans. In: Morrey B, ed. The Elbow and Its Disorders. Philadelphia: W.B. Saunders, 2000: 255–260

27. Vispo-Seara J, Loehr JF, Krauspe R, Gomlke F, Eulert J. Osteochondritis dissecans in children and adolescents. J Shoulder Elbow Surg 1995;4:S21

28. Holland P, Davies A, Cassar-Pulucino V. Computerized tomographic arthrography in the assessment of OCD of the elbow. Clin Radiol 1994;49:231–235

29. Bauer M, Jonsson K, Josefsson PO, Linden B. Osteochondritis dissecans of the elbow. A long term followup study. Clin Orthop Relat Res 1992;284:156–160

30. Schenck RJ, Athanasiou KA, Constantinides G, Gomez E. A biomechanical analysis of articular cartilage of the human elbow and potential relationship to osteochondritis dissecans. Clin Orthop Relat Res 1994;299:305–312

31. Bradley J, Dandy D. Results of drilling osteochondritis skeletal maturity. J Bone Joint Surg 1989;71-B:642–644

32. Hunter S. Little League elbow. In: Zarins B, Andrews J, Carson W, eds. Injuries to the Throwing Arm. Philadelphia: W.B. Saunders, 1985

33. Jobe F, Nuber G. Throwing injuries of the elbow. Clin Sports Med 1986;5:621–636

34. Indelicato P, Jobe F, Kerlin R. Correctable elbow lesions in professional baseball players. Am J Sports Med 1979;7:72–79

35. King J, Brelsford H, Tullos H. Analysis of the pitching arm of the professional baseball pitcher. Clin Ortho Relat Res 1969;67: 116–123

36. Tullos HS, Erwin WD, Woods GW, Wukasch DC, Cooley DA, King JW. Unusual lesions of the pitching arm. Clin Orthop RelatRes 1972;88:169–182

37. Tullos H, King J. Lesions of the pitching are in adolescents. JAMA 1972;220:264–271

38. Singer K, Roy S. Osteochondrosis of the humeral capitellum. Am J Sports Med 1984;12:351–360

39. Haraldsson S. On osteochondrosis deformans juvenilis capituli humeri including investigation of intra-osseous vasulature in the distal humersu. Acta Orthop Scand 1959;38(suppl):1–232

40. Peiss J, Adam G, Casser R, Urhahn R, Gunther RW. Gadopentate-dimeglumine-enhanced MRI imaging of osteonecrosis osteochondritis dissecans of the elbow: initial and experience. Skeletal Radiol 1995;24:17–20

41. Minami M, Nakashita K, Ishii S, Usui M, Muramatsu I. Twenty-five cases of osteochondritis dissecans of the elbow. Rinsho Seikei Geka 1979;14:805–810

42. Bradley J. Upper extremity: elbow injuries in children and adolescents. In: Stanitski C, De Lee J, Drez DJ, eds. Orthopaedic Sports Medicine Practice and Principles. Philadelphia: W.B. Saunders, 1994:242–261

43. Bunnell DH, Fisher DA, Bassett LW, Gold RH, Ellman H. Elbow joint: normal anatomy on MR images. Radiology 1987;165:527

44. Fritz R, Steinbach L. Magnetic resonance imaging of the musculoskeletal system. Part 3. The elbow. Clin Orthop Relat Res 1996;324:321–339

45. Fritz RC. MR imaging of osteochondral and articular lesions. MRI Clin North Am 1997;5:579–602

46. Middleton W, Macrander S, Kneeland JB, Froncisz W, Jesmanowicz A, Hyde JS. MR imaging of the normal elbow: anatomic correlations. Am J Radiol 1987;149:543–547

47. Steinbach LS, Fritz RC, Tirman PF, Uffman M. Magnetic resonance imaging of the elbow. Eur J Radiol 1997;25:223–241

48. Kramer J, Stiglbauer R, Engel A. MR Contrast (MRA) in osteochondritis dissecans. J Comput Assist Tomogr 1992;16: 254–260

49. Rosenberg Z, Beltran J, Cheng Y. Pseudodefect of the capitellum: potential MR imaging pitfall. Radiology 1994;191:821–823

50. Byrd JWT, Jones K. Arthroscopic surgery for isolated capitellar osteochondritis dissecans in adolescent baseball players. Am J Sports Med 2002;30:474–478

51. Cugat R, Garua M, Cuscuo X. Osteochondritis dissecans: a historical review and its treatment with cannulated screws. Arthroscopy 1993;9:675–684

52. Brittberg M, Lindahl A, Nilsson A. Treatment of deep cartilage defects in the knee with autologous chondrocyte implantation. N Engl J Med 1994;331:889–895

53. Caplan A, Elyaderani M, Mochizuki Y. Principles of cartilage repair and regeneration. Clin Orthop Relat Res 1997;342: 254–269

54. Brittberg M, Lindahl A, Nilsson A, Ohlsson C, Isaksson O, Peterson L. Treatment of deep cartilage defect in the knee with autologous chondrocyte transplantation. N Engl J Med 1994;331: 889–895

55. Bradley J, Petrie R. Osteochondritis dissecans of the humeral capitellum. In: Miller M, ed. Clinics in Sports Medicine. New York: W.B. Saunders, 2002

56. Boyd HB. Surgical exposure of the ulna and proximal third of the radius through one incision. Surg Gynecol Obstet 1940;71:86–88

57. Sellers RS, Zhang R, Glasson SS, et al. Repair of articular cartilage defects one year after treatment with recombinant human bone morphogenetic protein-2 (RHBMP-2). J Bone Joint Surg 2000;82-A:151–160

20

Cartilage Injuries in the Shoulder

JEFF A. FOX, BRIAN J. COLE, TAMARA K. PYLAWKA, AND ANTHONY A. ROMEO

Localized articular cartilage lesions of the glenohumeral joint in young athletes are a rare occurrence and are generally well tolerated. When symptomatic, however, they can be quite painful and limiting. Treatment recommendations remain difficult because there is little information to glean from our experience or from the literature to guide the decision-making process. Clearly, some analogies can be extrapolated from a relatively mature treatment algorithm used to treat chondral injury of the knee.[1–4] At this juncture, however, the application of existing and emerging technologies is largely anecdotal or relegated to case reports. This chapter provides the orthopaedic surgeon with guidance in treating these problems by summarizing the information available on this topic, and discusses how contemporary treatment in other joints may be applicable to the glenohumeral joint. This chapter does not address degenerative arthritis as seen in older individuals.

■ Classification and Etiology

There is no classification scheme designed specifically to describe articular cartilage lesions in the shoulder. The Outerbridge system[5] is one classification system commonly used in the knee and is acceptable for use in the shoulder as a tool to describe the general appearance of a chondral lesion. Grade 0 is normal cartilage, grade I is articular cartilage softening, grade II is fibrillation involving half the depth of the articular surface, grade III is fissur-ing involving more than half the depth of the articular surface, and grade IV is full-thickness loss reaching to or through the subchondral bone. Other factors such as location (glenoid or humerus), position (central or peripheral), size, degree of containment, depth (chondral or osteochondral), etiology (avascular necrosis, localized degenerative or posttraumatic), and defects that develop following surgical intervention (i.e., shoulder stabilization) also factor into the decision-making process and provide a common language to communicate the nature of these lesions.

■ Incidence

The incidence of articular cartilage lesions in the shoulder is unknown. Due to issues related to impact loading and weight bearing, one would expect it to occur less frequently than in the knee joint. It is probable that articular cartilage lesions of the glenohumeral joint are more likely to remain asymptomatic and quiescent relative to their counterparts that occur in the knee and therefore are more likely to remain unrecognized clinically. The authors believe that the incidence of these lesions in the knee is at best considered a worst-case scenario of what might be occurring in the shoulder.

Curl et al[6] reviewed 31,516 knee arthroscopies. They reported on the incidence of grade III lesions (41%) and grade IV lesions (19%). In patients less than 40 years of age, the incidence of grade IV lesions was only 5%. Hjelle et al[7] performed a prospective study consisting of 1000 patients and similarly found a 5% incidence of grades III and IV chondral defects. It must be understood that only a small percentage of these lesions were clinically symptomatic requiring treatment.

One small study using magnetic resonance arthrography (MRA) found glenohumeral cartilage lesions in up to one third of patients.[8] Some studies describe the incidence of chondral injury in association with specific pathology. In a cadaveric study, Hsu et al[9] demonstrated that the area of articular cartilage damage to the glenoid and humeral head in specimens with associated rotator cuff tears was 32% and 36%, respectively. This compared with 6% in the glenoid and 7% in the humeral head in specimens without rotator cuff tears. The location of the degeneration tended to be in the anterioinferior glenoid and posterior humeral head, and the degree of damage in the glenoid was correlated with that of the humeral head. Gartsman and Taverna[10] identified only nine significant cartilage lesions (grade IV) in 200 arthroscopies (4.5%) in association with full-thickness rotator cuff tears as incidental intraarticular abnormalities at the time of rotator cuff repair.

The incidence of chondral injury in patients with shoulder instability is well documented. Recently, Werner et al[11] demonstrated that patients with traumatic and atraumatic shoulder instability who came to surgery had approximately an 80% incidence of Hill-Sachs lesions in addition to chondral damage of the glenoid in many instances. Typically, in patients with atraumatic shoulder instability who respond to therapy, the incidence of Hill-Sachs lesions is significantly lower compared with patients with traumatically induced shoulder instability. In first-time traumatic dislocators, Taylor and Arciero[12] reported that 90% of the patients had a Hill-Sachs lesion, with 40% classified as a chondral lesion and 60% classified as an osteochondral lesion. In a large retrospective review published by Cameron et al,[13] the extent and presence of grade III and IV damage was associated with the time from injury to surgery. Patients with glenohumeral chondral damage were also significantly older than those without chondral damage (34.9 years versus 29.6 years). Hintermann and Gachter[14] reported a 23% incidence of glenoid and 8% incidence of humeral head degenerative arthritis in patients who sustained only one dislocation. This compared with a 36% incidence of humeral head and 27% incidence of glenoid degenerative arthritis in patients who sustained two or more dislocations.

The natural history of these lesions with or without associated pathology is completely unknown. The senior author (B.J.C.) believes that most chondral and osteochondral injuries of the glenohumeral joint are well tolerated. However, once they become symptomatic, they are unlikely to revert back to a quiescent state without effective treatment.

■ Patient Evaluation

A thorough history and physical examination is the first step in the decision-making process. The mechanism of injury and the chronicity of the symptoms are the initial factors determining the etiology of the patient's symptoms. A history of direct shoulder trauma, traumatic or atraumatic glenohumeral instability, or previous intraarticular surgery is a relevant issue to -explore. Patients may complain of mechanical symptoms, aching that may vary with barometric pressure change, discomfort at night, difficulty sleeping on the affected side, and pain with glenohumeral motion during activities of daily living. It is important that the surgeon obtain a realistic appraisal of the quality and severity of the patient's symptoms and discuss with the patient to what extent these symptoms interfere with daily activities as well as with higher level demands such as recreational or competitive sports. More than any other variable, managing patient expectations is critical to the ultimate success of the intervention chosen.

Physical examination includes assessment for atrophy, active and passive motion, scapulothoracic dyskinesis, stability testing, special testing to assess for labral pathology, and compression-rotation testing to assess for mechanical symptoms and pain. Unlike patients with osteoarthritis, these patients rarely have significant limitations in passive and active motion. The presence of motion loss is consistent with soft tissue contractures. Obvious cofactors, such as instability, superior labral anterior to posterior (SLAP) tears, and rotator cuff pathology, are usually apparent due to the patient's history and classic findings on examination.

Plain radiographs should be obtained consisting of a true anteroposterior, scapular-Y view, and an axillary view. Additional views such as the West Point axillary view, Stryker notch view, and supraspinatus outlet view facilitate more precise anatomic delineation. We commonly request magnetic resonance imaging (MRI) to evaluate the articular surface and to evaluate for any other intraarticular abnormalities. Carroll et al[15] have reported on MRI's use in detecting articular cartilage lesions on the humerus. The sensitivity varied between radiologists ranging from 53 to 100% and the specificity ranged from 51 to 87%.[8] Unfortunately, lesions can be missed by MRI as was demonstrated by Cameron et al,[16] where 45% of grade IV chondral lesions had no radiographic (MRI or plain radiographs) evidence preoperatively.

The same techniques used to identify chondral injuries in the knee are useful for the glenohumeral joint. Standard pulse sequences for articular cartilage frequently include a T2-weighted image with or without fat suppression and a T1-weighted fat-suppressed three-dimensional spoiled gradient-echo technique. These protocols benefit from the arthrogram-producing effect

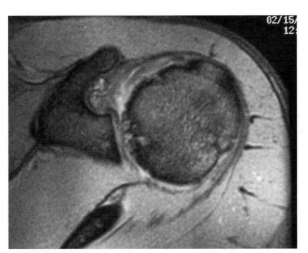

FIGURE 20–1 Axial-oblique T2-weighted magnetic resonance imaging (MRI) demonstrating significant articular cartilage loss involving primarily the humeral head with some subchondral cystic changes evident.

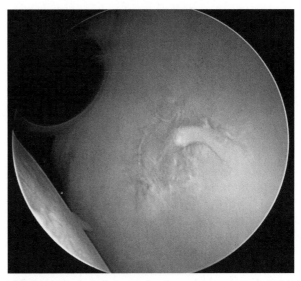

FIGURE 20–3 Arthroscopic view of a normal glenoid demonstrating the central-most portion to be nearly devoid of articular cartilage.

of the differential signal intensity on the joint fluid, which highlights irregularity or defects of the joint surface. On the T1-weighted images, cartilage is higher in signal intensity than joint fluid; the reverse is true for the T2-weighted images **(Fig. 20–1).**[17–20] A computed tomography (CT) scan is useful in situations where a significant osteochondral defect exists such as that following posttraumatic instability **(Fig. 20–2).**

It is not uncommon for patients in this age group (i.e., less than 40) to have concomitant pathology in addition to their chondral injury. Most commonly, these lesions are associated with a history of traumatic shoulder instability, SLAP tears, and rotator cuff pathology. Addressing these cofactors first with traditional treatment modalities is prudent, as it is likely that the associated chondral injury is nothing more than an incidental finding that will remain asymptomatic. However, the patient's symptom complex and history may provide an indication preoperatively to consider at least some form of initial treatment of these lesions (i.e., debridement,

marrow stimulation) at the time when the patient's primary pathology is addressed.

Arthroscopic evaluation of chondral injury is the most useful determinate as these lesions are generally occult when documented at the time of index treatment. The lesion itself must be carefully defined. Generally, the central portion of the glenoid is normally quite thin and may actually be translucent to the extent that subchondral bone is exposed **(Fig. 20–3).** It is also important to avoid confusing the bare area of the humeral head **(Fig. 20–4)** with a chondral lesion. This is an area of bare bone with remnants of old vascular channels. This area is juxtaposed with the rotator cuff insertion and completely devoid of cartilage on its most lateral extent. This bare

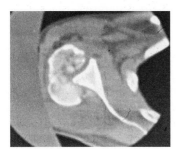

FIGURE 20–2 Computed tomography (CT) scan of a patient with a posterior fracture-dislocation involving the majority of the humeral head.

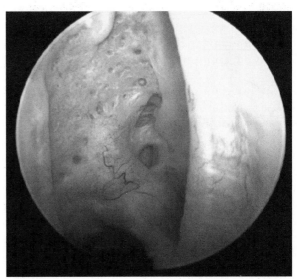

FIGURE 20–4 Arthroscopic view of the normal bare area of the humeral head.

area also correlates with the attachment of the infraspinatus tendon and can be used as a landmark in rotator cuff surgery to align the infraspinatus to its footprint.

Finally, the topography of the articular cartilage thickness of the humeral head has been studied by the authors in our laboratory and demonstrates mean thickness that ranges from 0.6 to 1.2 mm. The cartilage is thicker centrally and thins toward the periphery.[21] Although important, at this juncture, this finding has indeterminate significance when deciding on which treatment option is ultimately implemented.

Visualizing the lesion from opposite portals and during arm positioning facilitates a comprehensive evaluation of the defect, which is otherwise difficult to perform from a single portal due to the spherical nature of the humeral head. Palpating the lesion with a probe is important as the extent of the defect typically is beyond visible areas of exposed bone and should be documented to include any degenerated margins at the transition zone adjacent to healthy appearing cartilage. Measuring the lesion with a probe tip of specific length or a graduated instrument provides sizing to determine the surface area and depth of the defect.

■ Nonoperative Treatment

As with any shoulder pathology, conservative treatment is initially justified and should include nonsteroidal anti-inflammatory medications, physical therapy, glenohumeral steroid injections, and consideration for injectable viscosupplementation with hyaluronic acid compounds. Physical therapy should emphasize scapulothoracic and glenohumeral strengthening. Often, these patients have non-outlet or secondary impingement due to abnormal scapulothoracic kinematics. This can be predictably improved on with appropriate rehabilitation. Steroid injections may be appropriate, but we do not favor repeated use in younger patients. Patients typically become symptomatic once they resume physical activities. Finally, viscosupplementation, although currently approved for use in the knee, is considered for off-label usage in the shoulder and must be performed with explicit patient informed consent. The use of viscosupplementation is a promising alternative for patients with overt glenohumeral arthritis and is the subject of prospective study. However, similar to steroid injections, we rarely use this in the younger patient population with localized chondral disease.

■ Operative Treatment

Virtually any cartilage restoration option used in the knee can be applied to the glenohumeral joint.[22] There is a treatment continuum to consider when deciding which procedure to perform. The nature of these treatment options can be subcategorized into primary treatment, palliative treatment, reparative treatment, and restorative treatment. Primary treatment consists of repair of the cartilage. Palliative treatment consists of arthroscopic lavage and debridement. Reparative treatment consists of marrow stimulation techniques (abrasion, drilling or microfracture). Restorative options include osteochondral grafting (autograft and fresh allograft) and autologous chondrocyte implantation.

Decision Making

The decision making must take into account several factors. Treating obvious comorbidities first is essential, as most defects do not manifest in symptoms following repair of associated pathology such as rotator cuff tears, SLAP tears, or the pathoanatomy associated with instability. Initially, the presence of symptoms, not the mere identification or knowledge of an existing defect, must guide the decision to implement one of the treatment alternatives. Knowledge of previous treatments provided, the rehabilitation performed postoperatively, and the patient's response to this treatment facilitates decision making, as repeating the same option again is intuitively less desirable. In addition, managing and matching patient expectations must be considered in the context of the magnitude of improvement that might be expected with each treatment option.

Because the data available and our experience with these lesions is relatively limited, we recommend that initial treatment options be limited to those that will not compromise the implementation of future treatment options should they become necessary. In all situations, associated stiffness is managed with arthroscopic release with gentle manipulation. An examination under anesthesia enables the surgeon to ascertain the area of tightness and determine which portion of the capsule should be arthroscopically released. Subsequent decision making is implemented in the context of several patient- and defect-specific factors.

Synthesizing the findings from the patient's history, symptoms, and findings on examination may help to ascertain the exact etiology of the patient's pain and the subsequent level of treatment required. For example, pain at the extremes of motion may be due to capsular contracture and synovitis. Similarly, pain at rest may indicate synovitis. These patients may respond more favorably to guided capsular release and synovectomy. Pain from articular cartilage abnormalities more commonly occurs in the midranges of motion and may be associated with mechanical symptoms and crepitus made worse with loading of the glenohumeral joint. These patients may require specific attention to the articular cartilage defect to improve their function and reduce their pain.

The magnitude of the patient's symptoms is also a consideration, as first-line treatment with debridement and lavage or microfracture may suffice in patients with low-level symptoms or those who place relatively low physical demands on their shoulder. Similarly, the morbidity of the operation may be a factor considered by the patient in the decision making. Unlike autologous chondrocyte implantation, which requires a biopsy from the knee (preferred by the senior author, B.J.C.), or osteochondral autografting, which also requires harvesting of an osteochondral plug from the knee, fresh osteochondral allograft transplantation is a single-stage procedure limited to the glenohumeral joint, which may be preferable to some. Patients with large, uncontained defects with subchondral bone loss, independent of age, are excellent candidates for fresh osteochondral allograft transplantation. Patients with smaller contained superficial defects, especially when relatively young, are excellent candidates for autologous chondrocyte implantation.

Incidentally discovered defects that might be considered as a relative contributor to the patient's symptoms may be addressed at the same time any associated pathology is corrected (i.e., rotator cuff tears, SLAP tears, and instability patterns) with a marrow stimulation technique. Patients with deeper defects may more commonly complain of mechanical symptoms, and therefore will likely respond more favorably to solutions that can restore articular congruity such as osteochondral grafting. Smaller defects (i.e., less than 10 mm^2) may be amenable to osteochondral autograft transplantation, and larger defects may be more amenable to fresh osteochondral allograft transplantation.

Superficial lesions or surface lesions with minimal subchondral bone involvement, which fail first-line treatment using debridement and lavage or marrow stimulation, especially in young patients, are considered for revision with autologous chondrocyte implantation. The most difficult decision is for older patients with superficial defects. Because of the morbidity of two surgical procedures and the prolonged rehabilitation required of autologous chondrocyte implantation, we favor fresh osteochondral allograft in this population because if it fails, revision with arthroplasty is a plausible alternative.

The most advanced scenario includes young and active patients with opposing defects of the glenoid and humerus (i.e., bipolar disease). Clearly, this is the most challenging patient group and often requires salvage solutions as alternatives to arthroplasty. In this population, regaining motion is the first objective, and typically patients are managed initially with arthroscopic capsular release, lavage and debridement, and possibly microfracture of exposed surfaces. Second-line treatment options include biologic resurfacing with the posteriorly reflected anterior shoulder capsule, soft tissue allografts,

porcine small intestine submucosa (SIS), and meniscal allografts. These solutions may improve the patient's function and reduce pain without compromising future arthroplasty reconstruction.

■ Primary Treatment

Osteochondral fractures of the shoulder can occur following high-energy trauma and are most frequently seen with fracture dislocations of the shoulder **(Fig. 20–2)**. In relatively young patients, open reduction, fragment elevation, bone grafting, and fixation are attempted if possible. We recommend intraarticular fracture fixation with headless compression screws (Acumed, Inc., Beaverton, OR) that do not require removal.

Osteochondritis dissecans of the humeral head is a rare condition with only a few case series reported in the literature.[23–29] It is not uncommonly seen in relatively active individuals as the etiology is related to trauma with associated ischemia, although endocrine abnormalities, genetic influences, and the presence of anomalous centers of ossification have also been attributed to this entity.[23,24] Most commonly, it involves the humerus, but rarely may involve the glenoid.[25] It more commonly affects middle-aged and young males and typically involves the anterosuperior aspect of the humeral head.[26] Management may include drilling,[27,28] drilling with fragment removal,[26] or primary repair. Because of the risk for progressive degeneration following fragment removal, we recommend treatment with debridement, microfracture of the base, and primary repair using screws or bioabsorbable pins **(Fig. 20–5)**.

■ Palliative Treatment

Lavage and debridement improve congruence and remove debris and various enzymes and proteins such as metalloproteinases associated with the pathogenesis of arthrosis. The indications for arthroscopic lavage and debridement is as a first-line treatment and the outcome is technique and disease-level dependent. The principal components of arthroscopic debridement may include synovectomy, removal of loose bodies, and judicious use of capsular release for motion loss. In addition, if preoperative and arthroscopic findings implicate the subacromial space as a source of pain, a formal subacromial decompression should also be performed as supported by earlier studies.[30,31]

The objectives for the management of chondral and osteochondral defects include converting edges with gradual transition zones to those with vertical margins. The basic science supporting this technique was studied by Rudd et al,[29] with the recommendations from this investigation being widely accepted as a modality to

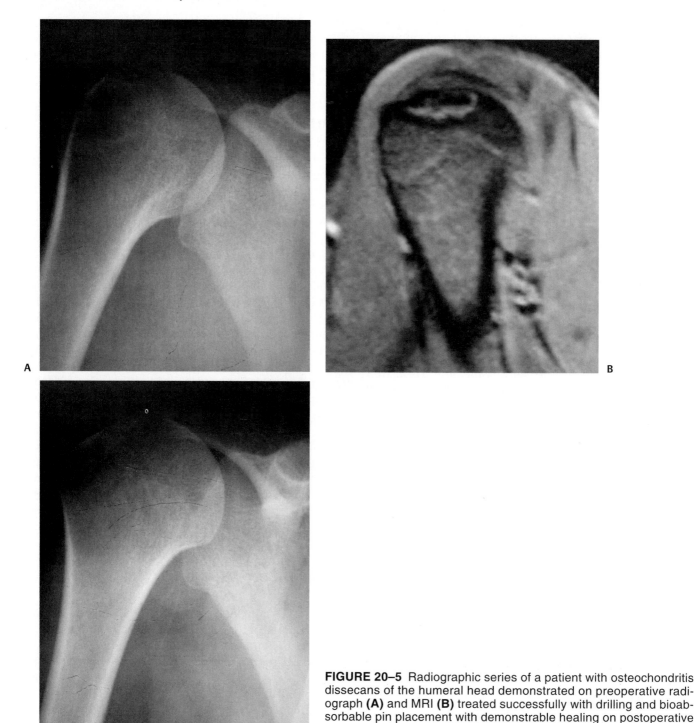

FIGURE 20–5 Radiographic series of a patient with osteochondritis dissecans of the humeral head demonstrated on preoperative radiograph **(A)** and MRI **(B)** treated successfully with drilling and bioabsorbable pin placement with demonstrable healing on postoperative anteroposterior radiograph **(C)** obtained at 12 months.

manage cartilage defects of any joint. In a canine model, humeral defects prepared with and without beveling of the margins of articular cartilage defects were compared over a 16-week period. The authors concluded that cartilage defects with beveled edges were significantly larger than those with perpendicular edges. In addition, chondral damage to the glenoid sur-

face occurred more frequently opposite beveled defects than opposing defects with vertical walls. Thus, if one chooses to modify the defect in any fashion, the combined use of curettes, motorized shavers run in a single direction, and arthroscopic hand instruments can change a gradual transition zone from the defect to the surrounding normal cartilage to one with a vertical wall of healthy articular cartilage. Intuitively, defects prepared in this fashion should be better suited to share load and provide relative protection to exposed subchondral surfaces.

Thermal chondroplasty should be used with great caution. It can result in a wide area of chondrocyte cell death, which might affect the subchondral bone, especially given the relatively thin articular surfaces of the glenohumeral joint.[32]

Similar to the results following arthroscopic lavage and debridement in the knee, the literature in the shoulder largely consists of patients with glenohumeral osteoarthritis, and the results tend to be relatively short-lived and incomplete.[16,33–39] The most relevant study to date is that published recently by Cameron et al.[16] In this investigation of patients diagnosed with shoulder instability, 61 patients with humeral or glenoid grade IV lesions were treated with arthroscopic debridement and capsular release where necessary.

Eighty-seven percent of the patients indicated that they would have the surgery again. Pain relief was obtained in 88% with a mean duration of pain relief of 28 months. Patients also demonstrated reductions in rest pain, and pain during light and strenuous activities. Negative prognostic factors leading to the return of pain and failure of the procedure included lesion size of greater than 2 cm^2. This is analogous to the cutoff used in the knee when lesion size is factored into the treatment algorithm.[1,3]

Arthroscopic debridement of the glenohumeral joint is a palliative measure that appears to be useful for short-term pain relief in patients who present with coexisting pathology without gross mechanical symptoms coming from the defect. The senior author (B.J.C.) most commonly uses arthroscopic debridement and modification of the lesion's transition zone for incidental lesions that do not seem to be categorically associated with the patient's symptoms **(Fig. 20–6).**

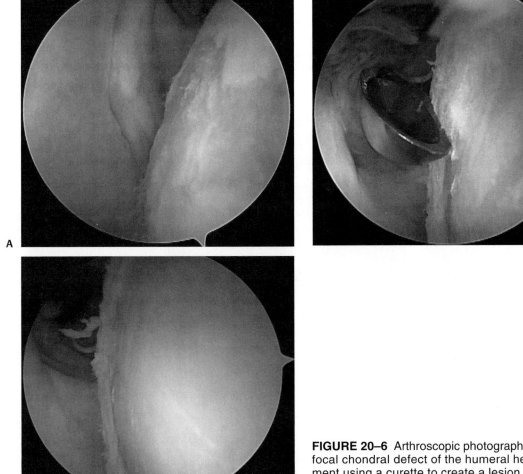

FIGURE 20–6 Arthroscopic photographs of a 28-year-old man with a focal chondral defect of the humeral head **(A)** treated with debridement using a curette to create a lesion **(B)** with well-defined vertical walls to facilitate more efficient load sharing with the normal surrounding articular cartilage **(C)**.

■ Reparative Techniques

Microfracture

Marrow stimulation involves penetration of the subchondral bone by one of three methods: abrasion, drilling, and microfracture. Microfracture, the author's preferred technique, was initially popularized by Steadman et al[37,40] and has been widely applied to the knee. The technique recently described by us for the treatment of chondral defects of the knee is exactly what we perform in the shoulder.[22,39] The basic steps include debridement through the calcified layer at the base of the defect, establishing vertical walls at the transition zone for reasons described previously, penetrating the base of the defect with a specialized awl with holes spaced 2 to 3 mm apart, and utilizing specific postoperative rehabilitation protocols.

The resultant tissue formed by the mesenchymal stem cells and growth factors is fibrocartilage, which is similar in appearance, but biomechanically inferior to hyaline cartilage.[41,42] There are no clinical series of patients with focal chondral defects of the glenohumeral joint treated with microfracture alone. Siebold et al[38] recently reported on five patients treated with a combination of microfracture and periosteal flap coverage at a mean follow-up of 25.8 months. Clinically, there were significant improvements in the Constant score and reductions in pain. Three patients underwent second-look arthroscopy at an average of 8 months, all with an improved appearance of the cartilage lesion.

The senior author (B.J.C.) has performed microfracture of the glenohumeral joint in 10 patients with localized chondral defects of the glenohumeral joint **(Fig. 20–7).** The average age of the patients was 28. Sixty percent had humeral lesions, and 40% had glenoid lesions. Only two had kissing lesions. The average size of the lesion was 2.0 cm². None of the patients had concomitant pathology. None were associated with instability. Postoperatively, these patients were treated with 4 to 6 weeks of pendulum exercises performed 600 times per day to mimic continuous passive motion. In all patients, there was a modest reduction in pain and improvements in function. However, no patients had complete elimination of their symptoms that were present preoperatively, and one patient is contemplating revision with a fresh osteochondral allograft transplant of the humeral head.

Microfracture of the glenohumeral joint is a measure that leads to fibrocartilage repair tissue. Although it may have some benefit in the knee, its usefulness in the shoulder is based on anecdotal implementation, with inferences that the same biologic milieu will occur in the glenohumeral joint that has been demonstrated in the knee joint. Nevertheless, the authors recommend microfracture as a first-line treatment of superficial defects believed to be associated with symptoms even in the setting where comorbidities are simultaneously corrected. Revision with restorative options is unlikely to be

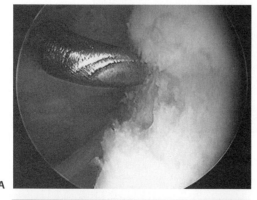
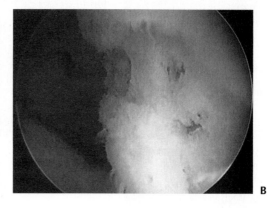
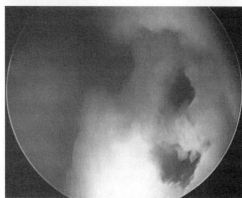

FIGURE 20–7 Arthroscopic photograph of an 18-year-old man with a focal chondral defect of the humeral head **(A)** treated with defect preparation and microfracture **(B)**, leading to blood return emanating from the subchondral bone **(C)**.

compromised following microfracture, and it can be performed entirely arthroscopically with very little morbidity. Osteochondral defects and mechanical symptoms are considered relative contraindications to microfracture, as these patients are unlikely to benefit. Practically speaking, for the reasons mentioned previously, smaller well-shouldered lesions should fare better clinically than larger unshouldered lesions with gradual transition zones.

■ Restorative Techniques

Osteochondral Autograft

Several authors have validated success with osteochondral autograft transplantation in the knee.[43-45] Intuitively, patients with smaller lesions (i.e., less than 1–1.5 cm²) of the humerus who have demonstrated failure of first-line treatment, including microfracture, may be excellent candidates for this procedure. The advantages include the ability to restore the glenohumeral architecture with a viable "organ" of bone and cartilage with a single-stage procedure. It results in osseous integration and preserves the articular cartilage tidemark. Practically, it is easiest to harvest a donor plug from the lateral trochlea of the knee just proximal to the sulcus terminalis, but it is also possible through further research that a relatively noncontact donor site may be present in an adjacent area of the humeral articular surface. This could be accomplished arthroscopically, but defect location might also warrant a formal arthrotomy. Laszlo Hangody (personal communication, 2003) has performed this procedure in two patients, each with an osteochondral lesion of the posterior surface of the humerus. The grafts were harvested arthroscopically from the knee. In a unique application of osteochondral autograft transplantation, Connor et al[46] reported on a patient with bilateral posterior fracture dislocations of the glenohumeral joint who was treated on one side with hemiarthroplasty, and on the contralateral side with a local autograft taken from the shoulder treated with arthroplasty, in a single-stage procedure where both shoulders where operated on simultaneously.

The use of osteochondral autografts as a restorative option is limited to patients with relatively small defects of the humerus who are willing to subject themselves to the potential complication of donor-site morbidity in an otherwise asymptomatic knee **(Fig. 20–8).** The best indication would be for patients with small osteochondral defects who complain of mechanical symptoms that would otherwise be poorly managed with palliative measures (i.e., microfracture). Fundamentally, osteochondral autografts represent an excellent solution, but the indications are narrow and are rarely present.

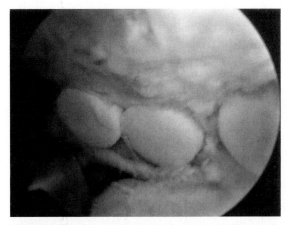

FIGURE 20–8 Arthroscopic photograph of an osteochondral autograft transplant performed for an isolated degenerative lesion of the humeral head. (Courtesy of Dr. John D. Kelly, IV, Department of Orthopedic Surgery, Temple University, Philadelphia.)

Fresh Osteochondral Allograft

Osteochondral allografting has been quite successful in the knee with the longest track record of any cartilage restoration procedure.[47-49] Like osteochondral autografts, osteochondral allografts restore the congruency of the articular surface with an intact osteochondral segment. Graft preservation is critical. Contemporary treatment includes fresh (i.e., within 72 hours of donor asystole) or prolonged-fresh osteochondral grafts (i.e., ideally, maintained cold with regular medium change for no more than 28 days).[50] The indications are for larger lesions (i.e., greater than 1.5–2.0 cm²) of the humeral head. As discussed earlier (see Decision Making), large uncontained lesions and osteochondral lesions in symptomatic patients are probably the best candidates. This is especially true for relatively older individuals who could also be considered as candidates for arthroplasty should the osteochondral allograft fail. There are only limited reports of the use of osteochondral allografts in the shoulder. In two case reports, fresh frozen humeral head allografts were used.[51,52] In another, frozen or autoclaved femoral head grafts were used.[53] Despite these limitations, very good outcomes were reported.

Osteochondral allografts are side- and size-matched using plain radiographs corrected for magnification. The technique is performed through a standard anterior deltopectoral approach. Technically, defects are treated using hand-fashioned grafts requiring supplemental fixation **(Fig. 20–9).** Newer instrumentation used in the knee (Arthrex, Inc., Naples, FL) in a technique recently described by the authors is another possibility that would potentially avoid the need for supplemental fixation.[54] It is critical that the grafts are implanted with a minimal amount of subchondral bone that is irrigated

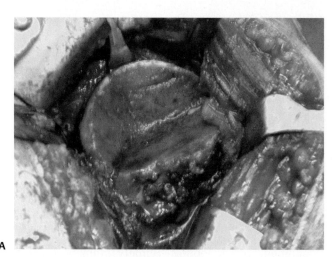
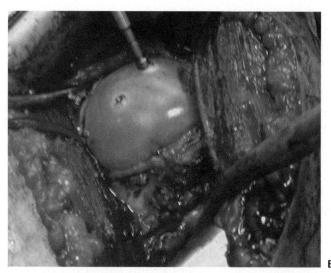

A   B

FIGURE 20–9 Case example of a large segmental defect of the proximal humerus treated by removing the fracture fragment and creating a wedge configuration of the recipient bed **(A)** and screw fixation of a fresh osteochondral allograft humeral head **(B)**.

copiously (i.e., no more than 6–8 mm) in an effort to minimize the immunogenic load contained in the osseous phase of the graft.

The use of osteochondral allografts as a restorative option is limited to patients with relatively large defects of the humerus who are willing to subject themselves to the infinitely low probability of the potential complication of donor disease transmission and the possibility of graft collapse. Osteochondral defects, such as those that occur with fracture-dislocations or engaging Hill-Sachs lesions, which lead to persistent instability despite standard stabilization techniques, are ideal lesions for this procedure. Because larger defects are more likely to become problematic and advances have occurred in terms of the availability of fresh osteochondral allograft transplant material, this solution represents an excellent first- or second-line option for appropriately selected patients.

Autogenous Chondrocyte Implantation

Autologous chondrocyte implantation (ACI) has a long track record for its implementation in the knee and the technique has been described by the senior author (B.J.C.) and others.[55–62] The use of ACI in the shoulder is considered an off-label usage, and strict patient informed consent must be obtained. In brief, this procedure involves the harvesting of healthy articular cartilage with subsequent culturing and expansion of the cells over a 3- to 4-week period prior to implantation. Thus, it requires two procedures. The biopsy is obtained arthroscopically from the knee, and the implantation is performed through a standard deltopectoral approach. At the time of implantation, the periosteum is harvested

from the proximal tibia in the standard location. As already mentioned,[21] the articular cartilage of the humeral head is substantially thinner than that found in the knee, and thus suturing of the periosteum is technically far more challenging compared with our experience in the knee.

The optimal indications are for contained unipolar superficial defects of the humerus or glenoid in relatively young patients who have failed first-line treatment including microfracture. It is useful in larger lesions (>2 cm^2) that are beyond the scope of osteochondral autograft transplantation and for superficial lesions where one would prefer to avoid violating the subchondral surface as is required of osteochondral allograft transplantation.

The authors recently published a case report of a young baseball player who had a defect develop in the anterosuperior humeral head following thermal capsulorrhaphy with a bipolar thermal device **(Fig. 20–10).**[63] Cell-based technology has several advantages over osteochondral grafting. It utilizes the patient's own tissue with minimal donor-site morbidity and does not violate the subchondral bone. The experience with this technology, however, is very limited and the indications are relatively small compared with some of the other technologies available.

Biologic Resurfacing

Unfortunately, a population of patients exists who have chondral lesions on both sides of the glenohumeral joint that ranges from localized to diffuse bipolar disease. The senior authors (B.J.C. and A.A.R.) have

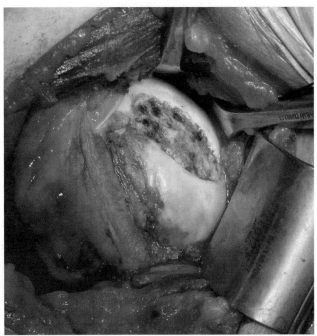

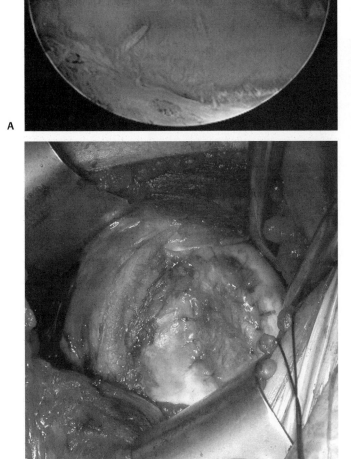

FIGURE 20–10 **(A)** Arthroscopic view of a focal chondral defect of the anterior humeral head in a 16-year-old boy treated previously with thermal capsulorrhaphy. **(B)** Intraoperative photograph showing the lesion covered by a thin layer of fibrous tissue. **(C)** Intraoperative photograph showing the periosteal patch sutured into place using 6–0 Vicryl suture and sealed with fibrin glue.

most commonly seen this in a population of patients referred following arthroscopic stabilization using suture anchors with and without the use of radiofrequency thermal capsulorraphy. These patients represent the most challenging treatment group as the treatment options are limited and relegated largely to anecdotal reports from surgeons interested in managing these problems with techniques considered investigational. Biologic resurfacing refers to solutions that provide some form of soft tissue interposition between the arthritic areas. This might include fascia lata, allograft tendon, the anterior shoulder capsule, periosteum, porcine small intestine submucosa or even allograft meniscus tissue.

Burkhead and Hutton[62] reported on the successful use of biologic resurfacing of the glenoid with fascia lata or anterior shoulder capsule in a relatively young population of patients who were treated with hemiarthroplasty in an effort to avoid glenoid replacement because of the significant risks for loosening in this at risk young population. Alternatives to this might include the use of porcine SIS (DePuy Orthopaedics, Inc., Warsaw, IN). Advantages of this material include the capability of inducing site-specific remodeling of various connective tissues.[64,65] This application is most similar to the use of periosteum and microfracture discussed previously as reported by Siebold et al.[38]

Similar to ACI, the application of SIS in the shoulder is considered an off-label usage and explicit patient informed consent must be obtained. The senior author (B.J.C.) has a single case where SIS was used to resurface a microfractured glenoid in a girl who, for reasons unknown, developed extensive chondrolysis following arthroscopic shoulder stabilization using a monopolar radiofrequency device **(Fig. 20–11).** This patient had already failed attempts at debridement and capsular release. Early follow-up of 12 months demonstrated significant reductions in pain and improvements in function.

Another option is to consider unloading the glenohumeral joint by placing an allograft meniscus along the periphery of the glenoid. This is the subject of a basic science study by the senior authors (B.J.C. and A.A.R.) as we have limited clinical experience with this technique **(Fig. 20–12).** Intuitively, glenoid lesions may respond favorably if reductions in contact area and force are

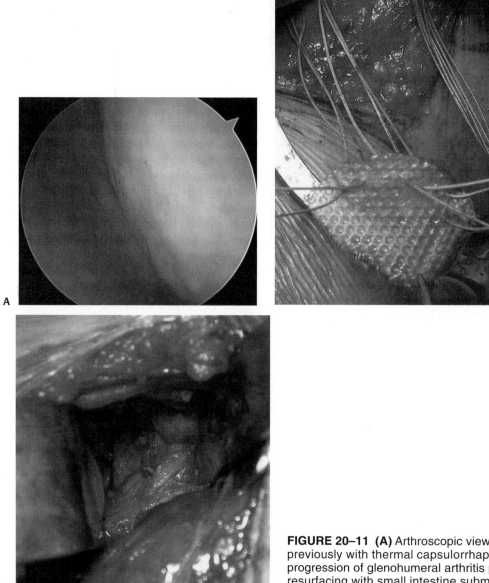

FIGURE 20–11 (A) Arthroscopic view of a 16-year-old girl treated previously with thermal capsulorrhaphy who demonstrated rapid progression of glenohumeral arthritis postoperatively. **(B)** Biologic resurfacing with small intestine submucosa (SIS) prepared to be sutured into place following microfracture of the glenoid. **(C)** SIS sewn into place.

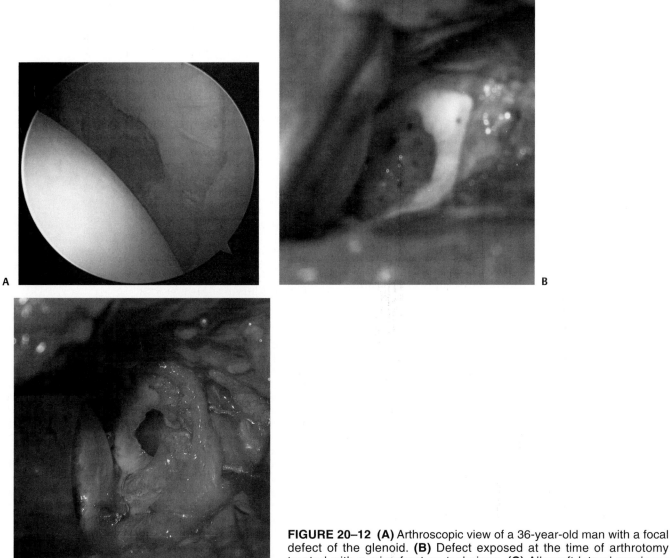

FIGURE 20–12 (A) Arthroscopic view of a 36-year-old man with a focal defect of the glenoid. **(B)** Defect exposed at the time of arthrotomy treated with a microfracture technique. **(C)** Allograft lateral meniscus sewn into place to the surrounding labrum.

achieved by suturing an allograft meniscus into the periphery of the glenoid. Similar to the use of SIS, this technique is considered investigational at this time, but offers a biomechanically attractive treatment alternative.

A high degree of caution must exist when offering patients biologic resurfacing alternatives to reduce pain and improve function in the setting of chondral damage to the glenohumeral joint. Decisions must be made in the context of other comorbidities including range-of-motion loss, the integrity of the rotator cuff, and the stability of the shoulder. The indications for these techniques remain rare and are likely to evolve as our understanding of the biology and biomechanics of these treatment options improves.

■ Postoperative Rehabilitation

The rehabilitation following all of these techniques is critical to their success. Postoperatively early range of motion is important.[66,67] Although we do not currently use continuous passive motion, patients begin with pendulum exercises the day after surgery with at least 600 cycles performed daily. Active range of motion is generally delayed until 6 weeks. Active range of motion and gentle strengthening begins at 6 to 8 weeks. Athletic endeavors are delayed until at least 6 months depending on the progress of the rehabilitation and the nature of the cartilage restoration procedure. The earliest time frame that patients can expect to get back to activities occurs following arthroscopic debridement. On the other hand, ACI and osteochondral allograft transplantation require the longest time frames postoperatively, and patients may not be permitted to engage in high-level activities for at least 12 months following their surgery.

■ Conclusion

One has to individualize the treatment of each lesion once it is certain that the cartilage lesion is the source of the patient's pain and impairment. A conservative approach is warranted given the lack of knowledge about the management of these defects. Beginning with palliative or reparative techniques may be the most prudent approach as patients may respond favorably and future treatment options are not compromised. If there is no or insufficient response to this initial treatment attempt, then one may consider a restorative option providing the level of the patient's symptoms warrant further treatment. For smaller defects, osteochondral autografts may suffice. For larger lesions, ACI or fresh osteochondral allograft transplantation may be required. Biologic resurfacing must be approached with caution and on a case-by-case basis. Lessons learned from the implementation of cartilage procedures in the knee will assuredly improve upon our capabilities in the shoulder, but only through further objective investigation in the clinical and laboratory setting will we further our understanding of the treatment algorithm for the management of chondral injury in the glenohumeral joint.

REFERENCES

1. Fox JA, Kalsi RS, Cole BJ. Update on articular cartilage restoration. Tech Knee Surg 2003;2:2–17
2. Sellards RA, Nho SJ, Cole BJ. Chondral injuries. Curr Opin Rheumatol 2002;14:134–141
3. Cole BJ, Farr J. Putting it all together. Orthop Tech 2001;11: 151–154
4. Miller M, Cole BJ. Atlas on chondral injury. Orthop Tech 2001;11: 145–150
5. Outerbridge GETRE. The etiology of chondromalacia patellae. J Bone Joint Surg Br 1961;43:742–757
6. Curl WW, Krome J, Gordon ES, Rushing J, Smith BP, Poehling GG. Cartilage injuries: a review of 31,516 knee arthroscopies. Arthroscopy 1997;13:456–460
7. Hjelle K, Solheim E, Torbjorn S, Rune M, Brittberg M. Articular cartilage defects in 1,000 knee arthroscopies. Arthroscopy 2002;18:730–734
8. Guntern DV, Pfirrmann CW, Schmid MR, et al. Articular cartilage lesions of the glenohumeral joint: diagnostic effectiveness of MR arthrography and prevalence in patients with subacromial impingement syndrome. Radiology 2003;226: 165–170
9. Hsu HC, Luo ZP, Stone JJ, Huang TH, An KN. Correlation between rotator cuff tear and glenohumeral degeneration. Acta Orthop Scand 2003;74:89–94
10. Gartsman GM, Taverna E. The incidence of glenohumeral joint abnormalities associated with full-thickness, reparable rotator cuff tears. Arthroscopy 1997;13:450–455
11. Werner A, Lichtenberg S, Nikolic A, Habermeyer P. Intraarticular pathology of atraumatic shoulder dislocations: an arthroscopic study. Unfallchirurg 2003;106:110–113
12. Taylor DC, Arciero RA. Pathologic changes associated with shoulder dislocations. Arthroscopic and physical examination findings in first-time, traumatic anterior dislocations. Am J Sports Med 1997;25:306–311
13. Cameron ML, Kocher MS, Briggs KK, Horan MP, Hawkins RJ. The prevalence of glenohumeral osteoarthritis in unstable shoulders. Am J Sports Med 2003;31:53–55
14. Hintermann B, Gachter A: Arthroscopic findings after shoulder dislocation. Am J Sports Med 1995;23:545–551
15. Carroll KW, Helms CA, Speer KP. Focal articular cartilage lesions of the superior humeral head: MR imaging findings in seven patients. AJR Am J Roentgenol 2001;176:393–397
16. Cameron BD, Galatz LM, Ramsey ML, et al. Non-prosthetic management of grade IV osteochondral lesions of the glenohumeral joint J Shoulder Elbow Surg 2002;11:25–32
17. Chung CB, Frank LR, Resnick D. Cartilage imaging techniques: current clinical applications and state of the art imaging. Clin Orthop 2001;391(suppl):S370–S378
18. Karantanas AH, Zibis AH, Kitsoulis P. Fat-suppressed 3D–T1-weighted-echo planar imaging: comparison with fat-suppressed 3D–T1-weighted-gradient echo in imaging the cartilage of the knee. Comput Med Imaging Graph 2002;6:159–165
19. Gold GE, Beaulieu CF. Future of MR imaging of articular cartilage. Semin Musculoskelet Radiol 2001;5:313–327
20. Matsui N, Kobayashi M. Application of MR imaging for internal derangement of the knee (orthopedic surgeon view). Semin Musculoskel Radiol 2001;5:139–141
21. Glenn RE, Cole BJ, Fox JA, Meininger AK, Romeo AA, Hayden JK. Articular cartilage thickness of the humeral head: an anatomic study. Review, Corr, September, 2005.
22. Fox J, Cole BJ. Update on articular cartilage restoration. Tech Knee Surg 2003;2:2–17
23. Ishikawa H, Ueba Y, Yonezawa T, Kurosaka M, Ohno O, Hirohata K. Osteochondritis dissecans of the shoulder in a tennis player. Am J Sports Med 1988;16:547–550
24. Pydisetty RV, Prasad SS, Kaye JC. Osteochondritis dissecans of the humeral head in an amateur boxer. J Shoulder Elbow Surg 2002;11:630–632
25. Shanley DJ, Mulligan ME. Osteochondrosis dissecans of the glenoid. Skeletal Radiol 1990;19:419–421
26. Hamada S, Hamada M, Nishiue S, Doi T. Osteochondritis dissecans of the humeral head. Arthroscopy 1992;8:132–137
27. Anderson WJ, Guilford BW. Osteochondritis dissecans of the humeral head. An unusual cause of shoulder pain. Clin Orthop 1983;173:166–168
28. Ganter M, Reichelt A. Osteochondrosis dissecans of the humeral head. Z Orthop Ihre Grenzgeb 1996;134:73–75
29. Rudd RG, Visco DM, Kincaid SA, Cantwell HD. The effects of beveling the margins of articular cartilage defects in immature dogs. Vet Surg 1987;16:378–383
30. Ellman H, Harris E, Kay SP. Early degenerative joint disease simulating impingement syndrome: arthroscopic findings. Arthroscopy 1992;8:482–487
31. Witwity T, Uhlmann R, Nagy MN, et al. Shoulder rheumatoid arthritis associated with chondromatosis, treated by arthroscopy Arthroscopy 1991;7:233–236
32. Lu Y, Edwards RB III, Cole BJ, Markel MD. Thermal chondroplasty with radiofrequency energy. An in vitro comparison of bipolar and monopolar radiofrequency devices. Am J Sports Med 2001;29: 42–49

33. Kelly E, O'Driscoll S, Steinmann S. Arthroscopic glenoidplasty and osteocapsular arthroplasty for advanced glenohumeral arthritis. Presented at the annual open meeting of the American Shoulder and Elbow Surgeons, 2001, San Francisco, CA.

34. Matthews LS, LaBudde JK. Arthroscopic treatment of synovial diseases of the shoulder Orthop Clin North Am 1993;24:101–109

35. Midorikawa K, Hara M, Emoto G, et al. Arthroscopic debridement for dialysis shoulders Arthroscopy 2001;17:685–693

36. Weinstein DM, Bucchieri JS, Pollock RG, et al. Arthroscopic debridement of the shoulder for osteoarthritis. Arthroscopy 2000;16:471–476

37. Steadman JR, Briggs KK, Rodrigo JJ, et al. Outcomes of microfracture for traumatic chondral defects of the knee: average 11-year follow-up. Arthroscopy 2003;19:477–484

38. Siebold R, Lichtenberg S, Habermeyer P. Combination of microfracture and periosteal flap for the treatment of focal full-thickness articular cartilage lesions of the shoulder: a prospective study. Knee Surg Sports Traumatol Arthrosc 2003;11:183–189

39. Freedman JB, Coleman SH, Olenac C, Cole BJ. The biology of articular cartilage injury and the microfracture technique for the treatment of articular cartilage lesions. Semin Arthroplasty 2002;13:202–209

40. Steadman JRR, WG, Singleton SB, Briggs KK. Microfracture technique for full-thickness chondral defects: technique and clinical results. Oper Tech Orthop 1997;7:300–304

41. Buckwalter JA, Mow VC. Cartilage repair in osteoarthritis. In: Moskowitz RW, Howell DS, Goldberg VM, Mankin HJ, eds. Osteoarthritis: Diagnosis and Management. Philadelphia: W.B. Saunders, 1992:71–107

42. Athanasiou KA, Rosenwasser MP, Spiker RL, Mow VC. Effects of passive motion on the material properties of healing articular cartilage. Trans Orthop Res Soc 1991;15:156

43. Hangody L, Feczki P, Bartha L, et al. Mosaicplasty for the treatment of articular defects of the knee and ankle. Clin Orthop 2001;391(suppl):S328–S336

44. Kish G, Modis L, Hangody L. Osteochondral mosaicplasty for the treatment of focal chondral and osteochondral lesions of the knee and talus in the athlete. Rationale, indications, techniques, and results. Clin Sports Med 1999;18:45–66

45. Hangody L, Kish G, Karpati Z, et al. Mosaicplasty for the treatment of articular cartilage defects: application in clinical practice. Orthopedics 1998;21:751–756

46. Connor PM, Boatright JR, D'Alessandro DF. Posterior fracture-dislocation of the shoulder: treatment with acute osteochondral grafting. J Shoulder Elbow Surg 1997;6:480–485

47. Bugbee WD. Fresh osteochondral allografting. Oper Tech Sports Med 2000;8:158–162

48. Gross AE, Aubin P, Cheah HK, Davis AM, Ghazavi MT. A fresh osteochondral allograft alternative. J Arthroplasty 2002;17(4, suppl 1) 50–53

49. Gross AE. Fresh osteochondral allografts for post-traumatic knee defects: surgical technique. Oper Tech Orthop 1997;7:334–339

50. Williams JM, Virdi AS, Pylawka TK, Edwards RB 3rd, Markel MD, Cole BJ. Prolonged-fresh preservation of intact whole eanine

femoral condyles for the potential use as osteochondral allografts. J Ortho Res 2005;23:831–837

51. Johnson DL, Warner JJ. Osteochondritis dissecans of the humeral head: treatment with a matched osteochondral allograft. J Shoulder Elbow Surg 1997;6:160–163

52. Yagishita K, Thomas BJ. Use of allograft for large Hill-Sachs lesion associated with anterior glenohumeral dislocation. A case report. Injury 2002;33:791–794

53. Gerber C, Lambert SM. Allograft reconstruction of segmental defects of the humeral head for the treatment of chronic locked posterior dislocation of the shoulder. J Bone Joint Surg 1996;78:376–382

54. Fox JA, Freedman KB, Lee JL, Cole BJ. Fresh osteochondral allograft transplantation for articular cartilage defects. Oper Tech Sports Med 2002;10:168–173

55. D'Amato M, Cole BJ. Autologous chondrocyte implantation. Orthop Tech 2001;11:115–131

56. Peterson L, Brittberg M, Kiviranta I, et al. Autologous chondrocyte transplantation. Biomechanics and long-term durability. Am J Sports Med 2002;30:2–12

57. Minas T. Autologous chondrocyte implantation for focal chondral defects of the knee. Clin Orthop 2001;391:S349–S361

58. Micheli LJ, Browne JE, Erggelet C, et al. Autologous chondrocyte implantation of the knee: multicenter experience and minimum 3-year follow-up. Clin J Sports Med 2001;11:223–228

59. Peterson L, Minas T, Brittberg M, et al. Two- to 9-year outcome after autologous chondrocyte transplantation of the knee. Clin Orthop 2000;374:212–234

60. Gillogly SD, Voight M, Blackburn T. Treatment of articular cartilage defects of the knee with autologous chondrocyte implantation. J Orthop Sports Phys Ther 1998;28:241–251

61. Brittberg M, Lindahl A, Nilsson A, et al. Treatment of deep cartilage defects in the knee with autologous chondrocyte transplantation. N Engl J Med 1994;331:889–895

62. Burkhead WZ, Hutton KS. Biologic resurfacing of the glenoid with hemiarthroplasty of the shoulder. J Shoulder Elbow Surg 1995;4:263–270

63. Romeo AA, Cole BJ, Mazzocca AD, Fox JA, Freeman KB, Joy E. Autologous chondrocyte repair of an articular defect in the humeral head. Arthroscopy 2002;18:925–929

64. Badylak SF, Tullius R, Kokini K, et al. The use of xenogeneic small intestinal submucosa as a biomaterial for Achilles tendon repair in a dog model. J Biomed Mater Res 1995;29:977–985

65. Dejardin LM, Arnoczky SP, Clarke RB. Use of small intestinal submucosal implants for regeneration of large fascial defects. An experimental study in dogs. J Biomed Mater Res 1999;46:203–211

66. Salter RB, Bell RS, Keeley FW. The protective effect of continuous passive motion in living articular cartilage in acute septic arthritis: an experimental investigation in the rabbit. Clin Orthop 1981;159:223–247

67. Williams JM, Moran M, Thonar EJ, Salter RB. Continuous passive motion stimulates repair of rabbit knee articular cartilage after matrix proteoglycan loss. Clin Orthop 1994;304:252–222

21

Cartilage Injury in the Skeletally Immature

CHRISTOPHER IOBST AND MININDER S. KOCHER

Chondral and osteochondral injuries are being diagnosed with increasing frequency in skeletally immature patients.[1] This is likely due to a combination of factors, including increased awareness of chondral injuries in general, increased participation of young children in organized sports at higher competitive levels, and improvements in magnetic resonance imaging (MRI) techniques for articular cartilage. Although chondral injuries in skeletally immature patients generally do not carry as grave a prognosis as similar injuries in skeletally mature patients, they are not inconsequential lesions. The consequences of childhood chondral injury have important long-term significance due to the young age of the patients.

This chapter reviews the diagnosis and management of juvenile osteochondritis dissecans, osteochondral fractures, and chondral injuries in skeletally immature patients.

■ Juvenile Osteochondritis Dissecans

Definition

Juvenile osteochondritis dissecans (JOCD) is a disorder involving the articular surface of a joint in a patient with open physes. Although it shares a similar pathophysiology with the adult form of osteochondritis dissecans (OCD), it is a distinct disease process that has a more favorable prognosis than the adult form and requires different management strategies.

Epidemiology

The onset of symptoms in JOCD can occur at any age during skeletal immaturity; however, adolescents are typically involved. The average age of patients at the time of diagnosis in published reports has ranged from 11.3 to 13.4 years, and there is some indication that this mean age is decreasing.[2,3] This may reflect the increased involvement of children at younger and younger ages in competitive sports. The prevalence of JOCD was found by Linden[4] to be 18/100,000 in females and 29/100,000 in males. A multicenter review found JOCD to affect 60% males and 40% females, although most previous reports have a male to female ratio of 2.5 to 4:1.[5] This ratio may continue to decrease because more young girls are participating in athletics today than in previous generations. The most commonly affected joints in JOCD are the knee (distal femur), elbow (capitellum), and rarely the ankle (talus) with the majority of cases (75–85%) involving the knee.[6,7] Both the right and left sides appear to be affected equally and lesions are bilateral 12 to 30% of the time.[6,7] This disease appears to be rare in African Americans with only two cases in Cahill's[2] series of 240 patients. JOCD has also been associated with many other musculoskeletal abnormalities including Legg-Calvé-Perthes, skeletal dysplasias, tibia vara, patellar malalignment, Sinding-Larsen-Johansson disease, Osgood-Schlatter disease, and Stickler's syndrome. These conditions may predispose the patient to developing JOCD by causing stress accumulation on the femoral condyles, which could provoke subchondral changes.

Pathology

The histopathologic processes involved in JOCD are similar to those of the adult form. The subchondral bone, not the articular cartilage, is the tissue that initiates the pathologic process. It is believed that a localized area of subchondral osseous elements suffers a stress fracture, which fails to heal to the adjacent normal bone due to continuing stresses upon it. Over time this area of subchondral bone demarcates from the surrounding normal bone. Resorption of bone at the site of the fracture leads to separation of the fragment from its underlying bed and eventual necrosis of the bone fragment as the blood supply is lost. Initially the overlying articular cartilage remains unaffected because it receives its nutrition by diffusion from the synovial fluid. However, as support for the overlying articular cartilage is lost due to the necrotic and collapsing subchondral bone, the cartilage softens and gradually breaks down as it is subjected to shear stresses. The overlying articular cartilage begins to demarcate from the surrounding normal articular cartilage and allows the osteochondral fragment to be defined. If the disease process is not arrested, this breakdown of cartilage leads to fragmentation and partial or complete separation of the osteochondral fragment from its bed. Once the underlying bone is exposed to synovial fluid, the stability of the osteochondral fragment is compromised and the physical separation of the bone makes spontaneous resolution unlikely. A completely separated lesion can detach into the joint, forming a loose body composed of viable articular cartilage and a variable-sized segment of subchondral bone with a compromised blood supply. The remaining crater in the femoral articular surface shows thickened subchondral bony trabeculae with avascular changes. Although this crater may heal with a fibrocartilaginous scar, it is more likely that the now-incongruous articular surface will progress to more advanced changes consistent with degenerative joint disease, especially in lesions involving the weight-bearing surface of the joint.

Etiology

Since its initial description over 100 years ago, there has been controversy regarding the etiology of OCD. Various hypotheses have been proposed, but there is no universally accepted cause of the disease process and no theory completely explains its occurrence. The primary causes that have been proposed are trauma, genetic predisposition, defects of ossification, and circulatory disturbances causing osteonecrosis.

The most commonly accepted cause of OCD is trauma, with most authors believing that a single acute episode is not at fault but rather multiple episodes of microtrauma. These accumulated stresses over months or years result in crushing or fissuring of the subchondral bone with subsequent bone necrosis. One theory to explain this is that each child has a different stress acceptance threshold in each joint related to his/her tissue maturity. If the child is given a large enough repetitive stress over enough time on his/her immature tissue, this threshold can be exceeded resulting in JOCD. This theory is supported by the fact that many children with JOCD have a long history of exercise or sports-related activity and do not recall a single traumatic event. Another theory is that the tibial spine repeatedly impinges on the lateral aspect of the medial femoral condyle, causing a subchondral stress fracture. This theory, however, does not explain how lesions can occur in other aspects of the knee or in other joints.

Direct trauma, such as a blow to the knee, certainly could create an osteochondral injury, and biomechanical studies have shown that there is a significant amount of shear force in the region of the lateral aspect of the medial femoral condyle when the loaded knee is flexed. The symptoms of OCD in an adolescent are preceded by a history of trauma to the knee in 40 to 60% of cases. However, because JOCD lesions have a predilection for the posterolateral portion of the medial femoral condyle and because affected sites are located at specific locations rather than randomly distributed, it is more likely that indirect microtrauma is responsible for the majority of JOCD lesions than direct trauma. Although most evidence seems to support direct or indirect trauma as the primary contributory factor, the lack of traumatic history in many instances and a reported incidence of bilaterality in up to 30% of cases prevents trauma from adequately explaining every lesion.

Unlike OCD in the skeletally mature, OCD in the skeletally immature must be differentiated from variations of ossification or hereditary epiphyseal abnormalities. The difference in clinical picture between JOCD and OCD has led some to conclude that OCD in young patients may simply be a variant of normal growth.[8,9] Some authors have proposed that OCD in young patients results from an abnormality of ossification that fails to heal. They believe that JOCD represents a basic disturbance of epiphyseal development with small accessory islets of bone being separated from the main osseous nucleus of the epiphysis. Because their blood supply is inadequate, minimal trauma may cause avascular necrosis of these bone islets leading to JOCD. Ribbing[9] wrote that the mechanism of OCD was an accessory bone nucleus that separates in childhood with subsequent partial reattachment. Caffey et al[8] also found marginal irregularities to be common in the regular epiphyseal outline of the distal femoral epiphysis with 66% of boys and 41% of girls having irregularities in the centers of ossification. Irregularity or roughening of the epiphyseal outline of the distal femoral physis may be a normal variant associated with periods of rapid skeletal growth. This seems to argue against the theory that abnormal ossification is a primary cause of OCD, as the epiphyseal defects seen in many patients with early lesions may have been a result of normal development.

Families with a predisposition for OCD in various joints have been documented in several studies but to date genetic factors have not been definitively shown to play a role in the development of OCD. Petrie[10] found no definite genetic etiology for OCD in his review of 34 families. The isolated reports of familial involvement may actually be unrecognized cases of multiple epiphyseal dysplasia. Multiple epiphyseal dysplasia must be considered in all patients with JOCD, especially if there is a family history of OCD. Because multiple epiphyseal dysplasia has autosomal dominant and recessive hereditary patterns, patients thought to have a familial form of OCD may actually have a variable expression of multiple epiphyseal dysplasia.

A final theory for the etiology of JOCD has been ischemia. Arterioles supplying small segments of subchondral bone become compromised by embolic phenomena, resulting in necrosis. This theory, although attractive, was refuted by the findings of Rogers and Gladstone (as reported by Cahill[2]), who revealed that the blood supply to the lower end of the femur is rich with numerous anastomoses in the cancellous bone, and that the subarticular areas of the distal femur are not supplied by end arteries.

■ The Juvenile Osteochondritis Dissecans Knee

Presentation

The most commonly affected joint in JOCD is the knee, with up to 85% of all cases being found there. The symptoms of OCD of the knee depend on the stage of presentation. Lesions early in their course are associated with poorly defined symptoms, and it may be difficult to differentiate a patient with osteochondral damage from a patient who has some other knee pathology, such as a meniscal tear, synovial problems, or extensor mechanism dysfunction. The presentation is often with vague, nonlocalized pain and ache. The initial disability often is only slight, but progresses before the diagnosis is made. The pain described is variable and intermittent, and typically increases with activity, especially running and jumping, but improves with rest. Parents may report a history of intermittent knee swelling associated with activity. Any degree of effusion after exercise should not be regarded as normal in this age group. As the lesion progresses, mechanical symptoms of catching, locking, and giving way are noted. The presence of loose bodies is associated with more constant symptoms of catching, locking, swelling, and pain. A patient rarely presents with an acutely locked knee due to a loose fragment as the initial manifestations of OCD.

Examination

The physical examination findings in JOCD also depend on the stage of the lesion at presentation. In the early stages, the physical examination can be nonspecific. There may be crepitus in the medial tibiofemoral compartment, and tenderness to palpation can be diffuse and poorly localized. As the lesion progresses, point tenderness may be present over the area of the lesion. The examiner should palpate both the medial and femoral condyles as well as the patella facet joint in an attempt localize the lesion. Axhausen described a sign of tenderness to palpation at the affected femoral condyle as the knee is brought into progressive degrees of flexion. The patient may also show loss of thigh circumference, antalgic gait, diminished range of motion, or an effusion. In a child with a lesion of the medial femoral condyle, careful examination of the child's gait may reveal that the affected leg is held in a position of external rotation. This is a learned behavior in an attempt to avoid impingement of the tibial spine on the lateral aspect of the medial femoral condyle. The classic physical examination finding associated with OCD was described by Wilson (as reported by Cahill[2]). The sign is elicited by flexing the knee to 90 degrees, internally rotating the tibia, and then slowly extending the knee. A positive Wilson sign is pain at ~30 degrees of flexion that is relieved by external rotation of the tibia. Although this maneuver is well known, it should not be relied on as a pathognomonic finding. In a series of 509 affected knees, this sign was positive in only 16% of patients.[2]

Radiographic Imaging

If the history and physical examination are suspicious for JOCD, then radiographic studies are necessary to confirm the diagnosis. Initial radiographic evaluation should consist of standing anteroposterior, lateral, and tunnel views of the affected knee. A tunnel view with the knee in flexion commonly demonstrates a lesion that is not as easily seen on a standard weight-bearing anteroposterior film (Fig. 21–1). If a lesion is suspected to involve the patella, then the skyline view is helpful to identify lesions.

Radiographically, the lesion typically appears as a well-circumscribed area of sclerotic subchondral bone separated from the remainder of the epiphysis by a radiolucent line. Many JOCD patients present with radiographic findings only in the lateral view. The classic location for JOCD of the knee is in the lateral non–weight-bearing mid- to posterior portion of the medial femoral condyle. This location accounts for ~75% of JOCD lesions in the knee. The remaining 25% of lesions are divided between the lateral femoral condyle and the patella. Multiple sites have been noted up to 40% of the time. Harding described two lines drawn on the lateral radiograph: one along the posterior femoral cortex and the other along

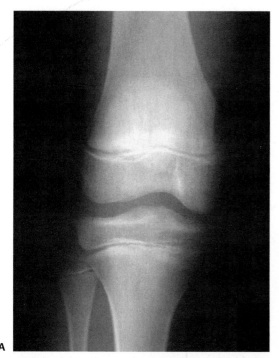
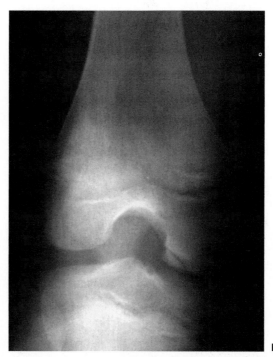

A   B

FIGURE 21–1 Anteroposterior (AP) **(A)** and notch view **(B)** radiographs of the knee in the same patient with juvenile osteochondritis dissecans (JOCD). The typical lesion involves the posterior weight-bearing portion of the lateral aspect of the medial femoral condyle and can be better appreciated on the notch view.

the Blumensaat line (intercondylar notch) **(Fig. 21–2)**. These lines divide the articular surface of the distal femur into three sections, and the arc of the articular surface between these two lines is the area where JOCD of the medial femoral condyle is commonly found. Lesions involving the lateral femoral condyle tend to be slightly more posteriorly located.

Prior to the introduction of MRI, a technetium-99m phosphate compound bone scan was used as the next step in the investigation of OCD **(Fig. 21–3)**. The bone

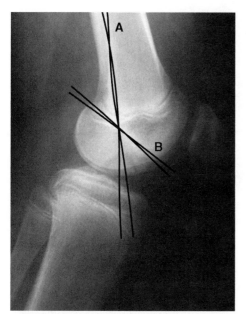

FIGURE 21–2 Lateral radiograph is useful in detecting osteochondritis dissecans (OCD). One line is drawn along the posterior cortex of the femur **(A)**, and another along Blumensaat's line **(B)**. (Adapted from Harding .)

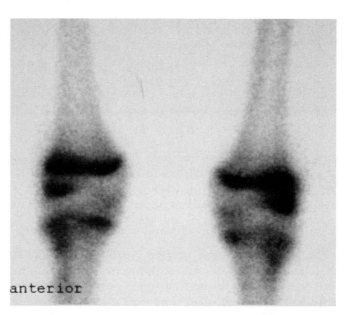

FIGURE 21–3 Bone scan of bilateral lateral femoral condyle JOCD demonstrating increased uptake within bilateral lateral distal femoral epiphyses.

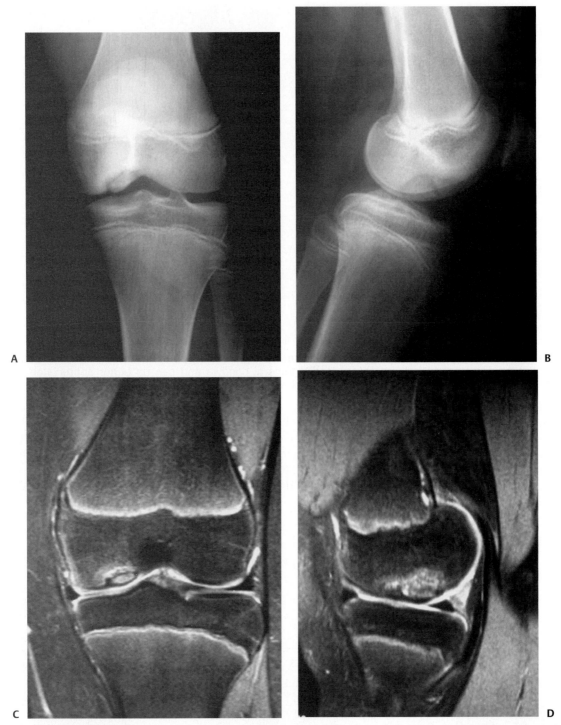

FIGURE 21–4 Magnetic resonance imaging (MRI) of JOCD of the knee. AP **(A)** and lateral **(B)** radiographs. Corresponding coronal **(C)** and sagittal **(D)** MRI images demonstrating an intact articular surface with clear demarcation of the underlying bony lesion.

scan is highly sensitive, can be positive as early as 12 hours after injury, identifies the presence of bilateral involvement, and is relatively inexpensive.[2] It is a helpful test in patients suspicious for OCD with negative radiographic findings. Cahill[2] recommends using the bone scan as the method of choice for following the progress of the disease. He has noted that the degree of osseous uptake on bone scan is related to the regional blood flow, and, therefore, the potential for healing of the fragment. He advises scanning the patient at 4-month intervals to monitor changes in the lesion's activity. Parallel-hole scans are to be obtained only with the initial scan with the much more sensitive and detailed pin-hole technique used thereafter. Paletta et al[11] also found the bone scan to be predictive for prognosis of nonsurgical treatment in patients with open physes. The patients with increased activity on bone scan went on to heal their lesions nonoperatively.

The disadvantages of a bone scan, however, are that it cannot quantify the exact size of the lesion or determine the condition of the articular cartilage. This is where an MRI can supply valuable information either as a supplement to the bone scan or as a primary study (**Fig. 21–4**). MRI is useful not only for identifying the location and extent of the suspected lesion, but also for determining the involvement and integrity of the articular cartilage.[12] It facilitates determining whether there is detachment of a fragment. If there is a joint effusion, the presence of fluid behind the fragment can clearly identify partial or complete detachment. If there is not an effusion, then intraarticular gadolinium can be used to enhance a detached lesion. This information is important clinically, because it can change the management of the patient. An MRI also provides important supplemental information such as the detection of subtle bone injuries, the integrity of the ligaments and menisci, and the presence or absence of any associated intraarticular osseous and cartilaginous bodies. Over the past 10 to 15 years, improvements in the techniques of acquiring images with MRI have increased our ability to diagnose articular cartilage injuries in the knee noninvasively. Loredo and Sanders[13] feel the optimal technique for evaluation of cartilage is a spoiled gradient-echo sequence using fat suppression and three-dimensional acquisition. With this sequence, spatial resolution is high, owing to the ability to obtain thin contiguous slices; the images can be reformatted in multiple planes, and there are high contrast-to-noise ratios between cartilage and fluid and between cartilage and bone. Despite these advancements, however, MRI is still not as sensitive or specific as arthroscopy in assessing articular cartilage injury.[12] Arthroscopy remains the gold standard and may be especially useful in the management of patients for whom MRI scans of good quality or intraarticular gadolinium arthrography is not available.

Classification

Radiographic studies have been used in an attempt to classify JOCD lesions. There have been multiple classification systems developed for JOCD, but there is no universally accepted system. Cahill[2] and Berg devised a classification based on the appearance of the lesion on bone scan (**Table 21–1**). MRI has also been used as the basis for a classification scheme with increasing stages indicating worsening of the lesion (**Table 21–2**). Finally, the lesions can be classified on the basis of surgical findings.[5] This classification is based on visual and palpable observations at surgery and is designed to allow accurate description of the lesion. The lesion is first classified under one of three categories: (1) intact cartilage, (2) disrupted cartilage, and (3) macerated cartilage. If there is intact cartilage, then one must determine if it is a stable or unstable lesion. If there is disrupted cartilage, then one can again examine to see if it is stable or unstable. If it is deemed to be unstable, then it falls into one of three types: predetachment, hinged, or loose body. Finally, if the cartilage is found to be macerated, then it can be subclassified as discolored, blistered, abraded, or fragmented.

Management

The management of JOCD is controversial. The data in the current literature regarding the ability of JOCD-involved femoral condyles to heal and be restored to normalcy is divided between those saying that no treatment is necessary and those believing that most patients need surgery.[14–17] Although it is true that all recent authors agree that children with open physes have a much higher frequency of spontaneous resolution of this condition than adults, JOCD is not an entirely benign condition.[14–17] The overall success rate of nonoperative treatment is ~50%.[14–17] Once the diagnosis of JOCD is confirmed, the race for healing of the lesion before the distal femoral physis closure begins. If the contest is lost,

TABLE 21–1 Bone Scan Classification of Juvenile Osteochondritis Dissecans Lesions

Stage 0: Normal radiographic and scintigraphic appearance.
Stage I: The lesion is visible on plain radiographs, but bone scans reveal normal findings.
Stage II: The scan reveals increased uptake in the area of the lesion.
Stage III: In addition, there is increased isotopic uptake in the entire femoral condyle.
Stage IV: In addition, there is uptake in the tibial plateau opposite the lesion.

TABLE 21–2 MRI Classification of Juvenile Osteochondritis Dissecans Lesions

Stage I: Small change of signal without clear margins of fragment.
Stage II: Osteochondral fragment with clear margins but without fluid between fragment and underlying bone.
Stage III: Fluid is visible partially between fragment and underlying bone.
Stage IV: Fluid is completely surrounding the fragment, but the fragment is still in situ.
Stage V: Fragment is completely detached and displaced (loose body).

and JOCD evolves into OCD with the potential for nonunion and detachment, then the favorable prognosis is lost. Consequently, for conservative treatment to have the best prognosis, JOCD must be diagnosed early. Two additional factors besides the age of the patient that have been found to affect the prognosis of JOCD are the size and location of the lesion. The larger the size of the lesion, the higher the likelihood of developing osteoarthritis according to Twyman et al.[16] Their work also agrees with that of Hefti et al,[5] who found that the chances of healing were better when the lesion was located at the classic site (lateral part of medial femoral condyle) rather than at other sites.

Most clinicians agree that initial treatment for patients with JOCD should be nonoperative unless the lesion is unstable, a loose body is present, or the patient is within 8 months of physis closure. The goal of conservative treatment is to obtain lesion healing before physis closure to prevent potential early-onset gonarthrosis. Provided the patient is compliant and the lesion remains stable, the success of conservative treatment of JOCD, as judged by radiographic healing of the lesion, has been reported to vary between 50% and 91%.[14–17] Therefore, a trial of adequate conservative treatment is appropriate. Nonoperative treatment options range from "watchful waiting" and activity modification to non–weight-bearing and immobilization with trials lasting from 6 to 18 months. The basic principle of nonoperative treatment is reduction of exercise to a level where symptom-free activities of daily living are possible.[18] In a report by Sales de Gauzy et al,[3] 30 of 31 lesions healed over an average of 11 months by simply discontinuing the child's involvement in sports activities until the pain had stopped.

If there is pain with ambulation, then crutches are used for 6 to 8 weeks with weight bearing as tolerated. During this time, no competitive sports or running is allowed. Because it can be difficult to restrict the activity of a child, removable splints or a knee immobilizer with intermittent knee motion may be used. Some clinicians utilize casts routinely; however, the deleterious effects of immobilization on cartilage nutrition and the potential for stiffness and atrophy should be considered. The results of unloader braces have not been established. Close clinical observation with serial radiographic studies is important. The choice of which radiographic study to use is clinician dependent. Radiographs or MRIs can be used to follow healing of the lesion. Cahill[2] recommends using a limited bone scan every 8 weeks in combination with physical examination until clinical and scintigraphic examinations demonstrate that healing has occurred.

Once the child has reached the symptom-free level, the crutches can be discarded. As healing progresses, activities such as recreational cycling, swimming, and lower extremity closed kinetic-chain strength training are added, provided the child remains asymptomatic.

Successful conservative treatment is indicated by a normal orthopaedic examination, especially the absence of swelling. If the child remains compliant, most lesions will heal within 10 months. However, some slow-healing lesions can take up to 18 months of nonoperative treatment to heal. Patient compliance with such prolonged activity restriction can be problematic. In Cahill's[2] experience, many of the 50% of patients that failed conservative treatment were noncompliant. He stresses the importance of educating the patient and the patient's family about the disease process and makes the point that both nonoperative and surgical treatments require similar periods of time restriction from sports participation. It is exceedingly difficult, however, in a society that demands instant gratification to convince young athletes and their parents to remain out of competitive sports for such an extended period of time. To suggest conservative treatment that could last for 1 year, and would eliminate competitive sports for that time, often surprises and disheartens the family. Consequently, many clinicians compromise and continue nonoperative management of stable JOCD lesions for approximately 6 months. At that point, if the child is still symptomatic, surgical intervention can be used. It can also be argued that excessive delay in operative intervention may allow some adolescents to approach skeletal maturity, thus giving them a worse prognosis for healing and eventual outcome.

Operative intervention is warranted if loose bodies are present, if detachment or instability of the fragment occurs while the patient is under conservative treatment, if there is persistence of symptoms for 6 to 12 months in a compliant patient undergoing conservative treatment, if epiphyseal closure is approaching, or if healing is unlikely as determined on the basis of bone scans, MRI, and clinical judgment.[14–17]

The basic tenets of operative treatment include anatomic restoration of the congruity of joint surfaces, enhancement of revascularization to the fragment or crater, and fixation of unstable fragments to permit early joint motion.[14–17] Surgical options depend on the lesions involved and include drilling (retrograde transarticular or antegrade through the distal femoral epiphysis), curettage, bone grafting, internal fixation, open or arthroscopic reduction of a loose fragment with internal fixation, fragment removal, autologous or allogenic osteochondral grafting, and autologous chondrocyte implantation.

Arthroscopy has become a valuable tool for evaluating the size, location, and stability of the fragment and is less invasive than open arthrotomy. Direct probe of the affected area under arthroscopic control reveals the character of the articular surface at the lesion margins and permits evaluation of the underlying bone's stability. The development of arthroscopic probes that measure the viscoelastic or electrostatic properties of

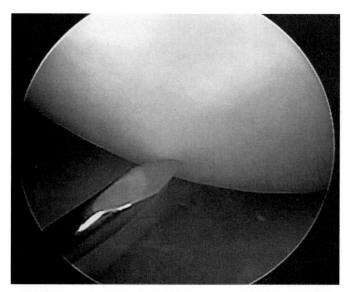

FIGURE 21–5 Arthroscopic transarticular drilling for a stable JOCD lesion of the knee with an intact articular surface.

articular cartilage holds promise. Each case should be decided on an individual basis depending on the lesion size and location. If at arthroscopy, the lesion is found to be stable, arthroscopic drilling without fixation is the treatment of choice. This treatment method theoretically offers the potential to create channels for revascularization and healing **(Fig. 21–5)**. Transarticular drilling is accurate and technically straightforward. Kocher et al[14] reported significant improvement in functional outcome after transarticular drilling, with radiographic healing occurring at an average of 4.4 months after drilling. The one drawback with this technique, however, is that it creates channels in the articular cartilage that heal with fibrocartilage, not hyaline cartilage. For this reason, the technique of antegrade drilling through the epiphysis has been advocated as a way to avoid this problem. This technique, unfortunately, has its own disadvantages, in that it is much more technically difficult, it tends to be inaccurate, and it can be hard to gauge the depth of penetration while drilling. Whichever drilling method is chosen, range of motion with protected weight bearing should be instituted immediately after surgery.

If the lesion is found at arthroscopy to be unstable or is partially detached, then the recommended treatment should be curettage of the femoral defect, drilling of the defect, and stable internal fixation of the lesion. Cancellous grafting may also be necessary to increase vascularity or to fill subchondral cavity defects. When the lesion has been partially detached or loose for months, a sclerotic rim of bone is common. In this instance, drilling alone will not improve the outcome. The crater base should be

curetted to bleeding bone and then drilled. The subchondral bone of the fragment may be sclerotic and require curetting, as well. These lesions should then undergo mechanical stabilization to increase the likelihood of maintaining joint congruity during healing, and to allow the potential benefit of early motion. Selection of the optimal device for stabilization of the lesion is debated. The options for internal fixation for JOCD include Kirschner wires, variable pitch compression screws, cannulated screws, bone pegs, absorbable compression devices, and absorbable pins **(Fig. 21–6)**. Postoperatively, range-of-motion exercises are started at once, but protected weight bearing is necessary for 3 months.

Skeletally immature patients with loose bodies should be managed in a manner similar to adults. If the lesion is from a weight-bearing area, it is imperative that it be replaced. For chronic loose bodies there may be a size mismatch between the loose body and the crater, making replacement challenging **(Fig. 21–7)**. The results of removal in long-term follow-up have been poor. The fibrous and fibrocartilaginous tissue that ultimately fills the JOCD crater after treatment is not hyaline cartilage and has a decreased ability to withstand weight-bearing stresses. If internal fixation of the lesion is impossible, either because it is too macerated or because the articular cartilage has been destroyed, then the lesion should be removed and chondral resurfacing should be considered. Resurfacing techniques include abrasion arthroplasty, microfracture, mosaicplasty, osteochondral allograft, and autologous chondrocyte implantation. To date, there are no published data regarding the outcome of allografts, autografts, or chondrocyte implantation specifically in skeletally immature patients. These methods, however, are recommended in salvage situations.

■ Epidemiology of Osteochondritis Dissecans of the Elbow

Osteochondral injury of the capitellum affects two different age groups in the skeletally immature. In children between the ages of 4 and 8 years, Panner's disease, an osteochondrosis often involving the entire capitellum, is seen. In adolescent athletes, the more traditional OCD lesion can be found.

Panner's Disease

Patients with Panner's disease present with a history of dull, aching pain in the elbow not associated with trauma.[19] There may also be decreased range of motion, swelling, and tenderness of the elbow. On exam, there are no specific findings, but an effusion, limited

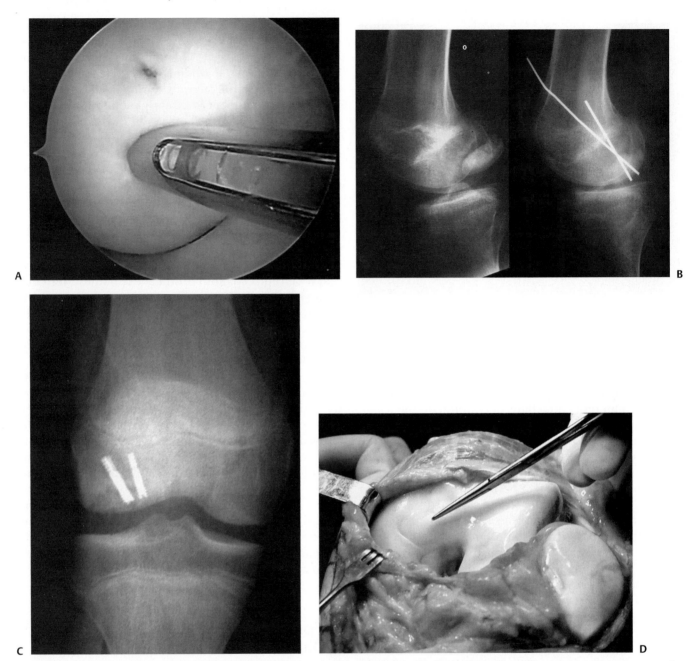

FIGURE 21–6 Surgical management of JOCD of the knee with absorbable implants **(A)**, wires **(B)**, variable-pitch compression screws **(C)**, and autologous chondrocyte implantation **(D)**.

motion, and tenderness over the lateral aspect of the elbow may be noted. The key to making a diagnosis is the radiographs, which reveal rarefaction and fragmentation of the entire ossific nucleus of the capitellum. The disease is thought to share a similar pathophysiology with Legg-Calvé-Perthes disease. Fortunately, Panner's disease is generally a self-limiting process that resolves with rest and splinting. In most cases, reconstitution of the capitellum occurs without late sequelae or limitations.

Osteochondritis Dissecans of the Capitellum

The typical patients are adolescent males involved in throwing sports and female gymnasts. The mechanism is thought to be repetitive microtrauma. Valgus overload results in tensile forces in the medial elbow and compressive forces in the lateral elbow.[19–23] The mechanical disparity of compressive stiffness between the radial head and the capitellum causes increased strain on the softer capitellar surface. This is thought to lead

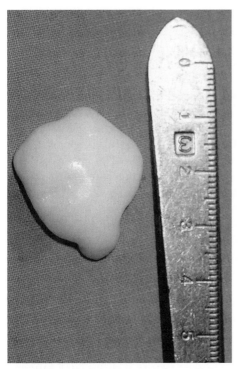

FIGURE 21–7 Loose body associated with juvenile osteochondritis dissecans of the knee.

to breakdown and avascularity of the subchondral bone of the capitellum producing an OCD lesion.[19–23] Ischemia has also been hypothesized to be a possible etiology of capitellar JOCD.[19–23] The blood supply to the capitellar chondroepiphysis enters posteriorly and has no communication with the metaphyseal vessels. This fragile arrangement may become compromised with the resulting ischemia producing OCD of the capitellum.

The presentation of capitellar OCD is one of insidious onset with poorly localized, diffuse joint pain. Symptoms are intermittent, increasing with activity and improving with rest. In patients who have more advanced irregularity of the articular surface, more dramatic symptoms, such as catching, clicking, giving way, and grinding may be reported. If loose bodies are present, true locking of the joint may occur. Physical examination can reveal an effusion and tenderness to palpation over the lateral elbow and capitellum. A decreased range of motion may be present with a lack of full extension being the most common finding.

Plain anteroposterior and lateral radiographs reveal the characteristic rarefaction or radiolucency of the lateral or central portion of the capitellum (**Fig. 21–8**). In contrast to Panner's disease, only a portion of the ossific nucleus of the capitellum is involved. Hypertrophy

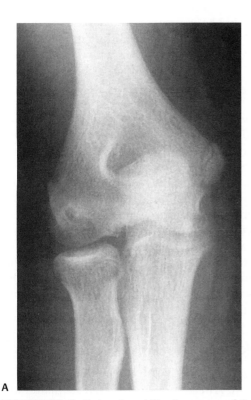

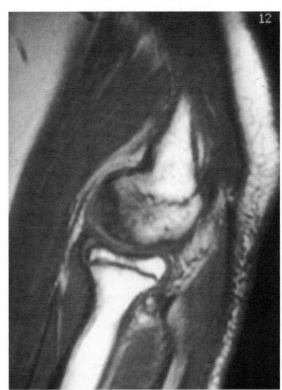

A

B

FIGURE 21–8 Osteochondritis dissecans of the capitellum: AP radiograph **(A)** and sagittal MRI **(B)**.

of the radial head and loose bodies are sometimes seen in the later stages. MRI can help make the diagnosis if there is still suspicion after obtaining plain radiographs. MRI also allows evaluation of the stage of the lesion (**Fig. 21–8**).

Treatment consists of rest and activity modification. Lesions that have not fragmented may heal if protected from additional trauma. The prognosis is improved if the patient is less than 13 years of age and if the lesion is not advanced. Loose fragments can be removed by arthroscopic or open methods, and the capitellar defect can be drilled. The results from fragment fixation have been disappointing.

■ Osteochondral Fractures

Osteochondral fractures in skeletally immature patients are more common than once thought. They most frequently involve the knee joint and are typically associated with acute patellar dislocations. The prevalence of osteochondral fractures associated with acute patella dislocation ranges from 25 to 50%.[24–29] Matelic et al[26] found 67% of children presenting with an acute hemarthrosis of the knee had an osteochondral fracture. The most common locations for these fractures are the medial patellar facet (**Fig. 21–9**) or the lateral femoral condyle.[24–29]

Etiology

A histopathologic study by Flachsmann et al[30] helps to explain the occurrence of osteochondral fractures in the skeletally immature at a cellular level. They noted that in the joint of a juvenile, interdigitating fingers of uncalcified cartilage penetrate deep into the subchondral bone, providing a relatively strong bond between the articular cartilage and the subchondral bone. In the adult, the articular cartilage is bonded to the subchondral bone by the well-defined calcified cartilage layer—the cement line. When shear stress is applied to the juvenile joint, the forces are transmitted into the subchondral bone by the interdigitating cartilage, with the resultant bending forces causing the open pore structure of the trabecular bone to fail. In mature tissue, the plane of failure occurs between the deep and calcified layers of the cartilage—the tidemark—leaving the osteochondral junction undisturbed. Although the juvenile and adult tissue patterns are different, they both provide adequate fracture toughness to the osteochondral region. As the tissue transitions, however, from the juvenile to the adult pattern during adolescence, the fracture toughness is lost. The calcified cartilage layer is only partially formed and the interdigitating cartilage fingers are progressively replaced with calcified matrix.

Consequently, the interface between the articular cartilage and the subchondral bone becomes a zone of potential weakness in the joint, which may explain why osteochondral fractures are seen frequently in adolescents and young adults.

There are two primary mechanisms for production of an osteochondral fracture.[24–30] First, a direct blow to the knee with a shearing force applied to either the medial or lateral femoral condyle can create an osteochondral fracture. The second mechanism involves a flexion-rotation injury of the knee in which an internal rotation force is placed on a fixed foot, usually coupled with a strong quadriceps contraction. The subsequent contact between the tibia and femur or patella and lateral femoral condyle causes the fracture. An example of this mechanism is an acute patellar dislocation. As the patella dislocates, the medial retinaculum tears but the remaining quadriceps muscle-patellar ligament complex still applies significant compressive forces as the patella dislocates laterally and shears across the lateral femoral condyle. The medial border of the patella then temporarily becomes impacted on the prominent edge of the lateral femoral condyle before it slides back tangentially over the surface of the lateral femoral condyle due to pull of the quadriceps. Either the dislocation or the relocation phase of this injury can cause an osteochondral fracture to the lateral femoral condyle, the medial facet of the patella, or both. Interestingly, osteochondral fractures are uncommon with chronic, recurrent subluxation or dislocation of the patella. In this situation, the laxity of the medial knee tissues and decreased compressive forces between the patella and the lateral femoral condyle prevents development of excessive shear forces.

History and Physical Examination

Osteochondral fractures present with severe pain, swelling, and difficulty with weight bearing. On examination, tenderness to palpation over the medial femoral condyle, lateral femoral condyle, or medial patella is exhibited. The patient usually resists attempts to flex or extend the knee and may hold the knee in 15 to 20 degrees of flexion for comfort. The large hemarthrosis is due to fracturing the highly vascular subchondral bone. A joint aspiration reveals a supernatant layer of fat, if allowed to stand for 15 minutes, indicating an intraarticular fracture. Late examination findings may be similar to those of a loose body with intermittent locking or catching of the knee.

Radiographic Imaging

Radiographic visualization of the osteochondral fracture should begin with anteroposterior and lateral plain radiographs. A skyline view of the patella is mandatory if the

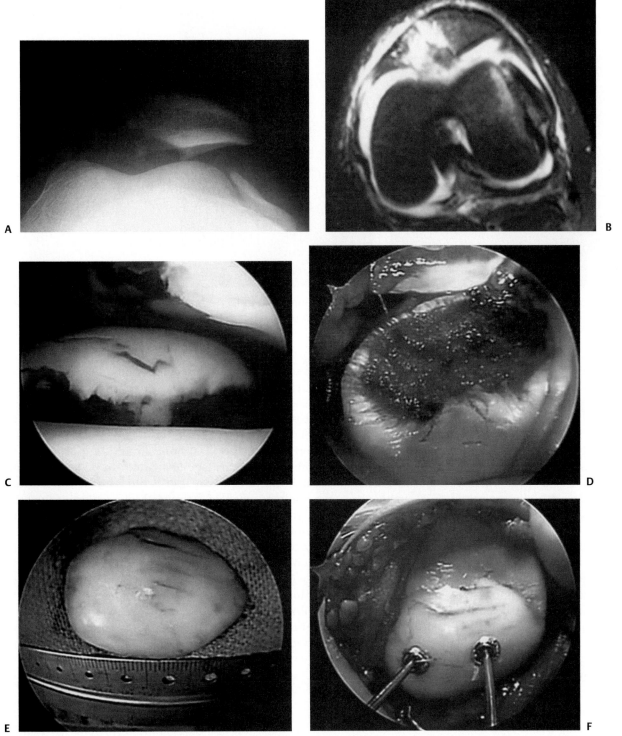

FIGURE 21–9 Osteochondral fracture of the medial patella facet associated with acute patella dislocation in a 12-year-old boy. Skyline radiograph **(A)** and axial MRI **(B)** demonstrating lateral patella subluxation with osteochondral fracture. **(C)** Arthroscopic appearance of osteochondral fragment. **(D)** Appearance of the medial patella defect through an open lateral retinacular release. The osteochondral fragment **(E)** was replaced and fixed using two 3.5-mm cannulated screws

(Continued)

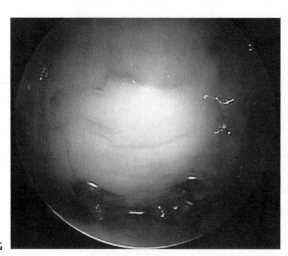
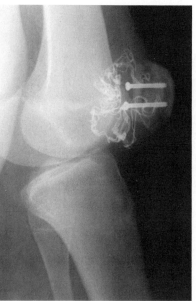

G   H

FIGURE 21–9 (*Continued*) **(F,G)**. Healed osteochondral fracture seen through the lateral arthrotomy at the time of screw removal, 6 weeks after fixation **(H)**.

patient has suffered an acute patellar dislocation. However, a roentgenographic diagnosis can be difficult because even a large osteochondral fragment may contain only a small ossified portion that is visible on plain radiographs. Matelic et al[26] report that standard radiographs failed to identify the osteochondral fracture in 36% of children who had an osteochondral fracture found during arthroscopy. For this reason, supplemental studies such as MRI or computed tomography (CT) arthrography may be necessary in cases where there is a high suspicion of osteochondral fracture despite negative radiographs.[31,32] Arthroscopic examination can also be done as the definitive diagnostic (and potentially therapeutic) test. With regard to plain film findings, two studies have reported that having a high-riding patella seems to have a protective effect against associated intraarticular osteochondral fractures. Patients with an Insall index >1.3 have a decreased chance of sustaining an osteochondral fracture compared with patients who have an Insall index within normal limits.[31]

Management

The recommended management of acute osteochondral fractures of the knee is either surgical removal of the fragment or fixation of the fragment to its anatomic location.[33] If the lesion is large (>1 cm), easily accessible, involves a weight-bearing area, and has adequate cortical bone attached to the chondral surface, then fixation should be attempted **(Fig. 21–9)**. This can be done via arthroscopy or arthrotomy with smooth or threaded

Steinmann pins or screws countersunk below the articular surface. If the fracture fragment is small, loose, and from a non–weight-bearing region of the knee, then arthroscopic excision is recommended. The fragment's crater should be debrided to stable edges, and the underlying subchondral bone should be perforated to encourage fibrocartilage formation. In patients with an osteochondral fracture after acute patellar dislocation, concomitant repair of the medial retinaculum at the time of fragment excision or fixation produces the best results. Postoperatively, patients treated by excision of the fragment can begin range-of-motion exercises immediately. Crutches may be necessary in the immediate postoperative period but patients can progress to weight bearing as tolerated. If the patient has the fragment fixed, initial immobilization with protected weight bearing is necessary. Weight bearing is gradually progressed and full weight bearing is allowed when the swelling has subsided and radiographs show evidence of fracture healing. Return to athletic activities is permitted when full range of motion is recovered and quadriceps strength is symmetric.

■ Chondral Injuries

Chondral injuries can occur in skeletally immature patients although the exact incidence of these injuries is unknown, because they can be difficult to diagnose. Chondral injuries are caused by major compression and shear forces at the articular surfaces such as occurs in acute patellar dislocations. Stanitski and Paletta[25] used four-view radiographs and arthroscopy to evaluate 48 adolescent patients with acute patellar dislocations and found only two purely chondral injuries (4%).

If after a complete history, physical exam, and plain radiographs, a chondral injury is suspected, then an MRI is recommended to evaluate the status of the articular cartilage. Gradient-echo sequences appear especially helpful in identifying chondral lesions and should be obtained when available.[31] Despite the improvements in imaging of articular cartilage, arthroscopy still remains the gold standard for identifying chondral injuries. Arthroscopy has the potential to be both diagnostic and therapeutic and can be used in situations where MRI is not available.

Treatment of chondral injuries in the skeletally immature generally uses the same management strategies as in adults, but there are a few differences that must be taken into consideration when managing a child with this injury. First, although the surgical procedures developed to repair cartilage damage in skeletally mature patients (abrasion chondroplasty, microfracture, transarticular drilling, articular cartilage autografting, autologous chondrocyte implantation, and allografting) have the same potential benefit in skeletally immature patients, there is little data in the literature to support one procedure over another in this age group. Our preference is to attempt microfracture first, and then, if this is unsuccessful, to use autologous chondrocyte implantation as a salvage procedure.

Second, when operating on the skeletally immature, there are a few technical points that must be remembered that are not ordinarily addressed in adults. When performing marrow stimulation techniques, such as drilling or microfracture, the surgeon must be cognizant of the proximity of the growth plate to prevent potential growth disturbances from inadvertent violation of the physis. Similarly, when autologous chondrocyte implantation is attempted, it is important not to disrupt the tibial tubercle apophysis while harvesting periosteum. Another difference in the management of skeletally immature chondral injuries is that most of these procedures require a period of protected weight bearing postoperatively. This can be difficult to enforce in younger children because they may not be able to follow complex rehabilitation programs. Consequently, the surgeon may need to modify the rehabilitation program to fit the patient's capabilities. Finally, although it is generally believed that children have greater reparative abilities than adults, they also have a longer remaining life span than adults. This means the implications of a full-thickness chondral injury and its repair are more important. Furthermore, the longevity of chondral resurfacing techniques is of utmost importance. It is especially important to attempt to re-create an anatomic articular surface with hyaline cartilage in a young patient who will need a lifetime of use from the joint.

REFERENCES

1. Kocher MS, Micheli LJ. The pediatric knee: evaluation and treatment. In: Insall JN, Scott WN, eds. Surgery of the Knee, 3rd ed. New York: Churchill-Livingstone, 2001:1356–1397
2. Cahill BR. Osteochondritis dissecans of the knee: treatment of juvenile and adult forms. J Am Acad Orthop Surg 1995;3:237–247
3. Sales de Gauzy J, Mansat C, Darodes PH, et al. Natural course of osteochondritis dissecans in children. J Pediatr Orthop 1999;8:26–28
4. Linden B. The incidence of osteochondritis dissecans in the condyles of the femur. Acta Orthop Scand 1976;47:664–667
5. Hefti F, Beguiristain J, Krauspe R, et al. Osteochondritis dissecans: a multicenter study of the European Pediatric Orthopaedic Society. J Pediatr Orthop 1999;8B:231–245
6. Schenk RC, Goodnight JM. Osteochondritis dissecans. J Bone Joint Surg 1996;78-A:439–456
7. Clanton TO, DeLee JC. Osteochondritis dissecans. Clin Orthop Relat Res 1982;167:50–64
8. Caffey J, Madell SH, Royer C, et al. Ossification of the distal femoral epiphysis. J Bone Joint Surg 1958;40-A:647–654
9. Ribbing S. The hereditary multiple epiphyseal disturbance and its consequences for the aetiogenesis of local malacias—particularly the osteochondrosis dissecans. Acta Orthop Scand 1955;24: 286–299
10. Petrie PW. Aetiology of osteochondritis dissecans. Failure to establish a familial background. J Bone Joint Surg Br 1977;59:366–367
11. Paletta GA Jr, Bednarz PA, Stanitski CL, et al. The prognostic value of quantitative bone scan in knee osteochondritis dissecans. A preliminary experience. Am J Sports Med 1998;26:7–14
12. Kocher MS, DiCanzio J, Zurakowski D, et al. Diagnostic performance of clinical examination and selective magnetic resonance imaging in the evaluation of intraarticular knee disorders in children and adolescents. Am J Sports Med 2001;29:292–296
13. Loredo R, Sanders TG. Imaging of osteochondral injuries. Clin Sports Med 2001;20:249–278
14. Kocher MS, Micheli LJ, Yaniv M, et al. Functional and radiographic outcome of juvenile osteochondritis dissecans of the knee treated with transarticular arthroscopic drilling. Am J Sports Med 2001;29:562–566
15. Carroll NC, Mubarak SJ. Juvenile osteochondritis dissecans of the knee. J Bone Joint Surg 1977;59-B:506
16. Twyman R, Desai K, Aichroth PM. Osteochondritis dissecans of the knee. J Bone Joint Surg 1991;73-B:461–464
17. Cain EL, Clancy WG. Treatment algorithm for osteochondral injuries of the knee. Clin Sports Med 2001;20:321–341
18. Cahill BR, Ahten SM. The three critical components in the conservative treatment of juvenile osteochondritis dissecans. Clin Sports Med 2001;20:287–298
19. Kocher MS, Waters PM, Micheli LJ. Upper extremity injuries in the paediatric athlete. Sports Med 2000;30:117–135
20. Baumgarten TE, Andrews JR, Satterwhite YE. The arthroscopic classification and treatment osteochondritis dissecans of the capitellum. Am J Sports Med 1998;26:520–523
21. Pappas AM. Elbow problems associated with baseball during childhood and adolescence. Clin Orthop 1982;164:30–41
22. Bauer M, Jonsson K, Josefsson PO, et al. Osteochondritis dissecans of the elbow: a long term follow-up study. Clin Orthop 1992;284:156–160
23. Ruch DS, Cory JW, Poehling GG. The arthroscopic management of osteochondritis dissecans of the adolescent elbow. Arthroscopy 1998;14:797–803
24. Nietosvaara Y, Aalto K, Kallio PE. Acute patellar dislocation in children: incidence and associated osteochondral fractures. J Pediatr Orthop 1994;14:513–515
25. Stanitski CL, Paletta GA. Articular cartilage injury with acute patellar dislocation in adolescents. Am J Sports Med 1998;26: 52–55

26. Matelic TM, Aronsson DD, Boyd DW, et al. Acute hemarthrosis of the knee in children. Am J Sports Med 1995;23:668–671

27. Farmer JM, Martin DF, Boles CA, et al. Chondral and osteochondral injuries. Clin Sports Med 2001;20:299–319

28. Alleyne KR, Galloway MT. Management of osteochondral injuries of the knee. Clin Sports Med 2001;20:343–363

29. Birk GT, DeLee JC. Osteochondral injuries. Clin Sports Med 2001;20:279–287

30. Flachsmann R, Broom ND, Hardy AE, et al. Why is the adolescent joint particularly susceptible to osteochondral shear fracture? Clin Orthop Relat Res 2000;381:212–221

31. Bohndorf K. Imaging of acute injuries of the articular surfaces (chondral, osteochondral, and subchondral fractures). Skeletal Radiol 1999;28:545–560

32. Wessel LM, Scholz S, Rusch M, et al. Hemarthrosis after trauma to the pediatric knee joint: what is the value of magnetic resonance imaging in the diagnostic algorithm? J Pediatr Orthop 2001;21:338–342

33. Menche DS, Vangsness CT, Pitman M, et al. The treatment of isolated articular cartilage lesions in the young individual. Instr Cours Lect 1998;47:505–515

Adjunctive Treatments with Cartilage Restoration

22

Corrective Osteotomies Around the Knee

GREGORY J. ADAMSON, JENNIFER R. MILLER,
AND PIERRE DURAND JR.

Historically, osteotomies about the knee have been performed to treat osteoarthritis or to correct a deformity in joint alignment. Early reports from Europe in the late 1950s, as well as Coventry's reports in North America in the 1960s, popularized both varus and valgus realignment osteotomies of the proximal tibia. Increased varus or valgus alignment has been shown to be associated with increased contact pressures in the knee.[1] Excessive pressure can lead to the breakdown of cartilage within the affected compartment. By redistributing the mechanical forces across the knee, a corrective osteotomy can potentially slow the progression of cartilage degeneration, provide pain relief, allow for return to sport or heavy labor, increase the life span of the joint, and delay the need for arthroplasty.

The prevalence of osteotomies for medial or lateral gonarthrosis has steadily decreased with the improved longevity and increased popularity of total or unicompartmental knee arthroplasty. The historic success rate of high tibial osteotomies for medial gonarthrosis in a meta-analysis of previously unpublished data are 76% at 5 years and 63% at 10 years,[2] whereas total knee arthroplasty is successful in up to 93% of patients at 10 years.[3] Yet, total knee arthroplasty requires activity modification and has a finite life span that may be incompatible with the needs of the young active patient.

With other good treatment options available for the arthritic knee, the indications for osteotomy have narrowed. The ideal patient has been described as a thin, active individual in the fifth or sixth decade of life with localized, activity-related, unicompartmental knee pain, and with at least 90 degrees of flexion and less than 10

to 15 degrees of flexion contracture.[4] They are best indicated in patients with only Ahlback I to II changes,[5] and should be overcorrected by 2 to 3 degrees to obtain lasting results.[6]

As the basic science and technology of cartilage restoration and meniscal transplantation have evolved, new indications for osteotomy of the proximal tibia, distal femur, and tibial tubercle have emerged. Physiologic genu varum or valgum is well tolerated in the knee with healthy cartilage. However, physiologic varus alignment in a knee with a medial compartment chondral or osteochondral defect creates a situation where excessive force is transmitted through the injured compartment. The same is true for a physiologic valgus aligned knee with a lateral compartment problem. Overload of the compartment undergoing cartilage repair is likely to lead to an unsatisfactory result. An osteotomy that maintains a level joint line and unloads the affected compartment prior to, or at the time of, meniscal allograft or articular cartilage restoration will enhance the success of the procedure.

■ Alignment

Alignment has traditionally been evaluated with both anatomic and mechanical axis measurements. The anatomic axis measures the tibiofemoral angle from standing anteroposterior (AP) radiographs using several centered points on the shafts of each bone. Normative data have shown the average tibiofemoral angle to be 5 to 7 degrees of valgus.[7] Height affects this angle, with taller individuals likely to be 5 degrees, medium tall individuals 7 degrees, and shorter individuals more likely to be up to 9 degrees.[8] Correspondingly, many generalize that men have a tibiofemoral axis of 6 degrees and women an axis of 7 degrees. The mechanical axis of the knee is the angle formed by lines connecting the center of the femoral head and the center of the tibiotalar joint to the center of the knee. Normative data show the axis ranges between 0 and 2.3 degrees of varus, with an average of 1.2 degrees.[7] Normal alignment results in ~60% of the load being transmitted through the medial compartment during weight bearing. The mechanical axis is measured on a full-length radiograph. The mechanical axis of the leg, which is often referred to as the "weight-bearing line," is derived from a line connecting the center of the femoral head to the center of the tibiotalar joint. Many believe the weight-bearing line more accurately defines load transmission forces across the knee joint.

Malalignment can come from extraarticular or intraarticular sources. Intraarticular causes such as cartilage loss and ligamentous laxity are of particular concern in the young adult athlete with gonarthralgia. This population may have physiologic varus or valgus that would otherwise be perfectly acceptable. Fortunately, this means that adjunctive osteotomies for these patients are usually of mild or moderate magnitude and only in one plane.

■ Preoperative Planning

A standard set of radiographs is helpful for preoperative planning. Many medical offices are not set up to obtain full-length films, so several combinations of the following radiographs are sufficient. If possible, obtain five different radiographs: (1) bilateral AP weight bearing in full extension, (2) bilateral posteroanterior (PA) weight bearing at 45 degrees flexion, and (3) lateral, (4) skyline, and (5) full-length standing of both lower extremities. It is important to remember that supine views may underestimate the correction required. Single-leg films may overestimate or underestimate the correction because of the soft tissue laxity not requiring bony correction, as well as malrotation of the extremity on the film.

Once the radiographs have been completed, measuring the alignment can help determine the appropriate location and magnitude of the osteotomy. Measure the mechanical axis and weight-bearing line from the full-length radiograph, and the anatomic axis from the weight-bearing AP in full extension. In knees with significant tibial or femoral deformity, consider measuring the individual articular angles of the tibia and femur. The joint congruency angles and posterior tibial slope

may also be helpful, especially in regard to anterior cruciate ligament (ACL) and posterior cruciate ligament (PCL) reconstructions.

The goal of osteotomy is to transfer the weight-bearing force to the healthy compartment of the knee. Several methods can be used to determine the appropriate angular correction to achieve this redistribution of forces. The general principle is to determine the desired postoperative anatomic axis, mechanical axis, or the location of the weight-bearing line, and calculate the angular correction necessary to achieve it. The optimal postoperative frontal/coronal plane alignment to unload the medial compartment should be 8 to 10 degrees of anatomic axis valgus,[6] 3 to 5 degrees of mechanical axis valgus, or a weight-bearing line passing through 62 to 66% of the tibial width (medial to lateral).[9] To unload the lateral compartment, postoperative alignment should place the weight-bearing line at slightly less than 50% of the tibial width, producing neutral anatomic alignment (6 degrees of mechanical axis varus).[10,11] Studies have shown good results with correction of up to 3 to 4 degrees of anatomic axis varus,[12] and as little as 4 degrees of mechanical axis varus.[13]

The weight-bearing line method divides the tibial plateau from 0 to 100% (medial to lateral) to determine the desired intersection of the mechanical axis through the knee joint. The weight-bearing line should not be corrected to greater than 75% of the tibial width (6 degrees of mechanical axis valgus) because it may result in medial lift-off. Noyes uses this technique, selecting 62% as the point on the joint line. An alternate technique for a high tibial osteotomy, described by Dugdale and Noyes,[9] uses a line drawn from the center of the femoral head to the 62% coordinate on the plateau. The radiograph is then cut through the osteotomy site, leaving the hinge intact, and the distal tibia is rotated until the weight-bearing line passes through the 62% coordinate. The correction angle is the lateral overlap for lateral closing wedge osteotomy or the medial gap for medial opening wedge osteotomy. The wedge height is calculated after correction for magnification of the radiograph if the operative technique does not utilize a jig that can be set at a particular angle. This angle or wedge height is the same for an opening or closing wedge osteotomy of the tibia or femur.

Miniaci et al[14] recommend using the weight-bearing line a different way, incorporating multiple lines. Line 1 connects the center of the femoral head to a point 60 to 70% of the tibial width. This line is continued beyond the knee joint for the length of the tibia. Line 2 connects the apex of the proposed osteotomy of the tibia to the center of the tibiotalar joint. Line 3 connects the apex to the point on line 1 where the ankle will intersect with the proposed long axis (line 1) when the osteotomy is performed. The angle formed between lines 2 and 3 corresponds to the angle of correction at the proximal tibia.

The rule of thumb method, described by Bauer et al,[15] estimates that for each millimeter of height, roughly 1 degree of angular correction will result. This method is accurate only when the actual width of the tibial flare is 56 mm and the radiographic magnification has been corrected. Typically, this method leads to undercorrection (due to the fact that the mean tibial width in women is 70 mm and in men is 80 mm).

A trigonometric method for determining the wedge height can be done, using the following equation: $y = x \tan(\theta)$, where y is the wedge height, x is the actual width of the tibia at the level of the planned osteotomy (2 cm below the joint line), and θ is the desired angle of correction.[16]

On a standing radiograph, attenuated ligaments or osseous defects can cause an overestimation of the magnitude of correction necessary. For a high tibial osteotomy, each millimeter of lateral tibiofemoral joint separation causes approximately 1 degree of varus angular deformity. Excessive deformity from soft tissue laxity is accounted for by comparing the amount of lateral joint space opening in millimeters on the standing AP radiograph with the contralateral knee and subtracting the difference from the calculated angular correction (1 degree/mm) to avoid overcorrection.[7]

Software programs, such as Osteotomy Analysis Simulation Software (OASIS), (Zona Japan, Inc.,) are also available to assist in preoperative planning and produce several options for correction.

The magnitude and direction of the coronal plane malalignment may dictate the location of the osteotomy or suggest the use of a particular technique. For mild or moderate corrections of varus, most valgus-producing osteotomies to augment cartilage restoration are best performed on the proximal tibia. Rarely are valgus producing osteotomies performed on the distal femur. For small degrees of valgus deformity (i.e., less than 12 degrees), proximal tibia varus osteotomies may be performed, but most varus producing osteotomies are preferentially performed on the distal femur. Based on historic results, osteotomies for correcting valgus deformities that exceed 12 degrees should be limited to supracondylar femoral osteotomy to avoid unacceptable joint line obliquity (>10 degrees).[17]

■ Valgus-Producing Osteotomies Proximal Tibial Osteotomies

Indications and Contraindications

Indications for a proximal tibial osteotomy include varus standing alignment associated with any of the following: medial compartment arthrosis in a stable or unstable knee, medial arthralgia with associated medial meniscus deficiency, and medial articular chondral or osteochondral lesions requiring repair or reconstruction. Proximal tibial osteotomies are traditionally reserved for younger patients, although older patients with high activity levels may also be candidates.

Contraindications include inflammatory arthritides, varus deformity greater than 15 degrees, flexion contracture greater than 10 to 15 degrees, lateral subluxation, significant patellofemoral symptoms that are not going to be addressed, excessive weight, unrealistic expectations, lack of tibial bone stock, and lateral compartment problems such as articular lesions or previous meniscectomy. The resulting valgus alignment may be cosmetically unacceptable to some patients and should be discussed prior to osteotomy.

Patient Selection

In 1979 Coventry[18] identified risk factors for failure that included undercorrection and an overweight patient. Patients with both risk factors had failure rates of 60% at 3 years and 80% at 9 years. Berman et al[4] identified factors that lead to increase success rates, including patient age less than 60, 90 degrees of knee motion, stability, and isolated unicompartmental involvement. The patient's history should be consistent with symptoms of localized pain in the medial compartment. The extremity should be examined for range of motion, fixed deformity, and stability.

Literature Review of Long-Term Results and Complications

The use of tibial osteotomies to correct genu varum from rickets was first reported by Sir Robert Jones (as reported by Wardle[19]). Jackson and Waugh[20] later published their results of tibial osteotomies distal to the tuberosity for the treatment of osteoarthritis secondary to varus and valgus knee alignment. In 1965, Coventry[21] described closing wedge osteotomies performed proximal to the tibial tuberosity for both varus (lateral approach) and valgus (medial approach) deformities. Coventry's technique was advantageous in that healing rates improved (osteotomy through cancellous bone) and the osteotomy was near the deformity. Furthermore, his use of staple fixation avoided the need for prolonged cast immobilization. There have been several modifications to Coventry's technique that have shown good results, including inferomedial excision of fibular head [maintaining lateral collateral ligament (LCL) attachment], use of an osteotomy jig, rigid fixation with a buttress plate, and early motion.

Results of high tibial osteotomy for medial compartment arthrosis have been best when the anatomic axis is corrected to 8 to 10 degrees of anatomic valgus[6] or when the weight-bearing line passes through the lateral plateau at 62 to 66% of the width of the plateau.[9] The reported recurrence rate of the deformity is 8% if the malalignment is undercorrected and 1% if it is overcorrected.[18] As noted above, a meta-analysis of proximal tibial osteotomies for varus gonarthrosis yields a success rate is 76% good or excellent results at 5 years and 63% at 10 years.[2]

Complications of Closing Wedge High Tibial Osteotomies

The overall complication rate from a meta-analysis of closing wedge osteotomies is 29%, with only 7% of those complications considered major.[2] Improper correction (more commonly undercorrection than overcorrection) is the most commonly reported complication. Patients with undercorrection generally have less pain relief, a lower satisfaction rate, and a higher reoperation rate. Infection has been reported in 5.1% of patients (6.3% if external fixation group is included), but only 1.6% of the patients required more than simple wound care. Peroneal nerve palsy was reported in 3.4% of patients, with only 0.55% having permanent impairment. An especially high risk of injury to the branch of the peroneal nerve to the extensor hallucis longus (between 7 and 15 cm distal to the head of the fibula) is associated with fibular osteotomies.[22] Delayed or nonunion was found in 2.9% of patients and were often related to technical errors such as loosening the medial hinge, inadequate immobilization, hardware failure, and poor placement of the osteotomy. Several intrinsic factors were also found to increase the risk of nonunion, including diabetes mellitus, infection, and obesity. Persistent instability (<5%), deep venous thrombosis/pulmonary embolism (DVT/PE) (4.6%), arterial injury (0.3%), and medial shift of the distal fragment (3.2%) have occurred.[2] In very few studies, compartment syndrome, avascular necrosis of the proximal segment, joint stiffness, and difficulty with conversion to total knee arthroplasty have been reported.[16,23] The risk of patella infra is decreased with the use of an osteotomy guide, rigid fixation, and early motion.[24,25]

Complications of Opening Wedge High Tibial Osteotomies

Potential complications of the opening wedge technique include inadequate or overcorrection of alignment, arthrofibrosis, patella infra, loss of correction over time, tibial plateau fracture, and arterial injury. The risk of peroneal nerve injury and compartment syndrome should be much less, as the lateral side is not violated. The risk of delayed union or nonunion may be higher than the closing wedge technique, as there is no compression at the osteotomy site. Bone grafting increases the likelihood of healing, but if autogenous graft is used it has its own morbidity.

Few studies report the results and complications of opening wedge proximal tibial osteotomies without concomitant procedures such as ACL reconstruction, meniscal allograft, or posterolateral corner injuries. Noyes[26] recently noted a 5% complication rate with staged high tibial osteotomy followed by ACL reconstruction. All of the osteotomies had autogenous iliac crest bone grafting. All of the osteotomies healed, and there were no infections, or cases of arthrofibrosis. Three percent lost correction and 3% had a delayed union, which healed with a bone stimulator.

Sterett[27] described his results with an opening wedge Puddu plate. Complications included delayed union, 17%; broken hardware, 12%; revision, 12%; infection, 9%; nonunion, 6%; and loss of correction, 4%. The study also reported on a distraction technique, which had complications of pin site infection, 46%; loss of correction, 6%; delayed union, 3%; and revision, 3%.

Tibial Opening Wedge: Medial

Instrumentation and Implants

Standard plates and screws can be used for opening-wedge proximal tibial osteotomies, but osteotomy systems are available that provide specialized plates with a block ("tooth") that sits inside the osteotomy opening, providing strength and reliable angular correction. These plates are now available in stainless steel and titanium. The titanium plate from Arthrex (Naples, FL) locks the screws to the plate for stronger fixation while maintaining a lightweight, low-profile design. The block on the plate is available in sizes from 3 to 17.5 mm in stainless steel, and 5 to 17.5 mm in titanium. The tibial plates are also available with an anterior/posterior slope built into the block. The systems use either a wedge, which, as it is inserted more deeply, increases the angle of the osteotomy, or an osteotome jack, which can be opened to the correct height and angle. Bone graft may be autologous, allogenic, or a combination of the two grafts. Autogenous cortical struts or cancellous graft can be obtained from the ipsilateral iliac crest at the time of surgery. Preshaped allograft wedges with cortical bone are available and can be easily inserted around the tines of the opening-wedge systems. Graft substitute putty with added bone morphogenic proteins can alternatively be used to fill the space and speed bone formation, but it offers no structural support.

Preparation

The patient is placed supine on a radiolucent table and a tourniquet is placed high on the thigh. Fluoroscopy is used to confirm that the center of the femoral head, knee, and talar dome are visible. An electrocardiogram marker is placed on the skin over the center of the femoral head and can be used as a palpable and radiographic landmark when evaluating alignment once the patient has been draped. A standard knee arthroscopy is performed to confirm isolated unicompartmental (medial) involvement. At this point the osteotomy portion is performed under tourniquet control.

Authors' Preferred Surgical Technique

A 5- to 6-cm longitudinal incision is made, beginning 2 cm distal to the medial joint line, and medial to the tibial tubercle. The knee is placed in a relaxed figure-four position and blunt dissection is performed over the capsule, patellar tendon, and pes anserinus. Just distal the joint line, an incision is made sharply along the medial border of the patellar tendon through the fascia and capsule down to bone. A Z-retractor is placed deep to the patellar tendon so that its insertion into the tibial tubercle can be visualized and protected. An incision is made near the upper border of the sartorius in line with its fibers. The semitendinosis and gracilis tendons are retracted distally, exposing the medial tibia.

Using fluoroscopy, a 3-mm guide pin is placed 1 to 1.5 cm distal to the joint and parallel to the joint line, from medial to lateral (maintaining the mid-anterior/posterior position) and advanced to within 1 cm of the lateral cortex **(Fig. 22–1A)**. A guide system (Arthrex, Naples, FL) is applied to the 3-mm guide pin, and two distal pins (2.4 mm) are placed and advanced so that the cut will be just proximal to the patellar tendon enthesis **(Fig. 22–1A)**. The guide system and the 3 mm guide pin are removed. The medial collateral ligament (MCL) is incised obliquely at the osteotomy site, and the periosteum is elevated 1 cm proximally and distally **(Fig. 22–1B)**. A hand-held retractor is placed posteriorly to protect the neurovascular structures. The cutting guide is placed on the two distal pins and a headed, central holding pin is placed through the cannulation of the guide to fix the cutting guide. The distal pins are broken off at their serrations and an oscillating saw is used to cut the medial, anterior, and posterior cortex with fluoroscopic assistance. Osteotomes are used to finish the cut to the tip of the first guide pin, being certain to leave the lateral cortex intact. An opening wedge device is inserted to the appropriate depth (determines amount of correction) as decided during preoperative planning **(Fig. 22–1C)**. This is performed slowly to allow for plastic deformation of the bone. Alternatively, an osteotome jack may be slowly opened to the desired wedge height. The two tines of the wedge are left in place, and the handle is removed **(Fig. 22–1D)**. The selected plate is placed between the wedge tines to the same measurement as the opening wedge device **(Fig. 22–1D)**. The position of the plate anterior to posterior and the selection of a straight or sloped block can affect the desired posterior slope. Alignment is checked with an alignment rod or an electrocautery cord with fluoroscopy. The weight-bearing line should cross the tibial plateau 62 to 66% of the way from medial to lateral. The plate is then secured with two 6.5-mm partially threaded cancellous screws proximally and 4.5-mm cortical screws distally **(Fig. 22–1E)**. If the titanium plate is used, there is an additional guide to ensure the screws lock into the plate. Optiform (Exactech, Gainesville, FL) bone graft substitute is packed into the osteotomy gap. Alignment and screw placement are confirmed with fluoroscopy **(Fig. 22–1F)**. The MCL and sartorius fibers are repaired and a Hemovac drain is placed prior to skin closure.

Closing Wedge: Lateral

Instrumentation and Implants

Coventry's[21] original technique used one or two stepped staples placed on the lateral side to compress the osteotomy site. This implant negated the need for prolonged cast immobilization. More recently, standard AO plating techniques with compression across the osteotomy site have been utilized for secure fixation with L- or T-shaped plates. New guide systems are also available. External fixators using fine wires (Ilizarov technique) or uniplanar fixators with larger pins have also been advocated because they allow for postoperative modifications of the angular correction, but they are cumbersome for the patient and have the potential for pin loosening and pin tract infections.

Surgical Technique

Preparation and arthroscopy are performed the same as in the opening wedge osteotomy. A lateral L-shaped skin incision is made anterior to the fibular head. The fascia of the anterior compartment is exposed and an incision is made along the anterolateral crest of tibia, leaving a 5-mm cuff of fascia for closure, and extending into the iliotibial band in line with its fibers. The muscle is elevated off the anterolateral tibia, and the posterior iliotibial tract fibers are elevated from Gerdy's tubercle. The peroneal nerve may be identified by palpation only or by careful dissection, but must be protected throughout the procedure.

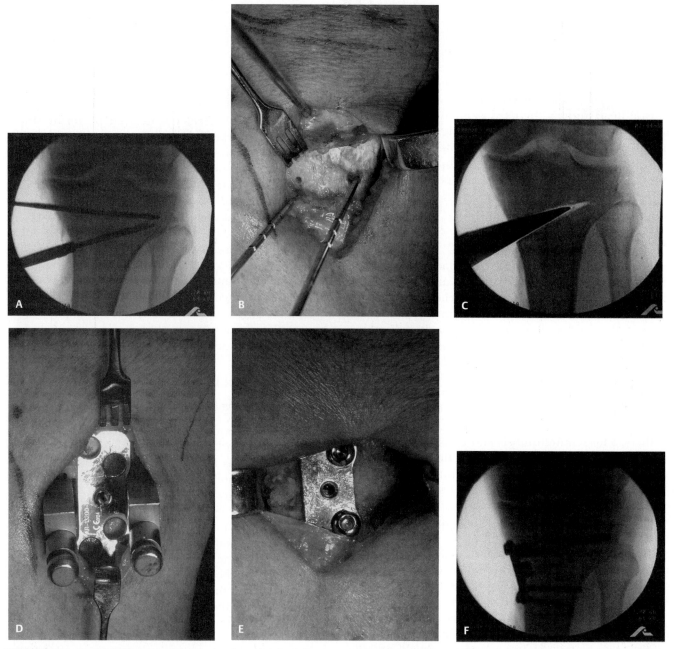

FIGURE 22–1 (A) A 3-mm guide pin is placed 1 to 1.5 cm distal to and parallel to the joint line, from medial to lateral and advanced to within 1 cm of the lateral cortex. Two distal pins (2.4 mm) are placed and advanced so that the cut will be just proximal to the patellar tendon enthesis. P, parallel guide pin; O, distal oblique pins. **(B)** The medial collateral ligament (MCL) is incised obliquely at the osteotomy site and the periosteum is elevated 1 cm proximally and distally. **(C)** An opening wedge device is inserted to the appropriate depth. **(D)** The two tines of the wedge are left in place, and the selected plate is placed between the wedge tines. **(E)** The plate is then secured with screws, and bone graft is packed into the osteotomy gap. **(F)** Final fluoroscopic view after correction, fixation, and bone grafting.

There are several options for addressing the fibula. The proximal tibiofibular joint may be excised or disrupted, a fibular osteotomy may be performed more distally, or the fibular head may be excised. We prefer to disrupt the joint but preserve the fibular head. The proximal tibiofibular joint is exposed, and the anterior capsule is excised using a curved osteotome directed posteromedially to disrupt the articulation and mobilize the fibula.

Next, the proximal tibia is exposed subperiosteally from the tibial tubercle to the posterolateral cortex for the osteotomy. A Z-shaped retractor is placed through the tibiofibular joint, directly against the posterior cortex of the tibia, to protect the posterior soft tissues and the peroneal nerve. A second Z-shaped retractor is placed underneath the lateral edge of the patellar tendon to protect the tendon from the saw blade.

A laterally based wedge is removed to correspond to a predetermined wedge height using a cutting guide or by cutting between pins that are placed free hand at a set distance. Up to two thirds of the wedge is cut with an oscillating saw, and then the most medial bone is removed with a curette, rongeur, or osteotome to decrease the complication risk of intraarticular fracture. Fluoroscopy is used to confirm adequate removal of bone medially to ensure the wedge will close. The defect is closed by applying a gentle, valgus stress. The medial cortex integrity and alignment are confirmed with fluoroscopy.

The compression plate (preferred) or staple fixation is completed, applying compression across the osteotomy site. A portion of the bone removed may be placed around the osteotomy site. An alignment rod or electrocautery cord along the weight-bearing line is used to confirm the final alignment. The wound is closed over a drain in layers with interrupted sutures.

Other Proximal Tibial Osteotomies

Dome Osteotomy

The dome osteotomy of the tibia was first reported on by Jackson and Waugh.[20] It is advocated for correction of large deformities, due to its main advantage of unrestricted correction. The position of the tibial tubercle in relation to the joint line is unaffected. Because most high tibial osteotomies performed for chondral lesions or meniscal deficiency do not have significant underlying varus deformities, this type of correction is rarely needed. Internal fixation is generally not required. An external fixator facilitates postoperative adjustment of alignment and early weight bearing, but runs the risk of a pin tract infection, scarring of the extensor mechanism, and intraarticular fracture, and is cumbersome to the patient. A recent study with 6-year follow-up comparing rigid internal fixation with a dome osteotomy and Ilizarov fixation reported better results for Hospital for Special Surgery scores, lower extremity alignment, and prevention of arthritis with the later technique.[28]

Medial Hemicallotasis

Schwartsman[29] has reported on the use of a circular external fixator (Ilizarov technique) with percutaneous osteotomy. He suggests that osteotomy below the tubercle decreases the likelihood of patella infera and decreased proximal tibial bone stock, both of which are believed to complicate subsequent total knee arthroplasty. This technique also allows for immediate weight bearing. A unilateral frame may also be employed. Disadvantages of this technique include large fixation devices, poor patient acceptance, pin loosening, and pin tract infection.

■ Varus-Producing Osteotomies: Distal Femoral Osteotomies

Indications and Contraindications

Varus-producing distal femoral osteotomies are indicated for situations involving symptomatic lateral gonarthrosis with or without anterior instability, lateral compartment arthralgia after meniscectomy, and valgus alignment with a concomitant cartilage restoration procedure or articular or meniscal transplant.

Contraindications include inflammatory arthritides, decreased range of motion, flexion contracture, and varus instability.

Patient Selection

Patient selection criteria are the same as for tibial osteotomies, except that patients should have lateral pathology on physical exam, radiographic studies, and at the time of arthroscopy.

Literature Review of Long-Term Results and Complications

There are only a few reports on the long-term results of distal femoral osteotomy, and most are for only closing-wedge techniques. The results have generally been good. McDermott et al[10] reported a 92% success rate at 4 years. Healy et al[30] reported 83% good or excellent results at 4 years and stated that osteotomies for osteoarthritis performed better than for rheumatoid arthritis or patients with decreased range of motion. Edgerton et al[31] reported a 71% success rate, while noting that overcorrection and undercorrection were associated with worse results and residual pain. Aglietti and Menchetti[32] reported a 9-year follow-up study in which 77% of patients had a good or excellent outcome, with an average correction to 6 degrees of anatomic valgus. Terry and Cimino[12] reported a series of both opening- and closing-wedge osteotomies in which the patients had a 60% decrease in pain and a 69% increase in functional activity. Most reports suggest obtaining at least neutral mechanical axis alignment. Some techniques suggest aiming for 4 degrees of mechanical axis varus. McDermott et al[10] recommends a 0-degree anatomic axis (6 degrees of mechanical axis varus), but they found no difference between the final clinical result and the alignment attained.

Morrey and Edgerton[11] recommend a weight-bearing line that is just medial to the midportion of the tibial plateau.

Staple fixation for distal femoral osteotomies has been largely abandoned because it has shown a high complication rate with up to a 25% nonunion rate, a 21% rate of fixation failure, as well as inadequate correction and subsequent decreased range of motion.[31] Studies on plate fixation of the femur have shown that a locked buttress plate is stronger than a standard plate or blade plate fixation.[33]

With the exception of peroneal nerve injury (which has not been a reported problem), complications with rigid fixation at the femur are essentially the same as for proximal tibial osteotomies, which include delayed union or nonunion, infection, arthrofibrosis, and under- or overcorrection. Conversions to total knee replacement have been acceptable after distal femoral osteotomy. McDermott et al's[10] study had one loss of fixation (4%), one pulmonary embolus (4%), and one patient with arthrofibrosis that required manipulation (4%). Matthews et al[34] study of 10 knees treated with a closing-wedge osteotomy had a 57% complication rate, with 48% requiring manipulation, 19% delayed/nonunion, 10% infection, and a 5% fixation failure. Better results were seen with rigid fixation than with staple fixation. Patella infera does not appear to be a problem after distal femoral osteotomy.[25] Unlike a valgus-producing osteotomy, a varus-producing osteotomy generally leads to a significant cosmetic improvement.

Closing Wedge: Medial

Instrumentation and Implants

Medial staples, T-shaped plate and screws, a blade plate or condylar screw/plate, intramedullary nails, or external fixation can be used depending on technique.

The osteotomy can be performed from either medial or lateral, with the wedge height based on the medial side. A well-known technique is cutting a medial wedge from the lateral side and applying a 95-degree blade plate from lateral, as would be done for fracture fixation. The main mechanical disadvantage of this technique is the loss of the tension band effect on the opposite site of the plate. The mechanical stress of all the varus/valgus forces and the flexion/extension forces is relying fully on the grip of the plate in the cancellous bone of the femoral condyles. A more stable construct is achieved by taking a two-thirds wedge from the medial supracondylar area, leaving the lateral cortex intact, and closing the osteotomy with a 90-degree blade plate on the medial side, creating compression and intrinsic stability.

Surgical Technique

The patient is positioned supine on the operating table and a tourniquet is applied. If the leg is too short, use a sterile tourniquet. The leg is prepped and draped free to allow knee movement during the procedure. A bump is placed under the knee to allow easy access to the medial side of the knee. Arthroscopy should confirm appropriate indications.

An incision 10 to 15 cm long is made straight medially or anteromedially (modified total knee incision) from the medial condyle proximally. The fascia of the vastus medialis muscle is identified and incised. The muscle is elevated anteriorly. Care is taken to avoid injury to the large medial neurovascular structures. The femur is exposed and the muscle is held anteriorly with a Hohmann retractor. Blunt dissection is performed posteriorly, and another retractor is placed directly on bone to protect the neurovascular structures.

Guidewires may be placed at the joint line and at the upper aspect of the trochlea to delineate the inclination of the patellofemoral joint so as to help avoid penetration of the chisel into the joint. A seating chisel is set up to the appropriate angle of correction (i.e., 80 degrees for a 10-degree correction). The insertion point is in the anterior part of the medial condyle. In the frontal plane, the chisel is running just proximal to the intercondylar notch, directed slightly downward. This direction is controlled by the flange of the seating chisel and thus is not normally parallel to the joint space.

With the seating chisel in place, the wedge is cut from the femur. The first cut is made 2 to 2.5 cm proximal to the chisel with an oscillating saw. The cut is usually parallel to the chisel and should stop two thirds to three quarters of the way across the femur, leaving the lateral cortex intact. A second cut is made proximally, based on the wedge height determined from the preoperative planning. The two cuts should meet at the apex. The wedge of bone is removed with curettes or a small osteotome.

The seating chisel is exchanged for a 90-degree, four-hole plate that has been contoured to fit the femur. There are usually several options for offset to ensure that the plate fits well along the femoral shaft. The lateral remaining bridge of bone is then weakened using a 2-mm drill. The osteotomy is closed and held in place with a Verbrugge clamp. The plate is fixed proximally with bicortical screws. Alignment is checked using an alignment rod or electrocautery cord and fluoroscopy.

Alternatively, a 95-degree blade plate can be inserted parallel to the joint line, and the wedge is cut with the distal cut parallel to the plate and the proximal cut the predetermined height above that cut, angled to intersect the first cut two thirds to three quarters of the way across the femur. When the wedge is closed down and impacted, the joint line should be level.

Opening Wedge: Lateral

Instrumentation and Implants

Manufacturers make specially designed T-shaped plates with a spacer block ("tooth") to hold the position of the osteotomy and prevent a later collapse of the bone. These plates come with systems that help to ensure that the correct wedge height and angle of correction are achieved. These plates are currently available only in stainless steel, but they should be available soon as a titanium locking plate as well. The block ranges from 5 to 17.5 mm in height. Alternatively, standard AO plates, locking plates, angled blade plates, or an external fixator could be used.

Authors' Preferred Surgical Technique

Preparation is the same as for a closing-wedge distal femoral osteotomy. A 6-cm longitudinal incision is made along the distal lateral femoral metaphyseal-diaphyseal region. The iliotibial band is identified and incised in line with its fibers. The vastus lateralis is retracted superior and medially. Blunt dissection posterior to the femoral shaft is performed, and a retractor is placed to protect neurovascular structures. Avoid exposure of, or injury to, the lateral collateral ligament.

Under fluoroscopic guidance, a 3-mm guide pin is placed parallel to the joint line, superior to the trochlea, aiming toward the origin of the medial collateral ligament. The pin is drilled into the medial cortex. The osteotomy guide assembly (Arthrex, Naples, FL) is placed on the pin to the laser mark and the parallel guide sleeve is attached proximally. If a biplanar osteotomy is needed, the parallel guide can be adjusted for flexion or extension. Select the appropriate angle of correction based on the preoperative planning. Two 2.4-mm guide pins are individually drilled obliquely under fluoroscopic control to intersect the transverse pin 10 mm from the medial cortex of the distal femur. The pins are serrated and are shortened so that they will not hinder the process of the osteotomy. The transverse pin and guide assembly are then removed. A cutting guide is placed over the oblique pins and is secured to the femur with a headed pin. With retractors protecting structures anterior and posterior to the femur, an oscillating saw is positioned superior to the guide pins and under fluoroscopic guidance is used to cut the cortex of the lateral, anterior, and posterior femur. The osteotomy is completed with osteotomes to the apex of the guide pins. The medial cortex is not violated. The guide pins are then removed.

A wedge with premarked depths to correspond with the desired wedge height and angle of correction is then carefully inserted into the osteotomy with a mallet while an assistant places gentle varus stress on the leg.

Advance the wedge slowly to allow for plastic deformation. Alternatively, small drill holes may be used at the medial cortex. Confirm placement and integrity of the medial cortex with fluoroscopy. A leg alignment rod or electrocautery cord should be used to confirm that the desired amount of correction has been achieved.

The T-shaped plate with an appropriate-sized block is placed and alignment is again confirmed. If the patient is very small, the opening wedge tibial plate may be used instead. The plate is fixed distally with three 6.5-mm partially threaded screws and proximally with four 4.5-mm fully threaded cortical screws. Bone graft from autologous and/or allogeneic sources is inserted into the defect anterior and posterior to the plate's position. Struts provide structural support, which may be advantageous for femoral osteotomies. The wound is closed over a drain in layers and a sterile dressing is placed.

Medial Closing Wedge Proximal Tibial Osteotomy

For small corrections (less than 12 degrees) some surgeons prefer a medial closing wedge osteotomy. Chambat et al[35] found that a medial closing wedge does increase joint line obliquity, but has a more positive effect in flexion than a distal femoral osteotomy, which is most efficient in decreasing lateral compartment stress in extension. External rotation of the epiphysis during a distal femoral osteotomy can correct the joint obliquity seen with distal femoral osteotomies at 90 degrees of flexion, if that is a concern. The closing-wedge medial osteotomy should not be used for large corrections, as the results have been very poor. Shoji and Insall[36] showed that the tibial osteotomy results were far worse for valgus disease than varus disease. They reported that the optimal position was 5 degrees of valgus and that overcorrection was bad. Knees with >15 degrees of medial tilting (joint line obliquity) did poorly. Coventry[37] described a 77% success rate, but recommended use of supracondylar femoral osteotomy for varus angulation in excess of 12 degrees or if the tilt that resulted would exceed 10 degrees. He recommended correction beyond the normal 5 to 7 degrees of anatomic valgus to a 0-degree anatomic axis.

Complications include fracture of the proximal fragment, DVT, and peroneal nerve palsy. Late complications of recurrent valgus deformity due to MCL laxity and loss of initially good correction during casting occurred.

Postoperative Rehabilitation Protocols

Tibial and Femoral Opening-Wedge Osteotomies

After surgery, the leg is placed in a locked brace in full extension. If the additional procedures require early motion, passive range of motion up to 90 degrees is started that day using a continuous passive motion (CPM) device. Quadriceps sets, isometrics, and straight leg raises are started on postoperative day 1. The patient should remain touch-down weight bearing for 4 weeks. Weight-bearing status may progress to partial weight bearing from 4 to 8 weeks. Postoperative radiographs are obtained at 8 weeks to assess the bony healing and alignment. If abundant callous is present at the osteotomy site, the patient may progress to full weight bearing. Long leg films should be obtained at 6 months to verify the final alignment.

Tibial and Femoral Closing-Wedge Osteotomies

Many surgeons use the same rehabilitation protocols for both closing wedge and opening wedge osteotomies. In theory, it may be safe to begin early partial weight bearing after a closing wedge osteotomy as long as the far cortex of the osteotomy remains intact.

Opening- Versus Closing-Wedge Osteotomies

Closing-wedge osteotomies have been the gold standard to which all osteotomy results are compared. New techniques and osteotomy guide systems have made opening-wedge osteotomies easier to perform with high accuracy. The theoretical advantages of an opening-wedge over a closing-wedge osteotomy are a single saw/osteotomy cut, a smaller incision with minimal soft tissue disruption, a higher degree of precision, maintenance of normal anatomy and bone stock, ability to adjust correction intraoperatively, and predictable correction in both the coronal and sagittal planes. With specific regard to tibial osteotomies, the avoidance of proximal tibiofemoral disruption or fibular osteotomy greatly reduces the risk of peroneal nerve injury. Also, in

patients with lateral ligamentous laxity, as is often seen in patients with posterolateral corner injuries, an opening-wedge tibial osteotomy allows for physiologic surgical repair of reconstruction. Disadvantages of opening-wedge osteotomies are that the procedure requires bone grafting (which adds harvest morbidity if autograft is used), a theoretically higher risk of nonunion, and a longer period of restricted weight bearing in the initial postoperative period.

■ Case Example

The patient is a 40-year-old, healthy, white male police officer who presented with a history of an injury to his right knee while attempting to take down a suspect. He described a twisting type injury in which his legs became entangled with the suspect's, followed by an impact to the ground. He developed an effusion over the ensuing 24 hours. His initial treatment with physical therapy was unsuccessful. He had ongoing recurrent sharp pain in the knee, predominantly anterior and medial, which became very limiting. He had some subjective feelings of instability, with no frank giving way. He had no mechanical locking. He had pain with prolonged sitting, as well as ascending and descending stairs. He had no history of previous knee injury. Magnetic resonance imaging (MRI) showed no evidence of meniscal tear or ligamentous injury. The hyaline cartilage surfaces did not show any obvious defects.

He underwent arthroscopy 3 months after his injury by the referring physician. He was reported to have a large grade III chondral defect of the femoral trochlea and a "quarter"-size grade IV defect of the medial femoral condyle (**Fig. 22–2**). Both of these defects were treated with a radiofrequency device. There were no

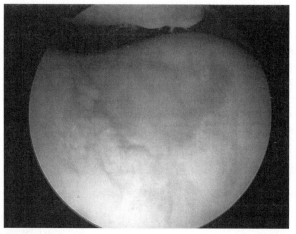
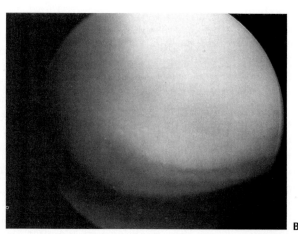

FIGURE 22–2 (A) A large grade III chondral defect of the femoral trochlea. (B) A "quarter"-size grade IV defect of the medial femoral condyle.

meniscal tears and the cruciate ligaments were intact. Despite surgery and physical therapy, his symptoms continued and he was referred for further treatment.

On physical exam, he stood 6'0" tall, weighing 205 pounds, with a level pelvis. He had apparent physiologic genu valgum, but bilateral tibial varum. His knees ranged from 0 to 135 degrees bilaterally. Patellar quadrant glide was 1.0 medially and laterally and his patella tracked normally. He had a minimal effusion. The knee was stable to varus and valgus stress testing at 0 and 30 degrees of flexion. Anterior and posterior drawer were negative at 20 and 70 degrees. He had tenderness over the anterior, medial joint line and over the medial femoral condyle. He had mild tenderness over the retropatellar surface and trochlea both medially and laterally. McMurray testing was negative.

Radiographs were obtained including AP standing, PA standing, both lower extremity standing, lateral, and Merchant views. He had an anatomic axis of 2 degrees of varus bilaterally on the standing AP views. His mechanical axis angle was 6 degrees of varus. His weight-bearing line crossed the tibia at 39% of the tibial width from medial to lateral. He had a Wyberg type III patella with no frank tilt or shift. His Merchant angle was 0 degrees on the right and 6 degrees medial on the other leg. He had mild disuse osteopenia at the patellofemoral articulation, noted on the Merchant and lateral views. His Insall-Salvati ratio was 0.92 bilaterally.

Operative options were reviewed with the patient. Given his ongoing discomfort it was felt to be worthwhile to reevaluate his knee arthroscopically. If he were found to have further problems with his chondral surface, the recommendation would be for cartilage biopsy for an autologous chondrocyte implantation. It was also recommended that he undergo an opening-wedge proximal tibial osteotomy to off-load his medial femoral condyle, due to his relative varus alignment. He had some mild patella baja, which was still within the range of normal, but if the proximal tibial osteotomy affected the patellar height, he may need a Fulkerson osteotomy at the time of his autologous chondrocyte implantation.

If, at the time of surgery, his lateral compartment is not intact, he would not be a good candidate for either proximal tibial osteotomy or autologous chondrocyte implantation. If the medial femoral defect was not suitable for cartilage restoration, but the lateral compartment was intact, a high tibial osteotomy could still be performed, giving him a 76% chance for good short-term success and a 63% chance for good long-term success. If he was not a candidate for osteotomy or cartilage restoration his options would be limited to continued treatment with rest, ice, elevation, antiinflammatory medication, injections of viscosupplementation or corticosteroids, and subsequent total knee arthroplasty when his symptoms did not respond to treatment.

Preoperative Planning for Opening-Wedge Proximal Tibial Osteotomy

The information in **Table 22–1** was then used to calculate the necessary angle of correction and corresponding wedge height for the opening wedge proximal tibial osteotomy using the methods described in the preoperative planning section (**Table 22–2**).

Based on the above calculations, a 10-degree opening-wedge proximal tibial osteotomy was to be performed to achieve a goal of 8 degrees of anatomic valgus alignment, which should place his weight-bearing line to ,62% of the distance from medial to lateral on his tibial plateau (**Fig. 22–3**). The rule-of-thumb method often underestimates the wedge height, as it is based on a tibial width of 56 mm. The trigonometric calculation is usually more accurate. We planned to choose between a 10- or 11-mm Arthrex osteotomy plate at the time of surgery, based on intraoperative fluoroscopic evaluation of the patient's weight-bearing line.

The patient was taken back to surgery 7 months after his initial injury. At arthroscopy he was found to have no chondromalacic changes on the medial or lateral side of the patella. He had a 3 × 2 cm² chondral defect of the trochlea with some fibrous repair at the base and stable surrounding edges. The medial femoral condyle

TABLE 22–1 Case Example of Preoperative Radiographic Data

Preoperative anatomic axis	2 degrees anatomic varus	Standing anteroposterior (AP)
Preoperative mechanical axis	6 degrees mechanical varus	Long leg standing AP
Preoperative weight-bearing line	39%	Long leg standing AP
Radiographic magnification	10%	All films
Tibial width at joint line	86 mm	77.4 mm after correction
Tibial width 2 cm distal along line of osteotomy	70 mm	63 mm after correction

TABLE 22–2 Case Example of Calculation of Degrees of Correction by Different Methods

Method	Angle Correction	Wedge Height
Coventry: $\theta = 10\ AA_{plan} - AA_{pre}$ $\theta = 10\ MA_{plan} - MA_{pre}$	AA: $\theta = 8 - (-2) = 10$ degrees MA: $\theta = 3 - (-6) = 9$ degrees	
WBL (Dugdale): angle formed connecting center of femoral head, center of talus and center of knee	$\theta = 10$ degrees	
WBL (Noyes): cut radiograph at osteotomy site and rotate until WBL crosses at 62%	$\theta = 10$ degrees	
WBL (Miniaci): 3 lines	$\theta = 10$ degrees	
Rule of thumb: 1 degree of angular correction = 1 mm wedge height	Goal: $\theta = 10$ degrees	10 mm
Trigonometric: $y = x\tan(\bullet)$, where y = wedge height, x = tibial width at 2 cm distal to joint line, and $\bullet$ = chosen angle of correction	Goal: $\theta = 10$ degrees	11 mm

WBL, weight-bearing line; AA, anatomic axis; MA, mechanical axis.

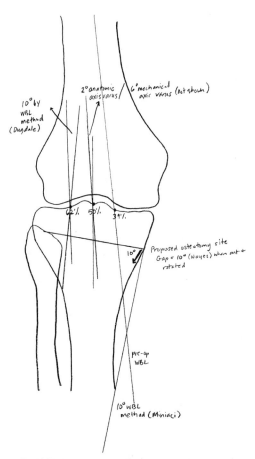

FIGURE 22–3 A 10-degree opening-wedge proximal tibial osteotomy was to be performed to achieve a goal of 8 degrees of anatomic valgus alignment, which should place the patient's weight-bearing line to ~62% of the distance from medial to lateral on his tibial plateau.

defect was 2×1.5 cm^2 and down into, but not through, the deep zone with friable tissue **(Fig. 22–4)**. The medial and lateral menisci and the cruciate ligaments were intact.

Based on these findings the patient was felt to be a candidate for autologous chondrocyte implantation. A chondral biopsy (300 mg) was taken from the medial edge of the lateral femoral condyle in the notch, and a 10-mm wedge height opening-wedge proximal tibial osteotomy was performed. Intraoperatively the alignment correction was checked with fluoroscopy to ensure the new weight-bearing line passed about 60 to 65% of the way across the tibial plateau. Optiform (Exactech, Gainesville, FL) was used for bone grafting. A femoral nerve block was used for postoperative pain control, along with oral narcotics.

Postoperatively, the patient was placed in a brace locked in extension. He started using a CPM machine that afternoon, and began quadriceps sets, isometrics, and straight leg raises the next day. He began formal physical therapy 1 week after surgery. He remained touch-down weight bearing for 4 weeks, at which time his motion was from 2 to 115 degrees of flexion. He slowly progressed to partial weight bearing over the next 4 weeks. At 8 weeks, his motion had improved to 2 to 130 degrees of flexion and his radiographs showed interval healing of his osteotomy. He was allowed to be weight bearing as tolerated, and he returned to light

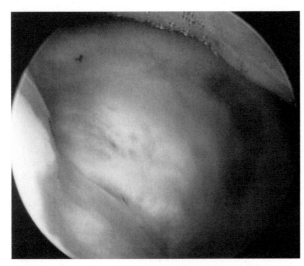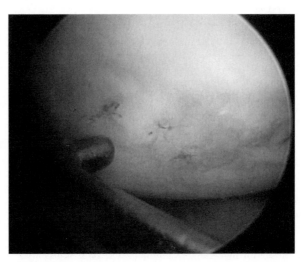

FIGURE 22–4 **(A)** On repeat arthroscopy, there was a 3 × 2 cm² chondral defect of the trochlea with fibrous repair at the base and stable surrounding edges. **(B)** The medial femoral condyle defect was 2 × 1.5 cm² and filled with friable tissue.

duty work. At 12 weeks, he had regained full motion and had healed his osteotomy. Repeat radiographs at 5 months showed his anatomic axis to be 8 degrees of valgus, his mechanical axis was 5 degrees of valgus, his weight-bearing line crossed at 66%, and his patellar height was unchanged from his preoperative measurements **(Fig. 22–5)**. He recently underwent autologous chondrocyte implantation for the trochlear and medial femoral condylar lesions, 1 year from his initial injury, and is progressing well.

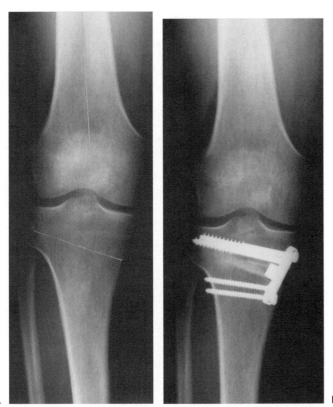

A   B

FIGURE 22–5 **(A)** Preoperative radiograph. **(B)** Postoperative radiograph at 5 months showing that the patient's anatomic axis was 8 degrees of valgus, his mechanical axis was 5 degrees of valgus, and his weight-bearing line crossed at 66%.

REFERENCES

1. Tetsworth K, Paley D. Malalignment and degenerative arthropathy. Orthop Clin North Am 1994;25:367–377
2. Adamson GJ, Tibone JE. Results and complications of high tibial osteotomy for varus gonarthrosis: a review of the literature. (Unpublished meta-analysis)
3. Font-Rodriguez DE, Scuderi GR, Insall JN. Survivorship of cemented total knee arthroplasty. Clin Orthop 1997;345:79–86
4. Berman AT, Bosacco SJ, Lorsjmer S, et al. Factors influencing long-term results in high tibial osteotomy. Clin Orthop 1991;272:192–198
5. Aglietti P, Rinonapoli E, Stringa G, Taviani A. Tibial osteotomy for the varus osteoarthritic knee. Clin Orthop 1983;176:239–251
6. Coventry MB, Ilstrup DM, Wallrichs SL. Proximal tibial osteotomy: a critical long term study of eighty-seven cases. J Bone Joint Surg Am 1993;75:196–201
7. Brown GA, Amendola A. Radiographic evaluation and preoperative planning for high tibial osteotomies. Op Tech Sports Med 2000;18:2–14
8. Muller W, Kentsch A, Schafer N. The elastic high tibia valgus osteotomy in the varus deformity. Op Tech Sports Med 2000;18:19–26
9. Dugdale TW, Noyes FR, Styer D. Preoperative planning for high tibial osteotomy: the effect of lateral tibiofemoral separation and tibiofemoral length. Clin Orthop 1992;274:248–264
10. McDermott AG, Finklestein JA, Farine I, et al. Distal femoral varus osteotomy for valgus deformity of the knee. J Bone Joint Surg 1988;70A:110–116
11. Morrey BF, Edgerton BC. Distal femoral osteotomy for lateral gonarthrosis. Instr Course Lect 1992;41:77–85
12. Terry GC, Cimino PM. Distal femoral osteotomy for valgus deformity of the knee. Orthopedics 1992;15:1283–1290
13. Phillips MJ, Krackow KA. Distal femoral varus osteotomy: indications and surgical technique. Instr Course Lect 1999;48:125–129
14. Miniaci A, Ballmer FT, Ballmer PM, Jakob RP. Proximal tibial osteotomy: a new fixation device. Clin Orthop 1989;246:250–259
15. Bauer GC, Insall J, Koshino T. Tibial osteotomy in gonarthrosis. J Bone Joint Surg 1969;51A:1545–1563
16. Hanssen AD. Osteotomy about the knee: American perspective. In: Insall JN, Scott WN, ed. Surgery of the Knee, 3rd ed. Philadelphia: Churchill Livingstone, 2001:1447–1464
17. Coventry MB. Proximal tibial varus osteotomy for osteoarthritis of the lateral compartment of the knee. J Bone Joint Surg 1987;69A:32–38
18. Coventry MB. Upper tibial osteotomy for gonarthrosis. The evolution of the operation in the last 18 years and long-term results. Orthop Clin North Am 1979;10:191–210
19. Wardle E. Osteotomy of the tibia and fibula. Surg Gynecol Obstet 1962;126:61–64
20. Jackson JP, Waugh W. Tibial osteotomy for osteoarthritis of the knee. J Bone Joint Surg 1961;43B:746–751
21. Coventry MB. Osteotomy of the upper portion of the tibia for degenerative arthritis of the knee. J Bone Joint Surg 1965;47A:984–990
22. Kirgis A, Albrecht S. Palsy of the deep peroneal nerve after proximal tibial osteotomy. An anatomical study. J Bone Joint Surg 1992;74A:1180–1185
23. Phillips MJ, Krackow KA. High tibial osteotomy and distal femoral osteotomy for valgus and varus deformity around the knee. Instr Course Lect 1998;47:429–436
24. Billings A, Scott DF, Camargo MP, Hofmann AA. High tibial osteotomy with a calibrated osteotomy guide, rigid internal fixation and early motion. Long-term follow-up. J Bone Joint Surg Am 2000;82A:70–79
25. Closkey RF, Windsor RE. Alterations in patella after high tibial or distal femoral osteotomy. Clin Orthop 2001;389:51–56
26. Noyes FR. Cruciate reconstruction and osteotomy. Presented at the American Orthopaedic Society for Sports Medicine Specialty Day, San Francisco, CA. 2004
27. Sterett WI. Posterior tibial slope following medial opening wedge proximal tibial osteotomy for varus arthrosis of the knee. Annual Meeting, American Orthopaedics Society for Sports Medicine, San Diego, CA, 2003
28. Sen C, Kacaoglu M, Eralp L. The advantages of circular external fixation used in high tibial osteotomy. Knee Surg Sports Traumatol Arthrosc 2003;11:139–144
29. Schwartsman V. Circular external fixation in high tibial osteotomy. Instr Course Lect 1995;44:469–474
30. Healy WL, Anglen JO, Wasilewski SA, Krackow KA. Distal femoral varus osteotomy. J Bone Joint Surg Am 1988;70A:102–109
31. Edgerton BC, Mariani EM, Morrey BF. Distal femoral varus osteotomy for painful genu valgum. A 5–11 year follow-up study. Clin Orthop 1993;288:263–269
32. Aglietti P, Menchetti PP. Distal femoral varus osteotomy in the valgus osteoarthritic knee. Am J Knee Surg 2000;13:89–95
33. Koval KJ, Hoehl JJ, Kummer FJ, Simon JA. Distal femoral fixation: a biomechanical comparison of the standard condylar buttress plate, a locked buttress plate, and the 95-degree blade plate. J Orthop Trauma 1997;11:521–524
34. Mathews J, Cobb AG, Richardson S, Bentley G. Distal femoral osteotomy for lateral compartment osteoarthritis of the knee. Orthopedics 1998;21:437–440
35. Chambat P, Selmi T, Dejour D, Denoyers J. Varus tibial osteotomy. Op Tech Sports Med 2000;8:44–47
36. Shoji H, Insall J. High tibial osteotomy for osteoarthritis of the knee with valgus deformity. J Bone Joint Surg 1973;55A:963–973
37. Coventry MB. Proximal tibial varus osteotomy for osteoarthritis of the lateral compartment of the knee. J Bone Joint Surg 1987;69A:32–38

23

Meniscal Transplantation

WAYNE K. GERSOFF

The meniscus was not always held in high esteem. In the early 1900s it was considered to be a functionless vestigial structure. It wasn't until Fairbanks's study in 1948 that the potential importance of the meniscus as a shock absorber was recognized. As more knowledge of the structure and function of the meniscus were obtained, its preservation became a prime concern. The development of arthroscopy created a procedure by which uninjured portions of the meniscus could be maintained. This ultimately led to the capability to repair the meniscus. Unfortunately, orthopaedic surgeons were confronted with patients who either had previous subtotal meniscectomies or irreparable tears requiring complete meniscectomies. The challenge was to maintain knee function in the postmeniscectomy knee. This challenge was answered by turning to the use of allograft meniscal tissue. The development of meniscal transplantation has evolved from a theoretical concept to an accepted surgical procedure that attempts to restore knee structure and function to near normal with a high degree of success.

■ Anatomy and Physiology of the Meniscus

The structure, biomechanics, and function of the meniscus are well documented in the literature; however, a basic review pertinent to meniscal transplantation is provided here.

The meniscus of the knee is a fibrocartilaginous structure represented by unique integration of cellular components and extracellular matrix. The cellular component, which is a minority portion, consists of structures termed *fibrochondrocytes*, reflecting the unique hybrid structure of fibroblasts and chondrocytes. They are responsible for the formation and maintenance of the extracellular matrix.

The extracellular matrix is largely composed of collagen fibers. It is the special orientation of these fibers that provides strength to the meniscus. The majority of these fibers are circumferential in nature. Intermixed with these circumferential fibers are radial fibers that link and bond the circumferential fibers (**Fig. 23–1**). This unique configuration is the foundation of the strength of the meniscus and its ability to resist compressive and rotational stress forces. This natural-occurring architecture is the challenge to replicate in a synthetic meniscus. Although the majority of the functional component is type I collagen, types II, III, and V have also been identified. The vascular supply to the meniscus is via the geniculate system. The anterior portion of the meniscus and peripheral capsule are supplied by the medial and lateral branches of the inferior and superior geniculates. The posterior portion is supplied by the middle geniculates. The vessel branch ultimately forms a perimeniscal capillary complex that then supplies the peripheral aspect of the menisci (**Fig. 23–1B** and **23–2**). On the medial side, the peripheral 10 to 30% of the meniscus is vascularized, whereas on the lateral aspect the peripheral 10 to 25% is vascularized. However, in children, up to 50% of the peripheral aspect of both menisci can be vascularized.

Grossly the menisci are semilunar in shape, being triangular in cross section with the thickened base

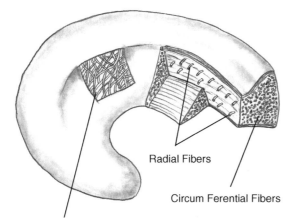

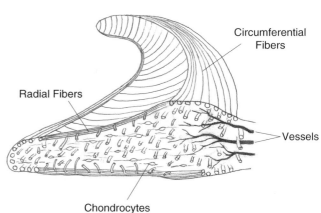

A Mesh network Fibers

B

Chondrocytes

FIGURE 23–1 **(A)** The meniscus is composed of circumferential and radial fibers, which are held together by meshed network of fibers. (From Bullough PG, Munuera L, Murphy J, Weinstein AM. The strength of the menisci of the knee as it relates to their fine structure. J Bone Joint Surg Br 1970; 52:564–567, with permission.) **(B)** The circumferential fibers are in the periphery, whereas the radial fibers extend from the circumferential fibers toward the central portion of the meniscus.

oriented peripherally. The medial meniscus is longer in the anteroposterior direction **(Fig. 23–3)**. An important factor when performing medial meniscal transplantation is that the anterior horn is in line with the medial tibial eminence, posterior to the fat pad and edge of the patellar tendon. The anterior fibers of the meniscus ultimately contribute to the formation of the transverse intermeniscal ligament. The attachment of the anterior horn may also go across the anterior slope of the tibia. The lateral meniscus is more circular in shape with a smaller anteroposterior length. The position of the anterior horn is anterior to the tibial spine and anterior cruciate ligament footprint, and must be replicated when

performing a lateral meniscal transplant **(Fig. 23–3)**. The lateral meniscal anatomy is further complicated by the presence of the popliteal hiatus and the meniscal femoral ligaments.

All these complexities allow the meniscus to achieve its function: load bearing, force distribution, joint stability, lubrication, and proprioception. The microstructure of the meniscus is an important component in meniscal function as the collagen forms circumferential fibers that are linked by regularly oriented collagen fibers, as previously noted. It is this network of fibers that helps to

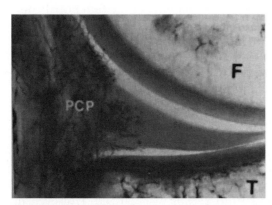

FIGURE 23–2 The perimeniscal capillary complex supplies the peripheral third of the meniscus. Also known as the "red-red" zone. (From Arnoczky SP, Warren RF. Microvasculature of the human meniscus. Am J Sports Med 1982;10:90–95, with permission.)

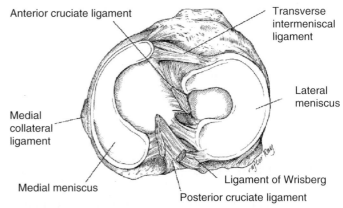

FIGURE 23–3 Topography of the proximal tibia showing the ligaments and menisci in their relevant relationships. (From Pagnani MJ, Warren RF, Arnoczky SP, Wickiewicz TL. Anatomy of the knee. In: Nicholas JA, Hershman EB, eds. The Lower Extremity and Spine in Sports Medicine, 2nd ed. St Louis:Mosby, 1995:581–614, with permission.)

resist tension, compression, and shear and ultimately contributes to the ability of the meniscus to bear load and distribute forces. The circumferential fibers run from bony horn attachment to bony horn attachment and resist the axial load and compression loads, converting radial forces to tension forces, termed hoop stresses. As stresses can be defined as force per unit area, it is then apparent that the meniscus can reduce stress to the articular cartilage by both redirecting the forces through the hoop stress and increasing the surface contact area.

■ Basic Science Considerations

The ability to utilize meniscal allograft as successful substitutes for the normal meniscus is founded in basic science considerations. The major factors that should be considered are immunology, chondroprotective potential, healing potential, and tissue preservation.

The relatively acellular nature of the meniscus allows it to be described as immunologically privileged.[1] Although the largest population of histocompatibility antigens are on the cellular components, the relatively low population and shielding by the extracellular matrix protects the tissue. Therefore, systemic rejection rarely occurs. However, it has been demonstrated that some form of immune response does occur.[2] The potential for a localized immune response exists: (1) even after deep freezing, histocompatibility antigens can be expressed on the cells of a meniscal allograft; (2) the bone and synovial attachments to the meniscal allograft will remain antigenic; and (3) the existence of immunoreactive cells in fresh frozen meniscal allograft has been demonstrated.[3] This localized response may have an affect on graft revascularization, repopulation, incorporation, and overall healing response. However, it appears that clinical results have not been compromised by this localized immune response.

It is generally accepted, based on multiple studies, that the meniscal allograft will heal, gradually repopulate with host cells, and not be systemically rejected.[4] One of the major concerns about meniscal transplantation is the chondroprotective potential, both short and long term. Several animal studies have demonstrated chondroprotective benefits of the meniscal allograft when compared with a total meniscectomy.[5] However, the studies did not demonstrate results identical to a normal meniscus. Similar improvements in contact/stress in a cadaveric model have also been demonstrated. These protective benefits are short term, and animal studies demonstrating long-term chondral protection are lacking.

■ Allograft Selection

Meniscal allograft tissue should only be obtained from a tissue-banking facility that is in compliance with the criteria established by the American Association of Tissue Banks.

This standardization maximizes the quality of the tissue (no evidence of degenerative change) and minimizes the risk of disease transmission.

At the present time, meniscal allograft tissue is processed by one of four techniques: fresh, cryopreserved, fresh frozen, or freeze dried. Fresh allograft tissue offers advantages regarding cell viability, but is not practical. Freeze dried tissue is associated with cell death. However, the major disadvantage of this process is the ultimate affect it has on the structural properties of the meniscal allograft, including graft shrinkage and potential damage to the collagen fibers. The processes of cryopreservation and fresh frozen tissue avoid the structural damage seen with freeze drying. Cryopreservation involves a slow freezing rate of the allograft tissue by utilizing a chemical cryoprotectant such as dimethylsulfoxide (DMSO). This method allows for a slight increase in cell viability and preservation of some degree of cell membrane integrity. The processes of cryopreservation and fresh frozen tissue both allow for prolonged storage. These processes of prolonged storage facilitate not only complete serologic testing, but also creation of a tissue bank of various subtle sizes, potentially improving tissue matching. Meniscal allograft tissue that undergoes fresh frozen processes undergoes a more rapid freezing process that results in slightly increased cell death, but without adversely affecting the structural properties of the graft. Cell viability, however, may not be an important issue, as has been shown by experimental studies that have suggested that there are no significant outcome differences between cryopreserved and deep frozen grafts. Indeed it has been demonstrated that the repopulation of meniscal allograft tissue by host-derived cells is extremely common and occurs within the first year of implantation. Future research will provide insight into the enhancement of the process of repopulation and incorporation. At the present time the utilization of fresh frozen tissue, compared with either fresh or cryopreserved, is simpler, less costly, and still provides the essential biologic scaffolding for successful function and incorporation.

■ Patient Selection and Indication

The general indications for meniscal transplantation are a history of documented total or subtotal meniscectomy with pain and/or disability relating to the affected compartment of the knee. However, other significant variables need to be considered. The duration of time since meniscectomy is important, especially as it relates to articular cartilage wear and possible alignment issues.

The patient's history should be correlated with the patient's symptoms and physical examination. As part of the general knee examination, attention should be paid to the nature of the previous surgical scars, the palpation of osteophytes, ligamentous laxity, standing alignment, and the observation of gait.

Radiographic evaluation should include at least the following: anteroposterior (AP) standing x-rays of both knees in full extension; non–weight-bearing, 45-degree flexion laterals; 45-degree flexion weight-bearing [posteroanterior (PA)]; and an axial view of the patellofemoral joint. Although magnetic resonance imaging (MRI) is not an imperative radiologic test, additional important information can be obtained regarding the status of the articular cartilage and the biologic activity of the subchondral bone, especially when performed with gadolinium enhancement. The ideal indications for meniscal transplantation are a symptomatic patient with (1) documented previous subtotal meniscectomy or absence of the major weight-bearing portion of the meniscus, (2) pain in the involved knee compartment, (3) less than grade 3 or correctable articular cartilage damage, (4) ligamentous stability or correctable stability, and (5) normal or correctable alignment.[6,7]

However, these indications will continue to evolve as the concept of cartilage restoration of the knee advances. Although the chronologic age most often referred to as a limit is 50 years, age is in reality a relative consideration. It is important to assess the biologic age, taking into consideration the environment of the knee, activity level, and ability to be compliant with the postoperative course and rehabilitation.

There are several contraindications to meniscal transplantation: degenerative arthritis, inflammatory arthritis, crystal deposition disease, and active infection. It is important to determine whether the articular cartilage changes that exist are secondary to the previous meniscectomy and can be restored or whether this truly represents advanced osteoarthritic changes. Obesity has the potential to compromise a normal knee joint. Based on articular cartilage-related studies, a body mass index (BMI) of over 35 should be considered a relative contraindication.

The patient who has recently undergone a subtotal meniscectomy and has not yet developed symptoms poses a significant challenge. The treatment and timing of treatment is certainly debatable as well as controversial. The natural history of the meniscal deficient knee is well documented. Nevertheless, not every postmeniscectomy patient develops degenerative arthrosis. There are several factors that are important in this treatment algorithm. Certainly these patients must undergo rigorous education about the signs and symptoms associated with knee degeneration. They should also be followed closely with standing 45-degree PA radiographs. Currently the measurement of articular cartilage degradation products is changing from a laboratory setting to the clinical realm, and may play an added role in early detection of postmeniscectomy articular cartilage damage. However, is that enough? The breakdown of articular cartilage can progress very rapidly in the meniscal-deficient joint. The factors that need to be considered are activity level, physiologic age, rehabilitative potential, and goals and expectations. In general, in the select postmeniscectomy individuals who have higher demands on their knee, rehabilitation potential, and realistic goals, there is a role for early consideration of meniscal allograft transplantation. The potential for articular cartilage breakdown in the younger patient and creation of a negative knee environment is too great to ignore. By the time the patient is symptomatic and has positive x-rays or a positive bone scan, the articular cartilage has already been damaged.

■ Surgical Technique

When the patient has been selected for meniscal transplantation by meeting the previous described criteria, the meniscus must be obtained. Prior to ordering the meniscus, sizing studies must be performed. The most commonly accepted method utilizes standard AP and lateral radiographs with magnification markers as described by Pollard et al.[8] It is important for both the surgeon and the tissue bank to measure these films and for the surgeon to comment on any special considerations that could alter accurate measurements, such as an osteophyte or previous trauma. It is also imperative to be certain of which side (right versus left) and which compartment (medial versus lateral) is being requested. This should be double-checked on the day of surgery prior to the patient's being anesthetized and prior to defrosting of the tissue.

The evolution of meniscal transplantation has allowed the procedure to advance to an arthroscopically assisted procedure with a miniarthrotomy. It may also be performed as an open procedure, especially when done concomitantly with a major articular cartilage restoration. Several different techniques have been developed for implantation. These include the double bone plug technique and the bone bridge techniques—keyhole, slot, trough, and dovetail. Regardless of which technique is selected, the essential foundation of successful meniscal transplantation is anatomic reduction and stable fixation of the meniscal allograft.

The fixation of the meniscal allograft is accomplished by the bony attachments and stabilization of the peripheral rim. Most recently developed all-inside meniscal repair devices are not well adapted for meniscal transplantation fixation. The majority of these devices are designed for meniscus-to-meniscus repair, not for meniscus to capsular soft tissue. In the situation where an adequate meniscal rim remains, the use of these devices may be considered. The most reliable method of fixation is by inside-out suture fixation.

The double bone plug technique[9,10] was developed for transplantation of the medial meniscus and represented the first bone-anchored procedure. The bone plug technique involved the creation of bone tunnels at the site of the anterior and posterior horn attachments of the meniscus **(Fig. 23–4)**. As compared with the medial meniscus, the anterior and posterior horn of the

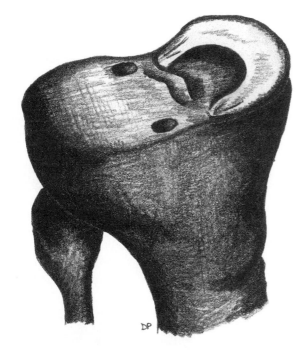

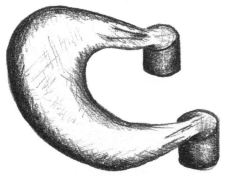

FIGURE 23–4 Bone plug technique. Note that although in this illustration, a bone plug is being used for a lateral meniscal allograft, this technique is recommended only for medial meniscal transplantation. See text for explanation.

lateral menisci are close enough that tibial tunnel creation and subsequent fixation could be compromised. Therefore, this technique is not indicated for lateral meniscal transplant. The medial meniscus is prepared by the creation of bone plugs at the anterior and posterior horn attachments of the allograft tissue. These bone plugs are then placed into the appropriately corresponding anterior and posterior tunnels. Placement of the posterior bone plug can often be difficult and can result in fracture of the bone plug, ultimately compromising fixation. As discussed earlier, it is imperative for anatomic reduction. Therefore, it must be remembered that the anterior horn attachment is usually on the anterior slope of the tibia. Therefore, creation of a true bony tunnel may not be possible and the anterior plug may be placed more as a press-fit. To compromise this anterior placement by simply placing the anterior horn where it lies best is certainly easier, but is unacceptable. This nonanatomic placement would compromise any chance of replicating normal biomechanical function[11] by creating abnormal stress and not establishing normal contact pressures. Although the use of this technique can be successful, careful attention must be given to maintaining the anatomic reduction to optimize function.

The utilization of a bone bridge between the anterior and posterior horn allows for maintenance of the normal anatomic alignment of the attachment points and for superior bone fixation along the bridge.

Several different bone bridge techniques have been developed: keyhole, slot, trough, and dovetail.[10,12] The keyhole technique **(Fig. 23–5)** was developed for placement of the lateral meniscal allograft. This technique involves the creation of a keyhole in the tibial plateau with subsequent creation of a key bridge corresponding to this tunnel. The procedure can be very demanding to perform because it requires fine-tuning of the key bridge to fit the slope and shape of the keyhole. In addition, the creation of the key bridge may be compromised by the initial harvest and preparation of the meniscal allograft.

The dovetail **(Fig. 23–6)**, slot **(Fig. 23–7)**,[7] and trough techniques **(Fig. 23–8)** have some basic similarities. They all utilize guide systems to create a trapezoidal or rectangular-shaped bone tunnel on the tibial plateau in an anteroposterior direction. This tunnel corresponds to the anatomic position of the anterior and posterior horn attachments. Both techniques can be used on either the medial or lateral side. The greatest difference in these two techniques is in the sizing of the bone bridge. For the trough technique, the bone bridge is created so that it is press-fit in the trough tunnel. The dovetail technique also creates a press-fit tunnel that allows for stabilization so that it will not ride up in the slot. The concept of press-fit is good only if there is extremely

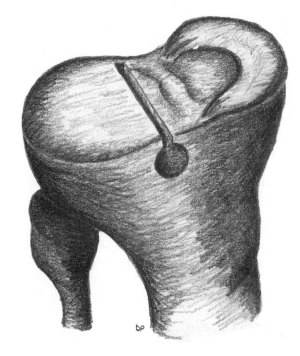

biomechanical alignment. The bone bridge can also be placed without impaction and removed for adjustment easily. The bone bridges can be fixated by suture, suture anchor, press-fit, interference fit with screws or bone dowels, or bone graft.

Meniscal transplantation is a complex multifactorial biologic process. Complications can range from the standardized risks associated with arthroscopic surgery and meniscal repair to failure of the procedure. With careful preoperative planning, intraoperative attention to detail, and postoperative monitoring and compliance, these potential complications and secondary morbidity can be minimized. The goal of the procedure is to restore a functional meniscus to the knee. Anything that will create suboptimal solutions is not acceptable. The allograft must be checked for sidedness and appropriate

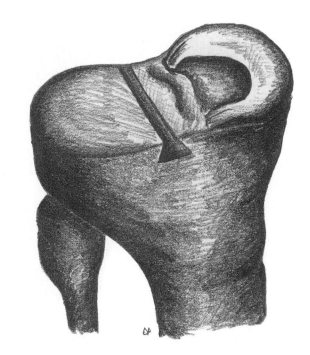

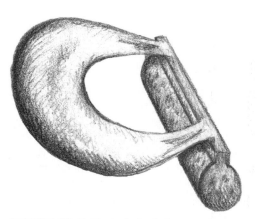

FIGURE 23–5 Keyhole technique.

accurate sizing and placement. These two factors are extremely important for appropriate function. The actual placement of a press-fit plug can also be difficult, and if impaction is utilized it has the potential for fracture of the bone bridge or damage to the anterior horn attachment site. In addition, once engaged, if removal of the bone bridge were required this could be extremely complicated.

The slot technique utilizes a slightly undersized graft, which allows for positioning and fixation to be considered independently. Once the bone bridge and meniscus tissue are reduced, the knee is cycled near extension, allowing the femoral condyle to capture the meniscus and fine tune the position of the bridge. At this point it is then fixated. This allows for the construct to be fixed in a position that provides appropriate

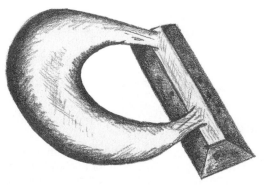

FIGURE 23–6 Dovetail technique.

compartment. Sizing can also be evaluated prior to initiating surgery. Unfortunately, defects in the actual tissue may not be realized until the tissue is thawed.

Again, it is extremely important to make certain the bone bridge is adequately seeded and the meniscus accurately fixed and aligned. The compromise of either factor will lead to early postoperative complications with long-term sequelae. Postoperative infection can occur and should be addressed appropriately based on the type of organism.

Arthrofibrosis can be a common complication due to the extensive nature of this surgery, especially if additional procedures are performed. It is important to recognize the development of extensive adhesions early and treat them aggressively by debridement and manipulation.

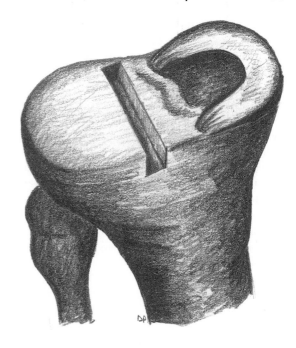

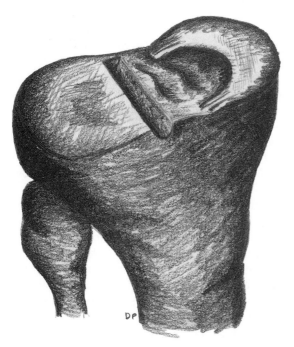

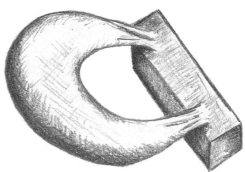

FIGURE 23–8 Trough technique.

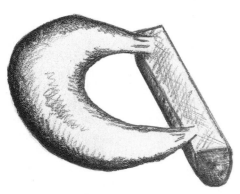

FIGURE 23–7 Slot technique.

■ Rehabilitation

The goal of rehabilitation is to allow early return to pain-free normal function without compromising the healing and remottling process. Rehabilitation from meniscal transplantation has had significant variability and evolution. Protocols have ranged from no motion to early motion, and non–weight-bearing to weightbearing as tolerated. It is important to recognize the need to protect the articular cartilage with early range of motion and mild loading to maintain the optimal matrix composition.

Initially weight bearing is limited to partial weight bearing for the first 4 weeks. After 4 weeks, weight bearing may be progressed to full weight bearing as tolerated. This progression corresponds to the increased metabolic activities of the meniscal cells and their ability to withstand stress. The requirement for loading and the positive influence and remodeling process then become a positive factor.

Range of motion is initially protected in a range-of-motion brace from full extension to 60 degrees of flexion for the first 2 weeks. After week 2 through week 4, flexion is increased to 90 degrees, and after 4 weeks there is progression to a full range of motion.

Standard knee rehabilitation is then initiated including strengthening, proprioception, and functional training. However, squatting should be avoided. The primary goals of range of motion, strengthening, and pain relief should be accomplished before progressing to more advanced activities. The full return to unrestricted activities requires 5 to 6 months.

■ Results

Although the basic concept of meniscal transplantation is similar to that originated in 1984, the basic and clinical science has undergone continuous improvement regarding understanding, application, and performance of the surgical procedure. When analyzing and comparing the results of any procedure, it is important to have minimal variables between the individual series. Unfortunately for meniscal transplantation, this is rarely the case. Since Milachowski et al's[13] first publication in 1989, multiple series have been reported. However, there are different variables in each study, such as patient population, knee arthrosis, graft preservation, surgical techniques, additional surgical procedures, rehabilitation, and parameters of follow-up. Therefore, it becomes challenging and difficult to make accurate conclusions about the role of meniscal transplantation. Though Milachowski et al were the first to perform a modern-type isolated meniscal transplant in 1984, their subsequent publication in 1989 on 22 patients with an average 14-month follow-up demonstrated healing of 15 to 18 (83%) grafts peripherally by arthroscopic evaluation. Milachowski et al had used both fresh frozen and freeze dried grafts, with the fresh frozen appearing more normal microscopically.

Garrett[14] in 1993 reported on the 7-year follow-up of 43 patients. The patient population in this study was certainly complex (salvage-type cases). Only six patients had an isolated meniscal transplant, and 28 patients underwent second-look arthroscopies, with 20 patients (71%) demonstrating healing of the meniscal allograft. The eight failures were attributed to grade 4 chondromalacia. The remaining 15 patients were asymptomatic and considered to have a good outcome.

Noyes and Barber-Westin[15] evaluated a large series of patients in 1995. This series reviewed 96 fresh frozen irradiated grafts in 82 patients. The results were extremely poor. Of the total 96 implants, 58% failed completely, 31% were partially healed, and 9% healed. Twenty-nine menisci had to be removed less than 2 years after surgery. The surgical technique involved attachment only of the posterior horn with bone plugs. No transplant was attached with bone both anteriorly and posteriorly. All grafts were irradiated. The presence of grade IV chondrosis was associated with 50% failure rate. Cameron and Seha[16] reported their results on 67 irradiated menisci without bone anchors in patients with generally advanced unicompartmental arthritis. These patients also underwent an osteotomy to unload that compartment at the time of surgery. At an average of 31 months' follow-up, 87% demonstrated a good or excellent result.

Van Arkel and deBoer[17] reported on 23 patients with a minimum of 2-year follow-up who underwent isolated meniscal transplantation. There were three failures at less than 24 months with uncorrected alignment. The remaining 20 patients (87%) were felt to have a satisfactory result.

Stollsteimer et al[18] reported a series of 22 patients with 23 cryopreserved allografts. Implantation was done arthroscopically assisted with bone plugs. The patients were followed for an average of 40 months. The most significant finding in this study was pain reduction in all patients. Although not associated with an adverse outcome, the allograft demonstrated a 37% shrinkage on MRI studies.

Carter[19] reported on 46 transplants with a minimum 2-year follow-up. Thirty-eight of the transplants underwent arthroscopic second looks between 3 and 48 months, with most occurring at 6 months. At the time of arthroscopy, four patients were considered failures, four had visible shrinkage, and two showed signs of progression of arthritis. Thirty-two of the 38 patients (84%) reported relief of pain and improvement in activities.

In 1999, Cole and Harner[20] reported the results of 22 fresh frozen menisci, and 95.5% of the patients reported improvement of pain, with associated improvement in knee function in all but one case. Rodeo et al[12] represented a comprehensive review of the literature at a national orthopedic meeting. In their review, as of March 2001, a total of 1599 meniscal transplants were performed in 1551 patients. Of these, direct objective evaluation of the transplanted tissue was done in only 366 menisci in 338 patients. Ages ranged from 10 to 68 and averaged 33. The series included fresh, fresh frozen, cryopreserved, freeze dried, irradiated, and non-irradiated menisci. The meniscus was implanted both with and without bone plugs. Concomitant procedures were performed in all but 136 cases. The degree of arthrosis in the knee varied from grade I to grade IV, and there was no consistent rehabilitation.

The author's personal experience (unpublished data) began in 1991. The current series consists of 94 meniscal transplants in 92 patients. During the time of this series there have been subtle changes in the surgical procedure, rehabilitation, and understanding of the associated basic science. Of these 92 patients, 36 had undergone concomitant procedures consisting of anterior cruciate ligament reconstruction, autologous cultured chondrocyte implantation, or tibial osteotomy. Sixty patients have been followed for greater than 2 years. Forty-seven (78%) of these patients can be considered to have a good or excellent result with improvement in pain and function. Nine patients would be considered failures, with the remaining patients having a fair result. The nine failures, seven of which were greater than 5 years postimplantation, were noted to have preexisting grade IV arthritic changes or uncorrected malalignment and were performed early in the series before these findings were known to be deleterious to the outcome of meniscal transplantation.

The present indications, techniques, and graft selection are based on the results of these earlier studies. Certain principles have achieved somewhat uniform acceptance. The grafts should be cryopreserved or fresh frozen. The procedure may be performed either open or arthroscopically assisted with the use of bone fixation, both anteriorly and posteriorly. The patient should have a subtotal meniscectomy with normal or correctable alignment, a ligamentously stable or correctable joint, and grade II changes or less chondrosis or restorable chondral defects in the affected compartment.

■ Concomitant Procedures

Ligamentous Reconstruction

The requirement for ligamentous stability of the knee joint is very important. If the knee is clinically unstable, the transplanted meniscus will be subjected to the same abnormal shear forces that often result in a native meniscal tear. This same philosophy applies to all ligamentous structures of the knee joint, whether it be the anterior or posterior cruciate ligaments, the collateral ligaments, or the posterolateral corner. Ligamentous reconstruction and meniscal transplantation may be done as a single-stage procedure, and it is not necessary to compromise placement of the cruciate ligament tunnel or of the bone slot when performing an anterior cruciate ligament procedure concomitantly. The bone bridge slot technique facilitates accurate placement of the bone trough with only minimal adjustment of the tibial tunnel and without compromise of the anatomic insertional point. If there is intersection between the tunnel and the slot, the bone of the allograft bone bridge and tendon of the anterior cruciate ligament graft will be in contact. This does not compromise the fixation, placement, or function of either graft in tissue.

Malalignment

The importance of alignment has been previously underestimated by many. Weight-bearing x-rays must be taken as part of the preoperative evaluation. If there is malalignment of even a few degrees of the affected extremity as compared with the normal extremity, realignment osteotomy should be considered. This is especially true on the medial side, which has greater stress even in normally aligned extremities. With newer techniques allowing for more distally placed osteotomies, intersection with the tunnels or slot to the meniscal allograft can be avoided with planning. This procedure can be done as a single-stage surgery. It should be remembered that the realignment procedure is not going to be similar to that done for an osteoarthritic knee.

Chondral Defects

The presence of a chondral defect has previously been a contraindication for meniscal transplantation in light of the study in which Noyes demonstrated poor results in knees with grade III to IV chondrosis. With the ability to restore articular cartilage by either osteochondral grafting or autologous chondrocyte implantation, the number of treatable patients can be expanded. The choice for articular cartilage restoration should follow guidelines based on size and location as highlighted in different publications. Regardless of the technique applied for articular cartilage restoration, the meniscal allograft should be placed and sutured prior to the full osteochondral plug placement or periosteal fixation. This will avoid damage to the graft or periosteum during reduction of the meniscus and suturing of the meniscal allograft peripherally. The author's experience with combined autologous chondrocyte implantation and meniscal transplantation has been very positive. This has resulted in the restoration of knee function and return to function in the majority of patients with minimal complications.

■ Conclusion

Meniscal transplantation has evolved as a successful procedure for the reconstruction of the meniscal deficient knee. This success will be further enhanced and improved by collaboration with basic science research. Although early results were promising, with the development and understanding of the technique, more recent studies have demonstrated improved results. As meniscal repair and preservation techniques continue to advance, the meniscal deficient knee will become less common. However, the technology of meniscal transplant will continue to be an integral procedure for the preservation of knee function.

REFERENCES

1. Arnoczky SP, Milachowski KA. Meniscal allografts: where do we stand? In: Ewing JW, ed. Articular Cartilage and Knee Joint Function: Basic Science and Arthroscopy. New York: Raven: 1990:129–136
2. Ochi M, Ishida O, Daisaku H, Ikuta Y, Akiyama M. Immune response to fresh meniscal allografts in mice J Surg Res 1995;58: 478–484
3. Rodeo SA, Seneviratne A, Suzuki K, Felker K, Wichiewicz TL, Warren RF. Histological analysis of human meniscal allografts. A preliminary report. J Bone Joint Surg Am 2000;82:1071–1082
4. Jackson DW, McDevitt CA, Simon TM, et al. Meniscal transplantation using fresh and cryopreserved allografts. An experimental study in goats. Am J Sports Med 1992;20:644–656
5. Szomor ZL, Martin RE, Bonar F, Murrell GA. The protective effects of meniscal transplantation on cartilage. An experimental study in sheep. J Bone Joint Surg Am 2000;82:80–88
6. Gersoff WK. Combined meniscal allograft transplantation and autologous chondrocyte implantation. Oper Tech Sports Med 2002; 10:165–167
7. Furr, J, Gersoff, WK. Current meniscal transplantation. Sports Med Arthrosc Rev 2004;12:69–82
8. Pollard ME, Knag Q, Berg EE. Radiographic sizing for meniscal transplantation. Arthroscopy 1995;11:684–687
9. Shelton WR, Dukes AD. Meniscus replacement with bone anchors. A surgical technique. Arthroscopy 1994;10:324–327
10. Cole BJ, Carter TR, Rodeo SA. Allograft meniscal transplantation background, techniques, and results. J Bone Joint Surg 2002;84-A:1236–1250
11. Paletta GA Jr, Manning T, Snell E, Parker R, Bergfeld J. The effect of allograft meniscal replacement on intraarticular contact area and pressures in the human knee. A biomechanical study. Am J Sports Med 1997;25:692–698
12. Rodeo SA, Senevirate A, Suziki K, Felker K, Wickiewicz TL, Warren RF. Histological analysis of human meniscal allografts. A preliminary report. J Bone Joint Surg Am 2000;82: 1071–1082
13. Milachowski KA, Weismeier K, Wirth CJ. Homologous meniscus transplantation. Experimental and clinical results. Int Orthop 1989;13:1–11
14. Garrett JC. Meniscal transplantation: a review of 43 cases with two-to seven-year follow-up. Sports Med Arthrosc Rev 1993;1:164–167
15. Noyes FR, Barber-Westin SD. Irradiated meniscus allografts in the human knee. A two- to five-year follow-up study Orthop Trans 1995;19:417
16. Cameron JC, Seha S. Meniscal allograft transplantation for unicompartmental arthritis of the knee. Clin Orthop 1997;33:164–171
17. Van Arkel ER, de Boer HH. Human meniscal transplantation. Preliminary results at 2- to 5-year follow-up. J Bone Joint Surg Br 1995;77:589–595
18. Stollsteimer GT, Shelton WR, Dukes A, Bomboy AL. Meniscal allograft transplantation. A one- to five-year follow-up of 22 patients. Arthroscopy 2000;16:343–347
19. Carter TR. Meniscal allograft transplantation. Sports Med Arthrosc Rev 1999;7:51–62
20. Cole BJ, Harner CD. Degenerative arthritis of the knee in active patients: evaluation and management. J Am Acad Orthop Surg 1999;7:389–402

24

Surgical Management of Patellofemoral Disease

TOM MINAS

This chapter offers the practicing orthopaedist a practical management approach to dealing with patellofemoral disease. The key to successful treatment relies on an accurate diagnosis of the underlying pathomechanics responsible for the pain resulting from patellofemoral pathology. Many factors have been implicated as a source of abnormal forces across the patellofemoral joint. These include patella alta; trochlear dysplasia; an abnormally increased quadriceps or Q angle, with secondary soft tissue problems; weakened or hypoplastic vastus medialis oblique quadriceps muscle with a contracted lateral retinaculum. These pathomechanics lead to abnormal forces across the patella, resulting in secondary degenerative changes or injury to the articular surfaces of the patellofemoral joint acutely or chronically.

Chronic patellofemoral pain is a common and problematic management issue. The term *chondromalacia*, which means soft cartilage, has often been applied to individuals suffering from anterior knee pain. Pain is a multifactorial perception. It is important to ensure that the pain is local and not referred. This is usually determined by a careful history and physical examination. The emotional well-being of the patient may modify the subjective response of pain. Even with obvious patellofemoral pathomechanics, if physical therapy has not been performed adequately to address these problems, then a repeated course of carefully directed physical therapy is worthwhile.

Physical therapy should address restoring soft tissue balance around the knee. This includes muscular and capsular balance; stretching to restore good flexibility of the quadriceps muscle, hamstrings muscle, and iliotibial band; as well as patellar mobilizations to loosen tight lateral capsular structures, proximal-distal quadriceps, and patellar tendon contractures. Patellar McConnell taping to centralize a maltracking patella is worthwhile, and possibly patellar bracing to perform the same centralized tracking as well. A strengthening program that does not overload the damaged patellofemoral articulation utilizing isometric and short arc closed chain concentric and eccentric muscle strengthening is valuable.

When standard conservative measures have failed, surgical intervention followed by a careful rehabilitation is often successful if the underlying pathomechanics are addressed surgically. The sensitivity of imaging studies has greatly increased to assess anatomic variations, articular cartilage damage, and joint homeostasis by radionucleotide scanning. In addition to a careful physical examination to determine underlying pathomechanics, preoperative imaging is useful. I use a management algorithm, which is largely evidence based on the literature[1] and new data from my use of autologous chondrocyte implantation (ACI) in the patellofemoral joint.[2]

■ Imaging Studies

Useful tests to assist in determining the diagnosis include standard radiographs to include standing anteroposterior (AP), 45 degree posteroanterior (PA) (Rosenberg views), lateral and skyline (Merchant views), and standard 54-inch axial alignment x-rays. Radiographs are useful with any patellofemoral joint to determine joint space

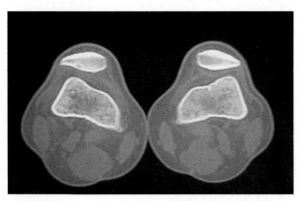

FIGURE 24–1 Bilateral subluxed patellae noted on computed tomography (CT) scan with quadriceps contracted.

Assessment of articular cartilage injury is receiving more attention with newly developed imaging protocols enhanced by intravenous gadolinium as an indirect arthrogram. Although the gold standard for assessing articular injury remains arthroscopy, sensitivity and specificity >90% can be obtained with high-resolution magnetic resonance imaging (MRI) scan using a standard 1.5-Tesla magnet, appropriate orthogonal gantry tilting to surfaces of the trochlea, and appropriate sequences. This is our preferred method of assessing articular cartilage injury to localize the site and size of chondrosis in the patellofemoral articulation. This work has been performed at our institution (Winalski) unpublished.

narrowing or osteoarthritis on a standard Merchant view. This view is taken at 45 degrees of flexion during which the patella is normally well engaged in the trochlea distally. It is not an effective view for assessing maltracking. Maltracking, when it occurs, is usually in the first 20 to 30 degrees of flexion from extension. The dislocated or subluxed patella in full extension travels medially as the knee is flexed, capturing the trochlea as it reduces. This is the clinical finding of a reverse J sign.

A spiral computed tomography (CT) scan with the leg in extension performed with the quadriceps both relaxed and contracted assists in evaluating subluxation or dislocation of patella in the trochlea **(Fig. 24–1)** or dysplasia of the bony patellofemoral joint **(Figs. 24–2 and 24–3)**. Accurate documentation of subluxation can be determined with a CT scan when clinical assessment is difficult, especially in the obese patient. When the pain pattern is suggestive of arising from the patellofemoral articulation, a bone scan is frequently useful to determine increased activity in that part of the joint.

■ Pathomechanics Assessment and Treatment Selection

In a patient with persistent patellofemoral pain and functional disability, there are certain factors that need to be determined prior to appropriate treatment of the patient with patellofemoral disease. These factors are determined after the history, physical examination, x-rays, MRI scan, and CT scan when indicated. The factors include patellar tilt, patellar tilt and subluxation, location on the patella of articular chondrosis, location on the trochlea of articular chondrosis, the quadriceps angle, vastus medialis oblique (VMO) quadriceps hypoplasia or atrophy, patella alta, and dysplasia of the trochlea. Once these factors are accurately determined, then the treatment algorithm in **Table 24-1** can be utilized.

Patellofemoral disease represents a spectrum with differing severities of subluxation, chondrosis, or arthrosis. This algorithm addresses the different stages of

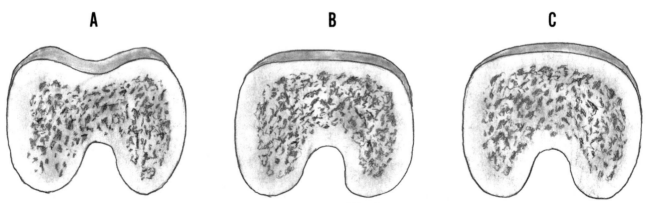

A　　　　　　　　　B　　　　　　　　　C

FIGURE 24–2 (A) Coronal view of a normal trochlea with a central concave groove. Variations of dysplasia may cause flattening of the groove **(B)** or a convex groove

(C). When this occurs developmentally, the sesamoid patellar articulation is congruent to the dysplastic trochlea.

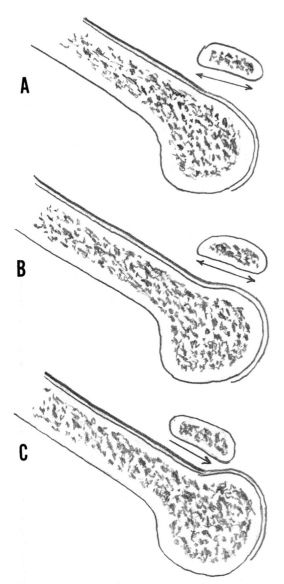

FIGURE 24–3 Dysplasia in the sagittal view may exhibit a smooth entry sulcus **(A,B)** or a prominence **(C)**, which drives the inferior pole of the patella into a "speed bump." If there is a commonly associated patella alta, it predisposes the patella to abnormal forces to subluxation and premature articular cartilage wear.

TABLE 24–1 Treatment Algorithm for the Surgical Management of Patellofemoral Disease

Patellar Status	Cartilage Status	Treatment
Patellar tilt only		Lateral release
Patellar tilt + subluxation	No chondrosis	Medial TTO
Tilt + sublux	Grade I, II chondrosis	AMZ, TTO (Fulkerson)
Tilt + sublux	Grade III, IV chondrosis	AMZ, TTO, ACI
Tilt + sublux	Loss of joint space	Patellofemoral arthoplasty and TTO

ACI, autologous chondrocyte implantation; AMZ, anteromedialization; TTO, tibial tubercle osteotomy.

disease in a stepwise fashion of increasing severity dependent on the findings.

Patellar Tilt

The procedure of arthroscopic lateral release is an overly utilized procedure. It is effective for isolated patellar tilt without subluxation of the patella when the lateral retinacular structures of the patella are contracted and mobility of the patella is limited. There may be early grade 2 Outerbridge chondromalacia associated with a chronically contracted and nonsubluxated patella. The procedure should be performed either arthroscopically or open from the superior lateral pole of the patella to the inferior lateral aspect of the patellar tendon. The superior-lateral and inferior-lateral geniculate arteries are cut with this procedure and must be isolated, coagulated or tied. It is important not to release the tendinous portion of the vastus lateralis muscle from the superior lateral patella because of the ensuing weakness that will develop. Any loose partial-thickness chondrosis flaps should be removed at the time of the lateral release to limit any pain resulting from mechanical causes.

If subluxation is associated with patellar tilt, arthroscopic lateral release as an isolated procedure should not be performed. Persistent subluxation and mechanical overload, with subsequent progressive chondral wear and pain, will persist, resulting in a failure of the procedure and unnecessary surgery for the patient (**Figs. 24–4 and 24–5**). The importance of an accurate diagnosis in differentiating tilt and subluxation can be seen in a case presentation (**Fig. 24–6**), as an isolated lateral release would not have been effective. Instead, an isolated medialization of the tibial tubercle with lateral release is indicated.

Patellar Tilt with Subluxation and with or Without Chondrosis

When there is a combination of patellar subluxation and tilting, the usual causes include a lateralized tibial tubercle patellar tendon insertion and an abnormally increased Q angle, with accompanying soft tissue medial attenuation and lateral retinacular contracture. Chondrosis may have developed and dysplasia of the trochlea may be present.

The surgical correction of the abnormal quadriceps vectors resulting from a lateralized tibial tubercle and lateral retinacular contracture need to be addressed. There have been various forms of tibial tubercle osteotomy (TTO) with lateral retinacular release performed over the years. The Fulkerson anteromedialization (AMZ) TTO has gained popularity in the United

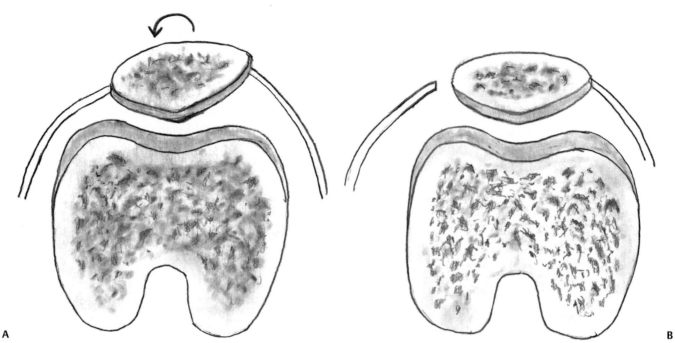

FIGURE 24–4 Isolated patellar tilt **(A)** is well managed by surgical release of the lateral retinaculum from the joint line to the superior lateral patellar tendon **(B)**.

States **(Fig. 24–7)** as a modification of the Elmslie-Trillat procedure in that it allows a more aggressive anterior translation than that provided by the latter. Soft tissue balancing, which is required to centralize the patella in the trochlea, may also be concomitantly performed

(Fig. 24–8). This procedure offloads the lateral and inferior poles of the patella by the anterior and medial translation of the tibial tubercle. Therefore, it loads off the proximal and medial poles of the patella. It has demonstrated successful clinical outcomes when the

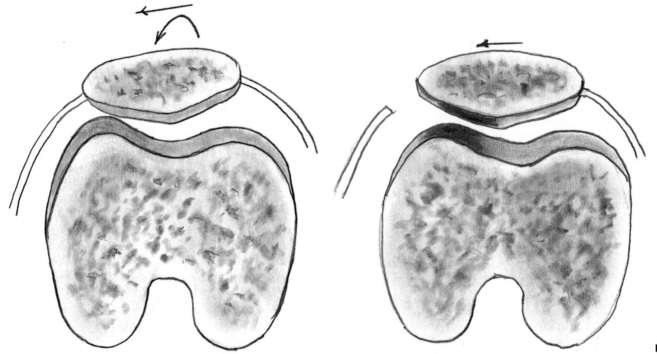

FIGURE 24–5 (A) When patellar tilt is accompanied by patellar subluxation, a lateral retinacular release does not correct the subluxation. **(B)** The overloaded lateral patellofemoral cartilage surfaces (open arrows) continue to experience overload with resultant progressive degeneration clinically manifested by persistent symptoms.

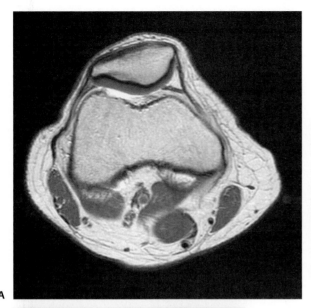

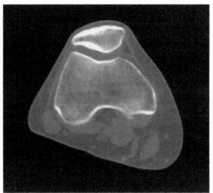

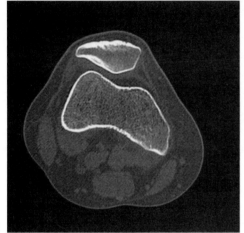

FIGURE 24–6 (A) A high-resolution magnetic resonance imaging (MRI) scan with intravenous gadolinium utilized as an effective indirect arthrogram. Notice the full-thickness nature of the lateral patellar articular cartilage. This 32-year-old woman has had a history of "chondromalacia" since the age of 12 years. She has undergone multiple courses of physical therapy, taping, and bracing. She has been offered a patellar lateral arthroscopic release and has sought another opinion. **(B)** A CT scan of the patella, which is well reduced to position. Notice the thickening of the subchondral bone to the lateral patellar facet. This is indicative of chronic lateral maltracking and overload with remodeling of the subchondral bone. **(C)** The patient contracting her quadriceps with the leg in extension. Notice the lateral subluxation of the patella. The patient requires isolated medial translation of the tibial tubercle accompanied by a patellar lateral retinacular release. The articular cartilage was normal; therefore, there was no need for anterior translation of the tubercle.

chondrosis involved with maltracking has been localized to the patella on the lateral facet or inferior patellar pole. Conversely, it has demonstrated poor clinical outcomes in the presence of articular damage to the proximal or medial patellar surfaces, or central trochlear involvement. This has led to the following classification of articular chondral injury to the patella locations: type 1, chondral injury to the inferior patella pole; type 2, chondral injury to the lateral patella facet; type 3, chondral injury to the medial patella facet; type 4, chondral injury to the proximal pole or panpatellar surface **(Fig. 24–9)**.

Presently, we are reviewing the clinical outcomes of the first 45 patients who have been treated by ACI with full-thickness chondral lesions involving the patellofemoral joint.[2] The follow-up has been 2 to 7 years. Our results when resurfacing type 3 and 4 chondral injuries to the patella have been successful with good clinical pain relief and improved function, whether or not there was preexisting patellofemoral maltracking requiring a Fulkerson osteotomy.

Trochlea Dysplasia

Dysplasia of the trochlea of the distal femur is an uncommon developmental abnormality leading to patellar instability and premature degeneration of the patellofemoral joint. It is occasionally associated with dysplasia of the lateral femoral condyle, leading to a valgus deformity accompanied by patellofemoral instability. The degree of dysplasia is variable, from subtle flattening of the proximal entry site to the trochlea, to a bulbous convex entry site leading to severe instability. As the

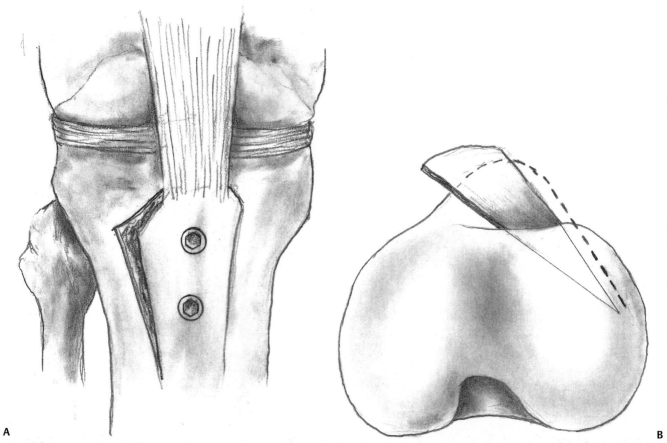

A

B

FIGURE 24–7 Diagrammatic illustration of an anterior medialization (Fulkerson) tibial tubercle osteotomy (AMZ TTO) **(A)** Anteroposterior view. **(B)** Axial view.

patella is a sesamoid bone that develops secondary to its congruity with the trochlea, it is frequently flattened or concave on its large lateral facet to match the shape of the trochlea. Like developmental dysplasia of the hip, leading to premature osteoarthritis in the fifth decade of life, dysplasia of the trochlea also usually presents with instability, anterior knee pain, a diagnosis of chondromalacia, and end-stage isolated patellofemoral arthritis (more commonly in women in the fifth decade of life).

The diagnosis requires attention to the possibility of dysplasia of the trochlea. If a patient has recurrent instability, a lateral x-ray may frequently demonstrate a prominent proximal cylinder-shaped trochlea. The diagnosis is made most accurately by a CT scan with three-dimensional reconstruction and may also be seen on MRI scan **(Fig. 24–10)**.

Patients frequently have undergone both open proximal soft tissue centralization of the patella and distal tubercle transfer with a failed clinical outcome and further instability episodes. The diagnosis is confirmed by clinical examination and demonstration of hypermobility in the medial to lateral direction, and a CT scan or MRI scan demonstrating a flattened or convex trochlea entry site.

Surgical correction by interposition soft tissue synovial trochleoplasty may be performed with good success.[3]

The procedure is outlined diagrammatically **(Fig. 24–11)**, and an intraoperative case is described in **Fig. 24–12**.

For a successful surgical outcome, an accurate assessment of patellofemoral maltracking should always include an assessment of trochlea dysplasia.

■ Treatment

Cartilage Repair with Autologous Chondrocyte Implantation

The Fulkerson osteotomy has demonstrated good and excellent clinical outcomes when the lateral patellofemoral maltracking is associated with chondral defects of type 1 or 2 locations **(Fig. 24–9)**. However, if patellar tracking is central and there are chondral defects located on the medial facet, and there is a proximal patellar pole or panpatellar crush type of injury, then the results are poor.[1]

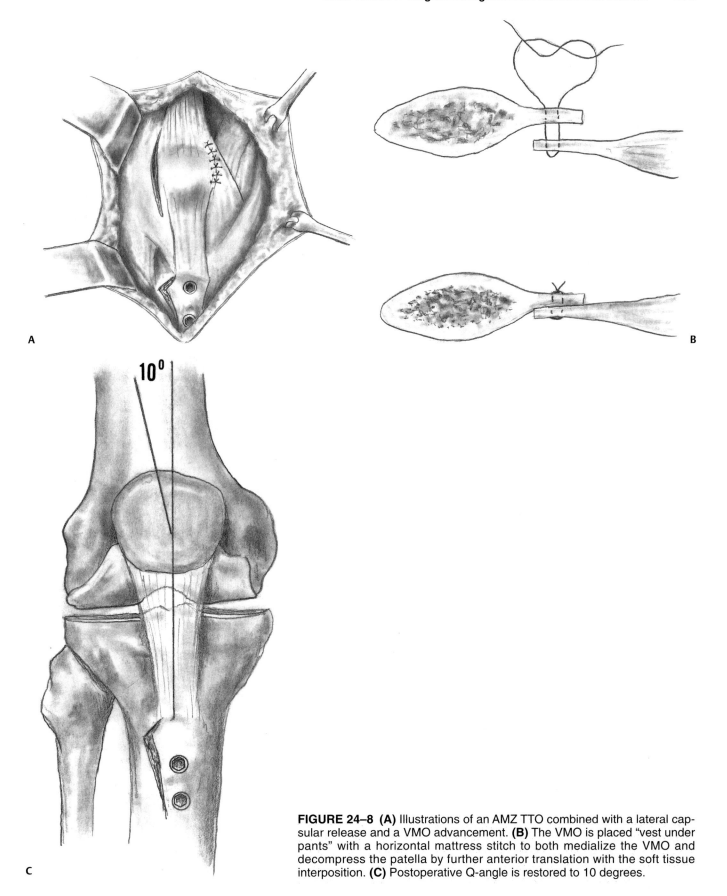

FIGURE 24–8 (A) Illustrations of an AMZ TTO combined with a lateral capsular release and a VMO advancement. **(B)** The VMO is placed "vest under pants" with a horizontal mattress stitch to both medialize the VMO and decompress the patella by further anterior translation with the soft tissue interposition. **(C)** Postoperative Q-angle is restored to 10 degrees.

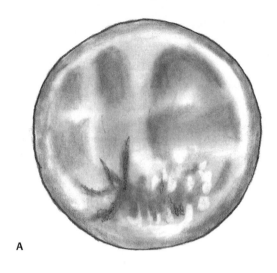

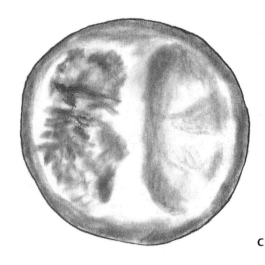

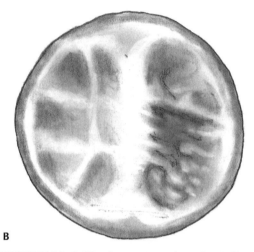

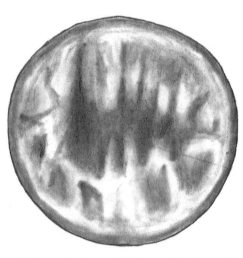

FIGURE 24–9 The four categories of patellar chondrosis as defined by Fulkerson. **(A)** Type 1 involves the inferior patellar pole. **(B)** Type 2 involves the lateral patella facet. **(C)** Type 3 involves the medial patella facet. **(D)** Type 4 involves the entire patella or the proximal pole.

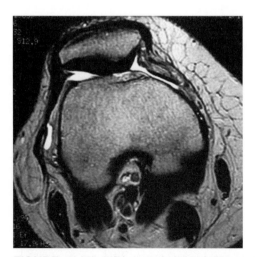

FIGURE 24–10 MRI scan demonstrating a patient with dysplastic trochlea. Note the flattened and convex nature of the proximal trochlea.

In this situation, the author has found that the use of cartilage repair with ACI has been extremely effective. The treatment is effective clinically and provides cartilage repair to the areas of loss. The standard factors previously mentioned in dealing with cartilage injury and degeneration with patellofemoral disease must be addressed prior to surgical repair of the articular cartilage injury, or at the same time as the ACI procedure.

The surgical technique of ACI, and the specific aspects relating to the patellofemoral disease are beyond the scope of this chapter and are discussed elsewhere.[4] Some of the technical considerations for ACI in the patellofemoral joint are illustrated in **Fig. 24–13**.

In my series of 45 patients (28 males and 17 females), the results of ACI in the patellofemoral joint have been encouraging. The average patient age was 37.5 years, with a range of 15 to 55 years. The average resurfacing

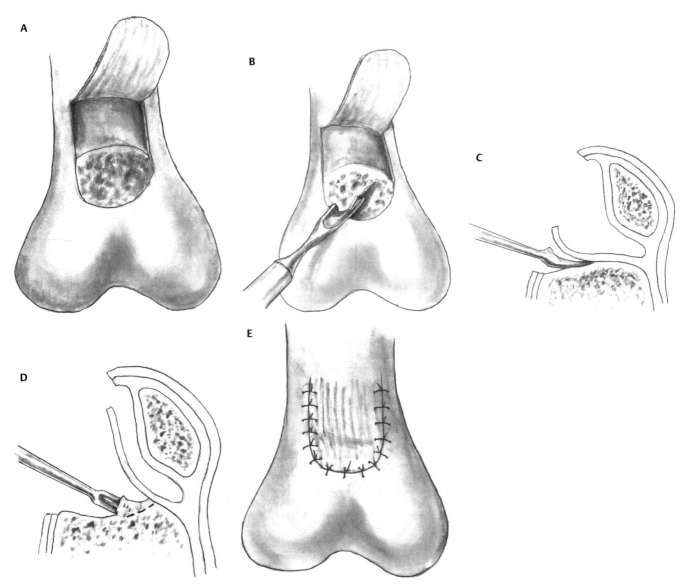

FIGURE 24–11 A diagrammatic illustration of a trochleoplasty. **(A)** The convex or flattened entry surface to the trochlea is identified centrally. The anterior supracondylar synovium is extraperiosteally reflected proximally. **(B–D)** The bulbous portion of the cartilage and bone is outlined with a sharp knife and removed with a sharp osteotome or curette. **(E)** The supracondylar synovium is then microsutured through the articular cartilage flush with the anterior femoral cortex acting as an interpositional soft tissue arthroplasty. After this procedure, the patella may capture and track centrally.

per knee was 2.18 defects, with a surface area of 10.45 cm² per knee. The patients had undergone an average of three surgeries prior to reconstruction with ACI. An example of a typical challenging ACI case of the patellofemoral joint, with a type 4 patella and trochlea defect pattern, is demonstrated in **Fig. 24–14**.

When assessing the first 45 patients treated with ACI for a patellofemoral joint, with a minimum 2-year follow-up, we have found patient satisfaction to be high. Overall 71% of the patients were satisfied, 16% were neutral, and 13% were dissatisfied. Compared with before surgery, 76% were better, 18% the same, and 6% were worse. Of patients who were asked if they would choose the surgery again, 87% said they would and 13% said they would not.

Overall, patients rated their results as follows: 71% good or excellent, 22% fair, and 7% poor. The average modified Cincinnati rating scale was 3.84 preoperative and 5.76 postoperative ($p < .0001$). Large clinical improvements and statistical significance were also encountered using the University of Western Ontario Macmaster Osteoarthritis Score (WOMAC) score, the Knee Society Score, and the Short Form (SF-36) score. These results are being prepared for peer review publication.

These results are similar to those found by Peterson et al[5,6] when patellar maltracking was addressed at the time of surgery or corrected prior to the time of ACI. When their earliest cohort of patients was removed from the group with ACI that had not undergone patellar realign-

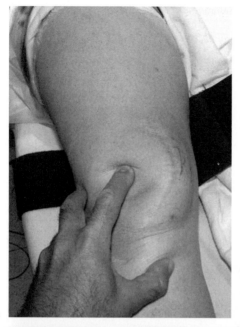

A

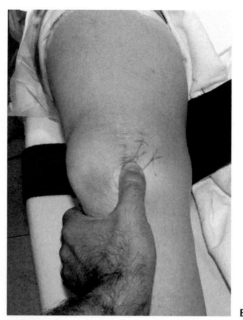

B

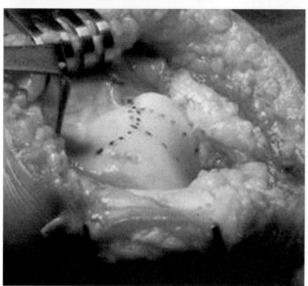

C

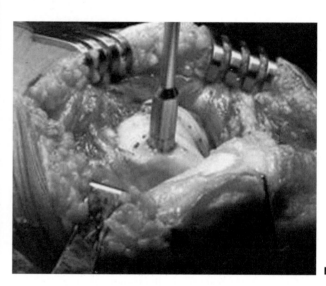

D

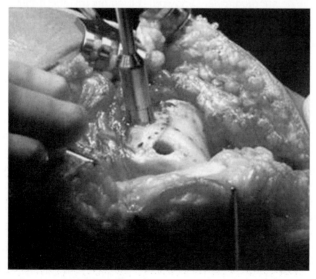

E

FIGURE 24–12 (A,B) Prior open proximal soft tissue realignment and prior tibial tubercle osteotomy have not successfully stabilized this patient with recurrent lateral dislocations and medial subluxations. Her diagnosis of trochlea dysplasia has not been addressed. **(C)** Open appearance with central markings into the intercondylar notch demonstrating the central tracking path of the patella. The proximal markings represent the cartilage and bone to be removed, centering on the distal tracking pathway. **(D)** A recipient area of full-thickness cartilage loss is removed with an osteochondral harvester. **(E)** A donor osteochondral plug is being harvested from the proposed area of discarded cartilage and bone. The donor osteochondral plug measures 1 mm and is oversized to ensure a good press fit into the recipient site, measured to the same recipient depth.

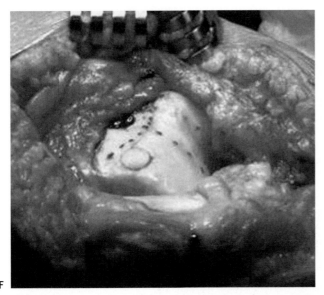

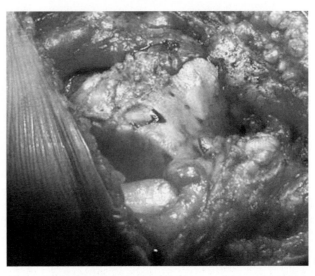

F

G

FIGURE 24–12 *(continued)* **(F)** The donor plug is transferred flush with the adjacent articular cartilage of the native trochlea; the proximal trochleoplasty can now be performed. **(G)** The final appearance of the joint after the synovium has been advanced to the area where the trochlcoplasty has been performed and where the donar plug was harvested from. The knee joint is closed with a medial advancement of the VMO. One year post-operatively the patient is asymptomatic with no recurrent insta-bility of patella and an absence of anterior knee pain. The oppo-site knee similarly has failed open proximal and distal realignment procedures. It will also undergo open trochleoplasty to ensure stability. Bilateral disease is common in this condition.

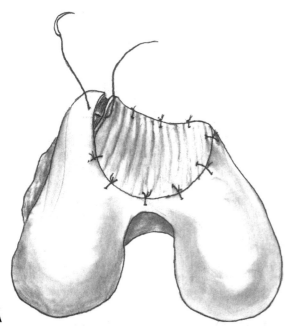

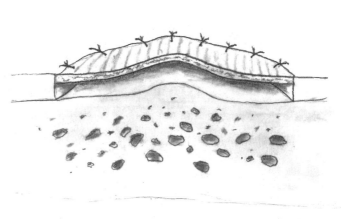

A

B

FIGURE 24–13 (A) Diagrammatic representation of the proper suture technique required to restore the concave ap-pearance of the trochlea when suturing the periosteum for autologous chondrocyte implantation (ACI). The suturing technique should start centrally at the depth of the trochlear sulcus and alternate medially and laterally to restore the concave nature of the trochlea so as not to flatten out the shape. A flattened periosteal cover puts the graft at prema-ture failure due to increased forces across the periosteal cover. **(B)** Diagrammatic representation of the proper suture technique required to restore the tent-like structure of the articular topography of the patella. The periosteal suturing must start at the apex of the patellar cartilage and then al-ternate medially and laterally until the periosteal cover is flush with the adjacent cartilage and the cartilage contour is restored. This prevents flattening of the periosteal cover and premature wear and failure of the ACI at the central bony apex.

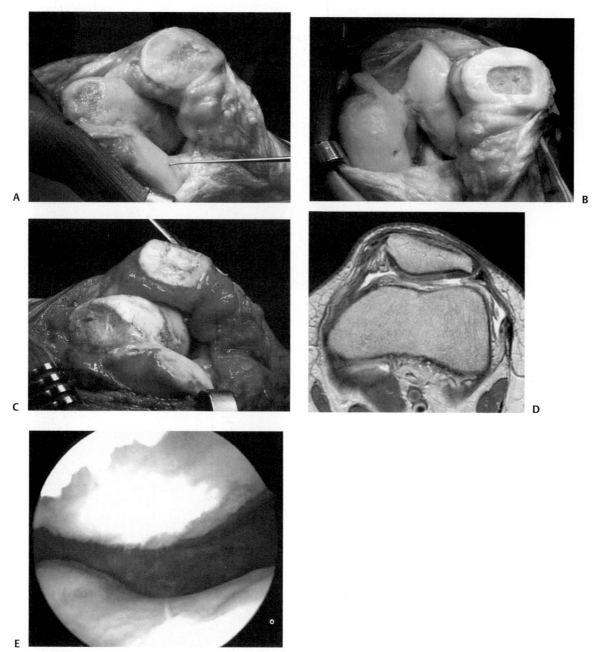

FIGURE 24–14 (A) Appearance of the full-thickness loss of cartilage of the central patella and trochlea. A 32-year-old woman who had undergone a prior AMZ TTO 6 years earlier. She had good pain relief for approximately 4 years prior to recurrent crepitations, effusions, and severe anterior knee pain, limiting her performance of activities of daily living. Sports were not possible. **(B)** Appearance of the knee after radical debridement of all damaged articular cartilage back to full-thickness normal cartilage margins. **(C)** Appearance after marker suturing of periosteum and ACI. **(D)** MRI in the coronal plane across the patella 7 months postoperatively. This demonstrates excellent repair and tissue fill. The density of the tissue is not yet isodense to the adjacent native patellar cartilage. The patient had developed mild catching secondary to periosteal remnants on the patella. **(E)** Arthroscopic appearance of the patella and trochlea 8 months after ACI for "kissing" lesions—patella and trochlea. Two years postoperatively, the patient is pain free. She no longer experiences effusions, catching, or locking. She is able to participate in recreational sports and play with her young child.

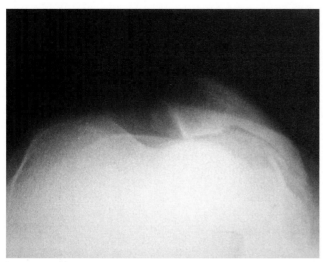

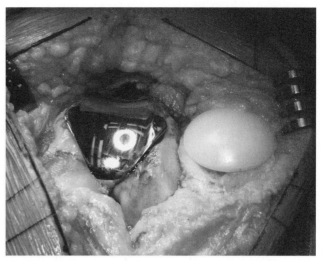

FIGURE 24–15 (A) Merchant x-ray view demonstrating obliteration of the articular joint space. **(B)** Intraoperative appearance of a patella femoral prosthetic resurfacing using a standard patella from an existing knee system with a custom designed inset trochlea metal surface.

ment surgery, their overall good and excellent results were 79%.[5] These results have remained durable up to 10 years after implantation.[6] These are excellent outcomes for a patient population that is difficult to treat.

Patellofemoral Prosthetic Arthroplasty

When collapse of the joint space radiographically has occurred, as viewed by the Merchant or skyline x-ray, cartilage repair by ACI is no longer possible. The procedure relies on intact, full-thickness cartilage margins to maintain the joint space so that the growing cartilage repair tissue may fill the defect. If the medial or proximal cartilage is absent, and there is no maltracking, then a tibial tubercle osteotomy with anterior and medial translation is also not effective. In this situation I have found that in the middle-aged patient who is too young for a total knee replacement, a unicompartmental patellofemoral prosthesis has been a useful interim solution. To date, a custom trochlea inset metal prosthesis with a standard polyethylene patella button has been used. The standard medial parapatellar arthrotomy is performed with a standard patellar resurfacing. The trochlea prosthesis is only 3 mm thick and removes little cartilage and bone. It is easily converted to a standard total knee replacement when the tibiofemoral cartilage becomes degenerated. It does not jeopardize future reconstructions, yet it allows adequate pain relief and functionality for activities of daily living **(Fig. 24–15)**.

■ Conclusion

Patellofemoral disease is one of the most problematic management issues for the orthopaedist dealing with knee reconstructive surgery. Once nonoperative management has failed in alleviating pain and improving functionality, a careful assessment to determine the underlying pathomechanics causing the degenerative process is necessary for successful management. These factors include patella alta, an increased quadriceps angle, dysplasia of the trochlea, secondary soft tissue imbalance, and the localization of cartilage damage to the patella and the trochlea.

The management algorithm presented here attempts to deal with these identified factors and the secondary degenerative processes. When used for the correct indications, the options of patellar lateral release, anteromedial tibial tubercle osteotomy, trochleoplasty, ACI, and a unicompartmental patellofemoral prosthesis provide improved functionality and pain relief for the young patient suffering with patellofemoral pain.

REFERENCES

1. Pidoriano AJ, Weinstein RN, Buuck DA, Fulkerson JP. Correlation of patellar articular lesions with results from amteromedial tibial tubercle transfer. AJSM 1997;25:533–537
2. Minas T, Bryant T. The role of antologous chondrocyte implantation in the patellofemoral joint. Clin orthop 2005, 436: 30–39
3. Peterson L, Karlsson J, Brittberg M, et al. Patellar instability with recurrent dislocation due to patellofemoral dysplasia results after surgical treatment. Bull Hosp Jt Dis Orthop Inst 1988;48: 130–139
4. Minas T, Peterson L. Advanced techniques in autologous chondrocyte transplantation. Clin Sports Med 1999;18:13–44
5. Peterson L, Minas T, Brittberg M, et al. Two- to 9- year outcome after autologous chondrocyte transplantation of the knee. Clin Orthop 2000;374:212–234
6. Peterson L, Brittberg M, Kiviranta I, et al. Autologous chondrocyte transplantation. Biomechanics and long-term durability. Am J Sports Med 2002;30:2–12

■ SECTION SEVEN ■

Future Directions

25

Future Directions in the Treatment of Cartilage Injury in the Athlete

CONSTANCE R. CHU, VOLKER MUSAHL, AND FREDDIE H. FU

Future advances in the treatment of articular cartilage defects will be based on improved understanding of chondrocyte biology, early detection of cartilage injury, and functional tissue engineering. Chondrocyte resuscitation following mechanical injury may assist in preventing net proteoglycan loss leading to structural breakdown. This can reduce both the incidence and the size of chondral defects. Larger, symptomatic defects will need reconstruction with tissue engineering methods that yield biomechanically sound neocartilage. New imaging methods allowing for nondestructive assessment of cartilage microarchitecture and metabolic capacity will assist in early diagnosis of compromised articular cartilage. These same methods can be used for longitudinal assessment of articular cartilage treatment modalities.

■ New Assessment Techniques

Advanced Magnetic Resonance Imaging

Magnetic resonance imaging (MRI) has revolutionized medical imaging of the musculoskeletal system.[1] Noninvasive and direct visualization of bone, marrow, and supporting soft tissue structures can be obtained with this technology, and the procedure is well tolerated by patients, especially after the development of open MRI systems. MRI offers a multiplanar tomographic viewing perspective, eliminating projectional distortion and magnification as well as the problem of superimposing of overlaying structures. Techniques describing articular cartilage with conventional MRI have been developed, and studies have shown that these techniques are both sensitive and specific for detecting articular cartilage defects in the knee.[2] A study revealed that in patients with hip dysplasia conventional radiography showed no evidence of joint space narrowing; however, MRI detected articular cartilage defects in almost half of the examined patients.[3] Furthermore, techniques for quantifying the volume of articular cartilage and for mapping its thickness have been developed and validated.[4–6]

However, the vast availability of MRI has affected the costs of health care in a significant manner, and studies have shown that a thorough clinical examination can be as successful in evaluating the status of articular cartilage as MRI. In one study, the diagnostic performance of clinical examination and MRI in the evaluation of intraarticular knee disorders was compared with intraoperative arthroscopic findings. The authors concluded that selective MRI does not provide enhanced diagnostic utility over clinical examination, particularly in children, and should be used cautiously.[7]

In recent years, more sensitive and specific MRI techniques have been developed for evaluating articular cartilage abnormalities. These techniques have focused on monitoring the concentration of glycosaminoglycans in articular cartilage, which are lost early in the course of osteoarthritis (OA) and, furthermore, are a major mechanical supporter of articular cartilage.[8] Gadolinium-enhanced MRI techniques rely on the fact that gadolinium diethylenetriamine pentaacetic acid

289

(Gd-DTPA^{2-}) distributes into degraded areas at a higher concentration than into nondegraded areas. This technique was validated in cadaveric specimens.[9]

Gadolinium-enhanced MRI has also been evaluated in vivo, and the technique was proven feasible for imaging of the glycosaminoglycan concentration of articular cartilage.[10] Studies have shown that T1 in the presence of Gd-DTPA^{2-} differs by more than twofold when comparing regions of normal and osteoarthritic tissue. The contrast agent can be administered intraarticularly or intravenously, whereby intravenous delivery is about four times faster and Gd-DTPA^{2-} is able to penetrate the articular cartilage both from the bone–cartilage as well as the synovial fluid–cartilage interfaces. Intravenous administration is associated with less patient discomfort. However, it involves a higher systemic dose and is more costly than intraarticular administration.

Triple-quantum-filtered sodium MRI has been proposed as a method to discriminate between intracellular and extracellular sodium. However, a low signal-to-noise ratio has been a major obstacle to triple-quantum-filtered sodium MRI. In one study, the results of phantom experiments showed that a gradient-echo multiple-quantum-filtered ^{23}Na imaging sequence produces the highest signal-to-noise ratio. The sensitivity of triple-quantum-filtered sodium MRI to ischemia was furthermore demonstrated in brains of live canines.[11] This technique was also applied in vivo in healthy volunteers to demonstrate its feasibility in imaging of human articular cartilage. Triple-quantum-filtered sodium MRI images clearly demarcated patellar cartilage and demonstrated fluid signal suppressed by the triple quantum filter.[12]

Optical Coherence Tomography

Optical coherence tomography (OCT) is an optical imaging technique that allows for nondestructive high-resolution cross-sectional imaging of articular cartilage.[13] Therefore, OCT has the potential to be used for early diagnosis of cartilage damage. OCT was first introduced to image the eye.[14] The technology can be described as similar to ultrasound except that the image generated is an echograph of infrared light instead of ultrasound. OCT has been applied to a wide variety of tissues to obtain high-resolution cross-sectional images comparable to low power histology and superior to both conventional MRI (150 μm) and ultrasound.[15]

When applied to assessment of tissue engineered cartilage repair, OCT imaging was found to be comparable to low-power histology (**Fig. 25–1**).[16] Unlike histology in which the diseased tissue must be removed for processing

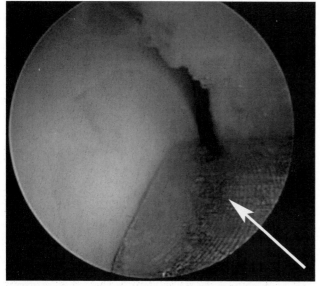

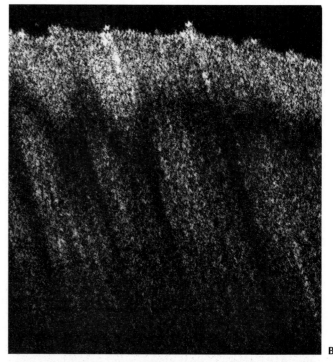

FIGURE 25–1 Optical coherence tomography (OCT) of articular cartilage. OCT is a new imaging technique that can be used arthroscopically to obtain histology resolution cross-sectional images of articular cartilage instantaneously. **(A)** Arthroscopic view of OCT probe (arrow). **(B)** Cross-sectional OCT image of healthy appearing articular cartilage (See Color Plate 25–1B).

and analysis, the OCT "biopsy" was obtained in situ and in near real time with no damage to the cartilage repair. The ability to obtain high-resolution nondestructive images of articular cartilage using OCT may result in earlier and more accurate diagnosis of articular cartilage injury.

Biomechanical Probes

Articular cartilage functions as a near frictionless, load-bearing tissue. Assessment of the compressive properties of the tissue may assist clinicians in determining the health of the articular cartilage. This information may also be useful in determining whether the repair tissue following a cartilage regenerative procedure is sufficiently strong to permit an athlete to return to sports. Indentation testing is a common method used to evaluate the compressive behavior of articular cartilage.[17]

Several handheld indentation probes have been developed to measure in situ compressive stiffness.[18,19] One electromechanical probe (Artscan 1000, Artscan, Ltd, Helsinki, Finland) has been used to assess repair tissue stiffness in patients after autologous chondrocyte implantation.[20] This device measures the resistance of the cartilage to a short deformation applied by an indenter. Although this type of indenter provides information on surface and subsurface stiffness, the device cannot measure or account for the important effects of cartilage thickness on the material properties of the tissue.[21–23]

Ultrasound devices enable measurement of cartilage thickness, and have some capacity to assess structure and composition.[24–27] A system that was developed at the University of Pittsburgh was validated utilizing bovine knee specimens. The true sound speed in articular cartilage was measured using a miniature ultrasound contact transducer and correlated with the indentation stiffness. The authors found a significant decrease in indentation stiffness for proteoglycan-depleted specimens compared with normal articular cartilage.[28]

■ Improved Injury Models

Chondrocyte injury and cartilage structural damage has been shown to occur following chemical, mechanical, and thermal injury. To evaluate the chondroprotective effects of interventions ranging from controlled passive motion to growth factors, antioxidants and heat treatment, appropriate models need to be developed at the cellular, tissue and organ levels. In relation to athletic injuries and arthroscopic surgery, the most relevant models involve impact injury and thermal stress.

Mechanical Injury Models

Early observations on decreased diffusion capacity of continuously compressed articular cartilage lead to the first impact injury models in articular cartilage research.[29] The classic impact injury model was described by Thompson and Bassett[30] in 1970. In this work, degeneration of articular cartilage was experimentally induced by compression immobilization and condylar resection. The survival of human articular cartilage was critically impaired by strains exceeding 20 to 25%.[31,32] By applying subfracture loads to human patellofemoral joints, horizontal split fractures in subchondral bone, and at the interface of calcified cartilage and subchondral bone could be observed.[33] The magnitude of cell damage was studied utilizing an impact injury model and is characterized by increased release of proteoglycans from the specimens subjected to stress.[34]

Excess mechanical stress has been shown to result in chondrocyte apoptosis, decreased proteoglycan synthesis, and matrix breakdown. Most current mechanical injury models focus on either static compression or cyclic loading. Although these models result in chondrocyte injury, it has been difficult to adequately model the effects of a single sudden impact similar to that of an anterior cruciate ligament (ACL) injury or subchondral fracture.

Controlled Thermal Injury

Thermal devices have gained widespread clinical use in the arthroscopic treatment of intraarticular pathology. There is great need for safe and effective arthroscopic methods to remove and stabilize damaged articular cartilage. The use of thermal energy to perform chondroplasty has sparked both interest and controversy. Histologically, radiofrequency energy (RFE) chondroplasty has been reported to deliver a smoother residual surface than mechanical shavers. Although RFE chondroplasty has been reported to deliver superior clinical results to shaver debridement in at least one study, the procedure has become increasingly controversial because of concerns over excessive collateral chondrocyte death from thermal injury. Quantifying the effects of thermal stress on articular cartilage is important both in evaluating the safety of intraarticular use of thermal devices and in the potential development of a well-defined chondrocyte injury model.

After examining the effects of time and temperature on both osteoarthritic and normal human articular cartilage, it has been determined that chondrocytes possess the ability to recover from short-term exposures to high temperatures. Arthritic cartilage was found to be more sensitive to increased thermal exposure than

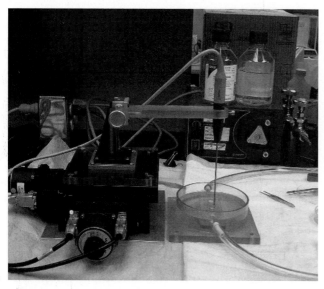
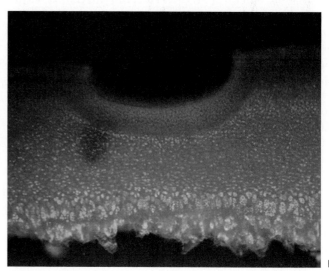

FIGURE 25–2 Computer-controlled treatment stage (See Color Plate 25–2B).

nonarthritic cartilage. Additionally, articular cartilage was found to transiently increase proteoglycan synthesis following mild temperature elevation.

The use of a computer-controlled treatment stage allows for the production of discrete, reproducible levels of articular cartilage injury (**Fig. 25–2**). Further development of this thermal injury model will allow for controlled in vitro and in vivo experiments to evaluate the effects of different depths of chondrocyte injury on the structural, metabolic and functional properties of articular cartilage. Controlled thermal stress also provides a means to study ways to optimize survival of the stressed chondrocyte.

■ Future Treatments

Although chondrocytes make up less than 10% of articular cartilage, they are responsible for maintenance of the glycosaminoglycan-rich matrix. Under normal physiologic conditions, chondrocytes exhibit low metabolic activity, divide infrequently, and have a long life. The stressed chondrocyte increases metabolic activity, clones itself, and may undergo apoptosis. Optimizing survival and recovery of the stressed chondrocyte represents an active area of research with long-ranging potential toward acute treatment of cartilage injury and the prevention of osteoarthritis.

Chondrocyte Resuscitation

The concept of chondroprotection is of great importance in reducing cartilage damage after injury and in slowing, perhaps even preventing or reversing, the

progression of degenerative arthritis. Recent studies from our laboratories demonstrate that the tolerance of articular cartilage for longer periods at higher temperatures may be improved in the presence of insulin-like growth factor-I (IGF-I) and an inhibitor of c-Jun N-terminal kinase (JNK) or stress activated protein kinase. The JNK pathway is considered important in stress-induced cell death through apoptosis. Both IGF-I and JNK inhibition improved metabolic recovery of human articular cartilage after thermal injury. In addition to having anabolic effects on articular cartilage, IGF-1 has been shown to have antiapoptotic effects.[35] Apoptosis is an ordered process known as "programmed cell death" important to morphogenesis and tissue homeostasis.[36] More recently, experimental evidence indicates that cells injured by environmental stress and cells in pathologic tissues such as osteoarthritic cartilage also undergo apoptosis.[37,38] The JNK pathway is an important signal transduction mechanism for converting stress signals into apoptosis signaling in a variety of cell types.[39,40] That improved recovery of cartilage metabolic activity after thermal stress was seen after the addition of two different antiapoptotic agents suggests that stress-induced apoptosis may be involved in chondrocyte necrosis following thermal injury. These studies demonstrate the great potential for the future use of substances such as JNK inhibitor and cartilage-friendly growth factors such as IGF-I to resuscitate damaged chondrocytes.

Gene Therapy

Growth factors are proteins that can be liberated by cells at the injury site (e.g., fibroblasts, endothelial cells, muscle cells, mesenchymal stem cells) and by the infiltrating reparatory or inflammatory cells (e.g., platelets, macrophages). They are capable of stimulating cells toward proliferation, migration, matrix synthesis, and differentiation.[41–49] With the help of recombinant DNA technology, using the specific gene encoding the proteins, it is now possible to synthesize large quantities of the therapeutic proteins for the purpose of treatment.

The direct application of human recombinant therapeutic proteins displays effects on the healing process; however, its application is limited by their short biologic half-life and by the need for repeated and high dosages. Therefore, the most difficult question to resolve prior to starting a gene therapy trial is what delivery method to choose. The goal of the delivery is to get the DNA that encodes for the specific protein into the target cell so that the cell will start expressing the growth factor. The most commonly used method is a viral insertion of the DNA into the target cell, which is called transduction.[50–52] Alternatively, there are nonviral methods, such as "naked DNA" or liposomal vectors. The transferred gene is either integrated into the chromosomal DNA (e.g., retroviral transfection) or maintained separately in the cell as an episome (e.g., adenoviral transfection).[53] For expression, the desired gene has to enter the pathways of transcription [copying the DNA into messenger RNA (mRNA)], translation (actual protein synthesis according to the mRNA template), and secretion of the therapeutic protein (e.g., growth factor). This process can be repeated so that the genetically manipulated cells serve as a reservoir for growth factors improving healing.

Gene therapy was originally for the manipulation of germline cells for treating inherited genetic disorders, but this application has been limited due to considerable ethical concern. Conversely, the manipulation of somatic cells has been widely accepted. However, the recently reported cases of the development of leukemia-like side effects of clinical trials for the treatment of children with severe combined immunodeficiency (SCID) have raised concerns about the risk-benefit ratio of gene therapy. Thus, research addressing safety issues is invaluable, especially in the field of orthopaedic sports medicine, where elective surgeries are performed on a relatively young population.[54,55]

Strategies for local gene therapy have been extensively investigated in the field of sports medicine. Vectors can be directly injected in the host tissue, or cells in culture can be genetically altered with a vector (ex vivo) and transplanted.[56] Although the direct method is technically easier to achieve, the cell-based ex vivo approach bares less risk, because gene manipulation occurs outside the body of the host. Furthermore, the genetically engineered and transplanted cells supply the host with the desired gene and with cells responding and participating in the healing process. Decreased gene expression over time is common and its mechanisms are not fully understood. However, in certain tissues such as articular discs of the spine, gene expression could be observed in rabbits for more than 12 months.[57] Currently research is focusing on regulating gene expression. Specifically, the induction of gene expression could help to control the gene expression and modulate implanted genes while turning them on and off. Certain promoter sequences that have been identified include a promoter that is activated only when animals have tetracycline in their diet and a promoter that is inducible by x-ray irradiation.[58,59]

At the experimental level, the feasibility of gene therapy was shown to the ligament insertion, meniscus, articular cartilage, and synovial tissue of the knee joint.[60,61] Beyond this stage, experimental research in animal models has revealed that ligament insertions can be enhanced through gene therapy, that muscle scarring can be diminished in muscle laceration, that knee joint arthritis can be decreased, and that muscle-derived stem cells promote the healing of cartilage lesions.

Cartilage has a low potential for healing. Injuries may lead to premature arthritis and a decrease in the quality of life, and it has enormous long-term health care costs. Growth factors such as bone morphogenetic protein–2 (BMP-2), basic fibroblast growth factor (bFGF), transforming growth factor-((TGF-(), IGF-I, and cartilage-derived morphogenetic protein (CDMP) have both demonstrated in vitro and in vivo beneficial effects on cartilage healing.[62,63] Muscle scaffolds in combination with myoblasts and IGF-I have been successfully used to induce healing in a rabbit articular cartilage injury model (**Fig. 25–3**).[64] In addition to autologous chondrocytes, stem cells from peripheral tissues such as muscle or bone marrow represent potential sources for cell transplantation, which can be used in conjunction with gene therapy approaches. Several gene therapy and tissue engineering approaches to cartilage lesions are currently under investigation. However, the most efficient methodology for healing of these lesions has not yet been established.

Meniscus tears can be treated with surgical techniques such as sutures, arrows, or staples when they occur in the vascularized peripheral third of the meniscus. Meniscal lesions in the avascular central part do not heal. Experimental studies have shown that healing in the central meniscus parts might be promoted by stimuli derived from a fibrin clot, synovial tissue, or growth factors (transforming growth factor-(, bFGF, epidermal-derived growth factor).[65,66] The aims of gene therapy approaches are to deliver these growth factors directly or with the help of cells. This could also be managed in a preconditioning approach.

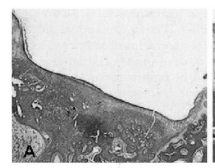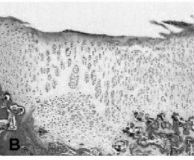

FIGURE 25–3 Cartilage full-thickness defect **(A),** after 6 weeks of healing with myoblasts and insulin-like growth factor-I.

Although gene therapy is not yet established as a clinical therapy, it has great potential for the treatment of musculoskeletal injuries in the future. Phase I of the first clinical trial in orthopedics was successfully completed for human joints.[56,67] It is believed that further tissue engineering with muscle-derived stem cells and gene therapy will lead to the development of new treatment strategies for tissues with low healing capacities such as articular cartilage. New techniques that address the biologic base of healing might further improve the outcome and create indications for surgical interventions in tissues with low healing potential. However, a large number of basic science studies and preclinical trials have to be completed to reach the necessary efficiency and safety for orthopedic applications.

Functional Tissue Engineering

Autologous chondrocyte implantation is the first Food and Drug Administration (FDA)-approved cell-based treatment for articular cartilage defects. The two-stage procedure involves arthroscopic harvest of ~200 mg of cartilage from the patient's knee. The chondrocytes are isolated from the biopsy and expanded ex vivo into several million cells, which are then reimplanted into the defect under a piece of periosteum at second-stage arthrotomy. Future improvements to the reimplantation of autologous chondrocytes include substituting both natural and synthetic membranes for the periosteum. Membranes under consideration include collagen membranes, biodegradable membranes, and porcine intestine submucosal tissue. Another strategy is to seed the autologous chondrocytes into collagen gels, hydrogels, hyaluronic acid, biodegradable scaffolds, or injectable pastes and glues.[68–75]

Coaxing stem cells into chondrogenic repair cells represent another promising line of research for the repair of chondral defects. Stem cells are cells that can turn into different tissue types, such as bone, cartilage, muscle, or tendon. For example, fetal umbilical cord cells are stem cells that display the ability to differentiate in various tissue types. Unfortunately, they are not available in adults. In contrast, bone marrow–derived stem cells and muscle-derived stem cells persist throughout life, are available in abundance, and easily accessible through a biopsy. A special stem cell population derived from muscle tissue was identified, and tissue-engineering approaches are currently under development, which means biologic substitutes for repair, reconstruction, regeneration, or replacement of musculoskeletal tissues with muscle-derived stem cells.[76]

Functional tissue engineering is a novel approach to enhance tissue regeneration and provides the possibility of producing tissue that is biomechanically, biochemically, and histomorphologically similar to the normal.[77,78] The basic concept of tissue engineering is based on the manipulation of cellular and biochemical mediators to affect protein synthesis and to improve tissue formation and remodeling. Ultimately, the process is expected to lead to a restoration of mechanical properties.[79] Examples of the available approaches are the use of growth factors, gene transfer technology to deliver genetic material, stem cell therapy, and the use of scaffolding as well as external mechanical factors. Each of these approaches, or their combinations, offers the opportunity to enhance the healing process.

■ Conclusion

Advances in regenerative medicine, cell biology, genomics, and biomaterials hold promise for development of effective treatment techniques for articular cartilage injuries. Although many partial solutions will likely make their way into clinical practice in the near future, treating cartilage-injured patients and athletes with arthritis will most likely remain a clinical challenge. It must be remembered that articular cartilage is an enigmatic tissue and that methods to repair articular cartilage have eluded scientists and physicians at least since Hippocrates's time. The future, however, belongs to those with vision. We foresee cartilage restoration through comprehensive assessment, chondrocyte resuscitation, and functional tissue engineering.

REFERENCES

1. Damadian R. Tumor detection by nuclear magnetic resonance. Biophys J 1971;11:739–760
2. Recht M, Pirraino D, Paletta G, Schils J, Belhobek G. Accuracy of fat-suppressed three-dimensional spoiled gradient-echo FLASH MR imaging in the detection of patellofemoral articular cartilage abnormalities. Radiology 1996;198:209–212
3. Nishii T, Sugano N, Tanako H, Nakarishi K, Ohzono K, Yoshikawa H. Articular cartilage abnormalities in dysplastic hips without joint space narrowing. Clin Orthop Relat Res 2001;383:183–190
4. Peterfy C, van Dijke CF, Janzen DL, et al. Quantification of articular cartilage in the knee with pulsed saturation transfer subtraction and fat-suppressed MR imaging: optimization and validation. Radiology 1994;192:485–491
5. Eckstein F, Winzheimer M, Hohe J, Englmeier K, Reiser M. Interindividual variability and correlation among morphological parameters of knee joint cartilage plates: analysis with three-dimensional MR imaging. Osteoarthritis Cartilage 2001;9:101–111
6. Cicuttini F, Forbes A, Asbeutah A, Morris K, Stuckey S. Comparison and reproducibility of fast and conventional spoiled gradient-echo magnetic resonance sequences in the determination of knee cartilage volume. J Orthop Res 2000;18:580–584
7. Kocher M, DiCanzio J, Zurakowski D, Micheli L. Diagnostic performance of clinical examination and selective magnetic resonance imaging in the evaluation of intraarticular knee disorders in children and adolescents. Am J Sports Med 2001;29: 292–296
8. Frank EH, Grodzinsky AJ. Cartilage electromechanics—I. Electrokinetic transduction and the effects of electrolyte pH and ionic strength. J Biomech 1987;20:615–627
9. Bashir A, Gray M, Burstein D. Gd(DTPA)2– as a measure of cartilage degradation. Magn Reson Med 1996;36:665–673
10. Bashir A, Gray M, Boutin R, Burstein D. Glycosaminoglycan in articular cartilage: in vivo assessment with delayed Gd(DTPA)2-enhanced MR imaging. Radiology 1997;205:551–558
11. Kalyanapuram R, Seshan V, Bansal N. Three-dimensional triple-quantum-filtered 23Na imaging of the dog head in vivo. J Magn Reson Imaging 1998;8:1182–1189
12. Borthakur A, Hancu I, Boada FE, Shen GX, Shapiro EM, Reddy R. In vivo triple quantum filtered twisted projection sodium MRI of human articular cartilage. J Magn Reson 1999;141: 286–290
13. Herrmann JM, Pitris C, Bouma BE, et al. High resolution imaging of normal and osteoarthritic cartilage with optical coherence tomography. J Rheumatol 1999;26:627–635
14. Huang D, et al. Optical coherence tomography. Science 1991; 254:1178–1181
15. Pan Y, Lavelle JP, Bastacky SI, et al. Detection of tumorigenesis in rat bladders with optical coherence tomography. Med Phys 2001;28:2432–2440
16. Han C, Chu CR, Adachi N, et al. Analysis of rabbit articular cartilage repair after chondrocyte implantation using optical coherence tomography. Osteoarthritis Cartilage 2003;11:111–121
17. Athanasiou KA, Niederauer GG, Schenck RC Jr. Biomechanical topography of human ankle cartilage. Effects of excimer laser on healing of articular cartilage in rabbits. Ann Biomed Eng 1995;23:697–704
18. Appleyard RC, Burkhardt D, Ghosh P, et al. Topographical analysis of the structural, biochemical and dynamic biomechanical properties of cartilage in an ovine model of osteoarthritis. Osteoarthritis Cartilage 2003;11:65–77
19. Toyras J, Lyyra-Laitinen T, Niinimaki M, et al. Estimation of the Young's modulus of articular cartilage using an arthroscopic indentation instrument and ultrasonic measurement of tissue thickness. J Biomech 2001;34:251–256
20. Peterson L, Lindahl A, Brittberg M, Nilsson A. Durability of autologous chondrocyte Transplantation of the knee. In: 67th annual meeting of the American Academy of Orthopaedic Surgeons, Orlando, FL, 2000
21. Jurvelin JS, Vaatainen U, Helminen HJ, Wong M. Volumetric changes of articular cartilage during stress relaxation in unconfined compression. Scand J Med Sci Sports 2000;10:186–198
22. Mow VC, Gibbs MC, Lai WM, Zhu WB, Athanasiou KA. Biphasic indentation of articular cartilage—II. A numerical algorithm and an experimental study. Material properties of the normal medial bovine meniscus. J Biomech 1989;22:853–861
23. Chen FS, Frenkel SR, Di Cesare PE. Chondrocyte transplantation and experimental treatment options for articular cartilage defects. Am J Orthop 1997;26:396–406
24. Cherin E, et al. Ultrasonic propagation properties of articular cartilage at 100 MHz. J Bone Miner Res 1997;12:1378–1386
25. Cherin E, Saied A, Pellaumail B, et al. Assessment of rat articular cartilage maturation using 50-MHz quantitative ultrasonography. Osteoarthritis Cartilage 2001;9:178–186
26. Seedhom BB, Yao JQ. Ultrasonic measurement of the thickness of human articular cartilage in situ. Clin Biomech (Bristol, Avon) 1999;14:166–176
27. Toyras J, et al. T2 relaxation reveals spatial collagen architecture in articular cartilage: a comparative quantitative MRI and polarized light microscopic study. Ultrasound Med Biol 2002;28: 519–525
28. Youn I, Fu F, Suh J. Determination of the indentation stiffness of articular cartilage using a high-frequency ultrasonic indentation technique. Pittsburgh Orthop J 1999;10:159–160
29. Salter RB, Field P. The effects of continous compression on living articular cartilage. An experimental investigation. J Bone Joint Surg 1960;42-A:31–90
30. Thompson RC Jr, Bassett CA. Histological observations on experimentally induced degeneration of articular cartilage. J Bone Joint Surg Am 1970;52:435–443
31. Repo RU, Finlay JB. Survival of articular cartilage after controlled impact. J Bone Joint Surg Am 1977;59:1068–1076
32. Radin EL, Paul IL, Lowy M. A comparison of the dynamic force transmitting properties of subchondral bone and articular cartilage. J Bone Joint Surg Am 1970;52:444–456
33. Atkinson PJ, Ewers BJ, Haut RC. Blunt injuries to the patellofemoral joint resulting from transarticular loading are influenced by impactor energy and mass. J Biomech Eng 2001;123: 293–295
34. Quinn TM, Allen RG, Schalet BJ, Perumbuli P, Hunziker EB. Matrix and cell injury due to sub-impact loading of adult bovine articular cartilage explants: effects of strain rate and peak stress. J Orthop Res 2001;19:242–249
35. Parrizas M, Saltiel AR, LeRoith D. Insulin-like growth factor 1 inhibits apoptosis using the phosphatidylinositol 3'-kinase and mitogen-activated protein kinase pathways. J Biol Chem 1997;272: 154–161
36. Majno G, Joris I. Apoptosis, oncosis, and necrosis. An overview of cell death. Am J Pathol 1995;146:3–15
37. Lotz M, Takahashi K. Effect of hyaluronan on chondrocyte apoptosis and nitric oxide production in experimentally induced osteoarthritis. Arthritis Rheum 2001;44:1644–1653
38. D'Lima DD, Hashimoto S, Chen PC, Lotz MK, Colwell CW Jr. In vitro and in vivo models of cartilage injury. Cartilage injury induces chondrocyte apoptosis. J Bone Joint Surg Am 2001;83-A(suppl 2):22–24
39. Davis RJ. Signal transduction by the JNK group of MAP kinases. [comment] Cell 2000;103:239–252
40. Zanke BW, Boudreau K< Pubie E, et al. The stress-activated protein kinase pathway mediates cell death following injury induced by cis-platinum, UV irradiation or heat. Curr Biol 1996;6:606–613

41. Yablonka-Reuveni Z, Balestreri TM, Bowen-Pope DF. Regulation of proliferation and differentiation of myoblasts derived from adult mouse skeletal muscle by specific isoforms of PDGF. J Cell Biol 1990;111:1623–1629

42. Menetrey J, Kasemkijwattana C, Day CS, et al. Growth factors improve muscle healing in vivo. J Bone Joint Surg Br 2000;82:131–137

43. Schofield JN, Wolpert L. Effect of TGF-beta 1, TGF-beta 2, and bFGF on chick cartilage and muscle cell differentiation. Exp Cell Res 1990;191:144–148

44. Shuler FD, Georgescu H, Niyibizi C, et al. Increased matrix synthesis following adenoviral transfer of a transforming growth factor beta-1 gene into articular chondrocytes. J Orthop Res 2000;18:585–592

45. Sellers RS, Zhang R, Glasson SS, et al. Repair of articular cartilage defects one year after treatment with recombinant human bone morphogenetic protein-2 (rhBMP-2). J Bone Joint Surg Am 2000;82:151–160

46. Hunziker EB, Rosenberg LC. Repair of partial-thickness defects in articular cartilage: cell recruitment from the synovial membrane. J Bone Joint Surg Am 1996;78:721–733

47. Isgaard J, Nilsson A, Lindahl A, Jansson JO, Isaksson OG. Effects of local administration of GH and IGF-1 on longitudinal bone growth in rats. Am J Physiol 1986;250:E367–E372

48. Kasemkijwattana C, Menetry J, Bosch P, et al. Use of growth factors to improve muscle healing after strain injury. Clin Orthop Relat Res 2000;370:272–285

49. Lieberman JR, Le LQ, WU L, et al. Regional gene therapy with a BMP-2-producing murine stromal cell line induces heterotopic and orthotopic bone formation in rodents. J Orthop Res 1998;16:330–339

50. Hannallah D, Peterson B, Lieberman JR, Fu F, Huard J. Gene therapy in orthopaedic surgery. J Bone Joint Surg Am 2002;84:1046–1061

51. Robbins PD, Ghivizzani SC. Viral vectors for gene therapy. Pharmacol Ther 1998;80:35–47

52. Robbins PD, et al. Retroviral vectors for use in human gene therapy for cancer, Gaucher disease, and arthritis. Ann N Y Acad Sci 1994;716:72–88; discussion 88–89

53. Musgrave DS, Bosch P, Ghivizzani S, Robbins PD, Evans CH, Huard J. Adenovirus-mediated direct gene therapy with bone morphogenetic protein-2 produces bone. Bone 1999;24:541–547

54. Marshall E. Gene therapy. Second child in French trial is found to have leukemia. Science 2003;299:320

55. Hacein-Bey-Abina S, von Kall C, Schmidt M, et al. A serious adverse event after successful gene therapy for X-linked severe combined immunodeficiency. N Engl J Med 2003;348:255–256

56. Evans C, Robbins P. Possible orthopaedic application of gene therapy. J Bone Joint Surg Am 1995;77:1103–1114

57. Kang R, Ghivizzani S, Muzzonigro TS, Herndon JH, Robbins PD, Evans CH. The Marshall R. Urist Young Investigator Award. Orthopaedic applications of gene therapy. From concept to clinic. Clin Orthop 2000;375:324–337

58. Gossen M, Bujard H. Tight control of gene expression in mammalian cells by tetracycline-responsive promoters. Proc Natl Acad Sci U S A 1992;89:5547–5551

59. Worthington J, Robson T, Murray M, O'Rourke M, Keilty G, Hirst DG. Modification of vascular tone using iNOS under the control of a radiation-inducible promoter. Gene Ther 2000;7:1126–1131

60. Martinek V, Latterman C, Usas A, et al. Enhancement of tendon-bone integration of anterior cruciate ligament grafts with bone morphogenetic protein-2 gene transfer: a histological and biomechanical study. J Bone Joint Surg Am 2002;84-A:1123–1131

61. Adachi N, Sato K, Usas A, et al. Muscle derived, cell based ex vivo gene therapy for treatment of full thickness articular cartilage defects. J Rheumatol 2002;29:1920–1930

62. Morales I, Roberts A. Transforming growth factor-β regulates the metabolism of proteoglycans in bovine cartilage organ cultures. J Biol Chem 1988;263:12828–12831

63. Tyler J. Insulin-like growth factor-1 can decrease degradation and promote synthesis in cartilage exposed to cytokines. Biochem J 1989;260:543–548

64. Lee CW, et al. Myoblast mediated gene therapy with muscle as a biological scaffold for the repair of full-thickness defects of articular cartilage. In: 25th annual meeting of the Orthopaedic Research Society, vol. 25. Orlando, FL, 2000:1068

65. Martinek V, Usas A, Pelinkovic D, Robbins P, Fu FH, Huard J. Genetic engineering of meniscal allografts. Tissue Eng 2002;8:107–117

66. van Tienen TG, Heijkants RG, Buma P, de Groot JH, Pennings AJ, Veth RP. Tissue ingrowth and degradation of two biodegradable porous polymers with different porosities and pore sizes. Biomaterials 2002;23:1731–1738

67. Evans CH, Ghivizzani SC, Herndon JH, et al. Clinical trials in the gene therapy of arthritis. Clin Orthop 2000;379:S300–S307

68. Freed LE, Marquis JC, Nohria A, mmanual J, Mikos AG, Langer R. Neocartilage formation in vitro and in vivo using cells cultured on synthetic biodegradable polymers. J Biomed Mater Res 1993;27:11–23

69. Badylak SF, Park K, Peppas N, McCabe G, Yoder M. Marrow-derived cells populate scaffolds composed of xenogeneic extracellular matrix. Exp Hematol 2001;29:1310–1318

70. Caplan AI. Tissue engineering designs for the future: new logics, old molecules. Tissue Eng 2000;6:1–7

71. Marcacci M, Zaffagnini S, Kon E, Visani A, Iacono F, Loreti I. Arthroscopic autologous chondrocyte transplantation: technical note. Knee Surg Sports Traumatol Arthrosc 2002;10:154–159

72. Knudson CB, Knudson W. Hyaluronan-binding proteins in development, tissue homeostasis, and disease. FASEB J 1993;7:1233–1241

73. Martin I, Shastri VP, Padera RF, et al. Selective differentiation of mammalian bone marrow stromal cells cultured on three-dimensional polymer foams. J Biomed Mater Res 2001;55:229–235

74. Kawamura S, Wakitani S, Kimura T, et al. Articular cartilage repair. Rabbit experiments with a collagen gel-biomatrix and chondrocytes cultured in it. Acta Orthop Scand 1998;69:56–62

75. Wakitani S, Goto T, Young RG, Mansour JM, Goldberg VM, Caplan AI. Repair of large full-thickness articular cartilage defects with allograft articular chondrocytes embedded in a collagen gel. Tissue Eng 1998;4:429–444

76. Huard J, Ascadi G, Jani A, et al. Gene transfer into skeletal muscles by isogenic myoblasts. Human Gene Ther 1994;5:949–958

77. van der Meulen MC, Huiskes R. Why mechanobiology? A survey article. J Biomech 2002;35:401–414

78. Guilak F. Functional tissue engineering: the role of biomechanics in reparative medicine. Ann N Y Acad Sci 2002;961:193–195

79. Woo SL, Hildebrand K, Watanabe N, Penwick JA, Papageorgiou CD. Tissue engineering of ligament and tendon healing. Clin Orthop 1999;367:S312–S323

80. Martinek V, Fu FH, Huard J. Gene Therapy and Tissue Engineering in Sports Medicine. Phys Sportsmed 2000;28:34–51

26

Gene Therapy in the Treatment of Cartilage Injury

ANDRE F. STEINERT, GLYN D. PALMER, STEVEN C. GHIVIZZANI,
AND CHRISTOPHER H. EVANS

■ Limitations of Current Treatments of Cartilage Injury

The specialized architecture and limited repair capacity of articular cartilage, coupled with the high physical demands placed upon this tissue, make it exceedingly difficult to treat cartilage injury medically. As outlined in other chapters of this book, several surgical treatment options are available for resurfacing chondral and osteochondral lesions. "Traditional" resurfacing procedures such as debridement, abrasion arthroplasty, drilling, and microfracture aim to promote natural fibrocartilage repair.[1] As fibrocartilaginous scar tissue has inferior mechanical and physical properties compared with normal articular cartilage, modern "resurfacement" tries to achieve a more hyaline-like cartilage repair. Such procedures include transplantation of periosteum or perichondrium, autologous osteochondral transfers, autologous chondrocyte implantation, and tissue engineering approaches, which deliver a space-filling entity composed of cells with or without matrix. Despite these advances, most surgical interventions result in improvement of clinical symptoms such as pain relief, but none of the current treatment options have regenerated long-lasting hyaline cartilage tissue to replace damaged cartilage.[1]

■ Cartilage Injury Versus Disease

Many who study cartilage repair fail to draw distinctions between lesions resulting from acute injury and those resulting from disease. Acute cartilage injury often arises in an otherwise healthy joint; the patient may be young, and the focal defect will likely require a localized treatment. In contrast, damage to cartilage that arises from an underlying disease process, such as in osteoarthritis (OA), where the patient is likely to be older, may require the treatment of the entire articulating region. In this case, repair of the lesion may provide symptomatic relief and delay of the progression of symptoms, but unless the underlying disease is also treated effectively, any improvement is likely to be temporary. Gene transfer approaches might be adapted for the treatment of both localized cartilage injury and diseased cartilage, but these should be recognized as different entities.

■ Why Can Gene Therapy Be Important for Cartilage Repair?

With the completion of the Human Genome Project, a new era of gene-based therapies is evolving, including applications in the field of orthopaedics. Beyond the goal of replacement of defective genes, gene therapy has become a tool for delivering individual proteins and other gene products to specific tissues and cells. It is conceivable that the above-stated limitations of cartilage repair may be overcome by adapting gene transfer technologies. In particular, it should be possible to develop techniques for transferring genes encoding the necessary gene products to the appropriate sites in the joint, and for expressing those genes locally for the intervals of time needed to achieve cartilage repair. Data are beginning to emerge that suggest delivery and expression of certain genes can influence a repair response toward the synthesis of normal articular cartilage in vivo. This chapter gives a systematic overview of the current status of gene delivery for cartilage healing, and presents some of the remaining challenges in the development of successful gene-based cartilage repair techniques.

■ Which Proteins Aid Cartilage Repair?

Research advances in cellular, molecular, and developmental biology have led to the identification of a variety factors that might be useful in the treatment of cartilage disease and injury. These molecules have a broad range of activities, among which are the capacity to induce the synthesis and deposition of cartilage extracellular matrix components by chondrocytes, stabilization of the extracellular matrix, induction of chondrogenesis by mesenchymal progenitor cells, and the ability to inhibit inflammatory processes **(Table 26–1)**. It is thought that the coordinated administration of the appropriate protein cocktail to chondrocytes, chondroprogenitors, or synovial lining cells could be used to improve treatment of injured or diseased cartilage. This could occur either by fostering differentiation into and/or maintenance of the appropriate chondrocyte phenotype for synthesis of repair tissue that functionally resembles normal articular cartilage, or by protecting the cartilage from inflammatory and degradative stimuli.[2]

Potentially useful in this respect are members of the transforming growth factor-ß (TGF-ß) superfamily, including TGF-β_1, -β_2, and -β_3, several of the bone morphogenetic proteins (BMPs), insulin-like growth factor-I (IGF-I), fibroblast growth factors (FGFs), and epidermal growth factor (EGF), among others (reviewed in Hickey et al[3]). Other secreted proteins, such as Indian (IHH) or sonic (SHH) hedgehog play key roles in regulating chondrogenic hypertrophy[4] and may also prove beneficial for modulating chondrogenesis of grafted cells. Another class of biologics that may be useful in cartilage repair is the transcription factors that promote chondrogenesis or the maintenance of the chondrocyte phenotype. Sox9 and related transcription factors such as L-Sox5, and Sox6 have been identified as essential for chondrocyte differentiation and cartilage formation.[5] Signal transduction molecules, such as SMADs, are also known to be important regulators of chondrogenesis.[6]

As an alternative to stimulating expression of endogenous chondrogenic genes, delivery and expression of complementary DNAs (cDNAs) encoding specific extracellular matrix (ECM) components may be used for maintenance of the proper hyaline cartilage phenotype.[7]

To treat cartilage loss due to diseases such as OA or rheumatoid arthritis (RA), inhibition of the actions of certain proinflammatory cytokines, such as interleukin-1 (IL-1) and tumor necrosis factor-α (TNF-α) may be required. These proteins, synthesized by synovial cells and chondrocytes, are found at elevated levels in arthritic joints and are important mediators of cartilage degradation. Administration of mediators that are antiinflammatory or immunomodulatory, such as IL-1 receptor antagonist (IL-1Ra), soluble receptors for TNF (sTNFR) or for IL-1 (sIL-1R), IL-4, or IL-10 may be effective in reducing cartilage loss.[8] Moreover, apoptosis inhibitors such as bcl-2 and nitric oxide (NO) antagonists could be employed to maintain chondrocyte populations.

Furthermore, various combinations of candidate growth factors may also be envisaged. For example a dual-axis therapy using an anabolic growth factor like TGF-β or IGF-I, and an inhibitor of the catabolic action of inflammatory cytokines such as IL-1Ra, has potential synergistic effects in the repair process.

TABLE 26–1 Classes of Chondroregenerative and Chondroprotective Gene Products

Gene Product	Examples
Stimulator of matrix synthesis	IGF-I, BMPs, TGF-ßs
Stimulator of chondrogenic differentiation	Cartilage growth and differentiation factors: BMPs, TGF-ßs, IGF-I, FGFs, EGF, SHH, IHH
	Transcription factors: L-SOX5, SOX6, SOX9
Signal transduction molecules	SMADs
ECM components	Type II procollagen
Cytokines and cytokine antagonists	Proinflammatory cytokine inhibitors IL-1Ra, sIL-1R, sTNFR
	Antiinflammatory cytokines IL-4, IL-10, IL-13
Apoptosis inhibitors	Bcl-2

However, as already mentioned, the clinical application of recombinant proteins is hindered by several obstacles. In vivo, many proteins have short half-lives and thus are difficult to maintain at functional concentrations for periods sufficient to facilitate an effective repair, making repeated administration or methods for timed-release necessary. Certain proteins, such as transcription factors or signal transduction molecules, function completely intracellularly, and because cells cannot normally import these molecules, they cannot be readily delivered in soluble form.

■ Gene Transfer as a Protein Delivery System

Gene transfer offers an alternative approach to protein delivery that may satisfactorily overcome the limitations of conventional methods.[2] By delivering cDNAs that code for various chondrogenic or therapeutic proteins to specific target cells and providing for sustained synthesis of the transgene products, the genetically modified cell is converted to a small factory for protein production (**Fig. 26–1**). Through the localized delivery of gene transfer vectors or genetically modified cells to specific sites of damage, protein synthesis can be concentrated at the site of injury or disease with minimal collateral exposure of nontarget tissues.

There are various ways to deliver exogenous cDNAs to joint tissues for treatment of cartilage lesions. In devising a useful strategy, several factors must be taken into account, including the specific disease, the extent of cartilage pathology, and the biologic activity of the gene product. A key component to any gene therapy application is a vector that efficiently delivers the cDNA of interest to the target cell, and enables transgene expression of a suitable level and duration to affect the desired biologic response. Furthermore, an understanding of the natural behavior of the target cell, such as its half-life, rate of division, and accessibility to the vector, is also essential to the effectiveness of the procedure.

■ Nucleic Acids that Directly Regulate Gene Expression

In addition to genes that encode messenger RNA (mRNA) leading to the synthesis of specific proteins, there are also those that give rise to RNA but no protein. Of particular interest are species of nucleic acids with the

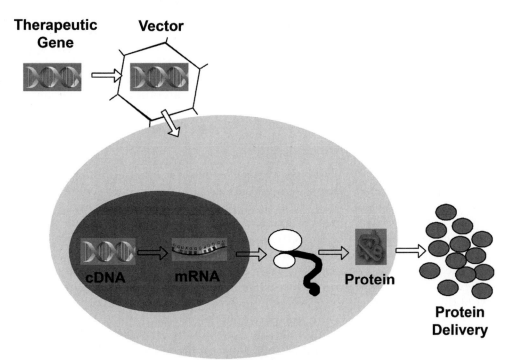

FIGURE 26–1 Gene transfer as protein delivery system. A therapeutic gene is inserted into a vector, which can be viral or nonviral in nature. The vector delivers its genetic material to the cell, where it is translocated to the nucleus of the host cell. In the nucleus the DNA stays either episomal (nonintegrating vector) or inserts its genetic material into chromosomes of the host cells (integrating vector). The complementary DNA (cDNA) encoding the protein then serves as a template for synthesis of the corresponding messenger ribonucleic acid (mRNA) by the endogenous transcriptional machinery of the cell. The mRNA leaves the nucleus and is translated into protein by the ribosomal machinery and, if a secreted protein, is released from the cell. In this way, the genetically modified host cell is converted into a small factory for protein production. Protein synthesis can be localized to the site of injury or disease, with minimal collateral exposure of nontarget tissues.

ability to directly regulate activities of other genes, and which may be harnessed for disease therapy and tissue regeneration by gene transfer methods.[9] These include antisense and "decoy" oligonucleotides, ribozymes, and small interfering RNAs (siRNAs). Antisense oligodeoxynucleotides (ODN) are short single-stranded nucleic acids that hybridize to specific mRNA molecules, resulting in the formation of RNA/DNA duplexes that are cleaved by nucleases leading to subsequent block of gene expression.[10] Decoy oligonucleotides are double-stranded nucleotides that are recognized and bound specifically by critical molecules, such as transcription factors. Thus, these decoys can completely inhibit the activities of proteins, necessary for the expression of particular endogenous genes.[11] Ribozymes are catalytic RNA molecules that cleave RNA substrates in a sequence-specific fashion. Various entities exist, and initial gene therapy clinical trials are currently underway, using this technique to treat various infectious diseases.[9] RNA interference (RNAi) is the term used to describe the blocking of gene expression by the introduction of small fragments of double-stranded RNA (dsRNA) into the cell cytoplasm. The mechanism involves the conversion of the added dsRNA into short interfering RNAs (siRNAs) that direct ribonucleases to homologous RNA targets.[12] Its actions are highly specific and very efficient in mammalian cells.

These techniques have potential use in diseases where overexpression of a normal or mutated gene contributes to pathology. For example, it might be beneficial for any cartilage regeneration process to limit expression of osteogenic genes such as osteocalcin or *Cbfa1,* or genes such as noggin that antagonize the actions of certain BMPs. The major advantage of the delivery of such genes is that they directly regulate gene expression, and are not translated into proteins, thus avoiding the potential risk of dissemination of stimulatory factors to nontarget sites and immune responses to allo- or xenogenic proteins.

Gene-based methods currently being explored for the treatment of articular cartilage injury range from those as simple as direct delivery of a vector to a defect, to synthesis of cartilaginous implants through genetically augmented tissue engineering procedures. In the next few paragraphs we give an overview of the properties of commonly used vectors in gene therapy applications and discuss their use in the context of the different delivery strategies to joint tissues.

■ Choosing a Strategy for Gene Delivery

Because exogenous cDNAs are not spontaneously taken up and expressed by cells, they have to be transferred to cells with the aid of a vector. The most commonly used and most effective methods to insert DNA into target cells are by way of a viral vector, which is termed "transduction." An alternative to the viral gene transfer systems are the nonviral methods of delivering DNA, termed "transfection," which are typically less efficient.

Viral Vectors for Orthopaedic Applications

To convert a virus into a gene transfer vector, the parts of the viral genome that enable it to replicate and cause disease are removed and replaced with therapeutic genes. This results in recombinant viruses that retain their infectivity and ability to transfer genes, minus any virulence they might have possessed. Vectors derived from several types of viruses have been used to transfer genes to joints, and have been reviewed extensively.[13] Some of the most important characteristics of each these viral vectors are summarized in **Table 26–2.** Viral vectors are generally categorized according to whether their genomes integrate into the host cells chromosomes (retroviruses, lentiviruses) or whether they do not integrate but persist in the cell nucleus predominantly as episomal DNA [recombinant adeno-associated virus (AAV), adenovirus, and herpes virus vectors]. Episomal DNA can be lost with time, especially if the cell divides. This distinction is one important determinant for the suitability of each vector system for a specific application; nonintegrating vectors can be harnessed for applications where transient expression of the transgene is desired, but integrating vectors are, at present, the tools of choice if stable genetic alteration needs to be maintained in dividing cells.

Adenoviral Vectors

Wild-type serotype 5 adenovirus causes mild respiratory and eye infections in humans. Vectors based on this virus are nonintegrating and have the advantage of being able to infect dividing and nondividing cells with excellent efficiency. Recombinant adenoviral vectors are easy to construct and purify[14] and can be grown in high titer to greater than 10^{14} particles per milliliter. Adenovirus vectors can be divided into three general categories—first generation, second generation, and gutless or high capacity—depending on the number of viral genes which have been inactivated. First-generation adenoviral vectors, deficient for one or two viral early genes (E1 and E3), have been used in several clinical trials (reviewed in Thomas et al[15]). First-generation adenovirus vectors transduce chondrocytes, synoviocytes, and chondroprogenitor cells very efficiently.

There are several disadvantages, however, associated with first-generation adenoviral vectors. Despite deletion of some of the critical early-phase genes, low levels of

TABLE 26–2 Viral Vectors for Orthopaedic Gene Therapy Applications

Vector	Description	Advantages	Disadvantages
Adenovirus	dsDNA virus 35-kb genome Episomal Divided in 100 map units (E1–E4) 7.5-kb capacity Multiple serotypes	Infects dividing and nondividing cells High transduction efficiency High levels of transgene expression Straightforward production High titer Approved for use in clinical trials	Transient transgene expression Immunogenicity of transduced cells Cytotoxic at high doses

Adeno-associated
virus (AAV)
	ssDNA virus
	8 serotypes, has AAV-2
	  has highest chondrocyte and
	  MSC tropism
	Wild-type AAV integrates
	  recombinant AAV appears to be
	  nonintegrating
	4-kb capacity
		Infects dividing and nondividing cells
		No viral protein expression in
		  infected cells
		Not known to cause disease in
		  humans
		Biologically relevant transgene
		  expression after direct Intra-
		  articular delivery
			Transient transgene expression
			Moderate transduction efficiency
			Moderate levels of transgene
			  expression
			
			Difficult to manufacture
			Small capacity

Herpes simplex virus (HSV)	dsDNA virus Episomal 40-kb capacity	Infects dividing and nondividing cells Very high transduction efficiency Very high levels of transgene expression Large capacity	Transient transgene expression Viral protein expression in infected cells Cytotoxic Immunogenic

Moloney murine
  leukemia virus
(MoMLV)
	RNA virus
	Integrating
	8-kb capacity
		Persistent transgene expression
		No viral protein expression in
		  infected cells
			Only infects dividing cells
			Possible insertional mutagenesis

Lentivirus	RNA virus
	Integrates in genome
	8-kb capacity
		Infects dividing and nondividing
		  cells
		High transduction efficiency and
		  persistent transgene expression
		No viral protein expression in
		  infected cells
			Possible insertional mutagenesis

the remaining viral proteins are expressed. This results in an immune response to the virally infected cell in vivo, which may ultimately lead to clearance of the infected cells. Further deletion of genes E2 and E4 in second-generation vectors reduces but does not eliminate the expression of viral genes. "Gutted" adenoviral vectors, also termed high-capacity adenoviral vectors, in contrast, contain no viral coding sequences and thus avoid this problem, while also enabling packing of up to 35 kilobase (kb) of exogenous DNA. Unfortunately, these vectors are considerably more difficult to manufacture and purify.[13]

Adeno-Associated Viral Vectors

Adeno-associated viruses (AAVs) are single-stranded, nonenveloped, small DNA viruses that require co-infection with a helper virus such as an adenovirus or a herpes simplex virus for replication. Wild-type AAV is not known to cause any disease in humans, and inserts its genetic material into a specific site on chromosome 19 of the host cell. The virus infects a wide variety of dividing and nondividing cells, but with varying levels of efficiency. Recently, recombinant AAV vectors have been designed that allow for generation of large scale, high-titer, and helper-virus free preparations. Further, the design of high-efficient self-complementary AAV-based vectors avoids problems associated with second-strand synthesis.[16] These AAV vectors are mainly nonintegrating and persist in many cell types as large episomal concatamers. Recombinant AAV vectors encode no viral gene products and may not generate neutralizing immune reactions. However, the main disadvantages are the small "cargo size" of ~4 kb, difficult production, and variable transduction efficiency. The use of AAV vectors to transfer genes to joints has been addressed with mixed results so far.[17] Synovium appears only modestly susceptible to transduction with recombinant AAV vectors, but chondrocytes are more readily transduced. There is evidence that the small size of AAV might allow it to transduce chondrocytes in situ, unlike the case with other viral vectors.

Herpes Simplex Virus Vectors

The herpes simplex virus (HSV) is a large enveloped, double-stranded DNA virus that can be engineered to hold up to 40 kb of foreign DNA, and stocks of 10^9 to

10^{12} infectious particles per milliliter can be generated. HSV can be used to infect both dividing and nondividing cells of many types. Major disadvantages are the difficulty in creating recombinant vectors, and the generation of HSV vectors is significantly more difficult and time-consuming than adenoviral or retroviral vector generation. Another disadvantage is that HSV is associated with transient gene expression and cytotoxicity. The use of HSV vectors has been reported in various in vivo applications including direct intraarticular injection,[18] leading to efficient transduction of synovium.

Retroviral Vectors

Retroviruses are enveloped single-stranded RNA viruses that replicate through a double-stranded DNA intermediate. By integrating into the host DNA, the viral genomes are maintained for the life of the cell and are passed on to all daughter cells after cell division.

Moloney Murine Leukemia Viral Vectors

The more common retrovirus systems are based on the Moloney murine leukemia virus (MoMLV), and have been used in a large number of gene therapy clinical trials.[15] MoMLV has been characterized extensively and has several attributes that make it attractive as a gene therapy vector: (a) the virus has no homology with human retroviruses, eliminating the possibility of recombination between the vector and resident human proviruses; (b) murine leukemia virus is nonpathogenic in humans; (c) the genome of the virus is relatively simple and amenable to molecular manipulation; (d) production is straightforward with moderately high titers; and (e) no viral proteins are contained in the vector, so infected cells are not antigenic. However, MoMLV requires division of the target cell for efficient transduction. MoMLV-based vectors can insert themselves randomly into the host DNA, resulting in stable modification of target cells, but also incurring the risk of insertional mutagenesis and activating a cell proto-oncogene or disrupting a tumor suppressor gene.[13] The safety of such vectors has recently been called into question because children in a clinical protocol receiving these vectors have developed leukemia.[15]

Lentiviral Vectors

Lentiviruses are a subclass of retroviruses that can infect both dividing and nondividing cells. Like other retroviral vectors, they can be engineered to express no viral proteins, so that transduced cells are not antigenic. They hold up to 8 kb of foreign genetic material. Lentiviruses are genetically more complex than murine leukemia-based retroviruses, which makes molecular manipulation of the lentiviral genome more difficult. But the powerful attributes of infecting slow or nondividing cells and the maintenance of the vector genome in dividing cell populations make these vectors appealing tools for certain orthopaedic gene transfer applications.[19] However, issues regarding their clinical applicability remain in question, due to the renewed fears about insertional mutagenesis.[15]

Vector Development Perspectives

It should be noted that vectorology is a rapidly developing field, and there have been significant efforts in the last few years to increase the safety and efficacy of the current viral vector systems. One area of interest involves the manipulation of promoters that drive transgene expression. To date, most investigations of gene transfer to cartilage have used vector systems with strong, viral promoters that provide constitutively high levels of transgene expression. This approach is useful during feasibility studies, where very high levels of transgene expression are used to overtly demonstrate the biologic effects that may be achieved with a particular gene and gene delivery method. However, for cartilage repair the stimulation of faithful synthesis of the complex architecture of articular cartilage, followed by its long-term maintenance, may require the use of more sophisticated types of tissue-specific regulatory elements.[20] Unfortunately, the promoter regions for most chondrogenic genes are large, not well characterized, and consequently not routinely used in gene therapy. But as our knowledge about the native promoter systems of specific cell types expands, we may be able to harness tissue-specific promoters for a local and endogenous regulated gene expression.

Another method of achieving regulated transgene expression is the use of extrinsically regulated promoters. For example, a promoter that is activated only in the presence of tetracycline has been developed,[21] and may be useful to turn off expression of the inserted gene after the therapeutic effect has been obtained.

Increasing the efficiency with which viral vectors infect specific cell populations may also increase the safety of gene therapy by allowing lower viral loads to be administered. Modifications on the vector capsid (including pseudotyping or molecular adaptors) to alter vector tropism away from its primary receptor is called "transductional targeting." It is an important focus of vector development, addressing the problem of nonspecific or inefficient uptake. In the field of musculoskeletal tissue repair, being able to target a specific cell type may prove beneficial for transduction of cell types that would otherwise not be amenable, and may also limit the transgene expression to selected tissues of interest. On the other hand, as there are mixed populations of

TABLE 26–3 Nonviral Vectors for Orthopaedic Gene Therapy Applications

Vector	Description	Advantages	Disadvantages
Naked DNA	Naked DNA or uncomplexed DNA	Easy to manufacture Noninfectious (safety)	Low transfection efficiency Transient transgene expression (less than 1 week) Inflammatory
Liposomes	Plasmid DNA delivered in a phospholipid vesicle that merges with host cell		
Others	DNA-injection Biolistics (gene gun) Electroporation Ca/P precipitation		

cell types in nearly all musculoskeletal repair tissues, it might not be necessary to target one specific cell type to facilitate repair. In the quest for better vectors, many researchers are attempting to combine the best features of different viruses in so-called hybrid or chimeric vectors, and there are many combinations of different beneficial vector features theoretically possible.

Nonviral Vector Systems for Orthopaedic Applications

In addition to viral vectors, several nonviral vectors (summarized in **Table 26–3**) have been used to transfer genes to joint tissues. Although certain cells such as myoblasts are able to take up naked DNA with some efficiency, complexion of DNA to different chemical formulations or to receptor/ligands increases DNA uptake and subsequent gene expression. Anionic and cationic liposomes are phospholipid vesicles that can fuse with cell membranes, and thus be used as gene transfer vehicles. Liposomes have been used to transfect chondrocytes in vitro, and also in various in vivo approaches for orthopaedic applications.[22] Additional nonviral methods of introducing genetic material into cells include direct injection of plasmid DNA, or by firing DNA-coated microprojectiles through the cell membrane (biolistics), electroporation, and calcium phosphate precipitation. Although these physical gene transfer methods are easy to use, the transfection efficiencies are low, and generally have not been proven to work sufficiently in vivo.

■ Choosing a Gene-Delivery Approach and a Target Cell

There are two general methods for delivering a therapeutic gene into a target cell: a direct in vivo approach, and an indirect ex vivo approach. The direct approach involves the application of the vector directly into the target tissue of the subject, whereas the indirect approach involves the genetic modification of cells outside the body, followed by transplantation of the modified cells into the host. The choice of which gene transfer method to use is based on numerous considerations, including the gene to be delivered, the disease to be treated, and the vector used. In general, adenovirus, HSV, AAV vectors, lentivirus, and nonviral vectors may be used for in vivo and ex vivo delivery. Retroviral vectors, because of their inability to infect nondividing cells, are more suited for ex vivo use. Ex vivo approaches are generally more invasive, expensive, and technically tedious. However, they permit control of the transduced cells and safety testing prior to reimplantation. In vivo approaches are simpler, cheaper, and less invasive, but viruses are introduced directly into the body, which limits safety testing.

Toward the treatment and repair of damaged articular cartilage, the three primary candidate cell types to target genetic modification are synovial lining cells, chondrocytes, and mesenchymal stem cells.

Intraarticular Injection

Direct intraarticular injection of a vector or genetically modified cells into the joint space is, at least conceptually, the simplest approach to gene transfer to joint tissues. Following delivery, the vector or cells are distributed throughout the joint space to interact with all available receptive cells and surfaces. Because the synovium lines all the internal surfaces of the joint space, except for cartilage, and is highly cellular, it is the primary site of vector interaction. Direct intraarticular injection of vector or modified cells results in synthesis and release of therapeutic proteins into the joint space, which then bathe all available tissues, including cartilage. Considerable progress has been made toward defining the parameters critical to effective gene transfer to synovium and prolonged intraarticular expression. Recent data suggest that the use of immunologically compatible vector systems and homologous transgenes allows sustained intraarticular transgene expression.[23] The effectiveness of synovial gene transfer of various transgenes is well documented in research directed toward rheumatoid arthritis,[8] and the safety of indirect IL-1Ra gene transfer via a retroviral vector has been demonstrated successfully in a human phase I clinical trial.[24] Data are beginning to emerge on its potential for treating OA with, for example, encouraging results for adenovirally delivered IL-1Ra to the joints of horses with experimental OA.[25]

There is a growing body of literature indicating that delivery of transgenes to synovium may not be compatible with many of the pleiotropic protein products considered for cartilage repair and regeneration. Gene transfer of TGF-β$_1$ or BMP-2 to the synovium, for example, has been reported to cause severe joint fibrosis, swelling, and osteophyte and ectopic cartilage formation.[26,27] This suggests caution when considering cDNAs for use in synovial gene transfer. Those selected should be safe when large amounts of gene product are expressed. Many antiinflammatory proteins have this property (see **Table 26–1**).

Gene Delivery to Cartilage Defects

For the gene-based delivery of certain factors to cartilage defects, a strategy whereby the transgenes are localized, and the gene products remain contained within the cartilage lesion, appears to be crucial. Possibly, the most direct manner by which to achieve this goal is by implantation of a three-dimensional matrix preloaded with a gene delivery vehicle into a defect **(Fig. 26–2A)**. Such a device would localize the vector to the lesion while forming a support structure for the attachment of infiltrating cells. Within the matrix, cells would acquire the vector and locally secrete the stimulating transgene products. Such matrix-associated gene transfer approaches have been explored to augment bone healing by delivery of plasmid DNA encoding BMP-4.[28] Recently, it was shown that collagen-glycosaminoglycan matrices incorporating plasmid-DNA at neutral pH were capable of transfecting seeded chondrocytes in culture, and enabling expression of a reporter gene for at least 28 days.[29] Similarly, hydrated collagen-glycosaminoglycan matrices containing adenoviral vectors have been found to promote localized transgene expression in vivo following implantation into osteochondral defects in rabbit knees.[30] In this system, bone marrow cells from the defect were infected by the virus within the matrix, and expressed the transgene locally for at least 21 days.[30]

Although transfer and expression of reporter genes has been observed by direct vector delivery to osteochondral lesions, it is not yet known whether this type of approach is capable of stimulating a sufficient biologic response for repair. One step toward a more cellular graft would be to supplement the vector-laden matrix with autologous cells that are intraoperatively readily available. Cells from bone marrow aspirates [bone marrow cells (BMCs)] fulfill this requirement and can be used in an abbreviated, genetically enhanced tissue engineering approach **(Fig. 26–2B)**. The advantage of direct, in vivo delivery systems of this type is that they can be conducted within one surgical setting, thus saving time and cost, while avoiding labor intensive ex vivo culture of cells. Their limitation, however, is the lack of control over gene transfer following implantation.

Gene transfer is also being explored as a mechanism for enhancing ex vivo cell delivery approaches for cartilage repair **(Fig. 26–2C)**. Although laborious and expensive, this indirect approach has several advantages: (a) a pure population of cells can be selected under controlled conditions; (b) it provides a highly cellular, space-filling entity; (c) it localizes transgene expression to the site of injury; (d) no free vector particles are administered to the subject; and (e) safety testing prior to reimplantation is possible. Various studies have been conducted to explore gene transfer to chondrocytes and mesenchymal progenitor cells to enhance ex vivo cell delivery approaches for cartilage repair.

Gene Transfer to Chondrocytes

Chondrocytes in monolayers are readily amenable to gene transfer by viral vectors such as MoMLV, lentivirus, adenovirus, and AAV. Adenoviral-mediated delivery of cDNAs for TGF-β$_1$, BMP-2, IGF-I, or BMP-7 has been shown to stimulate the expression of a cartilage-specific ECM, with increased proteoglycan and type II collagen production and a decreased tendency toward dedifferentiation.[31–35] Although chondrocytes have been somewhat resistant to transfection with plasmid DNA, formulations with certain commercially available lipid-based reagents such as FuGENE6 and Lipofectin have been found to enhance the efficiency of DNA uptake, especially if the surrounding matrix is subjected to mild enzymatic digestion.[22] Viral-based vectors, however, are capable of generating far higher levels of transgene expression with greater persistence.

Having shown the capacity of gene transfer approaches to beneficially alter the molecular properties of articular chondrocytes, the research focus has shifted toward exploring methods of delivery to cartilage defects. One approach would be to genetically augment the autologous chondrocyte implantation (ACI) procedure, with the given advantage that ACI is already clinically established and the associated infrastructure for its application is already in place. There is an accumulating body of literature that shows that genetically altered chondrocytes retain the ability to attach to and colonize cartilage explants in culture, and are capable of expressing

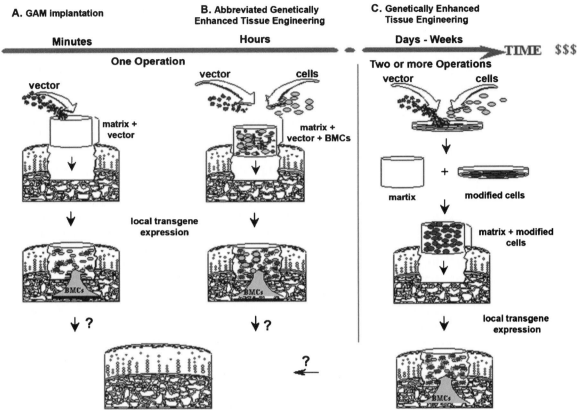

A. GAM implantation

B. Abbreviated Genetically Enhanced Tissue Engineering

C. Genetically Enhanced Tissue Engineering

FIGURE 26–2 Gene delivery approaches for the treatment of cartilage defects. **(A)** Matrix-associated in vivo gene transfer. In vivo gene transfer involves incorporation of the gene transfer vector into a biologically compatible matrix, which is implanted within an osteochondral defect. Bone marrow cells (BMCs) migrate into the matrix, encounter the vector, and acquire the desired gene. Genetically modified cells locally express and secrete the transgene products that influence mesenchymal progenitors toward chondrogenic pathways. This procedure does not require ex vivo cell manipulation. **(B)** Abbreviated ex vivo genetically enhanced tissue engineering. To facilitate this direct approach, the incorporation of a vector into the matrix can be conducted together with the incorporation of cells that could be harvested a single operative setting (like BMCs from bone marrow aspirates). **(C)** Traditional ex vivo genetically enhanced tissue engineering. For ex vivo gene transfer, target cells (e.g., chondrocytes or mesenchymal stem cells) are harvested in an initial surgical procedure. Then they are incubated with the vector of interest, selected, and amplified. The genetically modified cells are then seeded into a biologic matrix, which can be further cultured under controlled conditions. In a second surgical procedure the constructs are implanted into a cartilage lesion. This procedure may permit transgene expression to be concentrated within the cell types responsible for generating the repair tissue. In both approaches (B and C), locally secreted proteins could influence cartilage regeneration by implanted cells as well as those that may migrate into the defect after implantation of the matrix.

transgene products at functional levels following engraftment in vivo. Transplantation of transfected IGF-I expressing chondrocytes led to significant resurfacing and thicker tissue enriched with proteoglycans and type II collagen, compared with transplanted control cells.[22] In addition, adenoviral-mediated IL-1Ra gene transfer to chondrocytes resulted in resistance to IL-1–induced proteoglycan degradation after engraftment.[36]

As an alternative to delivery in suspension, efforts have also been made to augment tissue engineering procedures using genetically modified chondrocytes **(Fig. 26–2C).** For this, the cells are transduced/transfected in monolayer and then seeded into a matrix for subsequent implantation into chondral or osteochondral defects.[37]

Initial studies demonstrated that chondrocytes transduced with various vectors encoding marker genes, when embedded in collagenous matrices[38–40] or alginate microspheres[41] and delivered to osteochondral defects in rabbits, could support prolonged transgene expression for several weeks.

Results of efficacy studies are just beginning to emerge, showing the effects of genetically modified chondrocytes in cartilage lesions in vivo. In ex vivo approaches, adenovirally transduced chondrocytes expressing BMP-7,[42] incorporated in a matrix of autogenous fibrin, were implanted into full-thickness articular cartilage defects in horses. Four weeks after surgery, an increased tissue volume and accelerated formation of a proteoglycan and type II collagen–rich matrix could be observed in the BMP-7–treated defects compared with control defects treated with irrelevant marker genes. However, after 8 months, the levels of type II collagen and proteoglycan, and the mechanical characteristics of the treated defects compared with the controls were similar. This was attributed in part to the declining number of allografted chondrocytes that persisted in the defects after 8 months.[42] It is encouraging, however, that genetically modified chondrocytes can be used to augment a cartilage repair process in a large animal model.

Gene Transfer to Chondroprogenitor Cells

Major limitations for the use of autologous chondrocytes for cartilage repair are that they require the surgical removal of non–weight-bearing articular cartilage as a source of cells, of which there is a very limited supply, and that chondrocytes dedifferentiate during expansion with a subsequent loss of the chondrocytic phenotype. An alternative source of cells that can be harnessed for cartilage repair procedures are mesenchymal progenitor cells, also referred to as mesenchymal stem cells (MSCs). These cells have the capacity to differentiate into the various mesenchymal tissues including cartilage, bone, muscle, fat, and others.[43] MSCs have been isolated from several sources, including bone marrow,[44] bone chips,[45] adipose tissue,[46] periosteum, and perichondrium. MSCs have been shown to maintain their multilineage potential with passage in culture,[47] making them an attractive cell source for the repair of full-thickness osteochondral defects.

MSCs appear to be reasonably receptive to transduction with recombinant adenoviral vectors, retrovirus, lentivirus, and AAV[27,43,48,49] (and unpublished observations). Various in vitro systems have established that mesenchymal progenitor cells undergo chondrogenesis under certain three-dimensional culture conditions, provided that certain chondrogenic factors like TGF-β_1 or BMP-2 are present.[47,50,51] Following plasmid-mediated BMP-2 and BMP-4[52,53] and retrovirus-mediated BMP-2[54] gene transfer, the murine mesenchymal progenitor cell line C3H10T1/2 was able to differentiate along the chondrogenic lineage. Primary mesenchymal progenitor cells, genetically modified to express TGF-β_1 or BMP-2[48] were also found to undergo chondrogenesis in aggregate culture.

Initial studies have been conducted to apply gene transfer technologies to MSCs in vivo. One approach focuses on the delivery of genetically modified MSCs through tissue engineering methods **(Fig. 26–2C)**. In one study, retrovirally transduced periosteal cells expressing BMP-7, following selection and expansion, were seeded into polyglycolic acid scaffolds and implanted into rabbit osteochondral defects. Relative to control groups, the defects treated with the BMP-7 modified progenitors showed improved regeneration of bone and cartilage at 8 to 12 weeks postimplantation.[55,56] Using the same experimental approach, the delivery of sonic hedgehog (SHH) cDNA was recently found to result in superior overall repair after 12 weeks compared with BMP-7–treated defects, and both were superior to controls.[57] In another ex vivo approach, adenoviral-mediated BMP-2 and IGF-I gene transfer to mesenchymal progenitor cells from rib perichondrium was accomplished for the repair of partial-thickness lesions in rats. This resulted in a type II collagen and proteoglycan-rich repair tissue, compared with the fibrous tissue of the control defects after 8 weeks.[27]

In an effort to simplify these kinds of time-consuming and expensive ex vivo procedures, we have recently begun to explore methods for direct, in vivo gene transfer to sites of cartilage damage. In a matrix-associated gene transfer approach **(Fig. 26–2A)** to rabbit osteochondral defects, hydrated collagen-glycosaminoglycan matrices preloaded with adenoviral vectors have been found to promote localized expression of marker genes for at least 3 weeks by bone marrow cells that migrated into the matrix and became transduced.[30] In an attempt to take this approach a step further, we tried to find ways to facilitate this gene transfer approach with an endogenous cellular and space-filling entity **(Fig. 26–2B)**. Thus, in an abbreviated, genetically enhanced tissue engineering approach, we demonstrated that when fresh bone marrow aspirates were mixed with a solution of recombinant adenoviral vectors and allowed to coagulate, MSCs within the coagulum acquired and expressed the transgene for several weeks after implantation into osteochondral defects in rabbits.[30] Studies are underway to investigate how these advances can be harnessed to achieve cartilage repair.

■ Conclusions and Future Challenges

Gene transfer techniques are very powerful tools that might help us to overcome the limitations of the current treatments for damaged articular cartilage. This chapter summarized the progress toward the development of gene-based strategies for articular cartilage repair. It has been shown that exogenous genes can be delivered to cartilaginous defects by several methods, and that the corresponding transgenes can be expressed for extended periods of time. Nonetheless, what remains to be determined are the level and duration of gene expression needed, and the gene or combination of genes necessary to meet the complexities of treating this tissue. The results of recent efficacy studies provide evidence that vector-mediated delivery of certain growth factors can be used to elicit favorable biologic responses in vivo, and as more data surface, a clearer picture of the functional boundaries of these applications and the parameters critical for success will appear. However, much work remains to be done to establish the appropriate combination of cells, genes, and delivery methods for achieving long-term repair of articular cartilage.

The use of gene transfer techniques to facilitate musculoskeletal tissue repair offers what is perhaps an immediate opportunity for a clinical application of gene therapy. Compared with the treatment of genetic diseases, where lifelong expression of a corrective transgene is required, or cancer, where extraordinarily high efficiency and specificity of transgene delivery is required to eradicate tumor cells from the body, tissue repair may only require transient, localized expression of a specific transgene product. The use of integrating vector systems and lifelong expression of potent transgenes might thus not be necessary for most applications, and their associated risks could be avoided. Furthermore, because current medical and surgical procedures have limited effectiveness, a clinically useful gene-based repair system need not necessarily demonstrate complete regeneration of normal tissue. Because surgical procedures for cartilage repair are almost always elective, and cartilage injuries are not life-threatening, the safety of gene transfer approaches for repair is of particular importance.

REFERENCES

1. Buckwalter JA. Articular cartilage injuries. Clin Orthop 2002;402:21–37
2. Evans CH, Ghivizzani SC, Smith P, Shuler FD, Mi Z, Robbins PD. Using gene therapy to protect and restore cartilage. Clin Orthop 2000;379(suppl):S214–S219
3. Hickey DG, Frenkel SR, Di Cesare PE. Clinical applications of growth factors for articular cartilage repair. Am J Orthop 2003;32:70–76
4. Vortkamp A. Interaction of growth factors regulating chondrocyte differentiation in the developing embryo. Osteoarthritis Cartilage 2001;9(suppl A):S109–S117
5. Lefebvre V, Behringer RR, de Crombrugghe B. L-Sox5, Sox6 and Sox9 control essential steps of the chondrocyte differentiation pathway. Osteoarthritis Cartilage 2001;9(suppl A):S69–S75
6. Hoffmann A, Gross G. BMP signaling pathways in cartilage and bone formation. Crit Rev Eukaryot Gene Expr 2001;11:23–45
7. Dharmavaram RM, Liu G, Tuan RS, Stokes DG, Jimenez SA. Stable transfection of human fetal chondrocytes with a type II procollagen minigene: expression of the mutant protein and alterations in the structure of the extracellular matrix in vitro. Arthritis Rheum 1999;42:1433–1442
8. Robbins PD, Evans CH, Chernajovsky Y. Gene therapy for arthritis. Gene Ther 2003;10:902–911
9. Sullenger BA, Gilboa E. Emerging clinical applications of RNA. Nature 2002;418:252–258
10. Crooke ST. Molecular mechanisms of action of antisense drugs. Biochim Biophys Acta 1999;1489:31–44
11. Tomita N, Morishita R, Tomita T, Ogihara T. Potential therapeutic applications of decoy oligonucleotides. Curr Opin Mol Ther 2002;4:166–170
12. McManus MT, Sharp PA. Gene silencing in mammals by small interfering RNAs. Nat Rev Genet 2002;3:737–747
13. Oligino TJ, Yao Q, Ghivizzani SC, Robbins P. Vector systems for gene transfer to joints. Clin Orthop 2000;379(suppl):S17–S30
14. Hardy S, Kitamura M, Harris-Stansil T, Dai Y, Phipps ML. Construction of adenovirus vectors through Cre-lox recombination. J Virol 1997;71:1842–1849
15. Thomas CE, Ehrhardt A, Kay MA. Progress and problems with the use of viral vectors for gene therapy. Nat Rev Genet 2003;4:346–358
16. McCarty DM, Monahan PE, Samulski RJ. Self-complementary recombinant adeno-associated virus (scAAV) vectors promote efficient transduction independently of DNA synthesis. Gene Ther 2001;8:1248–1254
17. Madry H, Cucchiarini M, Terwilliger EF, Trippel SB. Recombinant adeno-associated virus vectors efficiently and persistently transduce chondrocytes in normal and osteoarthritic human articular cartilage. Hum Gene Ther 2003;14:393–402
18. Oligino T, Ghivizzani S, Wolfe D, et al. Intra-articular delivery of a herpes simplex virus IL-1Ra gene vector reduces inflammation in a rabbit model of arthritis. Gene Ther 1999;6:1713–1720
19. Gouze E, Pawliuk R, Pilapil C, et al. In vivo gene delivery to synovium by lentiviral vectors. Mol Ther 2002;5:397–404
20. Stein GS, Lian JB, Stein JL, van Wijnen AJ. Bone tissue specific transcriptional control: options for targeting gene therapy to the skeleton. Cancer 2000;88(suppl):2899–2902
21. Gossen M, Bujard H. Tight control of gene expression in mammalian cells by tetracycline-responsive promoters. Proc Natl Acad Sci U S A 1992;89:5547–5551
22. Madry H, Trippel SB. Efficient lipid-mediated gene transfer to articular chondrocytes. Gene Ther 2000;7:286–291
23. Gouze E, Pawliuk R, Gouze JN, et al. Lentiviral-mediated gene delivery to synovium: potent intra-articular expression with amplification by inflammation. Mol Ther 2003;7:460–466
24. Evans CH, Robbins PD, Ghivizzani SC, et al. Clinical trial to assess the safety, feasibility, and efficacy of transferring a potentially antiarthritic cytokine gene to human joints with rheumatoid arthritis. Hum Gene Ther 1996;7:1261–1280
25. Frisbie DD, Ghivizzani SC, Robbins PD, Evans CH, McIlwraith CW. Treatment of experimental equine osteoarthritis by in vivo delivery of the equine interleukin-1 receptor antagonist gene. Gene Ther 2002;9:12–20
26. Mi Z, Ghivizzani SC, Lechman E, Glorioso JC, Evans CH, Robbins PD. Adverse effects of adenovirus-mediated gene transfer of human transforming growth factor beta 1 into rabbit knees. Arthritis Res Ther 2003;5:R132–R139
27. Gelse K, von der Mark K, Aigner T, Park J, Schneider H. Articular cartilage repair by gene therapy using growth factor-producing mesenchymal cells. Arthritis Rheum 2003;48:430–441
28. Bonadio J, Smiley E, Patil P, Goldstein S. Localized, direct plasmid gene delivery in vivo: prolonged therapy results in reproducible tissue regeneration [see comments] Nat Med 1999;5:753–759
29. Samuel RE, Lee CR, Ghivizzani SC, et al. Delivery of plasmid DNA to articular chondrocytes via novel collagen-glycosaminoglycan matrices. Hum Gene Ther 2002;13:791–802
30. Pascher A, Palmer G, Steinert A, et al. Gene delivery to cartilage defects using coagulated bone marrow aspirate. Gene Ther 2004;11:133–141
31. Hidaka C, Quitoriano M, Warren RF, Crystal RG. Enhanced matrix synthesis and in vitro formation of cartilage-like tissue by genetically modified chondrocytes expressing BMP-7. J Orthop Res 2001;19:751–758
32. Brower-Toland BD, Saxer RA, Goodrich LR, et al. Direct adenovirus-mediated insulin-like growth factor I gene transfer enhances transplant chondrocyte function. Hum Gene Ther 2001;12:117–129
33. Nixon AJ, Fortier LA, Williams J, Mohammed H. Enhanced repair of extensive articular defects by insulin-like growth factor-I-laden fibrin composites. J Orthop Res 1999;17:475–487

34. Shuler FD, Georgescu HI, Niyibizi C, et al. Increased matrix synthesis following adenoviral transfer of a transforming growth factor beta1 gene into articular chondrocytes [In Process Citation]. J Orthop Res 2000;18:585–592

35. Smith P, Shuler FD, Georgescu HI, et al. Genetic enhancement of matrix synthesis by articular chondrocytes: comparison of different growth factor genes in the presence and absence of interleukin-1. Arthritis Rheum 2000;43:1156–1164

36. Baragi VM, Renkiewicz RR, Jordan H, Bonadio J, Hartman JW, Roessler BJ. Transplantation of transduced chondrocytes protects articular cartilage from interleukin 1-induced extracellular matrix degradation. J Clin Invest 1995;96:2454–2460

37. Kaps C, Bramlage C, Smolian H, et al. Bone morphogenetic proteins promote cartilage differentiation and protect engineered artificial cartilage from fibroblast invasion and destruction. Arthritis Rheum 2002;46:149–162

38. Ikeda T, Kubo T, Arai Y, et al. Adenovirus mediated gene delivery to the joints of guinea pigs. J Rheumatol 1998;25:1666–1673

39. Kang R, Marui T, Ghivizzani SC, et al. Ex vivo gene transfer to chondrocytes in full-thickness articular cartilage defects: a feasibility study. Osteoarthritis Cartilage 1997;5:139–143

40. Baragi VM, Renkiewicz RR, Qiu L, et al. Transplantation of adenovirally transduced allogeneic chondrocytes into articular cartilage defects in vivo. Osteoarthritis Cartilage 1997;5:275–282

41. Madry H, Cucchiarini M, Stein U, et al. Sustained transgene expression in cartilage defects in vivo after transplantation of articular chondrocytes modified by lipid-mediated gene transfer in a gel suspension delivery system. J Gene Med 2003;5:502–509

42. Hidaka C, Goodrich LR, Chen CT, Warren RF, Crystal RG, Nixon AJ. Acceleration of cartilage repair by genetically modified chondrocytes over expressing bone morphogenetic protein-7. J Orthop Res 2003;21:573–583

43. Caplan AI. Mesenchymal stem cells and gene therapy. Clin Orthop 2000;379(suppl):S67–S70

44. Prockop DJ. Marrow stromal cells as stem cells for nonhematopoietic tissues. Science 1997;276:71–74

45. Noth U, Osyczka AM, Tuli R, Hickok NJ, Danielson KG, Tuan RS. Multilineage mesenchymal differentiation potential of human trabecular bone-derived cells. J Orthop Res 2002;20:1060–1069

46. Zuk PA, Zhu M, Mizuno H, et al. Multilineage cells from human adipose tissue: implications for cell-based therapies. Tissue Eng 2001;7:211–228

47. Yoo JU, Barthel TS, Nishimura K, et al. The chondrogenic potential of human bone-marrow-derived mesenchymal progenitor cells. J Bone Joint Surg Am 1998;80:1745–1757

48. Yoo JU, Mandell I, Angele P, Johnstone B. Chondrogenitor cells and gene therapy. Clin Orthop 2000;379(suppl):S164–S170

49. Mosca JD, Hendricks JK, Buyaner D, et al. Mesenchymal stem cells as vehicles for gene delivery. Clin Orthop 2000;379(suppl):S71–S90

50. Haas AR, Tuan RS. Chondrogenic differentiation of murine C3H10T1/2 multipotential mesenchymal cells: II. Stimulation by bone morphogenetic protein-2 requires modulation of N-cadherin expression and function. Differentiation 1999;64:77–89

51. Johnstone B, Hering TM, Caplan AI, Goldberg VM, Yoo JU. In vitro chondrogenesis of bone marrow-derived mesenchymal progenitor cells. Exp Cell Res 1998;238:265–272

52. Steinert A, Weber M, Dimmler A, et al. Chondrogenic differentiation of mesenchymal progenitor cells encapsulated in ultrahigh-viscosity alginate. J Orthop Res 2003;21:1090–1097

53. Ahrens M, Ankenbauer T, Schroder D, Hollnagel A, Mayer H, Gross G. Expression of human bone morphogenetic proteins-2 or -4 in murine mesenchymal progenitor C3H10T1/2 cells induces differentiation into distinct mesenchymal cell lineages. DNA Cell Biol 1993;12:871–880

54. Carlberg AL, Pucci B, Rallapalli R, Tuan RS, Hall DJ. Efficient chondrogenic differentiation of mesenchymal cells in micromass culture by retroviral gene transfer of BMP-2. Differentiation 2001;67:128–138

55. Mason JM, Grande DA, Barcia M, Grant R, Pergolizzi RG, Breitbart AS. Expression of human bone morphogenic protein 7 in primary rabbit periosteal cells: potential utility in gene therapy for osteochondral repair. Gene Ther 1998;5:1098–1104

56. Mason JM, Breitbart AS, Barcia M, Porti D, Pergolizzi RG, Grande DA. Cartilage and bone regeneration using gene-enhanced tissue engineering. Clin Orthop 2000;379(suppl):S171–S178

57. Grande DA, Mason J, Light E, Dines D. Stem cells as platforms for delivery of genes to enhance cartilage repair. J Bone Joint Surg Am 2003;85-A(suppl 2):111–116

27

Hyaluronan-Based Autologous Chondrocyte Implantation

STEFANO ZAFFAGNINI, ELIZAVETA KON, LEONARDO
MARCHESINI, MARIA PIA NERI, FRANCESCO IACONO,
AND MAURILIO MARCACCI

The marked increase in sports participation and increased emphasis on physical activity in all age groups has increased both the incidence of articular cartilage lesions and the recovery expectations of the patients. However, articular cartilage lesions are difficult to treat due to the distinctive structure and function of hyaline cartilage and to the difficulty in determining which lesion will be symptomatic and will evolve in degenerative joint changes. Curl et al[1] found a 63% incidence of chondral lesion in a survey of 31,516 knee arthroscopies. Grade IV lesions were noted in 20% of patients and only 35% had no accompanying meniscal or ligamentous lesions. It is therefore difficult to determine which tissue injury is responsible for which symptoms and to what extent. Recently, Steadman et al[2] reported highly satisfactory results at 11 years' follow-up with the microfracture technique; however, patients may have to adjust their activity level to that of their knee function, and the authors stress the importance of a meticulous postoperative program that include the use of continuous passive motion (CPM) and 8 weeks of restricted weight bearing. Microfracture technique is simple and can be used in small lesions or in wide degenerative lesions; however, the repair tissue response can be unpredictable and variable, and it is unclear which stress is optimal for cartilage regeneration. Nehrer et al[3] frequently found fibrous soft, spongiform tissue combined with central degeneration in the defect. Moreover, the clinical failure has been observed at a mean time of 21 months after treatment.

Autologous chondrocyte implantation (ACI) has been developed as a reconstructive technique with the aim of replacing the cartilage defect with a new developed mature cartilage tissue, trying to restore a complete normal joint. The clinical use of autologous chondrocyte implantation was pioneered in Sweden in 1987 to treat patients with chronic symptoms of cartilage lesions.[4] The first clinical report in 1994 demonstrated highly satisfactory results with biopsy samples showing hyaline-like cartilage. Recently, Peterson et al[5] showed durability of the early results obtained with ACI technique. In fact, after 2 years, 50 of 61 patients had good to excellent results. At 5 to 11 years' follow-up, 51 of 61 patients had satisfactory results. Biomechanical evaluation of the grafted area by means of an indentation probe demonstrated stiffness measurements 90% that of normal cartilage. The outcome of these studies has demonstrated that 84 to 91% of the patients were able to achieve good to excellent results and return to active lifestyles. Therefore, we agree with Sgaglione et al[6] that ACI is a safe, effective, and reproducible treatment that should be considered a viable option for young patients with cartilage lesions greater than 2 cm^2 who want to resume an active lifestyle and restore so-called normal cartilage.

On the other hand, a recent study of Engebretsen[7] comparing prospectively microfracture versus ACI has shown that Lysholm and Visual Analog Scale (VAS) pain scores improved in both groups at 2 years, and the Tegner score improved only in the microfracture group. Microfracture patients had fewer failures and reoperations than ACI patients. However, ACI patients had a better histologic quality of the repair tissue than did microfracture patients. This study has demonstrated that the ACI technique can achieve the restoration of cartilage tissue in the defect in ~85% of the cases, but there are still many biologic and technical factors that influence the final clinical outcome and lead to comparable clinical results, especially at short-term follow-up with a simpler technique, as reported by Engebretsen.[7]

Our efforts have been utilized in the attempt to improve the efficacy and reduce the morbidity of ACI technique, which still remains for us one of the main concerns of this technique. In the original ACI technique, the liquid cell suspension is difficult to handle during surgery, as it needs to be covered by a periosteal flap, and the surgical technique is tedious, time-consuming, and initially technically difficult. Moreover, there is a need for an arthrotomy for joint exposure. This factor increases morbidity especially for young athletes, increasing the risk of joint stiffness and arthrofibrosis frequently observed with this procedure. Micheli and coauthors[8] in 2001, and other authors[9] more recently, have shown a reoperation rate of up to 42% due to joint stiffness or hypertrophic changes of the implanted graft owing to the intrinsic growth capacity of the cambium layer of the periosteal flap[9] with impingement syndrome as clinical findings. Another concern is whether the chondrocytes will be homogeneously distributed in the three-dimensional spaces of the defect[10] when used in liquid cell suspension.

To avoid these technical problems, we have used a new tissue-engineering technology to create a cartilage-like tissue in a three-dimensional culture system with the possibility to reduce morbidity and improve cell culture biology. HYAFF® (Fidia Farmaceutici s.p.a., Abano Terme, Italy) is the class of hyaluronan derivatives obtained by esterifying the glucuronic acid group with different types of alcohols.11 HYAFF-11®–based scaffolds can be used in skeletal tissue engineering both as a tissue-guiding device and as a delivery vehicle.[13] HYAFF-11 nonwoven matrix has been extensively characterized in a series of in vitro and in vivo studies in which it has been shown to effectively support growth of chondrocytes and to favor the expression of typical chondrocyte markers.[14] This three-dimensional scaffold allows the maintenance of different phenotypes during culture and after implant. The quality of this scaffold in the laboratory experimental tests has facilitated verifying this system in an experimental animal trial. Grigolo et al[13] in a rabbit model obtained

statistically significant differences in the quality of the regenerated tissue found between the grafts performed with biomaterial carrying chondrocyte cells compared with the biomaterial alone or controls, thus demonstrating the efficacy of HYAFF-11–based scaffold for autologous chondrocytes implantation.

With this scientific and promising background, we have started to use ACI with HYAFF in symptomatic cartilage lesions. Due to the easy handling capacity of this scaffold, the implant can be performed by the mini-open or arthroscopic technique[15] depending on the location of the defect.

Thanks to hydrophilic features of the scaffold, if the patch is correctly positioned inside the prepared defect, tensioactive pressure permits a natural fixation of the patch without the need of fibrin glue, or periosteal flap coverage. The avoidance of a periosteal flap enabled us to implant the chondrocyte-suspended scaffolds arthroscopically, simplifying and reducing the morbidity of this two-stage procedure.

■ Surgical Technique

The arthroscopic surgical technique for ACI involves two separate procedures. The arthroscopic biopsy of healthy cartilage for cell culture remains mandatory to evaluate the site of the lesion and cartilage quality. At this time associated procedures such as anterior cruciate ligament (ACL) reconstruction or meniscal surgeries are usually performed.

In the second arthroscopic procedure, the lesion is visualized and, using a motorized shaver, debridement and lavage of the chondral lesion is performed. All fibrous tissue is removed from the surface of the lesion. Mapping and sizing of the defect is then executed using a delivery device of variable diameters (6.5–8.5 mm) with a sharp edge to achieve the complete coverage of the defect (**Fig. 27–1**). A flipped cannula especially designed is then inserted in the anteromedial portal. The flip allows removal of the fat pad from the field of view of the camera, especially when you have to put the knee in a high degree of flexion. A specifically designed cannulated low profile drill (6.5–8.5 mm) is positioned according to the mapping previously performed (**Fig. 27–2**). The drill is maintained in the selected position by a Kirschner guide wire (0.9-mm diameter) fixed in the bone. This drill, which presents a safety stop at a 2-mm distance, has been developed specifically to avoid damage to the subchondral bone plate, which has to remain intact during debridement of the lesion. Only the Kirschner wire passes through the subchondral plate, but the amount of stem cells coming from this small hole is not significant enough to require modifying the action of cultured

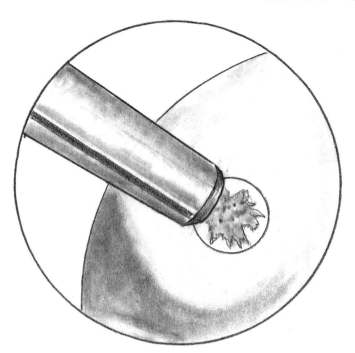

FIGURE 27–1 The sizing and mapping of the lesion is performed with the sharp edge of delivery system.

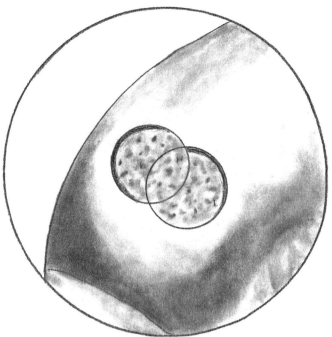

FIGURE 27–3 Prepared surface of the chondral lesion after drilling.

chondrocyte. The low-speed drilling of the cartilage surface enables the surgeon to create the predetermined circular area with regular margins for the graft **(Fig. 27–3)**. This step must be executed carefully to achieve stable and precise lesion contours.

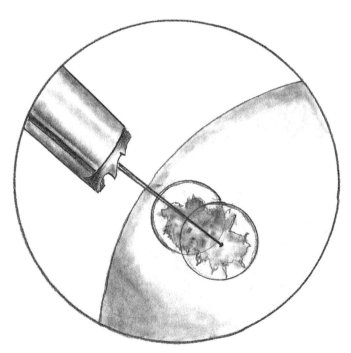

FIGURE 27–2 Preparation of the area is performed, with a low profile and slow speed drill, avoiding penetration of the subchondral bone.

The procedure is repeated to prepare the entire defect surface according to the previous sizing. From the same portal, it is usually possible to correctly prepare a wide area, changing the knee flexion and orientation of the cannula thanks also to the previously mentioned flipped cannula.

After drilling, the joint is lavaged with a motorized shaver. The inflow then is closed and suction from the cannula inserted in the anteromedial portal is applied to create a dry joint surface.

The delivery system with a sharp edge is put in contact with the hyaluronic acid patch containing the autologous chondrocyte culture **(Fig. 27–4)**. The stamp obtained remains automatically in the sheath of the delivery system, which is then transported through a cannula and positioned in the prepared area **(Fig. 27–5)**. The delivery tamp is pushed to advance the stamp into the defect. The procedure is repeated until the entire defect is entirely filled **(Fig. 27–6)**. It is important to cover the prepared area as much as possible without overhanging the margin of the defect with the implanted stamps. In this manner, the stamps do not move from the defect. This has been tested after repeated cycles of joint motion (with and without tourniquet) performed in open cases previously performed utilizing the same device.

Under arthroscopic visualization, the stability of implanted stamps is evaluated with a blunt probe. The tourniquet is released and the graft swelling is observed and the stability reevaluated. If the swelling of the patch increases its size in such way that the graft overhangs the

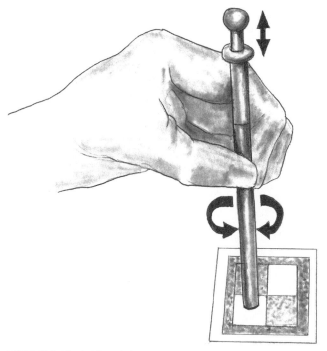

FIGURE 27–4 The delivery system with a sharp edge is put in contact with the hyaluronic acid patch containing the autologous chondrocyte culture.

margins of the defect, a smaller patch should be placed to prevent overhanging. For example, place a 6.5-mm diameter patch in a 8.5-mm diameter area. With the scope still in the joint, the knee is cycled several times, and the possibility of graft migration from the prepared defect is checked. Mobilization of the implanted patch has never been observed in our series. The arthroscopic implant has been developed for medial or lateral condyle lesions. With improving expertise and a long learning curve, we are now able to address almost any lesion, except for those in the patella.

Rehabilitation Protocol

Patients are discharged on postoperative day 1 after the arthroscopic procedure. In the first 2 weeks, continuous self-assisted passive motion is started from 0 to 90 degrees from the second postoperative day, promoting joint nutrition and preventing adhesions. Stretching exercise and quadriceps contractions are allowed if tolerated. Toe-touch weight bearing is permitted, whereas full weight bearing is avoided for the first 4 weeks. From the 4th to 5th week, weight bearing is increased, beginning in the swimming pool, to recover the normal

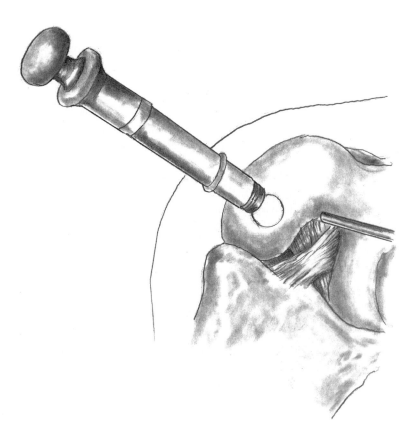

FIGURE 27–5 The tamp is pushed in the delivery system to precisely plug the stamp in the defect.

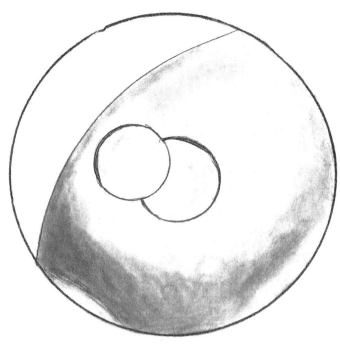

FIGURE 27–6 Complete coverage of the defect by two implanted patches after irrigation removal from the joint.

gait phases; muscle strengthening exercise is allowed from the 7th week. Increased strength and functional exercise is then gradually allowed. Return to contact sports should not be attempted before 8 to 12 months.

■ Patient Selection and Prospective Follow-Up Evaluation

The autologous chondrocyte transplantation on HYAFF scaffold has been used in Europe since 1999. At the moment, more than 3000 implants have been performed by the mini-open or arthroscopic techniques. At our institution, 139 patients have had this procedure since September 1999. Of these cases, 88 patients were treated arthroscopically (arthroscopic technique has been used since November 2000). The approval of the ethics committee of the Rizzoli Orthopaedic Institute was obtained for the clinical experimentation, and the informed consent of all the patients was obtained. All the patients were prospectively evaluated clinically according to the International Repair Cartilage Society score preoperatively and at 12, 24, and 36 months postoperatively. We were able to obtain CT or MRI scans for all patients at 12, 24, and 36 months of follow-up.

Among the patients who were treated by arthroscopic procedure, we have selected a group of 24 young athletes. Of these patients, 13 were soccer players, three skiers, three basketball players, one volleyball player, one rugby player, one body builder, one tennis player, and one biker. Of these athletes, eight practiced sports at the professional level. Twenty-four patients (23 male, one female) were analyzed at a minimum of 1-year follow-up. Twenty-two patients had isolated chondral lesions: 13 medial condyle, eight lateral condyle, and one trochlear lesion. Two patients had multiple knee lesions: one lateral compartment kissing lesion and one medial condyle and trochlea defect. All the defects were grade III to IV Outerbridge and the mean size was 2.9 cm2 (2–4.5 cm^2). Mean age of the patients at time of surgery was 25 years (range 16–37 years). The etiology was traumatic in 18 cases, osteochondritis dissecans (OCD) in one case, and degenerative (microtraumatic) in five cases. Of the 18 traumatic lesions, seven were treated acutely (within 3 months after traumatic event) and 11 chronically. In 17 patients, associated procedures were performed during the cartilage harvesting: 15 ACL and one posterior cruciate ligament (PCL) reconstruction, nine medial and three lateral meniscectomies, two medial and one lateral meniscal repairs, and one autologous bone grafting. Previous surgery in 10 of the patients included three meniscectomies; two ACL reconstructions; one patellar tendon repair; five cartilage reparative operations, such as shaving and debridement of chondral lesion and one mosaicplasty.

Patients were asked for a subjective evaluation of the knee symptoms and physical function using the International Knee Documentation Committee (IKDC) Subjective Knee Evaluation Form. According to this questionnaire, a higher score represents higher levels of function and lower levels of symptoms. Therefore, a score of 100 is interpreted to mean no limitations on activities of daily living or sports with the absence of symptoms. Patients were also asked to evaluate their quality of life using the EuroQol EQ-5D questionnaire. This is a recognized assessment of health–related quality of life based on self-care, mobility, usual activities, and pain/discomfort and anxiety/depression dimensions. It includes a 0 to 100 Visual Analogue Scale (EQ-VAS) for a self-rating of the global health state, in which the 100 value represents the best imaginable health state. A knee functional test was performed by the surgeon according to the IKDC Knee Examination Form. The lowest ratings in effusion, passive motion deficit, and ligament examination were used to determine the final functional grade of the knee (normal, nearly normal abnormal, or severely abnormal).

No complications related to the implant and no serious adverse events were observed during the treatment and follow up period. The International Cartilage Repair Society (ICRS) objective evaluation was normal or

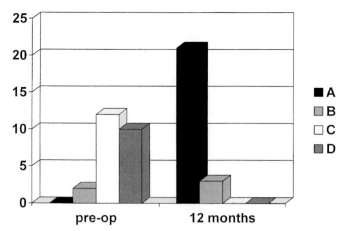

FIGURE 27–7 Clinical results in 24 patients at 12-month follow-up according to the ICRS objective evaluation.

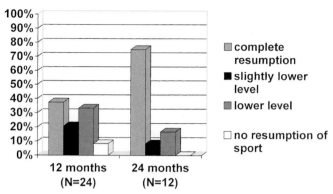

FIGURE 27–9 Resumption of sports activities of 24 patients at 12-month follow-up and of 12 patients at 24-month follow-up.

nearly normal in 100% of patients displaying knee conditions within the two best categories **(Fig. 27–7)**.

The mean IKDC subjective score increased from 42.0 [standard deviation (SD) = 15.6] preoperatively to 80.8 (SD = 12.5) at 12-month follow-up. Subjective improvement in knee function and symptoms was seen in 95.8% of the patients. Only one patient (4.2%) experienced an unchanged knee condition. An improvement in quality of life, as assessed by the EQ-VAS, was noted in 87.5% of patients.

Twelve patients were analyzed at 12 and 24 months. The mean IKDC subjective score of these patients was 39.9 (SD = 19.3) preoperatively and 78.1 (SD = 15.0) at 12 months of follow-up and 84.5 (SD = 10.7) at 24 months **(Fig. 27–8)**. None of these 12 patients worsened from 12 to 24 months' follow-up.

Resumption of sports participation at the same or a slightly lower level was obtained in 14 (58.3%) of 24 patients at 12 months' follow-up. Eight patients returned

to sports activity at a lower level. Only two patients were not able to return to sports activity at 12 months. However, one of these two patients achieved nearly complete resumption of sports activity after 24 months. At 24 months, the resumption of sports activity was complete or nearly complete in 10 (83.3%) of the 12 patients analyzed **(Fig. 27–9)**.

A second-look arthroscopy was performed in five patients at a 12-month follow-up. Visual inspection and probing for the consistency of the implanted cartilage revealed complete healing of the defect and the excellent quality of regenerated cartilage macroscopically. The biopsy of implanted cartilage was performed in two cases, and the histologic evaluation by an independent examiner showed a hyaline-like tissue with good integration within the host tissue **(Fig. 27–10)**. The re-

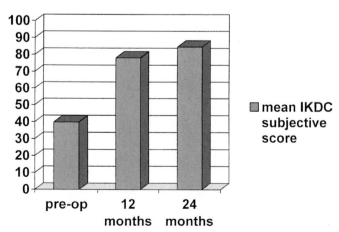

FIGURE 27–8 Clinical results in 12 patients at 12- and 24-month follow-up according to the IKDC subjective evaluation.

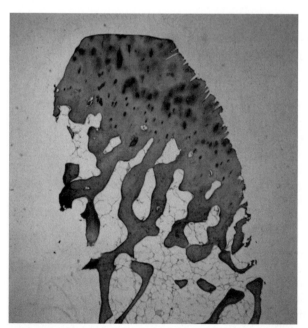

FIGURE 27–10 Histologic evaluation of regenerated tissue at 12-month follow-up. Excellent integration of the newly formed tissue with the subchondral bone. The tidemark is developing. (Courtesy of Prof. G. Abatangelo, University of Padova, Italy.)

sults of our series are in agreement with those of the original ACI technique.[4] The arthroscopic implant, however, has reduced the morbidity for the patient, the recovery time, and the rehabilitation protocol, allowing easier recovery for patients. This technique achieves clinical and histologic results comparable to those of traditional ACI, but reduces the morbidity for patients and improves the reliability of the procedure. Certainly, this technique is only one step forward from the original ACI technique. Several improvements will probably appear quickly as more knowledge on cell culture and chondrocyte behavior will permit a more reliable surgical technique and clinical outcome.

REFERENCES

1. Curl WW, Krome J, Gordon ES, Rushing J, Smith BP, Poehling GG. Cartilage injuries: a review of 31,516 knee arthroscopies. Arthroscopy 1997;13:456–460
2. Steadman JR, Briggs KK, Rodrigo JJ, Kocher MS, Gill TJ, Rodkey WG. Outcomes of microfracture for traumatic chondral defects of the knee: average 11-year follow-up. Arthroscopy 2003;19:477–484
3. Nehrer S, Spector M, Minas T. Histologic analysis of tissue after failed cartilage repair procedures. Clin Orthop 1999;365:149–162
4. Peterson L, Minas T, Brittberg M, Nilsson A, Sjogren-Jansson E, Lindahl A. Two- to 9-year outcome after autologous chondrocyte transplantation of the knee. Clin Orthop 2000;374:212–234
5. Peterson L, Brittberg M, Kiviranta I, Akerlund EL, Lindahl A. Autologous chondrocyte transplantation. Biomechanics and long-term durability. Am J Sports Med 2002;30:2–12
6. Sgaglione NA, Miniaci A, Gillogly SD, Carter TR. Update on advanced surgical techniques in the treatment of traumatic focal articular cartilage lesions in the knee. Arthroscopy 2002;18(suppl 1):9–32
7. Engebretsen L. Comparison ACT—microfractures. Proceedings of the International Symposium on Matrix-Assisted Chondrocyte Transplantation—a 2-year-update with hyalograft C. Bad Gastein, Austria, January 23–25, 2004
8. Micheli LJ, Browne JE, Erggelet C, et al. Autologous chondrocyte implantation of the knee: multicenter experience and minimum 3-year follow-up. Clin J Sport Med 2001;11:223–228
9. Anderson AF, Fu FH, Bert RM, et al. A controlled study of autologous chondrocyte implantation versus microfracture for articular cartilage lesions of the femur. 70th American Academy of Orthopaedic Surgeons (AAOS) annual meeting proceedings, New Orleans, February 5–9, 2003
10. Ochi M, Uchio Y, Kawasaki K, Wakitani S, Iwasa J. Transplantation of cartilage-like tissue made by tissue engineering in the treatment of cartilage defects of the knee. J Bone Joint Surg Br 2002;84:571–578
11. Campoccia D, Doherty P, Radice M, Brun P, Abatangelo G, Williams DF. Semi synthetic resorbable materials from hyaluronan esterification. Biomaterials 1998;19:2101–2127
12. New frontiers in medical sciences: redefining hyaluronan. In: Abatangelo G, Weigel PH, eds. Proceedings of the Symposium Held in Padua, Italy—17–19 June 1999. New York: Elsevier, 2000
13. Grigolo B, Roseti L, Fiorini M, et al. Transplantation of chondrocytes seeded on a hyaluronan derivative (HYAFF®11) into cartilage defects in rabbits. Biomaterials 2001;22:2417–2424
14. Brun P, Abatangelo G, Radice M, et al. Chondrocyte aggregation and reorganization into three-dimensional scaffolds. J Biomed Mater Res 1999;46:337–346
15. Marcacci M, Zaffagnini S, Kon E, Visani A, Iacono F, Loreti I. Arthroscopic autologous condrocyte transplantation: technical note. Knee Surg Sports Traumatol Arthrosc 2002;10:154–159

Index

Page numbers followed by f or t denote figures or tables, respectively.

A

Abrasion arthroplasty
  complications, 104
  early arthritic joint debridement, 103–104
Abrasion chondroplasty, acute osteochondral defects
    treatment, 194
Acetaminophen
  adverse effects and safety, 75
  dosage and administration, 74
  efficacy, 74–75
  mechanism of action, 74
Activities of daily living (ADL) assessment, microfracture
    technique, 121
Acute osteochondral defects, knee
  basic principles, 187–188
  classification, 188–189
  diagnosis, 189–190
  surgical treatment, 190–198
    complications, 198
    postoperative care, 198
    repair, 191, 192f–193f, 193–194
    replacement, 194–198, 195f–197f
    resectioning, 190–191
Adeno-associated vectors (AAV), orthopaedic
    applications, 301
Adenoviral vectors, orthopaedic applications, 300–301
Adverse effects
  cyclooxygenase-2-selective NSAIDs, 79–80
  hyaluronic acid viscosupplementation, 93
  nonsteroidal antiinflammatory drugs, 77–79
  opioids, 83–84
Alignment techniques, knee osteotomy, 249–250
Allografts. *See also* Graft implantation
  failure, osteochondral allograft transplantation, 163–164,
    164f
  meniscal transplantation, 265
  osteochondral allograft transplantation, 162, 162f
American Orthopaedic Foot and Ankle Society (AOFAS)
    score, osteochondral lesions of talus, 177–178

Analgesics
  acetaminophen, 74–75
  basic principles, 73–74
  opioids, 80–84, 82t
Animal studies, osteochondral autograft transfer
    (OATS/Mosaicplasty), 134–135, 136f
Ankle joint, osteochondral lesions of talus, 172
Anterior cruciate ligament (ACL)
  acute osteochondral defects, 188
  autologous chondrocyte implantation, clinical evaluation, 143
  knee osteotomy, 250–251
  microfracture technique, 117–119, 117f–119f
  osteochondral autograft transfer, 137
Antiinflammatory medications
  basic principles, 73–74
  nonsteroidal antiinflammatory drugs
    COX-2 selective, 79–80
    nonselective, 75, 75t–76t, 77–79
  opioids, 80–84, 82t
Apoptosis, acute osteochondral defects treatment, 198
ArthroCare 2000 RFE device, assessment of, 40–43
Arthrofibrosis
  autologous chondrocyte implantation, 154–155
  meniscal transplantation complication, 269
Arthroplasty
  failure rates, 141
  patellofemoral prosthetics, 285, 285f
Arthroscopic laser systems, articular cartilage repair, 34
Arthroscopic management, early arthritic joint
  abrasion arthroplasty, 103–104
  basic principles, 99
  categories of debridement, 100
  complications, 104
  cost-benefit debate over, 104, 106
  debridement history and results, 102–103
  evidence-based studies, 104, 105t
  indications for, 99–100, 100t
  lavage treatment, 102
  surgical debridement technique, 101–102, 101f

Arthroscopic technique
  acute osteochondral defects treatment, 190–191
  autologous chondrocyte implantation, 144–145, 144f
  juvenile osteochondritis dissecans, knee, 238–239
  osteochondral autograft transfer (OATS/Mosaicplasty),
    126–129
    defect preparation and templating, 126–128
    graft harvest, 128–129
    graft implantation, 129
    portal placement, 126
  osteochondral defects, elbow, 206–210
  shoulder cartilage injury, 219–220, 219f
    palliative treatment, 223, 223f
Arthroscopic visualization, articular cartilage injury and repair
    classification, 66–69, 67f–68f
Arthrotomy, osteochondral autograft transfer
    (OATS/Mosaicplasty), 129–130, 130f
Articular cartilage. See Cartilage
Athletes
  acute osteochondral defects treatment, 193f, 194
  cartilage injury, 289–294
    advanced magnetic resonance imaging, 289–229
    assessment techniques, 289–291
    biomechanical probes, 291
    chondrocyte resuscitation, 292
    functional tissue engineering, 294
    gene therapy, 292–294, 294f
    injury models, 291–292, 292f
    optical coherence tomography, 290–291, 290f
  glucosamine/chondroitin sulfate use in, 88–89
  hyaluronic acid viscosupplementation in
    acutely injured athletes, 95
    high-endurance applications, 94–95
  osteochondral autograft transfer, outcomes, 138–139
  osteochondral defects, elbow
    skeletally immature athletes, 210–214, 210t
    skeletally mature athletes, 214
    very early and early lesions, 211–213
Autologous chondrocyte implantation (ACI)
  acute osteochondral defects treatment, 197–198
  articular cartilage repair, 20
    outcomes, 28–29
  cartilage repair, 278, 280–281, 280f, 283f–284f, 285
  complications, 154–155
  future developments, 156
  gene transfer to chondrocytes, 304–305
  healing process, 142, 142t
  hyaluronan-based techniques
    basic principles, 309–310
    patient selection and follow-up, 313–315, 314f
    rehabilitation protocol, 312–313, 313f
    surgical techniques, 310–312, 311f–312f
  indications for, 145
  magnetic resonance imaging of, 57–58
  microfracture technique and, 122
  osteochondral lesions of talus, 180–182, 181f
  outcomes, 22, 155–156
  overview of, 141–142
  patient presentation and assessment, 143–145
    arthroscopic evaluation, 144–145, 144f
    clinical evaluation, 143
    radiographic evaluation, 143–144
  patient selection, 145, 146f, 147, 147f
  postoperative care, 151–154, 155f
  shoulder cartilage, 226, 226f
  surgical technique, 148, 148f–154f, 150–151
Autologous osteochondral transfer
  articular cartilage repair, 20–22, 21f
  outcomes, 22
Awls, for microfracture technique, 117–119

B
Bextra, adverse effects and safety, 79–80
Bioabsorbable implants, acute osteochondral defects
    treatment, 191, 192f–193f, 193–194
Biologic resurfacing, shoulder cartilage, 226–228, 227f–229f
Biomechanical probes, cartilage injury assessment, 291
Biomechanics
  acute osteochondral defects treatment, 197
  meniscus anatomy and physiology, 263–265, 264f
  osteochondral autograft transfer (OATS/Mosaicplasty), 130,
    131t–134t, 134, 135f–136f
Biphasic nature, articular cartilage biomechanics, 16–17, 16f,
    18f
Bipolar radiofrequency energy (bRFE)
  cartilage repair applications, 37–43, 38f–39f, 42f
  current systems, 35, 35f
  electrothermal chondroplasty, 109–113
  evolution of, 32
  outcomes assessment, 37
Body mass index (BMI), meniscal transplantation indications,
    266
Bone bridge techniques, meniscal transplantation, 267
Bone morphogenetic proteins (BMPs), cartilage repair with,
    298–299, 298t
Bone peg grafting, osteochondtritis dissecans, elbow, 208–209
Bone scans, juvenile osteochondritis dissecans, knee, 237, 237t
Boosted lubrication, cartilage, 19
Boyd approach, osteochondtritis dissecans, elbow, 208, 208f
Bronchospasm, nonsteroidal antiinflammatory drugs and risk
    of, 78–79
Buprenorphine, dosage/administration and indications,
    81–82

C
Calcified zone, articular cartilage, 6
Capitellum, osteochondritis dissecans, 240–242, 241f
Cardiovascular disease, nonsteroidal antiinflammatory drugs
    and risk of, 78–79
Cartilage
  articular
    function, 7–8
    structure-function relationships, 8
  biomechanics, 16–17, 16f, 18f
    joint loading, 19
  composition, 3–5, 13–16
    cellular cartilage, 5, 5f
    extracellular cartilage, 3, 4f, 5
  compression, 7
  defects, gene delivery to, 304, 305f

disease *vs.* injury, 297
electrothermal energy effects
  applications, 37–43, 38f–39f, 42f
  basic principles, 31–32
  composition, 32–33
  outcomes, 36–37
  principles and techniques, 33–36, 35f
function, 7–8
injury and repair classification
  assessment techniques, 60–69
  imaging techniques, 65–69
    arthroscopy, 66–69, 67f–68f
    magnetic resonance imaging, 66
    radiography, 65–66
  patient history, 60
  physical examination and functional assessment, 65
  subjective knee scores, 60–65, 61t, 62f, 63t–64t
injury response
  autologous chondrocyte implantation, 28–29
  chondrocyte orientation, 24, 25f
  collagen matrix composition, 24, 25f
  impact injuries, 27
  motion effects on cartilage repair, 28
  potential remedies, 28–29
  repair cartilage durability, 27–28, 27f
  subchondral bone lesions, 26–27, 26f
  superficial lesions, 26
lubrication theories, 18
magnetic resonance imaging, 50–58
  autologous chondrocyte implantation, 57–58
  contrast-enhanced imaging, 55
  diffusion-weighted imaging, 55
  driven equillibrium Fourier transfer imaging, 55
  fat-suppression and fast spin-echo sequences, 51–52
  high field strength and local gradient coils, 56
  magnetization transfer, 54
  microscopy, 56
  osteochondral autograft transplantation, 56–57, 57f–58f
  parameter mapping, 54
  postarthrography imaging, 52–54, 53f
  postsurgical cartilage repair, 56
  projection-reconstruction spectroscopic imaging, 54–55
  quantitative imaging volume measurement, 54
  short echo-time-projection-reconstruction imaging, 54
  sodium magnetic resonance imaging, 55
  T1-weighted fat suppressed three-dimensional spoiled gradient echo sequences, 52, 52f
  T1-weighted spin-echo images, 51
  T2-weighted spin-echo images, 51, 51f
osteochondral lesions of talus, repair procedures, 178–182
radiofrequency energy effects on, 40–41
repair techniques, 19–22
  autologous chondrocyte implantation, 20
  autologous osteochondral transfer, 20–22, 21f
replication process, 24–25
shear, 7
shear function, 7
structure, 5–7, 6f
  calcified zone, 6
  matrix compartmentalization, 5f, 6–7

  radial (deep) zone, 5–6
  tangential (superficial) zone, 5
  transitional (intermediate) zone, 5
structure-function relationships, 8
swelling of, 17
tension, 7–8, 7f
zones of, 14–16, 15f
Cartilage-derived morphogenetic protein (CDMP), cartilage injury in athletes, 293–294, 294f
Cartilage injury
  in athletes, future directions, 289–294
    advanced magnetic resonance imaging, 289–229
    assessment techniques, 289–291
    biomechanical probes, 291
    chondrocyte resuscitation, 292
    functional tissue engineering, 294
    gene therapy, 292–294, 294f
    injury models, 291–292, 292f
    optical coherence tomography, 290–291, 290f
  autologous chondrocyte implantation for repair of, 278, 280–281, 280f, 283f–284f, 285
  gene therapy
    applications, 297–298
    in athletes, 292–294
    delivery and cell targeting, 303–306
    disease *vs.*, 297
    limitations, 297
    nucleic acid regulation, 299–300
    protein classification, 298–299, 298t
    protein delivery system, 299
    vector development, 302–303
    viral vectors, 300–302
  magnetic resonance imaging, 50–58
    autologous chondrocyte implantation, 57–58
    contrast-enhanced imaging, 55
    diffusion-weighted imaging, 55
    driven equillibrium Fourier transfer imaging, 55
    fat-suppression and fast spin-echo sequences, 51–52
    high field strength and local gradient coils, 56
    magnetization transfer, 54
    microscopy, 56
    osteochondral autograft transplantation, 56–57, 57f–58f
    parameter mapping, 54
    postarthrography imaging, 52–54, 53f
    postsurgical cartilage repair, 56
    projection-reconstruction spectroscopic imaging, 54–55
    quantitative imaging volume measurement, 54
    short echo-time-projection-reconstruction imaging, 54
    sodium magnetic resonance imaging, 55
    T1-weighted fat suppressed three-dimensional spoiled gradient echo sequences, 52, 52f
    T1-weighted spin-echo images, 51
    T2-weighted spin-echo images, 51, 51f
  shoulder
    assessment, 217–218
    nonoperative treatment, 220
    operative treatment, 220–221
    palliative treatment, 221–223
    patient evaluation, 218–220, 219f
    postoperative rehabilitation, 229–230

Cartilage injury, shoulder (*Continued*)
  primary treatment, 221
  reparative techniques, 224–225, 224f
  restorative techniques, 225–229
    autogenous chondrocyte implantation, 226, 227f
    biologic resurfacing, 226–229, 228f–229f
    fresh osteochondral allograft, 225–226, 226f
    osteochondral autograft, 225, 225f
  in skeletally immature athlete
    chondral injuries, 244–245
    elbow osteochondritis dissecans, 239–242
    juvenile osteochondritis dissecans, 232–239
    osteochondral fractures, 242–244
Celcain-AM labeling, confocal laser microscopy, 37
Celebrex, adverse effects and safety, 79–80
Celecoxib, adverse effects and safety, 79–80
Cellular structure, cartilage composition, 5, 5f
Chemical expansion stress, articular cartilage swelling, 17
Chondral injury
  patient evaluation
    patient history, 47
    physical examination, 47–48
    radiographic evaluation, 48
  shoulder instability, 218
  skeletally immature cartilage, 244–245
Chondrocyte resuscitation, cartilage injury in athletes, 292
Chondrocytes
  articular cartilage
    composition, 13
    orientation and injury response, 24, 25f
  electrothermal energy effects on, 32–33
  gene transfer to, 304–305, 305f
  radiofrequency energy therapy, injury and death from, 39–43
  superficial articular lesions, injury response, 26
Chondroitin sulfate
  chemical composition, 87
  combined therapy with glucosamine, 87–88
  osteoarthritis management, 86
  use in athletes, 88–89
  in vitro studies, 89–90
Chondromalacia
  electrothermal energy effects on, 33, 33f
  radiofrequency energy effects on, 40–43
Chondropenia, articular cartilage injury and repair classification, 60
Chondroprogenitor cells, gene transfer to, 305f, 306
Chondroprotective potential, meniscal transplantation, 265
Chondrosis, patellar tilt subluxation, 275–277, 278f–280f
c-Jun N-terminal kinase (JNK) inhibitor, chondrocyte resuscitation, 292
Closing wedge osteotomy
  high tibial, complications, 252
  lateral tibial
    instrumentation and implants, 253
    surgical technique, 253–255
  medial, 256
Collagen
  acute osteochondral defects, 188
  articular cartilage matrix composition, 13–14, 13f
    injury response and, 24, 25f

composition, 3, 4f, 5
  electrothermal energy effects on, 32–33
Complementary DNA (cDNA), cartilage repair with, 298–299, 298t
Complete blood count (CBC), nonsteroidal antiinflammatory drugs, 77–78
Complications
  acute osteochondral defects treatment, 198
  arthroscopic surgery, 104
  autologous chondrocyte implantation, 154–155
  closing wedge high tibial osteotomy, 252
  meniscal transplantation, 268–269
  microfracture technique, 120
  opening wedge high tibial osteotomy, 252
  osteochondral allograft transplantation, 163–164
  proximal tibial osteotomies, 251–252
  varus-producing osteotomies, 255–256
Compression
  articular cartilage, 7
    biomechanics, 16, 16f
  synovial joints, 11
Computed tomography (CT)
  articular cartilage injury, postarthrography imaging, 52–54, 53f
  autologous chondrocyte implantation, 143–144
  chondral injury evaluation, 48
  osteochondral defects, elbow, 205
  osteochondral lesions of talus, 174–175, 174f–176f
  patellofemoral disease, 273–274, 274f
  shoulder cartilage injury, 219–220, 219f
Confocal laser microscopy (CLM), articular cartilage repair techniques, 37
  applications, 38–43, 38f–39f
Continuous passive motion (CPM)
  acute osteochondral defects treatment, 198
  articular cartilage joint loading, 19
  autologous chondrocyte implantation, postoperative therapy, 151–152
  microfracture technique
    outcomes assessment, 121
    postoperative protocol, 120
Contrast-enhanced imaging, articular cartilage injury, 55
Controlled thermal injury, 291–292
CoVac RFE device, assessment of, 40–43
Coventry's technique, proximal tibial osteotomies, 251–252
"Crabmeat" cartilage fibrillation, 27–28, 27f
  arthroscopic debridement, early arthritic joint, 101–102, 101f
Creep
  articular cartilage viscoelasticity, 17, 16f–17f
  synovial joint viscoelasticity, 12
Cryopreservation, meniscal transplantation allografts, 265
  outcomes, 270
Cyclooxygenase-2 (COX-2)-selective NSAIDs
  adverse effects and safety, 79–80
  dosage and indications, 79
  efficacy, 79
  mechanism of action, 79
  research background, 73–74
Cytokines, cartilage repair with, 298–299, 298t

D

Debridement technique
  acute osteochondral defects treatment, 190–191
  autologous chondrocyte implantation, 148, 148f–154f, 150–151
  early arthritic joint, 101–102, 101f
    history and outcomes, 102–103
    limitations of, 104–106
  osteochondral allograft transplantation, 164, 165f
  osteochondral lesions of talus, 176–178, 177f–178f
  shoulder joints, 104, 223
    cartilage injury, 221–223, 222f–223f
Defect preparation and templating, osteochondral autograft transfer (OATS/Mosaicplasty), 126–128
Degenerative joint disease (DJD), glucosamine/chondroitin sulfate and, 88–89
Dietary Supplement Health and Education Act (DSHEA), nutraceutical research, 87
Diffusion-weighted imaging, articular cartilage injury, 55
Distal femoral osteotomies
  indications and contraindications, 255
  patient selection, 255
  results and complications, 255–256
Distal femur, autologous osteochondral plugs, 21–22, 21f
Dome osteotomy, 255
Donnan ostmotic pressure, articular cartilage swelling, 17
Donor-site concerns, osteochondral autograft transfer, 135–136
Double bone plug technique, meniscal transplantation, 267, 267f
Double-stranded RNA (dsRNA), gene expression regulation, cartilage repair, 300
Dovetail bone bridge technique, meniscal transplantation, 267–268, 268f
Drilling procedures
  juvenile osteochondritis dissecans, knee, 239
  osteochondral lesions of talus, 176–178, 177f–178f
Driven equilibrium Fourier transfer (DEFT) imaging, articular cartilage injury, 55
Dynamics, synovial joints, 11

E

Elastohydrodynamic lubrication, cartilage, 18
Elbow
  osteochondral defects
    basic principles, 202
    diagnostic evaluation, 204–205, 204f–205f
    etiology, 202–203
    future research issues, 214–215
    literature review, 205–210, 207f–209f
    patient history, 203
    physical examination, 204
    skeletally immature athletes, 210–214, 210t
    skeletally mature athletes, 214
  osteochondritis dissecans, epidemiology, 239–242
Electrocautery, effects on cartilage, 33–34
  current research, 36–37
Electrothermal chondroplasty
  basic science, 110–111
  chondromalacia treatment, 109–113

clinical indications for, 111–112
historical background, 31–32
outcomes assessment, 36–37
Electrothermal energy effects
  articular cartilage
    applications, 37–43, 38f–39f, 42f
    basic principles, 31–32
    composition, 32–33
    outcomes, 36–37
    principles and techniques, 33–36, 35f
  chondromalacic cartilage, 33, 33f
Elmslie-Trillat procedure, patellar tilt subluxation, 276–277, 279f
Erbium:yttrium-aluminum-garnet (Er:YAG) laser
  articular cartilage repair, 34
  outcomes assessment, 36
Ethidium homodimer-1 (EthD-1), confocal laser microscopy, 37
Evidence-based medicine studies, arthroscopic debridement, 104, 105t
Extraarticular ligaments, synovial joints, 13
Extracellular cartilage, composition, 3, 4f, 5
Extracellular matrix (ECM)
  meniscus anatomy and physiology, 263, 264f
  water and, 13
"Extrinsic" injury response, articular cartilage, 26–27

F

Fast spin-echo techniques
  articular cartilage injury, 51–52
  chondral injury evaluation, 48
Fat-suppressed magnetic resonance imaging
  articular cartilage injury, 51–52
  autologous chondrocyte implantation, 144
Femoral condyle, osteochondral allograft transplantation, 160–162, 160f–161f
Femoral opening-wedge osteotomies, postoperative protocols, 257–258
Fentanyl, dosage/administration and indications, 81–82
Fibrillation, repair cartilage, 27–28, 27f
Fibrocartilage formation
  motion effects on cartilage repair, 28
  subchondral bone articular lesions, 26–27
Fibrochondrocytes, meniscus anatomy and physiology, 263
"Fingerprint" of articular cartilage, osteochondral autograft transfer (OATS/Mosaicplasty), 134
Flow-dependent viscoelasticity, articular cartilage, 17
Flow-independent viscoelasticity, articular cartilage, 17
Fluid-film lubrication models, cartilage lubrication, 18
Fluid retention effects, nonsteroidal antiinflammatory drugs, 78–79
Fluoroptic thermocouple devices, radiofrequency energy therapy, 41
Food and Drug Administration (FDA), nutraceutical regulation, 86–87
Fresh allograft tissue, osteochondral allograft transplantation, 166–167
  shoulder cartilage, 225–226, 226f
Fulkerson anteromedialization (AMZ), patellar tilt subluxation, 275–277, 278f–280f

Fulkerson osteotomy, cartilage repair with autologous chondrocyte implantation, 278, 280–281, 280f, 283f–284f, 285

Full-thickness chondral defects, subchondral bone articular lesions, 27

Functional assessment protocol, articular cartilage injury and repair classification, 65

Functional tissue engineering, cartilage injury in athletes, 294

G

Gadolinium-enhanced imaging
  advanced techniques, cartilage injury assessment, 289–290
  articular cartilage injury, 55

Gastrointestinal effects, nonsteroidal antiinflammatory drugs, 78–79

Gene therapy, cartilage injury
  applications, 297–298
  in athletes, 292–294
  delivery and cell targeting, 303–306
  disease *vs.*, 297
  limitations, 297
  nucleic acid regulation, 299–300
  protein classification, 298–299, 298t
  protein delivery system, 299
  vector development, 302–303
  viral vectors, 300–302

Glenohumeral joint. *See also* Shoulder
  allograft techniques, 228–229, 229f
  cartilage injury
    operative treatment, 220–221
    patient assessment, 218–220, 219f
  microfracture reparation, 224–225, 224f

Glucosamine
  chemical composition, 87
  combined therapy with chondroitin sulfate, 87–88
  osteoarthritis management, 86
  use in athletes, 88–89
  in vitro studies, 89–90

Glycosaminoglycans (GAG) chains
  articular cartilage composition, 14, 14f
  autologous osteochondral transfer, 20–22, 21f
  in chondroitin sulfate, 87
  in glucosamine, 87

Graft failure
  autologous chondrocyte implantation, 155
  osteochondral allograft transplantation, 163–164, 164f

Graft harvesting
  autologous chondrocyte implantation, 150–151, 151f–154f
  osteochondral autograft transfer (OATS/Mosaicplasty), 128–129

Graft implantation. *See also* Allografts
  closing wedge medial osteotomy, 256
  lateral tibial closing wedge, 253
  medial tibial opening wedge osteotomy, 252–253
  opening wedge lateral osteotomy, 257
  osteochondral autograft transfer (OATS/Mosaicplasty), 129

Growth factors
  cartilage injury in athletes, gene therapy, 293–294, 294f
  cartilage repair with, 298–299, 298t
  cartilage synthesis, 3, 5

H

Healing protocols
  autologous chondrocyte implantation, 142, 142t
  juvenile osteochondritis dissecans, knee, 238–239, 239f
  microfracture technique, 120–121, 120f

Health-related quality-of-life (HRQOL) instrument, articular cartilage injury and repair classification, 65

"Heath shock" to chondrocytes, radiofrequency energy therapy, 39–40

Heat loss, radiofrequency energy applications, articular cartilage repair, 34–35

Helicobacter pylori, nonsteroidal antiinflammatory drugs, 78–79

Hematoxylin and eosin staining (H&E), radiofrequency energy therapy assessment, 37–43

Herpes simplex virus vectors, orthopaedic applications, 301–302

High-resolution magnetic resonance imaging, articular cartilage injury, field strength and local gradient coils, 56

Hill-Sachs lesions, shoulder instability, 218

Holmium:yttrium-aluminum-garnet (Ho:YAG) laser
  articular cartilage repair, 34
  chondromalacia treatment, 109–111
  outcomes assessment, 36
  thermal chondroplasty, clinical indications for, 111–112

Hospital for Special Surgery (HSS) scores, osteochondral autograft transfer, 137

Human leukocyte antigen (HLA), osteochondral allograft transplantation, immunologic response, 167

HYAFF derivatives, hyaluronan-based autologous chondrocyte implantation (ACI), 310

Hyaluronan-based autologous chondrocyte implantation (ACI)
  basic principles, 309–310
  patient selection and follow-up, 313–315, 314f
  rehabilitation protocol, 312–313, 313f
  surgical techniques, 310–312, 311f–312f

Hyaluronic acid (HA)
  articular cartilage composition, 14, 14f
  cartilage composition, 3, 4f, 5
  viscosupplementation
    adverse effects, 93
    applications in acutely injured athletes, 95
    applications in high-endurance athletes, 94–95
    basic science, 92
    commercially available sources, 92–93
    osteoarthritis management and, 93–94

Hydrodynamic lubrication, cartilage, 18

I

"Ice-pick" microfracture technique, 121

Ilzarov technique, medial hemicallotasis, 255

Immobilization, articular cartilage atrophy, 19

Immunologic privilege, meniscus anatomy and physiology, 265

Immunologic response, osteochondral allograft transplantation, 167

Impact injuries, articular cartilage response, 27

Indentation probes, cartilage injury assessment, 291

Indian hedgehog (IHH) protein, cartilage repair with, 298–299, 298t

Injury models, cartilage injury in athletes, 291–292, 292f

Instrumentation, osteochondral allograft transplantation, 161, 161f

Insulin-like growth factor-1 (IGF-1), chondrocyte resuscitation, 292

Intercondylar notch, autologous chondrocyte implantation, 145, 145f

International Cartilage Repair Society (ICRS)
  acute osteochondral defects classification, 188–189
  articular cartilage injury and repair classification, 60–61, 62f
    cartilage repair assessment, 66, 68f, 69
      mapping grid and defect thickness assessmeny, 66–69, 67f
  hyaluronan-based autologous chondrocyte implantation (ACI) outcomes, 313–315, 314f
  osteochondral autograft transfer, 138

International Knee Documentation Committee (IKDC)
  articular cartilage injury and repair classification, 60, 61t
  hyaluronan-based autologous chondrocyte implantation (ACI), 313–315, 314f
  microfracture technique assessment, 122

Interstitial fluid, extracellular cartilage composition, 3, 4f, 5

Interterritorial matrix, articular cartilage, 6–7

Intraarticular injection, gene delivery approach, 303–304

Intraarticular ligaments, synovial joints, 13

"Intrinsic" injury response, articular cartilage, 26–27

In vitro studies, glucosamine/chondroitin sulfate, 89–90

Isotropy/anisotropy, synovial joints, 12

J

Joint loading, articular cartilage biomechanics,19

Joint space narrowing (JSN), hyaluronic acid and osteoarthritis, 93–94

Juvenile osteochondritis dissecans (JOCD)
  definition, 232
  epidemiology, 232
  etiology, 233–234
  knee, 234–239
    classification, 237t
    management, 237–239, 239f
    patient examination, 234
    presentation, 234
    radiographic imaging, 234–237, 235f–236f
  pathology, 232–233

K

Keyhole bone bridge techniques, meniscal transplantation, 267, 268f

Kinematics, synovial joints, 11

Kirschner wires, acute osteochondral defects treatment, 191, 192f–193f, 193–194

"Kissing" lesions, autologous chondrocyte implantation, 147, 147f

Knee
  acute osteochondral defects
    basic principles, 187–188
    classification, 188–189
    diagnosis, 189–190
    surgical treatment, 190–198
      complications, 198
      postoperative care, 198

      repair, 191, 192f–193f, 193–194
      replacement, 194–198, 195f–197f
      resectioning, 190–191
  juvenile osteochondritis dissecans, 234–239
    classification, 237t
    management, 237–239, 239f
    patient examination, 234
    presentation, 234
    radiographic imaging, 234–237, 235f–236f
  osteotomies
    alignment, 249–250
    background, 249
    case studies, 258–261
    preoperative planning, 250–251
    proximal tibial techniques, 251–255
    valgus-producing, 251–255
    varus-producing, distal femoral, 255–258

Knee Injury and Osteoarthritis Outcome Score (KOOS), articular cartilage injury and repair classification, 61, 62t–64t, 64–65

Knee scores, articular cartilage injury and repair classification, 60–65, 61t, 62f, 63t–64t

L

Laser energy techniques
  articular cartilage effects, 36–37
  effects on cartilage, 34

Lavage techniques, arthroscopic debridement, early arthritic joint, 102

Legg-Calvé-Perthes disease, epidemiology, 240

Lentiviral vectors, orthopaedic applications, 302

Lesquene Index of Severity of Osteoarthritis of the Knee (ISK), glucosamine/chondroitin sulfate and, 88–89

Levorphanol, dosage/administration and indications, 81–82

Ligamentous reconstruction
  autologous chondrocyte implantation, 143
  meniscal transplantation with, 271

Light microscopy, bipolar radiofrequency energy repair assessment, 38–39

Literature review, osteochondral defects, elbow, 205–210, 207f–209f

Load-elongation curve, synovial joints, 11, 12f

Lubrication theories, synovial joints, 17–19

M

Magnetic resonance angiography (MRA)
  autologous chondrocyte implantation, 144
  chondral injury evaluation, 48
  hyaluronic acid viscosupplementation protocols, 95
  shoulder cartilage injury, 218

Magnetic resonance imaging (MRI)
  acute osteochondral defects classification and diagnosis, 189–190
  advanced techniques, cartilage injury assessment, 289–290
  articular cartilage injury, 50–58
    autologous chondrocyte implantation, 57–58
    contrast-enhanced imaging, 55
    diffusion-weighted imaging, 55
    driven equillibrium Fourier transfer imaging, 55
    fat-suppression and fast spin-echo sequences, 51–52

Magnetic resonance imaging (MRI), articular cartilage
injury (*Continued*)
    high field strength and local gradient coils, 56
    magnetization transfer, 54
    microscopy, 56
    osteochondral autograft transplantation, 56–57, 57f–58f
    parameter mapping, 54
    postarthrography imaging, 52–54, 53f
    postsurgical cartilage repair, 56
    projection-reconstruction spectroscopic imaging, 54–55
    quantitative imaging volume measurement, 54
    short echo-time-projection-reconstruction imaging, 54
    sodium magnetic resonance imaging, 55
    T1-weighted fat suppressed three-dimensional spoiled
      gradient echo sequences, 52, 52f
    T1-weighted spin-echo images, 51
    T2-weighted spin-echo images, 51, 51f
  articular cartilage injury and repair classification, 65–66
  autologous chondrocyte implantation, 143–144
  chondral injury evaluation, 48
  osteochondral allograft transplantation, 159–160
  osteochondral defects, elbow, 204–205, 204f–205f
  osteochondral lesions of talus, 173–175, 173f–175f
  patellofemoral disease, 274
  shoulder cartilage injury, 218–220, 219f
  thermal chondroplasty, 112
Magnetic resonance microscopy (MRMICS), articular
    cartilage injury, 56
Magnetization transfer imaging, articular cartilage injury, 54
Malalignment
  arthroscopic debridement and, 100
  autologous chondrocyte implantation, 147, 147f
  meniscal transplantation with, 271
Marrow stimulation techniques (MSTs), microfracture
    technique and, 122
Matrix compartmentalization
  articular cartilage, 5f, 6–7
  osteochondral lesions of talus, 172
Mechanical injury models, cartilage injury in athletes, 291
Medial closing wedge
  instrumentation and implants, 256
  proximal tibial osteotomy, 257
  surgical techniques, 256
Medial hemicallotasis, 255
Medial malleolar osteotomy, osteochondral lesions of talus,
    182, 183f
Medial tibial opening wedge osteotomy, 252–253
Meniscal takedown, autologous chondrocyte implantation, 151
Meniscal transplantation
  allograft selection, 265
  basic science, 265
  concomitant procedures, 271
  overview, 263
  patient selection and indication, 265–266
  rehabilitation, 269–270
  results, 270–271
  surgical techniques, 266–269, 267f–269f
Meniscus
  anatomy and physiology, 263–265, 264f
  tears, in athletes, 293–294

Mesenchymal stem cells (MSCs), gene transfer to, 305f, 306
Messenger RNA (mRNA), gene expression regulation,
    cartilage repair, 299–300
Methadone, dosage/administration and indications, 81–82
Microfracture technique
  acute osteochondral defects treatment, 194–195
  complications, 120
  healing protocols, 120–121, 120f
  indications for, 116–117
  osteochondral lesions of talus, 176–178, 177f–178f
  patient evaluation, 116
  postoperative protocol, 119–120
  results evaluation, 121–122
  shoulder cartilage, 224–225, 224f
  surgical protocols, 117–119, 117f–119f
Miniarthrotomy, osteochondral allograft transplantation, 161,
    161f
Moloney murine leukemia vectors (MMLV), orthopaedic
    applications, 302
Monopolar radiofrequency energy (mRFE)
  cartilage repair applications, 37–43, 38f–39f, 42f
  current systems, 35, 35f
  electrothermal chondroplasty, 109–113
  evolution of, 32
  outcomes assessment, 37
Morphine, dosage/administration and indications, 81–82
Mosaicplasty. See Osteochondral autograft transfer
    (OATS/Mosaicplasty)

N

Neodymium:yttrium-aluminum-garnet (Nd:YAG) laser,
    articular cartilage repair, 31–32, 34
Newton's laws, synovial joint biomechanics, 10–11
Nonacetylated salicylates, adverse effects and safety, 78
Nonsteroidal antiinflammatory drugs (NSAIDS)
  adverse effects and safety, 77–79
  efficacy, 77
  mechanism of action, 77
  nonselective, 75, 75t–76t, 77–79
  opoids and, 81–84
  research background, 73–74
Nonviral vectors, orthopaedic applications, 302, 302t
Nucleic acids, gene expression regulation, cartilage repair,
    299–300
Nutraceuticals, FDA regulations and, 86–87

O

Oligodeoxynucleotides (ODN), gene expression regulation,
    cartilage repair, 300
Opening wedge osteotomy
  high tibial
    complications, 252
    postoperative protocols, 257–258
  lateral, 257
    postoperative protocols, 257
  proximal tibial, 259–261, 259t–260t, 260f–261f
Open mosaicplasty, osteochondral autograft transfer
    (OATS/Mosaicplasty), 129–130, 130f
Open reduction and internal fixation (ORIF), osteochondral
    autograft transfer, 138
Open surgical technique, osteochondral defects, elbow, 208f, 213

Opioids
  adverse effects and safety, 83–84
  agents, dosage/administration and indications, 81–82, 82t
  efficacy, 82–83
  mechanism of action, 81
Optical coherence tomography (OCT), cartilage injury assessment, 290–291, 290f
Orthoscopic categories, arthroscopic debridement, 100
Osteoarthritis (OA)
  arthroscopic management, early arthritic joint
    abrasion arthroplasty, 103–104
    basic principles, 99
    categories of debridement, 100
    complications, 104
    cost-benefit debate over, 104, 106
    debridement history and results, 102–103
    evidence-based studies, 104, 105t
    indications for, 99–100, 100t
    lavage treatment, 102
    surgical debridement technique, 101–102, 101f
  cartilage injury, gene therapy, 297–298
  glucosamine/chondroitin sulfate supplements, 86
    in athletes, 88–89
  hyaluronic acid viscosupplementation and, 93–94
  knee scores, 61
Osteochondral allograft transplantation
  acute osteochondral defects treatment, 197–198
  case study, 164, 165f
  complications, 163–164, 164f
  fresh allograft tissue, 166–167
  immunologic response, 167
  indications for, 159, 159t
  overview, 158–159
  patient selection, 159–160
  postoperative care, 163
  results, 165–166, 165t, 166f
  shoulder cartilage, 225–226, 226f
  surgical technique
    femoral condyle, 160–162, 160f–161f
    patellofemoral joint, 162, 162f
    tibial allografts, 162, 163f
Osteochondral autograft transfer (OATS/Mosaicplasty)
  acute osteochondral defects treatment, 195, 197
  animal studies, 134–135, 136f
  arthroscopic technique, 126–129
    defect preparation and templating, 126–128
    graft harvest, 128–129
    graft implantation, 129
    portal placement, 126
  basic principles, 124, 125f–129f
  biomechanics of, 130, 131t–134t, 134, 135f–136f
  clinical results, 136–139
  donor-site concerns, 135–136
  indications and patient selection, 124–125
  initial contact pressure, 134t, 135f–136f
  open mosaicplasty, 129–130, 130f
    postoperative protocol, 130
  osteochondral lesions of talus, 178–180, 179f–180f
  patient positioning, 126

preoperative evaluation, 125–126
shoulder cartilage, 225, 225f
Osteochondral autograft transplantation (OATS/Mosaicplasty)
  magnetic resonance imaging of, 56–57, 57f–58f
Osteochondral defects
  elbow
    basic principles, 202
    diagnostic evaluation, 204–205, 204f–205f
    etiology, 202–203
    future research issues, 214–215
    literature review, 205–210, 207f–209f
    patient history, 203
    physical examination, 204
    skeletally immature athletes, 210–214, 210t
    skeletally mature athletes, 214
  knee
    basic principles, 187–188
    classification, 188–189
    diagnosis, 189–190
    surgical treatment, 190–198
      complications, 198
      postoperative care, 198
      repair, 191, 192f–193f, 193–194
      replacement, 194–198, 195f–197f
      resectioning, 190–191
  meniscal transplantation with, 271
Osteochondral fractures
  etiology, 242
  management, 244, 244f
  patient history and physical examination, 242
  radiographic imaging, 242, 243f, 244
  shoulder, primary treatment, 221
Osteochondral injury, acute osteochondral defects treatment, 198
Osteochondral lesions, talus
  ankle joint characteristics, 172
  diagnosis and staging, 172–175, 173f–175f
  etiology, 171, 171f
  future research issues, 182–184
  nonsurgical treatment, 175–176
  osteotomies, 182, 183f
  overview, 171
  prevalence and pathophysiology, 171
  surgical treatment, 176–182
    autologous chondrocyte implantation, 180–182, 181f
    cartilage repair, 178–182
    debridement, drilling, and microfracture, 176–178, 177f–178f
    osteochondral autologous transfer/mosaicplasty/allograph, 178–180, 179f–180f
Osteochondral transfer, articular cartilage, 20–22, 21f
Osteochondritis dissecans (OCD)
  acute osteochondral defects, 188–189
  associated radial head osteochondral defects, 214
  autologous chondrocyte implantation, 144–145
  capitellum, 240–242
  elbow
    arthroscopic classification, 205–210, 207f–209f
    epidemiology, 239–240
    etiology, 202–203, 203f

Osteochondritis dissecans (OCD) (*Continued*)
  juvenile
    definition, 232
    epidemiology, 232
    etiology, 233–234
    knee, 234–239
    pathology, 232–233
  loose body lesions, surgical management, 214
  shoulder, primary treatment, 221
  in skeletally immature athletes, capitellum classification,
      210–214, 210t
  in skeletally mature athletes, 214
Osteotomies
  closing wedge
    high tibial, complications, 252
    lateral tibial
      instrumentation and implants, 253
      surgical technique, 253–255
    medial, 256
  Fulkerson osteotomy, cartilage repair with autologous
      chondrocyte implantation, 278, 280–281, 280f,
      283f–284f, 285
  knee
    alignment, 249–250
    background, 249
    case studies, 258–261
    preoperative planning, 250–251
    proximal tibial techniques, 251–255
    valgus-producing, 251–255
    varus-producing, distal femoral, 255–258
  opening-*versus*-closing-wedge, 258
  opening wedge osteotomy
    high tibial
      complications, 252
      postoperative protocols, 257–258
    lateral, 257
      postoperative protocols, 257
    proximal tibial, 259–261, 259t–260t, 260f–261f
  osteochondral lesions of talus, 182, 183f
  valgus-producing, proximal tibial, 251–255
    dome osteotomy, 255
    indications and contraindications, 251
    lateral closing wedge, 253–255
    medial hemicallotasis, 255
    patient selection, 251
    results and complications, literature review, 251–252
    tibial opening wedge, 252–253, 254f
  varus-producing
    indications and contraindications, 255
    patient selection, 255
    results and complications, 255–256
Outerbridge Classification, articular cartilage injury and repair
      classification, 66–69, 67f–68f
Oxycodone, dosage/administration and indications, 81–82

P
Panner's disease
  epidemiology, 239–240
  etiology, 203
"Parallelogram of forces" principle, synovial joints, 11

Parameter mapping, MRI techniques, 54
Patellar tilt, surgical technique, 275, 276f–277f
  subluxation with/without chondrosis, 275–277, 278f–280f
Patellofemoral joint
  abrasion arthroplasty, 103–104
  autologous chondrocyte implantation, postoperative
      therapy, 152–153
  fractures, treatment of, 193f, 194
  microfracture technique, 119
  osteochondral allograft transplantation, 163, 163f
  surgical management of disease
    autologous chondrocyte implantation, cartilage repair,
        278, 280–282, 280f–284f
    imaging studies, 273–274, 274f
    overview, 273
    patellar tilt, 275, 276f–277f
      subluxation with/without chondrosis, 275–277, 279f–280f
    patellofemoral prosthetic arthroplasty, 285, 285f
    pathomechanics assessment and treatment selection,
        274–275, 275f
    treatment algorthim, 275t
    trochlea dysplasia, 277–278, 280f–283f
Pathomechanics assessment, patellofemoral disease, 274–275,
      275f
Patient history
  acute osteochondral defects diagnosis, 189–190
  articular cartilage injury and repair classification, 60
  autologous chondrocyte implantation, 143–145
  chondral injury evaluation, 47
  microfracture technique, 116
  osteochondral autograft transfer (OATS/Mosaicplasty),
      124–126
  osteochondral defects, elbow, 203
  osteochondral fractures, 242
  shoulder cartilage injury, 218–220
Patient positioning
  medial tibial opening wedge osteotomy, 253
  osteochondral autograft transfer (OATS/Mosaicplasty), 126
Patient selection
  autologous chondrocyte implantation, 145, 146f, 147, 147f
  hyaluronan-based autologous chondrocyte implantation
      (ACI), 313–315
  meniscal transplantation, 265–266
  osteochondral allograft transplantation, 159–160
  proximal tibial osteotomies, 251
  varus-producing osteotomies, 255
Pericellular matrix, articular cartilage, 5f, 6–7
Periosteal graft hypertrophy, autologous chondrocyte
      implantation, 155
Periosteum harvesting
  acute osteochondral defects treatment, 197–198
  autologous chondrocyte implantation, 150, 151f
Physical examination protocol
  acute osteochondral defects diagnosis, 189–190
  articular cartilage injury and repair classification, 65
  chondral injury evaluation, 47–48
  juvenile osteochondritis dissecans, knee, 234–237, 235f–236f
  osteochondral defects, elbow, 204
  osteochondral fractures, 242
  shoulder cartilage injury, 218–220

Physical therapy, shoulder cartilage injury, 220
Plain radiography
    acute osteochondral defects diagnosis, 189–190
    articular cartilage injury and repair classification, 65–66
    chondral injury evaluation, 48
    meniscal transplantation, 266
    osteochondral defects, elbow, 204, 204f
    patellofemoral disease, 273–274, 274f
    shoulder cartilage injury, 218–220
Platelet aggregation, nonsteroidal antiinflammatory drugs, 77–78
Polysulfated glycosaminoglycans (PSGAGs), use in athletes, 89
Porcine SIS, biologic resurfacing, shoulder cartilage, 227–228, 227f–229f
Portal placement, osteochondral autograft transfer (OATS/Mosaicplasty), 126
Postarthrography imaging, articular cartilage injury, 52–54, 53f
Posterior cruciate ligament, knee osteotomy, 250–251
Postoperative protocol
    acute osteochondral defects treatment, 198
    autologous chondrocyte implantation, 151–154, 155f
    microfracture technique, 119–120
    osteochondral allograft transplantation, 163
    osteochondral autograft transfer (OATS/Mosaicplasty), 130, 131t–134t
    shoulder cartilage injuries, 229–230
    tibial and femoral closing-wedge osteotomies, 258
    tibial and femoral opening-wedge osteotomies, 257–258
Postsurgical cartilage repair, magnetic resonance imaging of, 56
Preoperative evaluation
    knee osteotomy, 250–251
    osteochondral autograft transfer (OATS/Mosaicplasty), 125–126
Pridie resurfacing technique
    abrasion arthroplasty, 103
    indications for, 100
Primary treatment, shoulder cartilage injury, 221
Programmed cell death (PCD), acute osteochondral defects treatment, 198
Projection-reconstruction spectroscopic imaging, articular cartilage injury, 54–55
Proportionality constant, articular cartilage tension, 7–8
Prosthetic arthroplasty, patellofemoral joint, 285, 285f
Proteins, cartilage repair, 298–299, 298t
    gene transfer delivery system, 299, 299f
Proteoglycan aggregates
    acute osteochondral defects, 187–188
    articular cartilage composition, 14, 14f
    articular cartilage swelling, 17
    cartilage composition, 3, 4f, 5
    electrothermal energy effects on, 32–33
    subchondral bone articular lesions, 26–27
Proximal tibial osteotomies, 251–255
    dome osteotomy, 255
    indications and contraindications, 251
    lateral closing wedge, 253–255
    medial closing wedge, 257
    medial hemicallotasis, 255
    patient selection, 251

    preoperative planning, 259–261, 260f–261f
    results and complications, literature review, 251–252
    tibial opening wedge, 252–253, 254f

Q

Quantitative imaging volume measurement, articular cartilage injury, 54

R

Radial (deep) zone, articular cartilage, 5–6, 15–16
Radial head osteochondral defects, surgical management, 214
Radiofrequency energy (RFE)
    articular cartilage repair
        applications, 37–43, 38f–39f, 42f
        current trends and techniques, 34–35
        historical background, 31–32
        outcomes assessment, 36–37
    cartilage injury in athletes, 291–292
    chondromalacia treatment, 109–110, 110f
    current systems, 35, 35f
    thermal chondroplasty, 110–111
Radiographic evaluation
    autologous chondrocyte implantation, 143–144
    chondral injury evaluation, 48
    juvenile osteochondritis dissecans, knee, 234–237, 235f–236f
    meniscal transplantation, 266
    osteochondral allograft transplantation, 159–160
    osteochondral fractures, 242, 243f–244f, 244
    osteotomies about knee, 259, 259t
    patellofemoral disease, 273–274, 274f
    shoulder cartilage injury, 221–223, 222f–223f
Rand Short Form (SF)-36, articular cartilage injury and repair classification, 61
Range of motion
    cartilage repair, effects on, 28
    meniscal transplantation, 270
    microfracture technique, postoperative protocol, 120
    synovial joints, 11
Recombinant human bone morphogenic protein-2 (rh-BMP-2)-impregnated collage sponge, osteochondral defects, elbow, 215
Rehabilitation
    hyaluronan-based autologous chondrocyte implantation (ACI), 312–313, 313f
    meniscal transplantation, 269–270
    shoulder cartilage injuries, 229–230
Renal toxicity, nonsteroidal antiinflammatory drugs, 78
Repair cartilage, durability, 27–28, 27f
Replication process, articular cartilage, 24–26
Resectioning techniques, acute osteochondral defects treatment, 190–191
Retroviral vectors, orthopaedic applications, 302
Ribozymes, gene expression regulation, cartilage repair, 300
Rib perichondrium, acute osteochondral defects treatment, 197–198
RNA interference (RNAi), gene expression regulation, cartilage repair, 300
Rofecoxib, adverse effects and safety, 79–80

S

Safety issues
  nonsteroidal antiinflammatory drugs, 77–79
  opoids, 83–84
Safranin O staining, radiofrequency energy therapy
      assessment, 37–43
Scanning electron microscopy (SEM), radiofrequency energy
      therapy assessment, 41–43, 42f
Screw fixation techniques, acute osteochondral defects
      treatment, 191, 192f–193f, 193–194
Second-look arthroscopy
  hyaluronan-based autologous chondrocyte implantation
      (ACI), 314–315, 314f
  osteochondral autograft transfer, 137–138
Shear force
  acute osteochondral defects, 188
  articular cartilage, 7
  flow-independent viscoelasticity, 17
  synovial joints, 11
Short echo-time-projection-reconstruction imaging, articular
      cartilage injury, 54
Short interfering RNAs (siRNAs), gene expression regulation,
      cartilage repair, 300
Shoulder. *See also* Glenohumeral joint
  abrasion arthroplasty, 104
  cartilage injury
    assessment, 217–218
    nonoperative treatment, 220
    operative treatment, 220–221
    palliative treatment, 221–223
    patient evaluation, 218–220, 219f
    postoperative rehabilitation, 229–230
    primary treatment, 221
    reparative techniques, 224–225, 224f
    restorative techniques, 225–229
      autogenous chondrocyte implantation, 226, 227f
      biologic resurfacing, 226–229, 228f–229f
      fresh osteochondral allograft, 225–226, 226f
      osteochondral autograft, 225, 225f
Signal transduction, motion effects on cartilage repair, 28
Slot bone bridge technique, meniscal transplantation,
      267–268, 269f
Sodium hyaluronic acid, osteoarthritis management, 94
Sodium magnetic resonance imaging, articular cartilage
      injury, 55
Sonic hedgehog (SHH)
  cartilage repair with, 298–299, 298t
  chondroprogenitor gene transfer, 305f, 306
Statics, synovial joints, 11
Stem cell techniques, cartilage injury in athletes, tissue
      engineering, 294
Stress relaxation
  articular cartilage viscoelasticity,17
  synovial joint viscoelasticity, 12
Stress-strain curve
  articular cartilage
    tension, 7–8, 7f
    viscoelasticity, 17
  synovial joints, 12
Structural matrix, articular cartilage composition, 14, 15f

Subchondral bone articular lesions, injury response, 26–27,
      26f
Subchondral drilling, acute osteochondral defects treatment,
      194
Subluxation, patellar tilt, with/without chondrosis, 275–277,
      278f–280f
Superficial articular lesions, injury response, 26
Superficial tangential zone (STZ), acute osteochondral
      defects, 188
Superficial zone, articular cartilage, 15
Superior labral anterior to posterior (SLAP) tears, shoulder
      cartilage injury, 218–221
Surgical techniques
  acute osteochondral defects treatment, 190–198
    repair, 191, 192f–193f, 193–194
    replacement, 194–198, 195f–197f
    resectioning, 190–191
  arthroscopic debridement, early arthritic joint, 101–102, 101f
  articular cartilage lesions, paradigms for, 28–29
  autologous chondrocyte implantation, 148, 148f–154f,
      150–151
  closing wedge medial osteotomy, 256
  electrothermal chondroplasty, 112–113, 112f–113f
  hyaluronan-based autologous chondrocyte implantation
      (ACI), 310–312, 311f–312f
  juvenile osteochondritis dissecans, knee, 239, 240f–242f
  lateral tibial closing wedge, 253–255
  medial tibial opening wedge osteotomy, 253, 254f
  meniscal transplantation indications, 266–269, 267f–269f
  microfracture, 117–119, 117f–119f
  opening wedge lateral osteotomy, 257
  osteochondral allograft transplantation
    femoral condyle, 160–162, 160f–161f
    patellofemoral joint, 162, 162f
    tibial allografts, 162, 163f
  osteochondral defects, elbow, 213–214
  patellofemoral joint
    autologous chondrocyte implantation, cartilage repair,
      278, 280–282, 280f–284f
    imaging studies, 273–274, 274f
    overview, 273
    patellar tilt, 275, 276f–277f
      subluxation with/without chondrosis, 275–277,
      279f–280f
    patellofemoral prosthetic arthroplasty, 285, 285f
    pathomechanics assessment and treatment selection,
      274–275, 275f
    treatment algorthim, 275t
    trochlea dysplasia, 277–278, 280f–283f
Symptomatic/disease modifying osteoarthritic drugs
      (S/DMOADs)
  current research in, 86
  use in athletes, 88–89
Synovial fluid
  hyaluronic acid viscosupplementation, 92
  synovial joint lubrication, 18
Synovial joints
  articular cartilage, repair techniques, 19–22
    autologous chondrocyte implantation,20
    autologous osteochondral transfer, 20–22, 21f

biomechanics, 10–11
  articular cartilage, 16–17
  dynamics, 11
  kinematics, 11
  Newton's laws, 10–11
  statics, 11
composition, 12–13
  articular cartilage, 13–16
isotropy/anisotropy, 12
material properties, 12
structural properties, 11, 12f
synovium and lubrication theories, 17–19
  cartilage, 18
  joint loading and biomechanical alteration,19
viscoelasticity, 12

T

Talus, osteochondral lesions
  ankle joint characteristics, 172
  diagnosis and staging, 172–175, 173f–175f
  etiology, 171, 171f
  future research issues, 182–184
  nonsurgical treatment, 175–176
  osteotomies, 182, 183f
  overview, 171
  prevalence and pathophysiology, 171
  surgical treatment, 176–182
    autologous chondrocyte implantation, 180–182, 181f
    cartilage repair, 178–182
    debridement, drilling, and microfracture, 176–178, 177f–178f
    osteochondral autologous transfer/mosaicplasty/ allograph, 178–180, 179f–180f
Tangential (superficial zone), articular cartilage, 5, 6f
Target cells, gene delivery approach, 303–306
Temperature thresholds, electrothermal effects on articular cartilage, 36–37
Tensile properties, articular cartilage, 17, 18f
Tension
  articular cartilage, 7–8, 7f
  synovial joints, 11
Territorial matrix, articular cartilage, 6
Thermal cautery, cartilage effects of, 33–34
Thermal chondroplasty. See Electrothermal chondroplasty
  shoulder cartilage injury, 223
Tibial allografts, osteochondral allograft transplantation, 162, 163f
Tibial opening wedge
  medial approach, 253, 254f
    instrumentation and implants, 252
    preparation, 253
  postoperative protocols, 257–258
Tibial tubercle osteotomy (TTO), patellar tilt subluxation, 275–277, 278f–280f
Torque, synovial joint, 11
Tramadol, efficacy, 83
Transforming growth factor-β family, cartilage repair with, 298–299, 298t
Transitional (intermediate) zone, articular cartilage, 5, 7f, 15

Triple-quantum-filtered sodium magnetic resonance imaging, cartilage injury assessment, 290
Trochlea dysplasia, surgical management, 277–278, 280f–283f
Trough bone bridge technique, meniscal transplantation, 267–268, 269f
T1-weighted fat-suppressed three-dimensional spoiled gradient echo sequences
  articular cartilage injury, 52, 52f
  chondral injury evaluation, 48
  postarthrography imaging, 52–54, 53f
T1-weighted spin-echo images, articular cartilage injury, 51
T2-weighted spin-echo images, articular cartilage injury, 51, 51f

U

Ultrasound devices, cartilage injury assessment, 291

V

Valdecoxib, adverse effects and safety, 79–80
Valgus-producing osteotomies, proximal tibial, 251–255
  dome osteotomy, 255
  indications and contraindications, 251
  lateral closing wedge, 253–255
  medial hemicallotasis, 255
  patient selection, 251
  results and complications, literature review, 251–252
  tibial opening wedge, 252–253, 254f
VAPR RFE device, assessment of, 40–43
Varus-producing osteotomies
  indications and contraindications, 255
  patient selection, 255
  results and complications, 255–256
Velocity vectors, synovial joints, 11
Vioxx, adverse effects and safety, 79–80
Viral vectors
  development perspectives, 302–303
  orthopaedic applications, 300–302, 301t
    adeno-associated vectors, 301
    adenoviral vectors, 300–301
    herpes simplex virus vectors, 301–302
    lentiviral vectors, 302
    Moloney murine leukemia vectors, 302
    retroviral vectors, 302
Viscoelasticity
  articular cartilage,17, 16f–17f
  synovial joints, 12
Viscosity coefficient, synovial joint lubrication, 17–18
Viscosupplementation, hyaluronic acid
  adverse effects, 93
  applications in acutely injured athletes, 95
  applications in high-endurance athletes, 94–95
  basic science, 92
  commercially available sources, 92–93
  osteoarthritis management and, 93–94
  shoulder cartilage injury, 220
Visual Analog Scale (VAS)
  articular cartilage injury and repair classification, 61
  osteoarthritis assessment, hyaluronic acid viscosupplementation and, 93–94
Vulcan EAS RFE device, assessment of, 40–43

W

Water, articular cartilage composition, 13

Weeping lubrication, cartilage, 18

Weight bearing, cartilage repair, effects on, 28

Western Ontario McMaster Universities Osteoarthritis Index (WOMAC)
  arthroscopic debridement outcome studies, 106

articular cartilage injury and repair classification, 61, 64–65

autologous chondrocyte implantation, cartilage repair outcomes, 281–282

hyaluronic acid managment of osteoarthritis, 94

Y

Young's modulus, articular cartilage tension, 7–8, 7f